Caring for the Vulnerable

Perspectives in Nursing Theory, Practice, and Research

W9-AUK-070

Editor

Mary de Chesnay, DSN, RN, CS, FAAN

N. Jean Bushman—Endowed Chair in Nursing
College of Nursing
Seattle University
Seattle, Washington

JONES AND BARTLETT PUBLISHERS

Sudbury, Massachusetts

BOSTON   TORONTO   LONDON   SINGAPORE

World Headquarters
Jones and Bartlett Publishers
40 Tall Pine Drive
Sudbury, MA 01776
978-443-5000
info@jbpub.com
www.jbpub.com

Jones and Bartlett Publishers Canada
2406 Nikanna Road
Mississauga, ON L5C 2W6
CANADA

Jones and Bartlett Publishers International
Barb House, Barb Mews
London W6 7PA
UK

Copyright © 2005 by Jones and Bartlett Publishers, Inc.
Cover Credits: (from top left clockwise) © Mel Curtis/Photodisc/Getty Images; © AbleStock; © AbleStock; © Ryan McVay/Photodisc/Getty Images; © Photodisc; © Photos.com

All rights reserved. No part of the material protected by this copyright may be reproduced or utilized in any form, electronic or mechanical, including photocopying, recording, or by any information storage and retrieval system, without written permission from the copyright owner.

Library of Congress Cataloging-in-Publication Data

Caring for the vulnerable : perspectives in nursing theory, practice,
and research / [edited by] Mary de Chesnay.— 1st ed.
    p. ; cm.
   Includes bibliographical references and index.
   ISBN 0-7637-4764-5 (pbk.)
  1. Nursing—Social aspects.   2. Transcultural nursing.   3. Nursing—
Cross-cultural studies.   4. Nursing—Philosophy.   5. Community health nursing.
  [DNLM: 1. Community Health Nursing.   2. Vulnerable Populations.
3. Nursing Theory.   4. Transcultural Nursing.   WY 106 C277 2004]   I. de Chesnay, Mary.
  RT86.5.C376 2004
  362.17′3—dc22

                              2004007484

Production Credits
Acquisitions Editor: Kevin Sullivan
Production Manager: Amy Rose
Associate Production Editor: Renée Sekerak
Editorial Assistant: Amy Sibley
Marketing Manager: Ed McKenna
Associate Marketing Manager: Emily Ekle
Manufacturing and Inventory Coordinator: Amy Bacus
Composition: ATLIS Graphics
Cover Design: Kristin E. Ohlin
Printing and Binding: Malloy Incorporated
Cover Printing: Malloy Incorporated

Printed in the United States of America
08 07 06 05   10 9 8 7 6 5 4 3 2

Dedication

For my mother who taught me to appreciate books
For my father who taught me to be a straight shooter

Contents

Contributors

Charles Barnes, SJ, MHA, MA
Instructor, College of Nursing
Seattle University
Seattle, WA

Carmen Benavides Mora, Lic, MS
Director, School of Nursing
Universidad Politecnica de Nicaragua
Managua, Nicaragua

Robyn Bennetts, BA
College of Nursing
Seattle University
Seattle, WA

Doris M. Boutain, PhD, RN
Assistant Professor
College of Nursing
Seattle University
Seattle, WA

Bonnie H. Bowie, RN, PhD, MBA
Lecturer, College of Nursing
Seattle University
Seattle, WA

Geraldine R. Britton, PhDc
Research Assistant
Decker School of Nursing
State University of New York
Binghamton, NY

Deborah Brown, MSN, RN
Family Nurse Practitioner
Seattle, WA

Kerry L. Clark, BS, BSN, RN
College of Nursing
Seattle University
Seattle, WA

Medrice Coluccio, RN, MN
Chief Executive Officer
PeaceHealth Lower Columbia Region
Longview, WA

Susan P. Colvin, RNC, MN (Retired)
School of Nursing
Duquesne University
Pittsburgh, PA

Mary de Chesnay, DSN, RN, CS, FAAN
Professor and Endowed Chair-Vulnerable
    Population, College of Nursing
Seattle University
Seattle, WA

Kathryn S. Deane, MSN, RN
Family Nurse Practitioner
Seattle, WA

Behice Erci, PhD
Associate Professor
School of Nursing
Atatürk University
Erzurum, Turkey

Jacquelyn H. Flaskerud, RN, PhD, FAAN
Professor Emerita, School of Nursing
UCLA
Los Angeles, CA

Clare Fontana, BSN
College of Nursing
Seattle University
Seattle, WA

Tyler Free, BA
College of Nursing
Seattle University
Seattle, WA

Jennifer Fritz-Millard, BS, BSN, RN
College of Nursing
Seattle University
Seattle, WA

Linda Frothinger, BA, BSN
College of Nursing
Seattle University
Seattle, WA

Beth Furlong, PhD, RN, JD
Associate Professor
School of Nursing
Creighton University
Omaha, NE

Jo Anne Latimer Grunow, DNSc, ARNP,
  FNP, CS
Assistant Professor
College of Nursing
Seattle University
Seattle, WA

Sarah Hall Gueldner, RN, DSN, FAAN
Dean and Professor
Decker School of Nursing
State University of New York
Binghamton, NY

Gladys L. Husted, PhD, RN
School of Nursing Distinguished Professor
Duquesne University
Pittsburgh, PA

James H. Husted, PhD
Independent Scholar
Pittsburgh, PA

Sharon Jensen, RN, MN
Instructor
College of Nursing
Seattle University
Seattle, WA

Natalie Keilholz, BA
College of Nursing
Seattle University
Seattle, WA

Deborah Koniak-Griffin, EdD, RNC, FAAN
Audrienne H. Moseley Professor in
  Women's Health Research
Director of the Center for Vulnerable
  Populations Research
UCLA School of Nursing
Los Angeles, CA

Kevin C. Krycka, PsyD
Chair, Department of Psychology
College of Arts and Sciences
Seattle University
Seattle, WA

Debra Kubinski, PhD, RN
Associate Professor
Department of Nursing
Edinboro University
Edinboro, PA

Cheryle G. Levitt, PhD, RN, MSN
Faculty, University of New England, Israel
  Branch and University of Phoenix Online
  College of Nursing
Tel Aviv, Israel

Hwey-Fang Liang, PhD, RN
Department of Nursing
Chung Hwa College of Medical Technology
Tainan City, Taiwan

Hanna Maijala, PhD, RN
Senior Lecturer, Häme Polytechnic
Health Care and Social Services
Degree Program in Nursing
Finland

Margaret McAllister, RN, BA, MEd, EdD
Deputy Head of School
School of Nursing
Griffith University
Queensland, Australia

Teodora Gáitan Mercado, MS
Faculty, School of Nursing
Universidad Politecnica de Nicaragua
Managua, Nicaragua

Jeri A. Milstead, PhD, RN, FAAN
Dean and Professor, School of Nursing
Medical College of Ohio
Toledo, OH

Keesha Morris, MSN, RN, ARNP
College of Nursing
Seattle University
Seattle, WA

Lynda P. Nauright, EdD, RN
Professor
Nell Hodgson Woodruff School of Nursing
Emory University
Atlanta, GA

Adeline Nyamathi, RN, ANP, PhD, FAAN
Audrienne H. Moseley Professor in
    Community Health Nursing
UCLA School of Nursing
Los Angeles, CA

Lauren E. Osterbur, BSN, RN
Jacksonville, NC

Christopher Pamp, MSN, MEd, RN
Family Nursing Practitioner
Seattle, WA

Deborah Parr, BA
College of Nursing
Seattle University
Seattle, WA

Nataly Pasumansky, MSN, ARNP
Family Nurse Practitioner
Seattle, WA

Carol M. Patton, DrPH, MSN, CRNP
Assistant Professor
School of Nursing
Duquesne University
Pittsburgh, PA

Jane W. Peterson, RN, PhD
Professor
College of Nursing
Seattle University
Seattle, WA

Debby A. Phillips, PhD, ARNP, CS
Assistant Professor
College of Nursing
Seattle University
Seattle, WA

Katharine Poinier, BSN
College of Nursing
Seattle University
Seattle, WA

Nick Polaschek, PhD, RN
Capital and Coast District Health Board
Wellington, New Zealand

Retha R. Porter, BA
Public Affairs Specialist
PeaceHealth, Lower Columbia Region
Longview, WA

Lenore K. Resick, MSN, RN, CRNP, BC
Associate Professor
Director of the Nurse-Managed Wellness
    Centers
Duquesne University
Pittsburgh, PA

Kathryn A. Robbins, RN
Parish Nurse Coordinator
PeaceHealth, Lower Columbia Region
Longview, WA

Carl A. Ross, PhD, RN, CRNP
Associate Professor and Director of the
    Center for International Nursing
Duquesne University
Pittsburgh, PA

Kelly Sehring, BSN
College of Nursing
Seattle University
Seattle, WA

Yvonne M. Sterling, DNSc, RN, C
Professor
Louisiana State University Health Sciences
    Center
School of Nursing
New Orleans, LA

Yukie Takemura, RN, PHN, MS
Department of Nursing Administration
Division of Health Sciences and Nursing
Faculty of Medicine
The University of Tokyo
Tokyo, Japan

Jenny Hsin-Chun Tsai, PhD, ARNP, CS
Assistant Professor
College of Nursing
Seattle University
Seattle, WA

Yun-Fang Tsai, PhD, RN
Professor, School of Nursing
Chang Gung University
Taiwan

Mari Van Court, MSN, RN
President-Van Court Associates, Inc.
Gig Harbor, WA

Toni M. Vezeau, PhD, RNC
Associate Professor
College of Nursing
Seattle University
Seattle, WA

Barbro Wadensten, RN, PhD
Senior Lecturer, Department of Caring
  Sciences
Örebro University
Örebro, Sweden

Jennifer Wagner, BSN, RN
College of Nursing
Seattle University
Seattle, WA

Rebecca Wharton, MSN, BA, RN
Family Nurse Practitioner
Seattle, WA

Thomas K.S. Wong, RN, PhD
Professor and Head
School of Nursing
The Hong Kong Polytechnic University
Hong Kong

Heather M. Young, PhD, GNP, FAAN
Professor, School of Nursing
Oregon Health Sciences University
Portland, OR

Anna Zisberg, PhDc, MA, RN
Fulbright Scholar and Doctoral Candidate
University of Washington School of Nursing
Seattle, WA

Roberta Zolkoski, PhD, RN, CRNP
Pittsburgh, PA

Rick Zoucha, APRN, BC, DNSc, CTN
Associate Professor
Duquesne University School of Nursing
Pittsburgh, PA

Leehu Zysberg, PhD
Organizational Psychologist
Faculty, Department of Psychology, College
  of Arts and Sciences and College of
  Nursing
Seattle University
Seattle, WA

Foreword

It is interesting to consider the mental images that the concept of *vulnerability* evokes. For some, the concept might be associated with people of color or those that are socially marginalized. For others, it might evoke images of those who are poor, those who are frail, or those who are without voice. *Vulnerability* is equally at home with those who rely on others to speak for them, as it is with those who are homeless or disenfranchised. *Vulnerability* might extend to those who experience violence as part and parcel of human existence or to those who go to bed hungry every night. Certainly, the term captures the notions of the global community better than most, amplifying our understanding of the struggles of those in the developing world to maximize their lives against tremendous odds.

The distinctiveness of *person* is often eroded in our imaging somehow. Try getting a clear picture of your own mental image of vulnerability. Mine would be stigma. Just as it seems to come into relief, it withdraws behind a curtain that hides the sharp edges of it. Stephen Bezruchka, MD, suggests that because the gap between those with resources and those without continues to widen in our society, health disparities are on the rise. Health disparities, then, are yet another image of vulnerability. In those disparities, persons are less visible. They will continue to be invisible as persons unless we actively seek to lift the curtain of public perception, and gaze on the private face of vulnerability.*

For many years, we thought that the notion of *safety net* applied to everyone who, for whatever reason, was unable to marshal the personal resources to overcome vulnerability. Yet, a close assessment of the health care industry, as one case in point, only magnifies the reality that 44.6 million people in our country alone have no health insurance—no safety net. We often thought of our *safety net* (federally funded social programs, for example) as strong mesh that held tight when people fell. That *safety net* did all kinds of things: held children who cried from hunger, held the hands of those who were dying, held those in circumstances of profound physical or social need. These days, the *safety net* does not seem quite so strong. As we examine our national economy, our health care industry, the elements of social support, and the capacities of each of us to reach out for one another, the *safety net* seems more fragile somehow, full of holes and shreds of a formally strong material substance. Indeed, if we look at that private face of vulnerability, we might be surprised to see our own face.

---

*Bezruchka, S. Is our society making you sick? *Newsweek,* February 26, 2001, p.14.

This book explores vulnerability from the perspective of individuals, groups, communities, and populations. The chapters address the many private faces of vulnerability and the implications of that vulnerability for nurses, nursing, and nursing care. Indeed, if we look around, it is often nurses who provide the single interface between those who are vulnerable on the one hand and access to solutions on the other. As practitioners, nurses buffer the many realities of vulnerability as they go about their appointed tasks with the people they serve and care for. As academicians, nurses embrace vulnerability and vulnerable populations as the frequent focus of their academic teaching, weaving threads of understanding into the fabric of the students' lives within their charge. As scientists, nurses explore the many faces of vulnerability from the perspective of thoughtful, reasoned, and reflective experiences, as well as from the quantitative perspectives of stress and coping, self-regulation, and self-efficacy, to name a few. Finally, as nurses, we stand in solidarity with those in need, fulfilling the social contract foundational to a life of caring.

This document is shared with the understanding that all of us are in this thing together—reflecting, if you will, the broader realities in which we find ourselves. Many of the chapters are eloquent, expressive examples of the realities of nursing and nursing care. Others advocate for individual and community strategies to address vulnerability as a common, lived experience. Still others are testaments to the professional and personal wisdom that is a hallmark of a mature discipline. Reflection is the process; understanding is the outcome. Both reflection and understanding are foundational to strengthening and supporting individuals and communities in our common quest for meaning and connection in our lives.

Mary K. Walker, PhD, RN, FAAN
Dean and Professor
Seattle University
College of Nursing
Seattle, WA

Preface

Caring for the vulnerable members of their society is a function nurses perform without regard for their own ambitions, personal safety, and financial security. They are driven to do this work by their desire to help the less fortunate and their profound commitment to social justice, regardless of religious orientation. *Vulnerability* is a trendy concept and *vulnerable populations* a term with specific meaning in the present political climate. Fashionableness in words comes and goes, but there will always be those who are poor and at risk and nurses will always define their role to care for them. This volume is an attempt to pull together papers from nurses who represent many different cultures—organized into six units designed to provide a sampling of the scope of nursing with vulnerable populations. Most of the chapters are written by nurses, but several other authors were included because they have something important to say about special populations and their ideas are relevant to nursing.

Unit 1 includes papers about key concepts that provide a basic structure for caring for the vulnerable. Unit 2 is an exploration of the relevance of nursing theories to vulnerable populations. In Unit 3, research reports show the kinds of phenomena nurses study and the methods they employ to examine questions of interest. It was not deliberate that the authors who submitted their research for consideration tended to use qualitative methods, but that they did is not surprising, since the nature of vulnerability lends itself to naturalistic research. The diverse papers in Unit 4 were selected because of their relevance to nursing practice. Unit 5 is about learning to work with vulnerable individuals and populations and is a set of chapters offering many ideas for learning experiences not only for nursing students, but also for practitioners who want to expand their ability to serve people of other cultures. Finally, Unit 6 provides ideas for how nurses might advocate for the vulnerable on a policy level.

The book was originally intended as a primary text for undergraduate and graduate courses on vulnerable populations, but it is also appropriate as a supplemental text for undergraduate community health courses and family nurse practitioner programs. The book might also be useful as a supplemental text for nursing theory courses, qualitative methods courses and doctoral courses that emphasize theory and research with vulnerable populations. The unit on teaching and learning might be useful to undergraduates to see examples of fieldwork and to graduate students who wish to teach. Finally, by representing the work of nurses in many countries, we hope that the book encourages interest in other cultures and might be appropriate for courses in international nursing. However the book is used, we hope that readers will be inspired to think more about the vulnerable within their own communities.

Mary de Chesnay, *DSN, RN, CS, FAAN*
Professor and Endowed Chair-Vulnerable Populations
Seattle University College of Nursing
Seattle, WA

Acknowledgments

Books are a team effort and thanks are due first and foremost to the contributing authors—nurses and others around the world who share the value of social justice and who care for and about the vulnerable members of their countries. Included among the contributors for the web-based Instructor Guide are Mari Van Court, who single-handedly designed the PowerPoints and seven undergraduate students who gave permission for their examinations to be used as samples: Linda Frothinger, Haeji Park, Pamela Gray, Tracey Shelton, Amanda Popik, Grace Williams, and Sunniva Zaratkjiewicz. Excellent editorial services were provided by Beth Branchaw and Rachel Wiseman of Seattle University College of Nursing, supervised by Mary Mainville. Tom Nally prevented several computer crises. Finally, Amy Sibley, Renée Sekerak, and Kevin Sullivan, the staff of Jones and Bartlett, were particularly helpful above the call of duty with the many questions that arose during the production of this work.

UNIT I

Concepts

The most profound wisdom they [my children] have given me is a respect for human vulnerability. I have known that people are resilient, but I didn't appreciate how fragile they are.

Shirley Nelson Garner

Source: Bartleby.com, retrieved 2/27/04.

CHAPTER 1

Vulnerable Populations: Vulnerable People

Mary de Chesnay

In this chapter, key concepts will be introduced to provide a frame of reference for examining health care issues related to vulnerability and vulnerable populations. The concepts presented in Unit I, as a whole, form a theoretical perspective on caring for the vulnerable within a cultural context in which nurses consider not only ethnicity as a cultural factor but also the culture of vulnerability. The goal is to provide culturally competent care.

VULNERABILITY

There are two aspects related to vulnerability, and it is important to distinguish between them. One is the individual focus (individuals viewed within a system context), and the other is an aggregate view of what would be termed "vulnerable populations." Much of the literature on vulnerability is targeted toward the aggregate view, and nurses certainly need to address the needs of groups; however, nurses also treat individuals, and this book is concerned with generating ideas about caring for both individuals and groups.

Vulnerability is a general concept meaning "susceptibility" and it has a specific connotation in health care as "at risk for health problems." According to Aday (2001), vulnerable populations are those at risk for poor physical, psychological, or social health. Anyone can be vulnerable at any given point in time as a result of life circumstances or response to illness or events. However, the notion of a vulnerable population is a public health concept that refers to vulnerability by virtue of status; that is, some groups are at risk at any given point in time relative to other individuals or groups.

To be a member of a vulnerable population does not necessarily mean one is vulnerable. In fact, many individuals within vulnerable populations would resist the notion that they are vulnerable because they prefer to focus on their strengths rather than their weaknesses. These people might argue that "vulnerable population" is just another label that health care professionals use to promote a system of health care that they, the consumers of care, consider patronizing. It is important to distinguish between a state of vulnerability at any given point in time and a labeling process in which groups of people at risk for certain health conditions are further marginalized.

Some members of society who are not members of the culturally defined vulnerable populations described in this book might be vulnerable only in certain contexts. For example, nurses who work in emergency rooms are vulnerable to violence. Hospital employees and visitors are vulnerable to infections. Teachers in preschool and daycare providers are vulnerable to a host of communicable diseases because of their daily contact with young children. Men who work with heavy machinery are at risk for certain injuries. Other examples might be people who pick up hitchhikers, drivers who drink, people who travel on airplanes during flu season, college students cramming for exams, and people caught in natural disasters.

VULNERABLE POPULATIONS

Who are the vulnerable in terms of health care? Vulnerable populations are those with a greater-than-average risk of developing health problems (Aday, 2001; Sebastian, 1996) by virtue of their marginalized sociocultural status, their limited access to economic resources, or personal characteristics such as age and gender. For example, members of ethnic minority groups have traditionally been marginalized even when they are highly educated and earning good salaries. Immigrants and the poor (including the working poor) have limited access to health care because of the way insurance is obtained. Children, women, and the elderly are vulnerable to a host of health care problems, notably violence, but also specific health problems associated with development or aging. Developmental examples might be susceptibility to poor influenza outcomes for children and the elderly, psychological issues of puberty and menopause, osteoporosis and fractures among older women, and Alzheimer's disease.

Bezruchka (2000, 2001), in his provocative work, addressed the correlation between poverty and illness but also asserted that inequalities in wealth distribution are responsible for the state of health of the American population. Bezruchka argued that the economic structure of a country is the single most powerful determinant of the health of its people. He noted that Japan, with its small gap between rich and poor, has a high percentage of smokers but a low percentage of mortality from smoking. Bezruchka advocated redistribution of wealth as a solution to health disparities.

Concepts and Theories

Aday (2001) published a framework for studying vulnerable populations that incorporated the World Health Organization's (1948) dimensions of health (physical, psychological, and social) into a model of relationships between individual and community on a variety of policy levels. In Aday's framework, the variables of access, cost, and quality are critical in understanding the nature of health care for vulnerable populations. Access refers to the ability of people to find, obtain, and pay for health care. Costs can be direct or indirect. Direct costs are the dollars spent by health care facilities to provide care. Indirect costs are losses resulting from decreased patient productivity (e.g., absenteeism from work.) Quality refers to the relative inadequacy, adequacy, or superiority of services.

Other authors who have addressed the conceptual basis of vulnerable populations include Sebastian (1996; Sebastian et al., 2002), who focused on marginalization as a factor in resource allocation, and Flaskerud & Winslow (1998), who emphasized resource availability in the broad sense of socioeconomic and environmental resources. Karpati, Galea, Awerbuch, & Levins (2002) argued for an ecological approach to understanding how social context influences health outcomes. Lessick, Woodring, Naber, & Halstead (1992) described the concept of vulnerability as applied to a person within a system context. Although this study applied the model to maternal—child nursing, the authors argued that the model is appropriate in any clinical settings.

Spiers (2000) argued that epidemiological views of vulnerability are insufficient to explain human experience and offered a new conceptualization based on perceptions that are both etic (externally defined by others) and emic (from the point of view of the person.). Etic approaches are helpful in understanding the nature of risk in a quantifiable way. Emic approaches enable one to understand the whole of human experience and, in so doing, help people capitalize on their capacity for action.

HEALTH DISPARITIES

In 1998, President Bill Clinton made a commitment to reduce health disparities that disproportionately affect racial and ethnic minorities by the year 2010. The Department of Health and Human Services selected six areas to target: infant mortality, cancer screening and management, cardiovascular disease, diabetes, HIV/AIDS, and immunization (National Institutes of Health [NIH], 2003). Subsequently, the NIH announced a strategic plan for 2002–2006 that committed funding for three major goals related to research, research infrastructure, and public information/community outreach (NIH, 2002).

Flaskerud et al. (2002) reviewed 79 research reports published in *Nursing Research* and concluded that although nurse researchers have systematically addressed health disparities, they have tended to ignore certain groups (indigenous peoples). They also inappropriately lump together as Hispanic members of disparate groups with their own cultural identity (e.g., Puerto Ricans, Mexicans, Cubans, Dominicans).

Aday (2001) emphasized certain groups as vulnerable populations, and the 2010 priorities showcase obvious needs within these groups.

- ☐ **High-risk mothers and infants-of-concern.** This population is a result of high rates of teenage pregnancy and poor prenatal care, leading to birth-weight problems and infant mortality. Affected groups include very young women, African American women, and poorly educated women, all of whom are less likely than middle-class white women to receive adequate prenatal care due to limited access to services.
- ☐ **Chronically ill and disabled.** Those in this category not only experience higher death rates than comparable middle-class white women as a result of heart disease, cancer, and stroke, but they are also subject to prevalent chronic conditions such as hypertension, arthritis, and asthma. The debilitating effects of such chronic diseases lead to lost income resulting from limitations in activities of daily living. African Americans are more likely to experience ill effects and to die from chronic diseases.
- ☐ **Persons living with HIV/AIDS.** Advances in tracing and treating AIDS have resulted in declines in deaths and increases in the number of people living with HIV/AIDS. This increase is also due, in part, to changes in transmission patterns from largely male homosexual or bisexual contact to transmission through heterosexual contact and sharing needles among IV drug users.
- ☐ **Mentally ill and disabled.** Mental illness is usually defined broadly to include even those with mild anxiety and depression. Prevalence rates are high with age-specific disorders, and severe emotional disorders seriously interfere with activities of daily living and interpersonal relationships.
- ☐ **Alcohol and other substance abusers.** The wide array of substances that are abused includes drugs, alcohol, cigarettes, and inhalants (such as glue). Intoxication results in

chronic disease, accidents, and, in some cases, criminal activity. Young male adults in their late teens and early twenties are more likely to smoke, drink, and take drugs.

☐ **Suicide- or homicide-prone behavior.** Rates differ by age, sex, and race, with elderly white and young Native American men most likely to kill themselves and young African American, Native American, and Hispanic men most likely to be killed by others.

☐ **Abusive families.** Children, the elderly, and spouses (overwhelmingly women) are likely targets of violence within the family, and although older children are more likely to be injured, young female children over 3 years old are consistently at risk for sexual abuse.

☐ **Homeless persons.** Because of problems in identifying this population, it is reasonably certain that the estimated prevalence rates at any given time are low and vary across the country. Generally, more young men are homeless, but all homeless are likely to suffer from chronic diseases and are vulnerable to violence.

☐ **Immigrants/refugees.** Health care for immigrants, refugees, and temporary residents is complicated by the diversity of languages, health practices, food choices, culturally based definitions of health, and previous experiences with American bureaucracies.

Aday (2001) provided much statistical information for these vulnerable groups, but prevalence rates for specific conditions change periodically, and readers are referred to the Web site of the National Center for Health Statistics at *www.cdc.gov/nchs* for updated information.

Trends in families over the last five decades (the lifetime of the baby boomers) show marked changes in the demographics of families, and these changes affect health disparities. At present, more men and women are delaying marriage, with more people choosing to live together first. Divorce rates are higher, with a concurrent increase in the single-parent family structure. Out-of-wedlock births have increased, partially due to decreases in marital fertility. There is a sharp and sustained increase in maternal employment (Hofferth, 2003).

Institute of Medicine Study

The US Congress directed the Institute of Medicine (IOM) to study the extent of racial and ethnic differences in health care and to recommend interventions to eliminate health disparities (IOM, 2003). The IOM found consistent evidence of disparities across a wide range of health services and illnesses: The IOM noted that although racial and ethnic disparities occur within a wider historical context, they are unacceptable.

The IOM urged a general public acknowledgement of the problem and specific cross-cultural training for health professionals. They recommended specific legal, regulatory, and policy interventions that speak to fairness in access, increases in the number of minority health professionals; and better enforcement of civil rights laws. IOM recommendations with regard to data collection should serve to monitor progress toward the goal of eliminating health disparities based upon different treatment for minorities.

VULNERABILITY TO SPECIFIC CONDITIONS OR DISEASES

Much of the research that has been done on specific conditions and diseases was generated from psychology data and predates much of the medical and nursing literature on disparities. Researchers on vulnerability to these specific conditions tend to take an individual approach in that conditions or diseases are treated from the point of view of how a particular individual responds to life stressors and how that response can cause the condition to develop or continue.

Researchers have focused on conditions too numerous to report here, but references were found to alcohol consumption in women and vulnerability to sexual aggression (Testa, Livingston, & Collins, 2000); rape myths and vulnerability to sexual assault (Bohner, Danner, Siebler, & Stamson, 2002); self-esteem and unplanned pregnancy (Smith, Gerrard, & Gibbons, 1997); lung transplantation (Kurz, 2002); coronary angioplasty (Edell-Gustafsson & Hetta, 2001); adjustment to lower limb amputation (Behel, Rybarczyk, Elliott, Nicholas, & Nyenhuis, 2002); reaction to natural disasters (Phifer, 1990); reaction to combat stress (Aldwin, Levensen, & Spiro, 1994; Ruef, Litz, & Schlenger, 2000); homelessness (Morrell-Bellai, Goering, & Boydell, 2000; Shinn, Knickman, & Weitzman, 1991); mental retardation (Nettlebeck, Wison, Potter, & Perry, 2000); anxiety (Calvo & Cano-Vindel, 1997; Strauman, 1992); and suicide (Schotte, Cools, & Payvar, 1990).

Depression

Many authors have focused on cognitive variables in an attempt to explain vulnerability to depression (Alloy & Clements, 1992; Alloy, Whitehouse, & Abramson, 2000; Hayes, Castonguay, & Goldfried, 1996; Ingram & Ritter, 2000). Others have explored gender differences (Bromberger & Mathews, 1996; Whiffen, 1988). In a major analysis of the existing literature on depression, Hankin and Abramson (2001) explored the development of gender differences in depression and noted that although both male and female rates rise during middle adolescence, rates in girls rise more sharply after age 13 or puberty. This model of general depression might account for gender differences based on developmentally specific stressors and implies possible treatment options.

Variables related to attitudes present a third area of focus in the literature (Brown, Hammen, Craske, & Wickens, 1995; Joiner, 1995; Zuroff, Blatt, Bondi, & Pilkonis, 1999). In a study of 75 college students, researchers found that a high level of "perfectionistic achievement attitudes," as indicated on the Dysfunctional Attitude Scale, correlated with a specific stressor (e.g., poorer than expected performance on a college exam) to predict an increase in symptoms of depression (Brown et al., 1995).

Schizophrenia

Smoking has been observed to be a problem in schizophrenics, and there is some evidence that smokers have a more serious course of mental illness than nonsmokers, the theory being that schizophrenics smoke as a way to self-medicate ((Lohr & Flynn, 1992). In a twin study investigating lifetime prevalence of smoking and nicotine withdrawal, Lyons et al. (2002) found that the association between smoking and schizophrenia may be related to familial vulnerability to schizophrenia. Other authors have examined the relationship between schizophrenia and personality and discovered that this relationship is largely unexplored and might provide a new direction in which to search for knowledge about vulnerability to schizophrenia. In their meta-analysis, Berenbaum and Fujita (1994) found a significant relationship between introversion and schizophrenia and suggested that studies on that relationship might provide new knowledge about the covariation of schizophrenia with mood disorders, particularly depression. In a thoughtful analysis of the literature on the role of the family in schizophrenia, Wuerker (2000) presented evidence for the biological view and concluded that there is a unique vulnerability to stress in schizophrenics and that communication difficulties within families with schizophrenic members may be due to a shared genetic heritage.

Eating Disorders

Acknowledgment of food as a common focus for anxiety has become a way of life. Canadian researchers refer to "food insecurity" to describe the phenomenon of nutritional vulnerability resulting from food scarcity and insufficient access to food by welfare recipients and low-income people who do not qualify for welfare (McIntyre, Glanville, Raine, Dayle, Anderson, & Battaglia, 2003; Tarasuk, 2003). In the United States, eating disorders are a growing set of outcomes related to patterns of eating behavior over time and body image problems that are particularly prevalent in gay men and heterosexual women (Siever, 1994). In a prospective study of gender and behavioral vulnerabilities related to eating disorders, Leon, Fulkerson, Perry, & Early-Zaid (1995) found significant differences for girls in the variables of weight loss, dieting patterns, vomiting, and use of diet pills. They reported a method for predicting the occurrence of eating disorders based on performance scores on risk-factor status tests early on.

HIV/AIDS

In a meta-analysis of 32 HIV/AIDS studies involving 15,440 participants, Gerrard, Gibbons, & Bushman (1996) found empirical evidence to support the commonly known motivational hypothesis. This hypothesis is derived from the Health Belief Model (Becker & Rosenstock, 1987). The authors found that perceived vulnerability was the major force behind prevention behavior in high-risk populations but cautioned that studies were not available for low-risk populations. They also found that risk behavior shapes perceptions of vulnerability; that is, people who engage in high-risk behavior tend to see themselves as more likely to contract HIV than those who engage in low-risk behavior. Evidence that high-risk men tend to relapse into unsafe sex behaviors is provided in a longitudinal study of results of an intervention in which researchers could successfully predict relapse behavior (Kelly, St. Lawrence, & Brasfield, 1991). In a gender study on emotional distress predictors, Van Servellen, Aguirre, Sarna, & Brecht (2002) found that although all subjects had scores indicating clinical anxiety levels, women had more HIV symptoms and poorer functioning than men.

In a study that used a vulnerable populations framework, Flaskerud and Lee (2001) considered the role that resource availability plays in the health status of informal female caregivers of people with HIV/AIDS ($n = 36$) and age-related dementias ($n = 40$). Not surprisingly, the caregivers experienced high levels of both physical and mental health problems. However, the use of the vulnerable populations framework explained the result that the resource variables of income and minority ethnicity contributed the most to understanding health status. In terms of the risk variables, anger was more common in HIV caregivers and was significantly related to depressive mood, which was also high among the HIV caregivers.

Substance Abuse

In a study of 288 undergraduates, Wild, Hinson, Cunningham, & Bacchiochi (2001) examined the inconsistencies between a person's perceived risk of alcohol-related harm and motivation to reduce that risk. They found a general tendency for people to view themselves as less vulnerable than peers regardless of their risk status, but the at-risk group rated themselves more likely to experience harm than the not-at-risk group. The authors concluded that motivational approaches to reducing risk should emphasize not only why people drink but also why they should reduce alcohol consumption. Additional support for the motivational hypothesis—that perceived vulnerability influences prevention behavior—extends to marijuana use (Simons & Carey, 2002) and to early onset of substance abuse among African American children (Wills, Gibbons, Gerrard, & Brody, 2000). Finally, in a study of family history of psychopathology in families of the offspring of alcoholics, researchers demonstrated that male college student offspring of these families are a heterogeneous group and that the patterns of heterogeneity are related to familial types in relation to vulnerability to alcoholism. Three different family types were identified:

- ☐ low levels of family pathology with moderate levels of alcoholism
- ☐ high levels of family antisocial personality and violence with moderate levels of family drug abuse and depression, and
- ☐ high levels of familial depression, mania, anxiety disorder, and alcoholism with moderate levels of familial drug abuse (Finn, Sharkansky, Viken, West, Sandy, & Bufferd, 1997).

CONCLUSION

This concludes an overview of the concept of vulnerability and models that incorporate vulnerability. There is a growing body of literature pertaining to vulnerability as a key factor of concern to practitioners who work with clients with many different kinds of presenting problems. The concept of vulnerability is explored on two levels in that vulnerability is both an individual and a group concept. In public health, the group concept is dominant, and intervention is directed toward aggregates. Other practitioners and researchers focus on individual vulnerabilities to specific conditions or diseases.

REFERENCES

Aday, L. (2001). *At risk in America.* San Francisco, CA: Jossey-Bass.

Aldwin, C., Levensen, M., & Spiro, A. (1994). Vulnerability and resilience to combat exposure: Can stress have lifelong effects? *Psychology and Aging, 9,* 34–44.

Alloy, L., & Clements, C. (1992). Illusion of control invulnerability to negative affect and depressive symptoms after laboratory and natural stressors. *Journal of Abnormal Psychology, 101,* 234–245.

Alloy, L., Whitehouse, W., & Abramson, J. (2000). The Temple-Wisconsin Cognitive Vulnerability to Depression Project: Lifetime history of axis I psychopathology in individuals at high and low cognitive risk for depression. *Journal of Abnormal Psychology, 109,* 403–418.

Becker, M., & Rosenstock, I. (1987). Comparing social learning theory and the health belief model. In W. B. Ward (Ed.), *Advances in health education and promotion* (Vol. 2, pp. 245–249). Greenwich, CT: JAI Press.

Behel, J., Rybarczyk, B., Elliott, T., Nicholas, J., & Nyenhuis, D. (2002). The role of perceived vulnerability in adjustment to lower extremity amputation: A preliminary investigation. *Rehabilitation Psychology, 47*(1), 92–105.

Berenbaum, H., & Fujita, F. (1994). Schizophrenia and personality: Exploring the boundaries and connections between vulnerability and outcome. *Journal of Abnormal Psychology, 103,* 148–158.

Bezruchka, S. (2000). Culture and medicine: Is globalization dangerous to our health? *Western Journal of Medicine, 172,* 332–334.

Bezruchka, S. (2001). Societal hierarchy and the health Olympics. *Canadian Medical Association Journal, 164,* 1701–1703.

Bohner, G., Danner, U., Siebler, F., & Stamson, G. (2002). Rape myth acceptance and judgments of vulnerability to sexual assault: An Internet experiment. *Experimental Psychology, 49,* 257–269.

Bromberger, J., & Mathews, K. (1996). A "feminine" model of vulnerability to depressive symptoms: A longitudinal investigation of middle-aged women. *Journal of Personality and Social Psychology, 70,* 591–598.

Brown, G., Hammen, C., Craske, M., Wickens, T. (1995). Dimensions of dysfunctional attitudes as vulnerabilities to depressive symptoms. *Journal of Abnormal Psychology, 104,* 431–435.

Calvo, M., & Cano-Vindel, A. (1997). The nature of trait anxiety: Cognitive and biological vulnerability. *European Psychologist, 2,* 301–312.

Edell-Gustafsson, U., & Hetta, J. (2001). Fragmented sleep and tiredness in males and females one year after percutaneous transluminal coronary angioplasty (PTCA). *Journal of Advanced Nursing, 34*(2), 203–211.

Finn, P., Sharkansky, E., Viken, R., West, T., Sandy, J., & Bufferd, G. (1997). Heterogeneity in the families of sons of alcoholics: The impact of familial vulnerability type on offspring characteristics. *Journal of Abnormal Psychology, 106,* 26–36.

Flaskerud, J., & Lee, P. (2001). Vulnerability to health problems in female informal caregivers of persons with HIV/AIDS and age-related dementias. *Journal of Advanced Nursing, 33*(1), 60–68.

Flaskerud, J., Lesser, J., Dixon, E., Anderson, N., Conde, F., Kim, S., et al. (2002). Health disparities among vulnerable populations: Evolution of knowledge over five decades in *Nursing Research* publications. *Nursing Research, 51*(2), 74–85.

Flaskerud, J., & Winslow, B. (1998). Conceptualizing vulnerable populations in health-related research. *Nursing Research, 47*(2), 69–78.

Gerrard, M., Gibbons, F., & Bushman, B. (1996). Relation between perceived vulnerability to HIV and precautionary sexual behavior. *Psychological Bulletin, 119,* 390–409.

Hankin, B., & Abramson, L. (2001). Development of gender differences in depression: An elaborated cognitive vulnerability-transactional stress theory. *Psychological Bulletin, 127,* 773–796.

Hayes, A., Castonguay, L., & Goldfried, M. (1996). Effectiveness of targeting the vulnerability factors of depression in cognitive therapy. *Journal of Consulting and Clinical Psychology, 64,* 623–627.

Hofferth, S. (2003). The American family: Changes and challenges for the 21st century. In H. Wallace, G. Green, & K. Jaros (Eds.). *Health and welfare for families in the 21st century.* Sudbury, MA: Jones and Bartlett.

Ingram, R., & Ritter, J. (2000). Vulnerability to depression: Cognitive reactivity and parental bonding in high-risk individuals. *Journal of Abnormal Psychology, 109,* 588–596.

Institute of Medicine-National Academy of Sciences. (2003) *Unequal treatment: Confronting racial and ethnic disparities in health care.* Retrieved Feb. 20, 2004, from *www.nap.edu.*

Joiner, T. (1995). The price of soliciting and receiving negative feedback: Self-verification theory as a vulnerability to depression. *Journal of Abnormal Psychology, 104,* 364–372.

Karpati, A, Galea, S., Awerbuch, T., & Levins, R. (2002). Variability and vulnerability at the ecological level: Implications for understanding the social determinants of health. *American Journal of Public Health, 92,* 1768–1773.

Kelly, J., St. Lawrence, J., & Brasfield, T. (1991). Predictors of vulnerability to AIDS risk behavior relapse. *Journal of Consulting and Clinical Psychology, 59*(1), 163–166.

Kurz, J. M. (2002). Vulnerability of well spouses involved in lung transplantation. *Journal of Family Nursing, 8,* 353–370.

Leon, G., Fulkerson, J., Perry, C., & Early-Zaid, M. (1995). Prospective analysis of personality and behavioral vulnerabilities and gender influences in the later development of disordered eating. *Journal of Abnormal Psychology, 104*(1), 140–149.

Lessick, M., Woodring, B., Naber, S., & Halstead, L. (1992). Vulnerability: A conceptual model. *Perinatal and Neonatal Nursing, 6,* 1–14.

Lohr, J., & Flynn, K. (1992). Smoking and schizophrenia. *Schizophrenia Research, 8,* 93–102.

Lyons, M., Bar, J., Kremen, W., Toomey, R., Eisen, S., Goldberg, J., et al. (2002). Nicotine and familial vulnerability to schizophrenia: A discordant twin study. *Journal of Abnormal Psychology, 111,* 687–693.

McIntyre, L., Glanville, N., Raine, K., Dayle, J., Anderson, B., & Battaglia, N. (2003). Do low-income lone mothers compromise their nutrition to feed their children? *Canadian Medical Association Journal, 168*(6), 686–691.

Morrell-Bellai, T., Goering, P., & Boydell, K. (2000). Becoming and remaining homeless: Qualitative investigation. *Issues in Mental Health Nursing, 21,* 581–604.

National Institutes of Health. *Addressing health disparities: The NIH program of action.* Retrieved December 4, 2003, from *http://healthdisparities.nih.gov/whatare.html.*

National Institutes of Health (2002). *Strategic research plan and budget to reduce and ultimately eliminate health disparities.* Washington, DC: US Department of Health and Human Services.

Nettlebeck, T., Wison, C., Potter, R., & Perry, C. (2000). The influence of interpersonal competence on personal vulnerability of persons with mental retardation. *Journal of Interpersonal Violence, 15*(1), 46–62.

Phifer, J. (1990). Psychological distress and somatic symptoms after natural disaster: Differential vulnerability among older adults. *Psychology and Aging, 5,* 412–420.

Ruef, A., Litz, B., & Schlenger, W. (2000). Hispanic ethnicity and risk for combat-related posttraumatic stress disorder. *Cultural Diversity and Ethnic Minority Psychology, 6*(3), 235–251.

Schotte, D., Cools, J., & Payvar, S. (1990). Problem-solving deficits in suicidal patients: Trait vulnerability or state phenomenon? *Journal of Consulting and Clinical Psychology, 58,* 562–564.

Sebastian, J. (1996). Vulnerability and vulnerable populations. In M. Stanhope & J. Lancaster (Eds.). *Community health nursing: Promoting health of individuals, aggregates and communities* (4th ed.). St. Louis, MO: Mosby.

Sebastian, J., Bolla, C. D., Aretakis, D., Jones, K. J., Schenk, C., Napolitano, M., et al. (2002). Vulnerability and selected vulnerable populations. In M. Stanhope & J. Lancaster (Eds.). *Foundations of community health nursing* (pp. 349–364). St. Louis, MO: Mosby.

Shinn, M., Knickman, J., & Weitzman, B. (1991). Social relationships and vulnerability to becoming homeless among poor families. *American Psychologist, 46,* 1180–1187.

Siever, M. (1994). Sexual orientation and gender as factors in socioculturally acquired vulnerability to body dissatisfaction and eating disorders. *Journal of Consulting and Clinical Psychology, 62*(2), 252–260.

Simons, J., & Carey, K. (2002). Risk and vulnerability for marijuana use: Problems and the role of affect dysregulation. *Psychology of Addictive Behaviors, 16*(1), 72–75.

Smith, G., Gerrard, M., & Gibbons, F. (1997). Self-esteem and the relation between risk behavior and perceptions of vulnerability to unplanned pregnancy in college women. *Health Psychology, 16*(2), 137–146.

Spiers, J. (2000). New perspectives on vulnerability using etic and emic approaches. *Journal of Advanced Nursing, 31*(3), 715–721.

Strauman, T. (1992). Self-guides, autobiographical memory, and anxiety and dysphoria: Toward a cognitive model of vulnerability to emotional distress. *Journal of Abnormal Psychology, 101,* 87–95.

Tarasuk, V. (2003). Low income, welfare and nutritional vulnerability. *Canadian Medical Association Journal, 168,* 709–710.

Testa, M., Livingston, J., & Collins, R. (2000). The role of women's alcohol consumption in evaluation of vulnerability to sexual aggression. *Experimental and Clinical Psychopharmacology, 8*(2), 185–191.

Van Servellen, G., Aguirre, M., Sarna, L., & Brecht, M. (2002). Differential predictors of emotional distress in HIV-infected men and women. *Western Journal of Nursing Research, 24*(1), 49–72.

Whiffen, V. (1988). Vulnerability to post-partum depression: A prospective multivariate study. *Journal of Abnormal Psychology, 97,* 467–474.

Wild, T. C., Hinson, R., Cunningham, J., & Bacchiochi, J. (2001). Perceived vulnerability to alcohol-related harm in young adults: Independent effects of risky alcohol use and drinking motives. *Experimental and Clinical Psychopharmacology, 9,* 1064–1297.

Wills, T. A., Gibbons, F., Gerrard, M., & Brody, G. (2000). Protection and vulnerability processes relevant for early onset of substance use: A test among African American children. *Health Psychology, 19*(3), 253–263.

World Health Organization. (1948). Constitution of the World Health Organization. In *Handbook of basic documents.* Geneva: Author.

Wuerker, A. (2000). The family and schizophrenia. *Issues in Mental Health Nursing, 21,* 127–141.

Zuroff, D., Blatt, S., Bondi, C., & Pilkonis, P. (1999). Vulnerability to depression: Reexamining state dependence and relative stability. *Journal of Abnormal Psychology, 108,* 76–89.

CHAPTER 2

The Nature of Social Justice

Charles Barnes

Hardly a day goes by that we do not open a newspaper or watch television and learn of the problems that plague the delivery of health care in the United States. Increasing costs, scaling back of benefits, seeming arbitrary rationing, and the inability of a significant number of Americans to gain access to even basic health care bespeak a health care system plagued with inefficiency and waste. We also see stories from further afield chronicling poverty, starvation, and disease. We read of public health crises such as AIDS in Africa, but we often do not hear about the lack of even basic levels of public health services or about the limited access to care that would, in many instances, inexpensively and effectively prevent or eradicate illnesses that are easily treatable.

The nurse who has frequent contact with underserved and deprived populations confronts these realities on a frequent, if not daily, basis. Although working with these populations is certainly rewarding and fulfills a pressing social need, it is only part of the picture when talking about notions of social justice, particularly in the delivery of health care and the restoration of health. This is because nursing is also about working to eliminate the underlying structural causes that cause the high incidence of illness and disease among the poor.

Yet social justice remains an elusive term that can be difficult to define and even more difficult to apply in practice. The purpose of this chapter is to describe the concept of social justice within the context of nursing by first defining the term and its relationship to more general notions of justice. We will then look at how the concept of social justice can be applied to the practice of nursing, particularly in service to underserved populations.

Prior to embarking on our discussion it should be noted that the promotion of justice is frequently tied to religious precepts and teachings, especially in most mainstream churches. Yet because of the diverse world we live in and the overwhelming nature of the task at hand, we cannot look upon justice as solely the purview of any particular religion if we are to truly realize a more just global society. The articulate, well-developed principles of the social teachings of the Roman Catholic church can, however, act as a bridge to connect both religious and secular notions of justice through a common language meant to transcend both religious boundaries and political ideology.

DEFINITIONS OF JUSTICE

Beauchamp and Childress (2001) identify interpretations of the term "justice," which has variously been described as "fairness," "desert" (i.e., that which one deserves), "entitlement," or "equity." Although these various descriptions may at first glance appear to be competing or attempting to achieve different goals, we can unify them by treating justice primarily as a virtue. In this context, virtue is a habit that advances both an individual and society toward the end or goal of human flourishing or human fulfillment (Aristotle, trans. 1941). The term "habit" in this context comes from the Greek *habitus,* which is a predictable disposition to choose the good whenever one is confronted with a choice. In other words, we will naturally gravitate toward whatever decision will advance the good of all, and this desire to choose the good is innate within us, with the end goal of human flourishing.

WHAT IS SOCIAL JUSTICE?

Social justice is a very broad term that is primarily concerned with how we relate to each other as persons, communities, and nations. The underlying concept bespeaks several factors that, together, color how we should act in relation to our fellow human beings and, more to the point, the basic human rights that underpin these relationships. They should act as a guide to how we form public policy, deliver services and social goods, and, for purposes of this discussion, how the practice of nursing should be conducted to ensure these human rights are respected and encouraged in others.

Some of the most comprehensive treatment of social justice issues, as mentioned previously, comes from the Catholic church. Catholics view part of the Christian mission on Earth as the promotion of justice and the healing of pain and suffering caused by the prevalence of injustices and oppression. Although it is true that working for justice is not solely a Catholic or even Christian endeavor, it is helpful to examine the social teachings of the Catholic church to help define and frame why nursing concerns itself with social justice, and why it is such an important element for the practice of nursing.

Part of the reason for this, as we will see a bit later, is that nursing began as a predominantly religion-sponsored work. Catholic nuns and affiliated lay people were a dominant force in the provision of health care in the early 1900s, both in North America and in Europe. Together, alongside asylums, schools, orphanages, and other institutions they founded and ran, Catholic health care providers accounted for half of all North American health care facilities by 1915 (Nelson, 2003). It is from this Catholic tradition that social justice as a value in nursing evolved, and that is why it makes sense to define social justice in light of Catholic social teaching.

The social teaching of the Catholic church rests on two conceptual principles: human dignity and the common good. From these wider notions of human solidarity, the preferential option for the poor, human rights, and other manifestations of social justice are drawn. In a health care context, promotion and restoration of health is seen not only in terms of being a social good but also as a basic human right that is interrelated with other issues of social justice such as poverty and oppression.

The promotion of human dignity has evolved over the last century to encompass issues relating to the right to life as well as social and economic well-being. The source of this teaching is the biblical statement in the book of Genesis that we are made in the image and likeness of God. Therefore, according to Brodeur (1995, p. 31), one is to be "valued for him or herself" and should be accorded basic rights that allow one to flourish as a human being.

Furthermore, it is important to point out that these rights and freedoms are not to be exercised in isolation but rather in community. This, according to Lustig (1993), enriches and places the inherent demands for liberty and equality in context, carrying rights to a deeper level, particularly in regard to health care. Liberty and equality are not viewed in this context as mutually exclusive principles where one has priority over the other but rather as being "mutually accommodating," where the person is able to exercise freedom and autonomy but does so as one among other human beings who are also endowed with the same rights.

This is because human beings are, at their most basic, social animals who naturally exhibit a desire to live in community with one another. Although it may seem as if notions of individualism and self-centeredness are highly prevalent in today's society, the reality is that we are far more interdependent and in need of being in relationship with others in community than we often realize. To deny this communal dimension of our lives or place primacy of the individual over the community is an exercise in futility. As Granfield (1988) insists, our entire human history "attest(s) to our state of continuous interdependence," where the attainment of common goals such as human dignity are only possible by working together.

Furthermore, it is equally problematic to submerge the dignity of the individual or place the needs of the community over and above the needs of the individuals who inhabit it. Doing so runs the risk of denying individual human dignity for a supposed greater good, which ultimately defeats the purpose of working to ensure a more just society through consequences that may be laudable while the actions themselves may be ethically problematic. The blanket refusal to pay for certain complex health care interventions solely on the basis of age, for example, may be aimed at a more efficient distribution of health dollars to ensure they are spent on illness with potentially more successful outcomes, but this also runs the risk of denying elderly individuals the right to restoration of a certain quality of life.

A possible resolution between individual rights and collective responsibility is found in a concept described by feminist health care ethicists as "agency." In this context, one is able to make autonomous decisions but does so within a web of interpersonal relationships (Sherwin, 1992). In this way, the dignity of the individual is preserved while, at the same time, the role of the individual as part of a wider group playing a role in helping to attain the goals of human life for all is promoted and recognized.

The notion of the common good is a Thomistic concept—one that is inspired by the philosophical methods and principles used by Thomas Aquinas (1224/5–1274) that forms the end or ultimate goal of our work on Earth. Thomas Aquinas, as noted by Bouchard (1999), viewed the common good as "the good of any being, as the good of a political community, and, finally as God's own self, to whom all creation tends."

In its application to health care, Hamel (1999) points out that the promotion of the common good finds its basis in such diverse areas as providing just and fair working conditions for employees, respect for the dignity of the individual, and the provision of high-quality care that affirms "our common solidarity and interdependency, without neglecting individual rights." Organizationally, the common good is promoted by a health care institution through the way such interdependency is extended both within and outside the health care facility. Responsibility toward the community, shown by providing services for the most vulnerable, promoting healthy lifestyles in the community and beyond, and espousing clinical practices that are both ethical and moral, are but a few ways the common good can be promoted.

Dioceses and religious orders that founded health care institutions did so primarily to serve the poor and those otherwise shunned or neglected by society. Although the circumstances may have changed, the problems have not. They have, in fact, been exacerbated by the increasing gap between rich and poor in the last 20 years, the numbers of poor people suffering from HIV and AIDS, and the inability of an estimated 48 million Americans to obtain access to health care because they are ineligible for public assistance or work low-paying part-time or temporary jobs.

The cornerstone of social justice lies in the Church's preferential option for the poor. Such a concept is born of a need to advocate for those who are poor and marginalized because they are frequently denied the means necessary to live with dignity. Such an option mandates that social change take place so the basic rights of these people are respected, along with their entitlement to fully participate in the life of the community. In the absence of such rights, they must be accorded "special consideration," as Curran (2002, p. 183) states, in order that their dignity and rights may be respected.

It is important to point out, however, that any discussion of rights carries with it an acknowledgment that the poor themselves should share in the work to "overcome the devastating and evil effects of poverty" (Brodeur, 1995). Acknowledging such responsibility wards off the dangers of falling into the trap of mere "victim blaming." Such victimization itself denies people the dignity they aspire to by instilling a sense of hopelessness or cynicism that they are completely at the mercy of outside forces and are therefore unable to assume any kind of ownership or empowerment of their own lives. The end result of such victimization is a vicious circle in which the oppression is perpetuated.

This is not to say, however, that individuals assuming responsibility for their own actions will alone solve problems of poverty and oppression as some libertarians would have us believe. It requires an effective mobilization by all to eliminate poverty and its systemic or structural causes. Or, as McCormick (1998, p. 258) asserts in the context of justice in health care, "Healthcare is a right only to the extent that individual responsibility is not enough."

SOCIAL JUSTICE AND NURSING PRACTICE

From the outset, the evolution of nursing as a profession has been intertwined with goals of social justice, namely, the basic right of humans to live with dignity regardless of economic status. These goals and, more specifically, a passion for social justice are what motivated Florence Nightingale to work with the poor and oppressed. Webb (2002) remarks that Nightingale was horrified by the visibly suffering poor of Victorian England and outraged by an institutionalized civil and religious infrastructure that viewed the nature of life as predestined by God as part of an "eternally decreed plan." This Calvinistic outlook on life, known as predestinationism, extended to all facets of English life, including the class system, which condemned the poor to a life of squalor and misery as part of God's divine plan. It was Nightingale's refusal to accept this status quo that motivated her to embark on a life of service to the poor and the suffering.

Nightingale learned the importance of justice as inherent in the practice of nursing from the Daughters of Charity of St. Vincent de Paul, an order of nuns whose apostolate was to care for the sick and the dying. Mother Mary Xavier Clark, writing in 1841, insisted that "our charity must be extended to all." The Daughters of Charity not only trained Florence but accompanied her to the Crimea to assist her in caring for those wounded in the fighting (Farren, 2003, pp. 38–39).

In the United States the Sisters were also instrumental in providing care to those as diverse as Civil War soldiers, elderly slaves, and poor urban immigrants, concentrating on those shunned by society or ignored because of their poverty and disease. Yet caring for the poor in their illness was not the only manifestation of the work of the Sisters. They realized early on that in order to improve health they must tackle the underlying causes of illness and disease. Friedman (1997, pp. 51–52) states that the Sisters made no distinction in their nursing care between what was clinical and what was social and did so because they knew that health entailed more than just the cure of illness. "They understood the concept of social medicine, of population-based healthcare, of health communities long before those ideas became commonplace."

In this respect, social justice has been the cornerstone of nursing practice from its inception. The values and virtues of caring for the whole person, client advocacy, and the imperative to work for social change in not only the delivery of health care but also the improvement of health (American Nurses Association, 2001) bespeak a long tradition of caring for all, particularly the poor and vulnerable.

Still, the question arises, what role does modern nursing play in efforts to eliminate structural inequality and advocate for a fairer and more equitable society? The essentials of baccalaureate education for professional nursing practice (American Association of Colleges of Nursing, 1998) mandate that nurses

- ☐ support fairness and nondiscrimination in the delivery of care,
- ☐ promote universal access to health care, and
- ☐ encourage legislation and policy consistent with the advancement of nursing care and health care.

How nurses achieve these goals is, on one level, directly related to the talents, abilities, and motivations of each individual nurse. As a practice, nursing is far more than just the technical aspects of patient care. It is first and foremost about the realization of certain social goods, which the application of technical skills helps to bring about. McIntyre (1981) suggests that such technical aspects are "transformed and enriched" by one's participation in the realization of these social goods. In other words, by both desiring and achieving excellence in our own practice of nursing, we are using the talents, skills, and abilities, both innate and learned, to play an individual role in promoting and restoring health to our clients and, in turn, working to realize the wider goals of nursing.

At the same time, it is also important to remember that nursing is a social practice that has impact far beyond the locus of care. Roth & Harrison (1991, p. 344) advocate for a balance in nursing practice between private duties (obligations to individual clients, groups of clients, and so-called interest groups) and public duties (those that serve the common good and are variously attained through legislative advocacy, policy formation, a voice in the "allocation of resources," and the preservation of human dignity). To integrate social justice in nursing, therefore, we must expand our definitions of excellence in nursing to include the ways in which we promote and restore health, not only to individual clients, but also to the populations in which those clients reside.

Leuning (2001) suggests a different perspective whereby we "adopt a pattern of thought and action that challenges institutionalized power relations or relations of domination." The emphasis on culturally competent care and the experience of caring for clients from other countries and cultures is one way of challenging such power insofar as it builds a bridge to a shared human experience that never loses sight of the need for people to live and die with dignity.

Furthermore, it is important that nurses understand the global perspective of their profession in a way that "challenges conventional roles, values and boundaries" (Hilfinger-Messias, 2001, p. 10). Nursing education that focuses on the global environment is another way to realize this challenge. Yet Hilfinger-Messias also advocates the building of "collaborative partnerships" and "fostering bridges across disparate worlds" as a means of linking local nursing practice to the wider global community (p. 11).

None of this can be achieved, however, without the commitment of nurses at all levels of the profession. That nurse leaders exhibit leadership in promoting social justice as a virtue in nursing testifies to the importance of working to achieve social change. Through the stated commitment of nursing to serve vulnerable populations, nursing displays a preferential option for the poor that works hard to promote personal autonomy and improve the social conditions necessary to restore human dignity.

CONCLUSION

The end goal of nursing, in this context, is to be aware of and to be responsive to the needs of clients within the locus of professional practice but also in terms of the wider context of the promotion and restoration of health, along with other colleagues who share the same goals and desire for excellence. Social justice in nursing is, therefore, about how we break down barriers and work to end inequality through our work as individuals participating in a profession as well as through the collective profession itself.

Through this conception of nursing as both a private and a public practice that is understood in a global context we can each play our part commensurate with our talents and our abilities to enact social change. We challenge these unequal power relationships by approaching nursing with a deliberate sense that the profession is about fostering human dignity and the common good through the restoration of health. This imperative has implications far beyond the bedside or individual client and finds itself in the collective actions of nurses as a whole.

REFERENCES

American Association of Colleges of Nursing. (1998). *The essentials of baccalaureate nursing education for professional nursing practice* (p. 9). Washington, DC: American Association of Colleges of Nursing.

American Nurses Association (2001). *Code of ethics for nurses with interpretive statements.* Washington, DC: American Nurses Association.

Aristotle. Nicomacean ethics (W. D. Ross, Trans., 1941). In R. McKeon (Ed.). *The basic works of Aristotle* (pp. 927–1112). New York, NY: Random House.

Beauchamp, T. L., & Childress, J. F. (2001). *Principles of biomedical ethics* (5th ed., p. 226). New York, NY: Oxford University Press.

Bouchard, C. (1999). Catholic healthcare and the common good. *Health Progress, 80*(3), 34–40.

Brodeur, D. (1995, September–October). Guidance for a failing system: Catholic social teachings provide the needed principles. *Health Progress, 76*(7), 30–35, 40.

Curran, C. E. (2002). *Catholic social teaching: A historical, theological and ethical analysis* (p. 183). Washington, DC: Georgetown University Press.

Farren, S. (2003, March–April). The sister nurses. *Health Progress, 84*(2), 38–42, 65.

Friedman, E. (1997, January–February). Fulfilling the Sisters' promise. *Health Progress, 78*(1), 50–55.

Granfield, D. (1988). *The inner experience of law: A jurisprudence of subjectivity* (p. 129). Washington, DC: Catholic University of America Press.

Hamel, R. (1999). Of what good is the common good? *Health Progress, 80*(3), 45–47.

Hilfinger-Messias, D. K. (2001). Globalization, nursing and health for all. *Journal of Nursing Scholarship, 33*(1), 9–11.

Leuning, C. J. (2001). Advancing a global perspective: The world as classroom. *Nursing Science Quarterly, 14*(4), 298–303.

Lustig, B. A. (1993). The common good in a secular society: The relevance of a Roman Catholic notion to the health care allocation debate. *Journal of Medicine and Philosophy, 18,* 569–587.

Macintyre, A. (1981). *After virtue* (2nd ed., p. 193). South Bend, IN: University of Notre Dame Press.

McCormick, R. A. (1998). A Catholic perspective on access to healthcare. *Cambridge Quarterly of Healthcare Ethics, 7,* 254–259.

Nelson, S. (2003, March–April). Invisible radicals. *Health Progress, 84*(2), 27–28.

Roth, P. A., & Harrison, J. K. (1991). Orchestrating social change: An imperative in the care of the chronically ill. *Journal of Medicine and Philosophy, 16,* 343–359.

Sherwin, S. (1992). *No longer patient: Feminist ethics and healthcare* (p. 156). Philadelphia, PA: Temple University Press.

Webb, V. (2002). *Florence Nightingale: The making of a radical theologian* (pp. 30–32). St. Louis, MO: Chalice Press.

CHAPTER 3

Social Justice in Nursing: A Review of the Literature

Doris M. Boutain

The purpose of this chapter is to explore how social justice is described in the nursing literature. Analysis has revealed that authors ascribe to social, distributive, and market views of justice. Most authors, however, do not explicitly attend to the differences among these concepts.

The three predominant models of justice will be reviewed first, then we will provide a framework for how nurses can focus on injustice awareness, amelioration, and transformation as forms of social justice. The multiple methods of promoting a social justice agenda, from consciousness raising to the re-creation of social policies, will also be delineated. Recognizing the many ways to promote social justice can have a transformational impact on how nurses teach, research, and practice.

Although social justice is not a new concept, the nursing literature lacks a coherent and complex understanding of its implications for studying societal health (Drevdahl, Kneipp, Canales, & Dorcy, 2001; Liaschenko, 1999). Social justice is often briefly mentioned after elaborate discussions about ethics. When ethics is defined in the forefront, the concept of social justice is often written in the conclusion section of articles as if it is a related afterthought. Inattention to the subtle variations in how social justice is conceived can inadvertently result in nursing practice, research, and education that are antithetical to a social justice agenda.

LITERATURE SEARCH METHODOLOGY

A search of the Cumulative Index of Nursing and Allied Health (CINAHL) literature from 1990 to 2003 revealed 142 articles, book chapters, commentaries, and abstracts categorized with the key words "social justice" and "nursing." Of this number, thirty-two articles, two book chapters, and three dissertations were classified using those key words as major descriptors. A major descriptor is a term that the manuscript authors view as a main focus of their work. Literature using the major descriptors of social justice and nursing form the basis of this review, while the other 105 publications supplement the literature analysis.

DEFINING JUSTICE IN NURSING

The ethical principle of justice was referred to frequently in the nursing literature surveyed. Ninety-two of the 142 publications (65%) retrieved equated justice with what is fair or what is deserved or "giving to others what is their due" (Lamke, 1996, p. 55). Authors discussed ethics, which is primarily viewed as a framework for understanding how values, duties, principles, and obligations inform people's sense of societal fairness, as the basis for moral decision making (Aroskar, 1995; Harper, 1994).

Although many authors mentioned justice, only seven articles actually defined justice beyond notions of ethical fairness (Drevdahl, 1999; Drevdahl et al., 2001; Kneipp & Snider, 2001; Liaschenko, 1999; Thorne, 1999; Vonthron Good & Rodrigues-Fisher, 1993). Liaschenko (1999) outlined the relationship between personal values and justice in an effort to describe how justice can guide nursing practice. Vonthron Good & Rodrigues-Fisher (1993) considered how justice was useful in assessing if vulnerability is compromised or protected in research. Exploring the philosophical underpinning of justice, Drevdahl et al. (2001) compared the concepts of social justice, distributive justice, and market justice. Like other scholars (Sellers & Haag, 1992), they posited that most nurses do not consider the distinction among concepts related to justice (Drevdahl et al., 2001). Without an intricate understanding of the different views of justice, nurses may limit their problem-solving abilities when it comes to understanding how unjust social conditions influence health status, access, and delivery. It is therefore important to explore the most prominent forms of justice in nursing literature today.

Social, Distributive, and Market Justice

Social, distributive, and market justice are the most common forms of justice referenced in the nursing literature. Social justice is often defined as a concern for "the equitable distribution of benefits and burdens in society" (Redman & Clark, 2002). Social justice is also, but less often, defined as changing social relationships and institutions to promote equitable relationships (Drevdahl et al., 2001). Distributive justice is discussed in reference to the equal distribution of goods and services in society (Schroeder & Ward, 1998). Market justice posits that people are entitled only to goods and services that they acquire according to guidelines of entitlement (Young, 1990).

Although these forms of justice appear similar, there are distinct differences (Beauchamp, 1986; Whitehead, 1992). Social justice is concerned with making equitable the balance between societal benefits and burdens. Social justice posits that there are social rights and collateral responsibilities with those rights (Lebacqz, 1986). Social beings are to both give and receive, using equity as a framework for relating to one another. Equity, derived from the Greek word *epiky,* means that persons must conduct themselves with reasonableness and moderation when exercising their rights (Whitehead, 1992). Distributive justice involves equality more than equity and is used most often to discuss the allocation or distribution of goods and services in society (Young, 1990). Equality focuses on giving the same access and resources to different groups (Sellers & Haag, 1992).

Social justice advocates explore social relationships and how those relationships form the basis for the allocation of goods and services (Young, 1990). Social justice focuses on equity because many theories of social justice assert that equal does not mean just (Lebacqz, 1986). Thus the concepts of social and distributive justice are somewhat parallel yet have different primary foci of study (Drevdahl et al., 2001).

Market justice is also viewed as a form of justice in nursing (Drevdahl, 2002). It is based on honoring the rights of those who have earned entitlement to those privileges. Market justice permits inequality as long as those inequalities result from a fair market system. That is, only those who earn rights are secured their entitled privileges in a market system. Those who earn no rights are not secured privileges.

Critics of the market justice agenda note that using the word market as an adjective for justice is itself an oxymoron (Beauchamp, 1986). "Justice" is a word most often used to discuss fairness. The term "market" is most often concerned with the balance between monetary value and goods allocation. The two terms do not work together when discussing equity. Simply "applying the word 'justice' to 'market' does not bring the concept into the realm of justice" (Drevdahl et al., 2001, p. 24). Social justice is not a parallel model to market justice; social justice is antithetical to a market model (Beauchamp, 1986). These two ways of viewing the world, therefore, diametrically oppose each other and simultaneously coexist.

An example may clarify the difference between social, distributive, and market justice. Using a social justice framework, everyone in the United States would be entitled to health care as needed if health care was deemed a right of citizenship. Health care, using a social justice view, is a moral obligation and a right of citizenship. A distributive justice framework would give a certain level of health care to everyone as a result of citizenship. The leveling of health care is needed to make sure that there are enough health care services for all to receive at least minimal benefit. Using distributive justice, health is a right of citizens but not necessarily a moral responsibility. Persons can receive health care as a result of how much they can pay for those services in a market system. The focus of a market system is not on moral or citizenship rights but on making sure those who want the good of health care, for example, can pay for those services.

All forms of justice, although somewhat distinct, may coexist to varying degrees. There are health care services in the United States that are given as needed, such as the care given to children who are orphaned. Then there are incidences when minimal health care is given, such as the medical and dental benefits associated with Medicaid. Persons who can afford more treatment or faster treatment may get those services as well if they can pay a particular price. An example may be health care clinics that are designed to give expanded services if clients pay certain access fees. Although these three forms of justice are noted in the nursing literature to varying degrees, seldom is it discussed how these views of justice guide nursing education, research, or practice.

Views of Justice in Articles About Nursing Education

Most manuscripts about nursing education and justice focus on the clinical preparation of undergraduate students to meet the needs of a culturally diverse population (Herman & Sassatelli, 2002; Leuning, 2001; Redman & Clark, 2002; Scanlan, Care, & Gessler, 2001). Other articles proclaim the need for a global consciousness among nurses as the starting point for injustice awareness (Leuning, 2001; Messias, 2001). Also present in the nursing literature are teaching models (Leuning, 2001), case examples (Thompson, 1991), and service-learning experiences (Herman & Sassatelli, 2002; Redman & Clark, 2002) that use justice as a framework to educate undergraduate students.

Although some nurse educators discussed the practical application of justice principles, no distinction was made between the use of social justice and distributive justice as concepts. For instance, authors defined social justice using distributive justice principles of equality (Thompson, 1991) or defined it as working with vulnerable populations (Redman & Clark, 2002). Another manuscript introduced justice in terms of contractual justice, the fair and honest contract between equals (Oddi & Oddi, 2000). In one instance, the words "social justice" were used but never defined (Herman & Sassatelli, 2002). Rarely is social justice used as a framework to critique nursing education models (Sellers & Haag, 1992) and student—faculty relationships (Oddi & Oddi, 2000; Scanlan, Care, & Gessler, 2001).

Views of Justice in Articles About Nursing Research

Most articles about justice and nursing research focus on how to protect vulnerable populations in research or understand the implications of working with those who are marginalized in society (Alderson, 2001; Lamke, 1996; McKane, 2000; Mill & Ogilvie, 2002; Rew, Taylor-Seehafer, & Thomas, 2000; Vonthron Good & Rodrigues-Fisher, 1993). Only a few authors explicitly stated that social justice was used as a theoretical framework for conducting research (Blondeau, Lavoie, Valois, Keyserlingk, Hebert, & Martineau, 2000; Clark, Barton, & Brown, 2002) or as a measurement parameter for understanding concepts related to nursing (Altun, 2002). Overall, in the literature, social justice is infrequently used as an explicit framework to guide the development of nursing research.

Views of Justice in Articles About Nursing Practice

Articles about how justice relates to nursing practice focus on how ethics is useful in making moral judgments about the care of individuals (Peter & Morgan, 2001). Justice is often defined as "treating people fairly" (Aroskar, 1995) in clinical practice. Other authors view justice as related to fairness but also as a social obligation for nurses to understand how practice is influenced by social inequalities in the design of health care and communities (Drevdahl, 2002; Leung, 2002; Ludwick & Silva, 2003; Russell, 2002). Most authors agree that discussions of justice are needed to assess how the work of individual nurses and the profession at large contribute to the formation of a just health care system and society (Schroeder & Ward, 1998; Haddad, 2002).

Despite the recognition that exploring justice is needed, most articles on this topic do not define justice beyond notions about fairness. Or if justice is defined more elaborately in relationship to nursing practice, authors often use a distributive justice framework (Schroeder & Ward, 1998). Authors using a distributive justice viewpoint assert that "all humans are born with equal opportunities and equal political agency and efficacy" (Schroeder & Ward, 1998, p. 230). The belief that persons are equal forms the basis for the even allocation of goods and services. A main limitation of the distributive view of justice is the lack of acknowledgment that social groups are often regarded unequally on the basis of gender, class, and race; thus the allocation of goods and services is also unequal in US society (Young, 1990).

Acknowledging the limitations of the distributive paradigm, a few authors explore the practice of nurses as embedded in the concept of the just state (Harper, 1994; Kikuchi & Simmons, 1999). The just state is concerned with how laws, public institutions, and communities act to limit or promote social inequalities in society. This view of the just state most closely parallels the concept of social justice.

Social Justice: Definitional Limitations in the Nursing Literature

The main concern with definitions of social justice in nursing is that injustice is viewed as a personal act, and justice is seen as an individual response to that act (Liaschenko, 1999; Olsen,

1993). The individualization of social justice is historically related to how nurses conceive the person as the primary site of, and remedy to, unjust conditions (Allen, 1996). Rarely is it highlighted how injustice nationally or globally (Austin, 2001) is created by power imbalances in the distribution of wealth, resources, and access. Seldom is it noted how unequal distribution in resources and access influences health care delivery, health status, and health actualization or achievement of optimum health. Often the articles about health and social justice in nursing limit the focus to underrepresented groups or people of color populations (Herman & Sassatelli, 2002; Redman & Clark, 2002). Nursing literature fails to address how inequitable conditions contribute to diminished health actualization in majority groups as well.

Deaton & Lubotsky (2003), for example, identified that death rates in US states with more income inequality were higher for all groups than in states with more equal income distributions. After considering the racial and ethnic composition of those US states, it remained unclear why the mortality of the majority group of white Americans was related to racial composition and income inequality (Deaton & Lubotsky, 2003). In part, this is due to the lack of research studying how inequality contributes to poor health outcomes for both minority and majority members of society. Despite this consideration, there is a growing body of literature suggesting that injustice lessens the presence of optimal health for all (Kawachi & Kennedy, 1999; Subramanian, Blakely, & Kawachi, 2003). Even on a global level, poor environments foster poor health locally and nationally (World Health Organization, 1997).

Considerations such as this remain underdocumented in the nursing literature for several reasons. Nurses have a limited view of social justice (Drevdahl, 2002). As justice is defined in relationship to individual equality and fairness, the social dimensions of justice and injustice are minimized. What is fair, however, does not necessary need to be equal or vice versa (Thorne, 1999). Given the historic disadvantages encountered by underrepresented groups in the United States, for instance, to give equal treatment would not remedy current or past ills.

Social justice asserts that vulnerable persons should be protected from harm and promoted to achieve full status in society. The dynamics of being perceived as privileged or vulnerable would require exploration. Particularly relevant would be an investigation of how nurses themselves are influenced by privilege as they espouse their role as social justice advocates. One question becomes focal: Can nurses really promote a social justice agenda when that promotion will result in the critique and dismantlement of their own advantage?

Social justice critique means, for example, that one must recognize the social factors that construe persons as privileged and/or vulnerable at different points in time. A social justice agenda necessitates transforming systems that promote subordination or disadvantage in the long term and the immediate conditions that limit self-actualization in the short term (Kirkham & Anderson, 2002). The focus on multiple simultaneous sites of social justice action is needed to begin to address the short- and long-term oppressive situations that create social injustice and limit access to health care. A multifocal approach to social justice is needed but is not, as of yet, fully articulated in the nursing literature.

ALTERNATIVE VIEWS OF SOCIAL JUSTICE

Definitions of social justice vary across disciplines and over time. Theories about social justice are espoused in philosophy (Young, 1990), public health science (Beauchamp, 1986), and religious studies (Lebacquz, 1986). The use of social justice by nurses as a research framework gained momentum in the early 1990s with the application of womanist, feminist, and social critical theories (Boutain, 1999) and in the late 1990s with the use of postcolonial perspectives (Kirkham & Anderson, 2002). Authors who use critical theories to critique nursing education, research, and practice help guide the nursing profession toward a social justice agenda (Boutain, 1999). However, these works were not developed to give explicit attention to the multiple ways to understand social justice as a concept.

One useful framework for nurses to consider is based on the work of Holland (1983). He argues that to be effective in promoting justice, scholars must think of addressing injustice on many fronts. Scholars must deal with the causes of injustice, the results of injustice, and the antecedents to injustice in society. Nurses can then focus on social justice in terms of social justice awareness, amelioration, or transformation.

SOCIAL JUSTICE AWARENESS, AMELIORATION, AND TRANSFORMATION

Social justice awareness entails exploring how one creates others as vulnerable or privileged. Awareness involves asking critical questions about how systems of domination and oppression foster categorizations such as "vulnerability" and "privilege." An example may be helpful in understanding social justice awareness.

Homelessness is a major health and social concern. A focus on social justice awareness may involve conducting a self- and client interview on how housing influences health. Think of what you know about how health is related to housing. Write your thoughts prior to interviewing clients with and without a home. Talk with clients who have homes and those who do not. Ask them about how having or not having a home influences their health. Record their thoughts.

Conduct a literature review on housing, home ownership, and health. Questions to consider include: How does having a home relate to health? What is the health status of those who have homes? What is the health status of those who do not have homes? Compare your initial thoughts to the knowledge gained in the interview and review of relevant literature. You may discover that your awareness of the relationship between housing and health increases.

Social justice awareness is an ongoing process. To alter the analogy as described by Lebacquz (1986), injustice is like a proverbial elephant standing right next to you. You cannot appreciate the entire view. You may not fully recognize how you are affected by or are affecting the elephant. You must continue to move, sensing each part of the elephant at different angles and with different senses. Social justice awareness is temporal and dependent on your frame of reference. Being aware is a start; however, it is not enough.

Social justice amelioration involves addressing the immediate results or antecedents to unjust conditions. To continue with the example of health and homelessness, amelioration entails a direct attempt to address the situation of the clients who are homeless. How that situation is addressed, however, is often to treat the most immediately seen concerns of that person. Getting grants to provide temporary shelter, food, clothing, or health care to the homeless, for example, is an illustration of social justice amelioration. In the short term, amelioration remedies urgent or semi-urgent concerns. However, social justice amelioration does not really change the conditions that will create others as homeless over and over again.

Social justice transformation also involves critically deliberating about the conditions of home dwelling and homelessness in relationship to health. Who are the most likely to have homes? What conditions were present that allowed them to have homes? Who are the most likely to be homeless? What conditions led them to become known as homeless? How does housing relate to health services allocation, current health status, or future health attainment? Social justice transformation advocates seek to answer these questions in attempts to change or develop just housing and health policies. Their aim is to eliminate or limit the conditions that result in homeless. Social justice transformation is devoted to redressing unjust conditions by changing the structures that foster those unjust situations. Transformation focuses individual actions toward long-range systematic solutions to unjust situations.

The work of Iris Young (1990) is helpful in further understanding social justice transformation. She argues that the distributive justice (similar to social justice amelioration) is based on a false system of distributing services and rights to those who are already marginalized. Thus, the rendering of service recreates the system of privilege by allowing those who give the services (the privileged) to remain in a position of power over those who receive those services (the needy). In the short term it addresses the needs of the most vulnerable, but simultaneously, in the long term, there is no change in the system because those privileged few in power remain so. Instead, Young believes it is most helpful to restructure systems so that certain services, such as homeless shelters, are no longer needed or are needed infrequently. System restructuring is accomplished by recognizing, confronting, and diminishing entrenched inequalities associated with gender, class, and racial inequalities in society (Young, 1990).

CONCLUSION

A social justice agenda recognizes that social groups are not treated equally in society. Social justice gives moral privilege to the needs of the most vulnerable group in an effort to promote justice within the society at large. As vulnerability among persons is eliminated or minimized, the moral agency of the privileged can also be elevated. This view of social justice is not clearly articulated in the literature on nursing education, research, and practice, however.

Discussions about social justice remain conceptually limited in the majority of published works in nursing. Without a more complex and nuanced view of social justice, nurses are less able to fully utilize this concept as a framework to redress unjust conditions in health care delivery and health attainment. Social justice is regarded as central to the nursing profession despite the need to critically revisit discussions about social justice. Nurses can contribute much to understanding how the interdisciplinary concept of social justice is useful in promoting just health and social relationships in society.

ACKNOWLEDGMENTS

Manuscript support was provided by grants from the National Institute of Child Health and Human Development (HD-41682); the National Institute of Nursing Research (F31 NR07249-01); and the Centers for Disease Control and Prevention (U48/CCU009654-06).

The author wishes to thank Joseph Fletcher III.

REFERENCES

Alderson, P. (2001). Prenatal screening, ethics, and Down's syndrome: A literature review. *Nursing Ethics, 8,* 360–374.

Allen, D. (1996). Knowledge, politics, culture, and gender: A discourse perspective. *Canadian Journal of Nursing Research, 28,* 95–102.

Altun, I. (2002). Burnout and nurses' personal and professional values. *Nursing Ethics, 9,* 269–278.

Aroskar, M. (1995). Envisioning nursing as a moral community. *Nursing Outlook, 43,* 134–138.

Austin, W. (2001). Nursing ethics in an era of globalization. *Advances in Nursing Science, 24,* 1–18.

Beauchamp, D. (1986). Public health as social justice: In T. Mappes & J. Zembaty (Eds.). *Biomedical ethics* (pp. 585–593). New York, NY: McGraw-Hill.

Blondeau, D., Lavoie, M., Valois, P., Keyserlingk, E., Hebert, M., & Martineau, I. (2000). The attitude of Canadian nurses towards advance directives. *Nursing Ethics, 7,* 399–411.

Boutain, D. (1999). Critical nursing scholarship: Exploring critical social theory with African-American studies. *Advances in Nursing Science, 21,* 37–47.

Clark, L., Barton, J., & Brown, N. (2002). Assessment of community contamination: A critical approach. *Public Health Nursing, 19,* 354–365.

Deaton, A., & Lubotsky, D. (2003). Mortality, inequality and race in American cities and states. *Social Science and Medicine, 56,* 1139–1153.

Drevdahl, D., Kneipp, S., Canales, M., & Dorcy, K. (2001). Reinvesting in social justice: A capital idea for public health nursing. *Advances in Nursing Science, 24,* 19–31.

Drevdahl, D. (1999). Sailing beyond: Nursing theory and the person. *Advances in Nursing Science, 21*(4), 1–13.

Drevdahl, D. (2002). Social justice or market justice? The paradoxes of public health partnerships with managed care. *Public Health Nursing, 19*(3), 161–169.

Haddad, A. (2002). Fairness, respect, and foreign nurses. *RN, 65*(7), 25–28.

Herman, C., & Sassatelli, J. (2002). DARING to reach the heartland: A collaborative faith-based partnership in nursing education. *Journal of Nursing Education, 41*(10), 443–445.

Harper, J. (1994). For-profit entities and continuing education: A nursing perspective. *Nursing Outlook, 42,* 217–222.

Holland, J. (1983). *Social analysis: Linking faith and justice.* Maryknoll, NY: Orbis Books.

Kawachi, I., & Kennedy, B. (1999). Income inequality and health: Pathways and mechanisms. *Health Services Research, 34*(1) Pt 2, 215–227.

Kikuchi, J., & Simmons, H. (1999). Practical nursing judgment: A moderate realist conception. *Scholarly Inquiry in Nursing Practice, 13*(1), 43–55.

Kirkham, S., & Anderson, J. (2002). Postcolonial nursing scholarship: From epistemology to method. *Advances in Nursing Science, 25*(1), 1–17.

Kneipp, S., & Snider, M. (2001). Social justice in a market model world. *Journal of Professional Nursing, 17*(3), 113.

Lamke, C. (1996). Distributive justice and HIV disease in intensive care. *Critical Care Nursing Quarterly, 19*(1), 55–64.

Lebacqz, K. (1986). *Six theories of justice.* Minneapolis, MN: Augsburg.

Leung, W. (2002). Why the professional-client ethic is inadequate in mental health care. *Nursing Ethics, 9*(1), 51–60.

Leuning, C. (2001). Advancing a global perspective: The world as classroom. *Nursing Science Quarterly, 14*(4), 298–303.

Liaschenko, J. (1999). Can justice coexist with the supremacy of personal values in nursing practice? *Western Journal of Nursing Research, 21*(1), 35–50.

Ludwick, R., & Silva, M. (2000, August). Nursing around the world: Cultural values and ethical conflicts. *Online Journal of Issues in Nursing.* Retrieved October 21, 2003, from *http://www.nursingworld.org/ ojin/ethical/ethics_4.htm.*

McKane, M. (2000). Research, ethics and the data protection legislation. *Nursing Standard, 2*(14), 36–41.

Messias, D. (2001). Globalization, nursing, and health for all. *Journal of Nursing Scholarship, 33*(1), 9–11.

Mill, J., & Ogilvie, L. (2002). Ethical decision making in international nursing research. *Qualitative Health Research, 12*(6), 807–815.

Oddi, L., & Oddi, S. (2000). Student-faculty joint authorship: Ethical and legal concerns. *Journal of Professional Nursing, 16*(4), 219–227.

Olsen, D. (1993). Populations vulnerable to the ethics of caring. *Journal of Advanced Nursing, 18,* 1696–1700.

Olsen, D. (2001). Empathetic maturity: Theory of moral point of view in clinical relations. *Advances in Nursing Science, 24*(1), 36–46.

Peter, E., & Morgan, K. (2001). Explorations of a trust approach to nursing ethics. *Nursing Inquiry, 8,* 3–10.

Redman, R., & Clark, L. (2002). Service-learning as a model for integrating social justice in the nursing curriculum. *Journal of Nursing Education, 41,* 446–449.

Rew, L, Taylor-Seehafer, M., & Thomas, N. (2000). Without parental consent: Conducting research with homeless adolescents. *Journal of the Society of Pediatric Nurses, 5,* 131–138.

Russell, K. (2002) Silent voices. *Public Health Nursing, 19*(4), 233–234.

Scanlan, J., Care, W., & Gessler, S. (2001). Dealing with unsafe students in clinical practice. *Nurse Educator, 26*(1), 23–27.

Schroeder, C., & Ward, D. (1998). Women, welfare, and work: One view of the debate, *Nursing Outlook, 46*(5), 226–232.

Sellers, S., & Haag, B. (1992). Achieving equity in nursing education. *Nursing & Health Care, 13*(3), 134–137.

Subramanian, S., Blakely, T., & Kawachi, I. (2003). Income inequality as a public health concern: Where do we stand? *Health Services Research, 38,* 153–167.

Thompson, D. (1991). Ethical case analysis using a hospital bill. *Nurse Educator, 16*(4), 20–23.

Thorne, S. (1999). Are egalitarian relationships a desirable ideal in nursing? *Western Journal of Nursing Research, 21*(1), 16–34.

Vonthron Good, B., & Rodrigues-Fisher, L. (1993). Vulnerability: An ethical consideration in research with older adults. *Western Journal of Nursing Research, 15*(6), 780–783.

Whitehead, M. (1992). The concepts and principles of equity and health. *International Journal of Health Services, 22*(3), 429–445.

World Health Organization (1997). *Health and environments in sustainable development: Five years after the Earth Summit.* Geneva: World Health Organization.

Young, I. (1990). *Justice and the politics of difference.* Princeton, NJ: Princeton University Press.

CHAPTER 4

Cultural Competence, Resilience, and Advocacy

Mary de Chesnay, Rebecca Wharton, and Christopher Pamp

The purpose of this chapter is to provide three key concepts that are particularly useful in the care of people who are vulnerable. The first, cultural competence, is a way of providing care that takes into account cultural differences between the nurse and patient while meeting the health needs of the patient. Resilience, the second, is both a characteristic and a desired outcome. Resilience is understood as the capacity for transcending obstacles, which is present to some degree in all human beings. A goal of nursing is to enhance resilience. The third concept, advocacy, is presented as a way to take cultural competence to a level beyond the nurse–patient relationship by having the nurse serve as the person who fights for or at least supports the patient when the patient is incapacitated. The central idea of this chapter is that these three concepts relate in specific ways that enable nurses to frame care within a cultural context, not just for vulnerable populations but also for all clients.

CULTURAL COMPETENCE

Cultural competence in any profession is a way of being sensitive to the differences in culture of constituents and acting in a way that is respectful of the values and traditions of the client while performing those activities or procedures necessary for the client's well-being. In nursing, the desired outcomes of care are positive changes in health status or lifestyle changes that can help overcome or prevent disease. A social justice view of cultural competence should take into account what Hall (Hall, Stevens, & Meleis, 1994; Hall, 1999) described as marginalization. Marginalized people experience discrimination, poor access to health care, and resultant illnesses and traumas from environmental dangers (or violence) that make them vulnerable to a wide range of health problems. Culturally competent practitioners, then, would seem to concern themselves not only with learning about other cultures but would view marginalized patients within a wider system context and intervene within that context.

Historically, nursing has moved from a view of cultural sensitivity (focus on awareness) to one of cultural competence (focus on behavior). That is to say that nurses aspire to cultural competence not because the concept is trendy or politically correct, as described by Poole (1998), but because nurses are pragmatists who understand that recognizing cultural differences enables them to act with patients and their families in ways that enable them to heal.

Zoucha (2001) urged that we put aside deep-seated feelings of ethnocentrism and accept the value that every health worldview is equally valid. Locsin (2000) proposed that cultural blurring might be a technique that bridges the gaps in cultural differences by enabling the practitioner to merge the best of both worlds. Cultural competence then becomes a practice with broad appeal in all the service professions. Teachers, social workers, and physicians understand the usefulness of the concept as good practice, not just politically correct (Bonder, Martin, & Miracle, 2001; Dana & Matheson, 1992; Fahrenwald et. al., 2001; Gutierrez & Alvarez, 1996; Leavitt, 2003; Sutton, 2000).

Models of Cultural Competence

Because cultural competence is an exciting theoretical development in nursing, several models have been developed to explore its dimensions. In reference to community health nursing, Kim-Godwin, Clarke, & Barton (2001) constructed a model derived from concept analysis that focuses on the relationship between cultural competence and health outcomes for diverse populations. They suggested that the four dimensions of cultural competence are caring, cultural sensitivity, cultural knowledge, and cultural skills. They developed a cultural competence scale that measures all of these dimensions except that of caring. Items include affective (emotional) and cognitive domains. The authors tested the model in a sample of 192 senior undergraduate and graduate nursing students and found factors that loaded on two dimensions, sensitivity and skill, explaining 72% of the variance and providing evidence of construct validity.

A second model portrayed cultural competence as a process in which the health care provider integrates cultural awareness, cultural knowledge, cultural skill, cultural encounters, and cultural desire (Campinha-Bacote, 2002). This model assumes variation within groups as well as between groups, an important distinction for those who would treat members of ethnic groups as if they are exactly like everyone else within their group, thereby constructing new stereotypes instead of developing cultural knowledge. Critiqued by Braithwaite (2003), Campinha-Bacote's model meets the criteria for good theory and is applicable to nursing education, practice, and research.

Taking a different direction, Purnell (2000, 2002) integrated the concepts of biocultural ecology and workforce issues into his model for cultural competence. Purnell asserted that health care providers and recipients of care have a mutual obligation to share information in order to obtain beneficial outcomes. In this sense, the patient is a teacher of culture as well as a client of the provider, and the provider becomes a teacher of the culture of health care. Derived from many disciplines and including many domains, the Purnell model might be seen as a diagram encompassing the patient within a series of concentric circles that include family, community, and global society.

A third view of cultural competence is that existing models are insufficient and the term itself is limiting. Wells (2000) argued for extending the concept of cultural competence into "cultural proficiency." Wells claimed that cultural competence is not adequate and that proficiency is a higher-order concept for institutions in that proficiency indicates mastery of a complex set of skills. The process of moving toward proficiency involves barriers that are both affective and cognitive. The most serious barrier is the unwillingness to examine our own assumptions about those who are different. Wells would say that the most effective way to develop cultural proficiency is to maintain an open attitude and interact with people who are different, allowing them to become our teachers or coaches.

Except for the extensive work of Leininger (1970, 1995), most of the nursing theories published to date do not include cultural competence because they were published long before its emergence as a major concept for nursing. The application of several of the nursing theories to caring for vulnerable populations is discussed elsewhere in this book. However, Watson's theory of caring deserves special note. In a theoretical review, Mendyka (2000) explored the relationship of culture and care, providing a clinical example of how the nurse and patient become more human through their interaction. In his description of a sample case of a Native American who was HIV positive, Mendyka showed how a nurse practitioner trying to treat the patient with a traditional Western medical approach came into conflict with the cultural belief system of the patient. On one hand, the nurse wanted to see the patient more often and suggested pharmacotherapy to prevent full-blown AIDS. The patient, however, wanted to use the healing practices of his tribe: sweat baths, herbs, and prayer. In this situation, unless the nurse practitioner can find a way to work with the tribe's medicine man, she is doomed to failure because the patient will place his own cultural belief system above the uncertainties of Western medical practice.

Other authors have recognized the need for institutional change to develop culturally competent models of intervention for the populations served by diverse providers. Home care nurses manage cultural issues with patients (DiCicco-Bloom & Cohen, 2003). Andrews (1998) applied the process of developing cultural competence to administration in an assessment process leading to organizational change in cultural competence. Holistic nursing, which views patients within their social and cultural contexts, makes cultural competence a core value. Yet, in a review of the concept in the holistic nursing literature, Barnes, Craig, & Chambers (2000) found that only 9.6% of the abstracts made reference to concepts of culture or ethnicity, and these authors raised the question as to whether the sample sizes were large enough to address cultural differences or whether the researchers lacked awareness. Finally, authors in psychiatric nursing (Craig, 1999; Kennedy, 1999) and oncology (Kagawa-Singer, 2000) spoke to the need for practitioners to develop cultural competence at both an individual and institutional level.

Learning Cultural Competence

Many methods and ideas for developing cultural competence are available in the literature, but there is general agreement that cultural competence happens on affective, cognitive, and behavioral levels and that self-awareness is a critical indicator of success. Simulation activities provide a setting in which participants can practice communication and problem solving as well as develop self-awareness (Meltzoff & Lenssen, 2000). Cross-cultural communication exercises for physicians can help them develop the skills needed to overcome barriers (Shapiro, Hollingshead, & Morrison, 2002).

Immersion programs are powerful learning experiences at all levels because they enable the learners to experience different cultures outside of their usual safe context. Immersion programs are probably the best learning tool, although they are costly and time-consuming. There are several examples in Unit 5 which also explore in detail how undergraduate and graduate nursing students can conduct fieldwork that leads to cultural competence.

One example of an immersion program used in nutrition studies was a food travel course in which participants learned diverse diet preferences and practices (Kuczmarski & Cole, 1999). Another example was a population-based program with the Hutterites, an isolationist religious sect found in the United States and Canada (Fahrenwals, 2001).

Didactic materials can be prepared for developing knowledge about groups and are a useful point of reference for practitioners who are under enormous pressure to function with diverse patients in high-acuity settings. An innovative program at the University of Washington in Seattle used action research as the basis for developing Culture Clues, which are documents that enable practitioners to see at a glance the dominant preferences of the diverse cultural groups served by the hospital. The documents cover perception of illness, patterns of kinship and decision making, and comfort with touch and were written for a variety of cultures, including Korean, Russian, Latino, Albanian, Vietnamese, and African American (Abbot, Short, Dodson, Garcia, Perkins, & Wyant, 2002). The didactic approach was also used in Sweden, a country that is becoming more diverse as immigration increases, largely from eastern Europe and Iraq. The researchers used Leininger's theory to guide development of a curriculum for undergraduate nursing students with specific content areas at all levels (Gebru & Willman, 2003).

Didactic programs are easier and less costly to operate than immersion programs, perhaps because cognitive outcomes are easier to measure than affective ones. In a multicultural training course for counseling students, outcomes included development of multicultural knowledge and skill and increased comfort with discussing differing worldviews. However, the program was less successful at getting participants to examine themselves as racial–cultural beings (Tomlinson-Clark, 2000).

RESILIENCE

Resilience has been defined as "the process of adapting well in the face of adversity, trauma, tragedy, or even significant sources of stress. These stressors can include family and relationship problems and workplace and financial stressors" (Newman, 2003, p. 42). Other descriptions include "the ability to 'bounce back' in spite of significant stress or adversity" (Place, Reynolds, Cousins, & O'Neill, 2002, p. 162; Stewart, Reid, & Mangham, 1997) and to "spring back" (Place et al., 2002, p. 162; Jacelon, 1997). Hope is essential for resilience to exist (Perry, 2002; Perry, 2002). Resilience is a concept that has been researched in both qualitative and quantitative studies across cultures and in many contexts. Frameworks have been developed and campaigns have been launched to help boost this concept of "bouncing back." A common theme in the literature is shifting negatives to positives, that is, figuring out how to rebound from adversity. The concept of increasing resilience through good coping skills has been researched thoroughly in recent years. Topics range from the prevention of physical injuries among high school athletes through social support to what factors help children overcome the death of a parent (Greef & Human, 2004; Smith, Smoll, & Ptacek, 1990).

A newly developed family resilience framework encourages a shift from focus on family deficits to family challenges, placing an emphasis on growth from adversity toward hope and strengthened family bonds. This framework uses three areas of family resilience: family belief systems, organizational patterns, and communication/problem-solving (Walsh, 2003). Newman (2003) describes "the road to resilience," a multimedia campaign launched in August 2002 by the American Psychological Association to help Americans bounce back from significant life stressors, hardships, threats, and uncertainty. Its messages focus on the principles that resilience is a journey rather than a single event, each journey is individual, and resilience can be learned by almost anyone (Newman, 2003).

Much current research focuses on the resilience of children, the factors that contribute to their resilience, and programs that help them overcome adversity. Although children are not born resilient, many factors contribute to whether or not they master resilience, including temperament, attentive care giving, healthy attachments, and opportunities to practice resilience using small stressors that promote flexibility (Perry, 2002; Perry, 2002). A current intervention program seeks to increase mental health resilience among children of depressed parents by providing them with educational sessions, community resources, and personal skill development (Place et al., 2002). Among victims of childhood cancers, the concept of uncertainty has traditionally been published with reference to its adverse effects (Parry, 2003). However, Parry (2003) found that uncertainty can also foster the development of confidence and resilience, among other positive effects.

Factors that contribute to resilience after the loss of a parent include intrafamilial emotional and practical support, internal strength of the family unit, support from extended family and friends, religious and spiritual beliefs and activities, and individual personality traits such as optimism (Greeff & Human, 2004). Similarly, a study of persons with chronic disabilities found that social support, perseverance, determination, and spiritual beliefs all were protective factors in creating turning points. These factors, along with processes such as transcendence (replacing loss with gain), accommodating (deciding to relinquish), and self-understanding, served to help persons with disabilities gain meaning in their lives (King et al., 2003). Resilience is a key concept in the idea of transformative aging, which emphasizes the importance of transcending the loss, pain, and uncertainty of growing older to create wholeness out of a fragmented life (Walker, 2002). Walker (2002) found that health care needs may be better met when mature adults are able to come to a point of "self-transcendence," wherein they have mastered their stress. He also found that women acknowledge and come to terms with their stressors more effectively than men.

Similar factors are found to contribute to resilience across cultural and national boundaries. In a study of several young survivors of the Ethiopian famine of 1984–1985, significant resilience factors were found to be faith and hope, having memories of one's roots, and having a living relative. Not surprisingly, the authors also found that after surviving such horrendous circumstances during childhood, these young adults struggled with depression and anxiety, alternating between hope and depression, dreams and fears (Lothe & Heggen, 2003). A stress-coping model of Ethiopian women's health focuses on the moderators of identity, enculturation, spiritual coping, and traditional healing (Walters & Simoni, 2002). Within the Latino youth population of the United States, researchers have described the cultural-community factors of family, *respeto* (respect for the authority of elders), and *personalismo* (the value of relationships for their own merit) as resilience factors against community violence (Clauss-Ehlers & Levi, 2002). A recent examination highlights the positive influences of farming communities on children, such as family cohesion, being raised by satisfied married couples, participation in community activities, and extended family networks nearby (Larson & Dearmont, 2002).

In a series of semistructured interviews conducted with a woman who was widowed in her 30s, one may gain further insight into the concept of resilience after the death of a spouse. Nora (not her real name) is a white woman in her early 50s who, after being widowed approximately 15 years earlier, went on to counsel others who have also suffered the death of a partner. These interviews were part of a larger study on success (de Chesnay, 2004). Although Nora does not explicitly mention resilience in her interviews she does elaborate extensively on the factors that have helped her successfully overcome grief, which she defines as, "the ability to move through the intense part of the pain coping with the situation until the point at which I reinvested in life I'm not living in the pain anymore. I'm happy in my life. I'm fulfilled." Nora's view corresponds well to the intent of the following quote: "to adapt successfully despite the presence of significant adversity" (Place et al, 2002; Beardslee, Versage, & Gladstone, 1998).

Nora credits a wide variety of supports as those that helped her overcome her own grief. "I feel like my therapist saved my life I can't even imagine doing it without a support group I had a wonderful group of friends I couldn't have gotten through it without them either and I couldn't have gotten through it without [my husband's] family I could *never* have gotten through without my sense of humor."

At least as important as the support of other people, Nora emphasizes spirituality, in a broad sense, as among the most important of factors that help widows overcome the death of a spouse. She views spirituality as the belief that "There's something more than just chaos, something greater than just us as individuals." Spirituality is "people caring about other people. It's loving each other." Many authors have cited the support factors of family, friends, and spirituality, all of which Nora credits for her resilience (Clauss-Ehlers & Levi, 2002; Greef & Human, 2004; Larson & Dearmont, 2002; Walters & Simoni, 2002).

No matter what the obstacle, protective factors such as social support, spirituality, and effective individual coping mechanisms are factors that increase resilience among people. The implications for nursing are to help clients shift their focus from despair to hope when confronting adversity and, in so doing, develop inner strength.

ADVOCACY AND ADVANCED-PRACTICE NURSING

This section is primarily concerned with how nurses advocate for their patients in clinical practice and how that might change as they transition into the advanced-practice role. A great deal of recent literature, much of it from the United Kingdom, has challenged many of the traditional assumptions of advocacy as an intrinsic part of "the moral art of nursing" (Hewitt, 2002; Mallik, 1997; Willard, 1996). In contrast, there is a paucity of research that examines patient advocacy in advanced-practice nursing.

Emergence of Nursing Advocacy

In the formative years of the nursing profession, nursing training was modeled on military training. There was complete obedience to the physician, which ultimately overarched the interests of the patient (Bernal, 1992; Nelson, 1988; Yarling & McElmurry, 1986). However, as nursing evolved and developed a theoretical base, advocating for patients came to be considered a fundamental and integral part of nursing (Nelson, 1988). The concepts of advocacy, accountability, cooperation, and caring are considered moral and ethical foundations of nursing (Fry, 2001, pp. 276). Accordingly, the American Nurses Association's (ANA) *Code of Ethics for Nurses with Interpretive Statements* delineates several advocacy duties of nurses, including protecting the patient's right to self-determination (ANA, 2001).

As nursing began to distinguish itself from medicine as being more about caring than curing and as having a unique nurse–patient relationship, several theories of nursing advocacy emerged (Mallik, 1997). Gadow (1980) proposed in her theory of existential advocacy that the nurse was "in the ideal position among health providers to experience the patient as a unique human being with individual strengths and complexities—a precondition for advocacy" (p. 81). From this unique position, nurses were enjoined to assist patients in "authentically" exercising their right of self-determination in making health care decisions. Curtain (1979) embedded advocacy in the moral art of nursing where advocacy evolves from the shared vulnerability, experience, and humanity of the nurse–patient relationship. Kohnke (1982) defined the role of the nurse advocate as simply to inform the patient and then support whatever decision he or she makes. In order to better inform the patient, Kohnke's theory of advocacy describes a framework of 10 intersecting areas of knowledge which, taken together, form a "gestalt" for nursing advocacy.

Reexamination of Advocacy

Recently, critics have argued that many pitfalls exist in the moral concept of nursing advocacy not the least of which is the danger of paternalism or imposing on patient autonomy (Melia, 1994). Many assumptions have been challenged. Are nurses uniquely positioned to advocate when other health care professionals such as physicians and social workers also have a fiduciary responsibility to the patient (Hyland, 2002)? Do nurses have the autonomy and power to effectively advocate for patients within the health care system (Hewitt, 2002; Hyland, 2002; Yarling & McElmurry, 1986)? Is advocacy even possible in today's health care environment of short hospital stays, nursing shortages, and nonexistent institutional rewards for performing advocacy (Hamric, 2000)?

Another criticism of advocacy is that it has not been operationalized as a concept, and therefore few empirical studies of the role have been done. Because of this inherent complexity, advocacy is not formally taught as a didactic subject in the classroom (Kohnke, 1982; Mallik, 1997). However, the nursing literature has long-standing reference to the idea that experience may be the best teacher, and there are examples of how nurse educators have integrated various advocacy activities into clinical experiences where students actually encounter vulnerable patients within the complexity of the health care system (Fay, 1978; Namerow, 1982).

The dimensions of nursing advocacy appear to be primarily focused at the individual patient level. Politically, nurses tend not to get involved with consumer advocacy groups or engage in collective legislative action in the cause of patient rights (Mallik, 1997).

Advocacy and the Advanced Nurse Practitioner

A question arises. As nurses move to a more autonomous role as advanced nurse practitioners, how much of their practice is influenced by nursing and how much by medicine? Thrasher (2002) considered the role of the primary care nurse practitioner as an advocate in promoting self-care and clearly chose the nursing model. Supporting her theoretical framework for this role are critical social theory and nursing theories of self-care. Prominent among these theories is Gadow's (1980) philosophy of existential advocacy, which includes caring and understanding the lived experience of the patients and assisting them to self-determination.

To gain an understanding of the meaning and application of advocacy in advanced-practice nursing, a semistructured interview was conducted with an experienced pediatric nurse practitioner. The informant, whose pseudonym is Star, was an African American female of about 30 years of age who practiced in an urban clinic where patients are predominately lower income and African American. This interview was part of de Chesnay's (2004) larger study of life histories of successful African Americans.

Thematically, Star identified responsibility and empowerment as elements that changed when she transitioned from bedside nursing to an independent advanced-practice role that enabled her to more effectively advocate for her patients. However, she did not see that the essence of her nursing advocacy or, as she called it, "looking out for patients," had changed as a result

of her expanded role, a fact that is illustrated by the following. "I think a lot of it was I was trying to get what I wanted from a doctor and at this point I can do those things myself. I don't have
to wait for an order to give a med. I just give it. You know, I just write a prescription. I do it myself. And so that way it's very different. I think in terms of just looking out for patients overall,
no, there's no difference."

Star pointed out how patient advocacy does differ in the advanced-practice nursing role in
that it is informed by the higher level of responsibility and accountability of being the primary
care provider. "I think I feel more responsible for my patients now because they're my patients.
In the hospital [where] I worked [before] they were the doctors' patients; they were their responsibility." These statements appear to support views presented earlier that power and autonomy are prerequisites for nurses to effectively advocate for their patients (Hewitt, 2002; Hyland,
2002; Yarling & McElmurry, 1986).

In terms of learning the advocacy role, Star intimated that her hospital experience trained
her for her role of a patient advocate as is consistent with other observations (Mallik, 1997). She
states: "you do discharge planning in the hospital. You have to connect with outside agencies,
home care, so that type of stuff."

Lastly, as with most nurses (Mallik, 1997), Star's focus is advocacy at the individual and local level and is not directed toward the macro view of consumer advocacy or political health reform: "I'm not so much interested in politics but in the health and well-being of children and the
health and well-being of my community."

CONCLUSION

The ideas presented here have much relevance to nursing practice, and the concepts relate in several specific ways. First, cultural competence is a set of behaviors that transcends mere good intentions. Accepting that cultural differences exist reflects an open mind, which in turn leads to
exploring the client's own strengths and adaptive capabilities. Using cultural resources at the
client's disposal concurrently with "best practices" in nursing and medicine is not only culturally
appropriate but also likely to develop resilience. Nurses who practice in a culturally competent
way serve as better advocates for their clients because they work from a point of view of mobilizing resources in collaboration with others who are knowledgeable about the culture.

REFERENCES

Abbot, P., Short, E., Dodson, S., Garcia, C., Perkins, J., Wyant, S. (2002). Improving your cultural awareness with culture clues. *Nurse Practitioner, 27*(2), 44–49.

American Nurses Association. (2001). *Code of ethics for nurses with interpretive statements.* Washington,
DC: American Nurses Association.

American Nurses Association Code of Ethics Project Task Force. (2000). A new code of ethics for nurses:
Combining an unchanged mission with the challenges of contemporary nursing. *American Journal of
Nursing, 100*(7), 72–73.

Andrews, M. (1998). A model for cultural change. *Nursing Management, 29*(10), 62–66.

Barnes, D., Craig, K., & Chambers, K. (2000). A review of the concept of culture in holistic nursing literature. *Journal of Holistic Nursing, 18*(3), 207–221.

Bernal, E. W. (1992). The nurse as patient advocate. *Hastings Center Report 22*(1) 18–23.

Bonder, B., Martin, L., & Miracle, A. (2001). Achieving cultural competence: The challenge for clients and healthcare workers in a multicultural society. *Generations, 25*(1), 35–43.

Campinha-Bacote, J. (2002). The process of cultural competence in the delivery of health care services: A model of care. *Journal of Transcultural Nursing, 13*(3), 180–84.

Clauss-Ehlers, C. S., & Levi, L. L. (2002). Violence and community, terms in conflict: An ecological approach to resilience. *Journal of Social Distress and the Homeless, 11*(4), 265–278.

Craig, A. B. (1999). Mental health nursing and cultural diversity. *Australian and New Zealand Journal of Mental Health Nursing, 8,* 93–99.

Curtain, L. L. (1979). The nurse as advocate: a philosophical foundation for nursing. *Advances in Nursing Science, 1*(3), 1–10.

Dana, R., & Matheson, L. (1992). An application of the agency cultural competence checklist to a program serving small and diverse ethnic communities. *Psychosocial Rehabilitation Journal, 15*(4), 101–106.

de Chesnay, M. (personal communication, January, 2003).

DiCicco-Bloom, B., & Cohen, D. (2003). Home care nurses: A study of the occurrence of culturally competent care. *Journal of Transcultural Nursing, 14*(1), 25–31.

Fahrenwald, N., Boysen, R., Fischer, C., & Maurer, R. (2001). Developing cultural competence in the baccalaureate nursing student: A populations-based project with the Hutterites. *Journal of Transcultural Nursing, 12*(1), 48–55.

Fay. P. (1978). Sounding board-in support of patient advocacy as a nursing role. *Nursing Outlook, 26*(4), 252–253.

Fry, S. T. (2001). Ethical dimensions of nursing and health care. In J. L. Creasia & B. Parker (Eds.). *The bridge to professional nursing practice* (3rd ed., pp. 272–293). St. Louis, MO: Mosby.

Gadow, S. (1980). Existential advocacy: Philosophical foundation of nursing. In S. F. Spicker & S. Gadow (Eds.). *Nursing: Images and ideals* (pp.79–101). New York, NY: Springer.

Gebru, K., & Willman, A. (2003). A research-based didactic model for education to promote culturally competent nursing care in Sweden. *Journal of Transcultural Nursing, 14*(1), 55–61.

Greeff, A. P., & Human, B. (2004). Resilience in families in which a parent has died. *American Journal of Family Therapy, 32*(1), 27–42.

Gutierrez, L., & Alvarez, A. (1996). Multicultural community organizing: A strategy for change. *Social Work, 41*(5), 501–509.

Hall, J. M. (1999). Marginalization revisited: Critical, postmodern and liberation perspectives. *Advances in Nursing Science, 22*(1), 88–102.

Hall, J. M., Stevens, P., & Meleis, A. (1994). Marginalization: A guiding concept for valuing diversity in nursing knowledge development. *Advances in Nursing Science, 16*(4), 23–41.

Hamric, A. B. (2000). What is happening to advocacy? *Nursing Outlook, 48,* 103–104.

Hewitt, J. (2002). A critical review of the arguments debating the role of the nurse advocate. *Journal of Advanced Nursing, 37*(5), 439–445.

Hyland, D. (2002). An exploration of the relationship between patient autonomy and patient advocacy: Implications for nursing practice. *Nursing Ethics, 9*(5), 472–482.

Kagawa-Singer, M. (2000). Addressing issues for early detection and screening in ethnic populations. *Oncology Nursing Forum, 27*(9), 55–61.

Kennedy, M. (1999). Cultural competence and psychiatric nursing. *Journal of Transcultural Nursing, 10*(1), 11–18.

Kim-Godwin, Y. S., Clarke, P., & Barton, L. (2001). *Journal of Advanced Nursing, 35*(6), 918–926.

King, G., Cathers, T., Brown, E., Specht, J. A., Willoughby, C., Polgar, J. M., et al. (2003). Turning points and protective processes in the lives of people with chronic disabilities. *Qualitative Health Research, 13*(2), 184–206.

Kohnke, M.F. (1982). *Advocacy: Risk and reality.* St. Louis, MO: C.V. Mosby.

Kuczmarski, M., & Cole, R. (1999). Transcultural food habits travel courses: An interdisciplinary approach to teaching cultural diversity. *Topics in Clinical Nutrition, 15*(1), 59–71.

Larson, N. C., & Dearmont, M. (2002). Strengths of farming communities in fostering resilience in children. *Child Welfare, 81*(5), 821–835.

Leavitt., R. L. (2003). Developing cultural competence in a multicultural world—Part II. *Magazine of Physical Therapy, 11*(1), 56–70.

Leininger, M. (1970). *Nursing and anthropology: Two worlds to blend.* New York, NY: John Wiley and Sons.

Leininger, M. (1995). *Transcultural nursing: Concepts, theories, research and practice.* New York, NY: McGraw-Hill.

Locsin, R. (2000). Building bridges: Affirming culture in health and nursing. *Holistic Nursing Practice, 15*(1), 1–4.

Lothe, E. A., & Heggen, K. (2003). A study of resilience in young Ethiopian famine survivors. *Journal of Transcultural Nursing, 14*(4), 313–320.

Mallik, M (1997). Advocacy in nursing: A review of the literature. *Journal of Advanced Nursing, 25,* 130–138.

Melia, K. M. (1994). The task of nursing ethics. *Journal of Medical Ethics, 20*(1), 7–11.

Meltzof, N., & Lenssen, J. (2000). Enhancing cultural competence through simulation activities. *Multicultural Perspectives, 2*(1), 29–35.

Mendycka, B. (2000). Exploring culture in nursing: A theory-driven practice. *Holistic Nursing Practice, 15*(1), 32–41.

Namerow, M. J. (1982). Integrating advocacy into the gerontological nusing major. *Journal of Gerontological Nursing, 8*(3), 149–151.

Nelson, M. L. (1988). Advocacy in nursing. *Nursing Outlook, 36*(3), 136–141.

Newman, R. (2003). Providing direction on the road to resilience. *Behavioral Health Management, 23*(4), 42–43.

Parry, C. (2003). Embracing uncertainty: An exploration of the experiences of childhood cancer survivors. *Qualitative Health Research, 13*(1), 227–246.

Perry, B. D. (2002). How children become resilient. *Scholastic Parent & Child, 10*(2), 33–34.

Perry, B. D. (2002). Resilience: Where does it come from?. *Early Childhood Today, 17*(2), 24–25.

Place, M., Reynolds, J., Cousins, A., O'Neill, S. (2002). Developing a resilience package for vulnerable children. *Child and Adolescent Mental Health, 7*(4), 162–167.

Poole, D. (1998). Politically correct or culturally competent? *Health and Social Work, 23*(3), 163–167.

Purnell, L. (2000). A description of the Purnell model for cultural competence. *Journal of Transcultural Nursing, 11*(1), 40–46.

Purnell, L. (2002). The Purnell model for cultural competence. *Journal of Transcultural Nursing, 13*(3), 193–196.

Shapiro, J., Hollingshead, J., & Morrison, E. (2002). Primary care resident, faculty and patient views of barriers to cultural competence and the skills needed to overcome them. *Medical Education, 36,* 749–759.

Smith, R. E., Smoll, F. L., & Ptacek, J. T. (1990). Conjunctive moderator variables in vulnerability and resiliency research life stress, social support and coping skills, and adolescent sport injuries. *Journal of Personality and Social Psychology, 58*(2), 360–370.

Sutton, M. (2000). Cultural competence. *Family Practice Management, 7*(9), 58–61.

Thrasher, C. (2002). The primary care nurse practitioner: Advocate for self care. *Journal of the American Academy of Nurse Practitioners, 14*(3), 113–117.

Tomlinson-Clark, S. (2000). Assessing outcomes in a multicultural training course: A qualitative study. *Counselling Psychology Quarterly, 13*(2), 221–232.

Walker, C. A. (2002). Transformative aging: How mature adults respond to growing older. *Journal of Theory Construction & Testing, 6*(2), 109–116.

Walsh, F. (2003). Family resilience: A framework for clinical practice. *Family Process, 42*(1), 1–18.

Walters, K. L., & Simoni, J. M. (2002). Reconceptualizing Native women's health: An 'indigenist' stress-coping model. *American Journal of Public Health, 92,* 520–524.

Wells, M. (2000). Beyond cultural competence: A model for individual and institutional cultural development. *Journal of Community Health Nursing, 17*(4), 189–200.

Willard, C. (1996). The nurse's role as patient advocate: Obligation or imposition? *Journal of Advanced Nursing, 24*(1), 60–66.

Yarling, R. R., & McElmurry, B. J. (1986). The moral foundation of nursing. *Advances in Nursing Science 8*(2), 63–73.

Zoucha, R. (2001). President's message. *Journal of Transcultural Nursing, 12*(2), 157.

UNIT II
NURSING THEORIES

There is at work a slow but steady growth of educated intelligence in nursing that is developing nursing science and working aggressively toward use of the capabilities of professional nurses in the health fields.

Hildegard Peplau

Source: Peplau, H. (1999). Nurse-doctor relationships. Reprinted in *Nursing Forum, 34*(3), 31–36.

CHAPTER 5

Nursing Theories Applied to Vulnerable Populations: Examples from Turkey

Behice Erci

This chapter presents the areas in which nursing models and theories guide nursing practice as it relates to vulnerable populations. Nine nursing theories are presented, with detailed clinical examples for several because these theories were thought more applicable. Readers are referred to the primary sources for complete descriptions and explanations of the theoretical concepts.

IMPORTANCE OF THEORIES IN ADVANCED NURSING PRACTICE

The dilemma for nurse educators is how best to prepare nurses for advanced-practice roles. Is nursing theory important? Does it contribute to clinical practice? Which theories provide sound foundations for advanced practice? Theories exist to challenge existing practice, create new approaches to practice, and remodel the structure of rules and principles. Furthermore, theories ought ultimately to improve nursing practice. Usually this goal is achieved by using theory or portions of theory to guide practice. Defining the scope of advanced practice requires that the role of nurse practitioners be considered unique. For nursing practice to be viewed as professional, it is essential that practice be based on theory. Theory and theoretical frameworks are intended to provide guidance and a rationale for professional practice, but as advanced-practice roles evolve in nursing, the incorporation of nursing theory becomes problematic. It has been suggested that the wide variety of definitions and concepts discussed in most nursing theories do not explain or predict anything. Therefore, they cannot practically be applied to clinical situations and are of little use to nurses in advanced practice.

OREM'S GENERAL THEORY OF NURSING

The self-care theory (Berbiglia, 1997; Orem, 1995) linked patient assessments with nursing diagnosis, expected patient outcomes, discharge planning, quality assurance, clinical research, and external agency reports. There are three subtheories within Orem's theory. The **theory of self-care deficit** details how individuals can benefit from nursing because they are subject to health-related or self-derived limitations. The **theory of self-care** states that care is a learned behavior that purposely regulates human structural integrity, functioning, and development. The **theory of nursing systems** describes how nurses use their abilities to prescribe, design, and provide nursing care.

Application to Vulnerable Populations

In nursing care, Orem identifies operations that are specifically professional and/or technological, including diagnostic, prescriptive, treatment or regulatory, and case management operations. The application of Orem's theory to nursing practice is relevant as a framework in a variety of settings, including acute care units, ambulatory clinics, community health programs, senior centers, nursing homes, hospices, and rehabilitation centers. The theory is applied to patients with specific diseases or conditions, alcoholics, the chronically ill, those undergoing head and neck surgery, and those who suffer from rheumatoid arthritis. The theory is also applied to selected age groups, including the aged, children, and mothers with newborns.

Example

Yeliz is 29 years old, married, and five months pregnant. She has anemia, is underweight, and is under the care of a primary health care center. Complete data have been compiled from the client's records and a home visit. The nurses are concerned that her self-care requisites (or requirements) are not being met. These are food, healthy activity, and rest. She requires assistance in food preparation, but can eat on her own. Her priority diagnoses are inadequate food intake, low activity level and fatigue due to inadequate rest.

Diagnostic and Prescriptive Operations

All three priority diagnoses previously listed are related to preventing health deterioration. In this client's case, the self-care deficit theory of nursing proposes a supportive–educational nursing system that is designed to individualize her care. The individualization of the nursing system is accomplished through the overlay of basic conditioning factors and developmental self-care requisites (or requirements for life and health) on the therapeutic self-care demands (those processes necessary to maintain life or health). The expected outcome is health status maintenance, health promotion, and prevention of further health deterioriation through the strengthening of the self-care agency. Unless expected outcomes are provided, the nursing system design will change.

Regulatory Operations

The self-care deficit theory of nursing is especially useful with this client. The theory changes the focus away from disease to the strengths and/or weaknesses of the self-care agent. It is evident that the client does seek to prevent and/or manage the conditions threatening her health, yet she requires assistance in this area. The most significant self-care deficit is in the area of nutrition. Guided by the theory, the nurse analyzed the self-care agency from the perspective of the basic conditioning factors. Cultural variety should be considered in reaching for the expected outcome.

Data collection for the client in terms of self-care requisites led to the following proposed outcomes: 1) maintenance of the healthy environment, 2) ability of the client to feed herself, and 3) discussion of her condition and medical regimen with the home health nurse and aide and the client's family. The nursing diagnosis showed a potential for anemic complications such as falls and decreased mobility. Methods of help and/or intervention included teaching, guiding, and providing and/or maintaining direction in an environment that supported personal development. Self-care agency is inadequate and implies the necessity to gain better understanding of the cause and subsequent prevention of problems. Nursing diagnosis is "potential for exacerbation and increased disability related to knowledge deficits concerning problems.

Again, teaching, guiding, and directing are methods of helping. For the nursing diagnosis, "inability to maintain ideal body weight related to cultural attitudes toward eating and weight gain and meal preparation by aide," the methods of helping are to provide and maintain an environment that supports personal development.

Roy's Adaptation Model

Roy drew upon expanded insights in relating spirituality and science to present a new definition of adaptation and related scientific and philosophical assumptions (Connerley et al, 1999; Roy, 1976). Her philosophical stance articulates that nurses see persons as co-extensive with their physical and social environments. Furthermore, nurse scholars take a value-based stance rooted in beliefs and hopes about the human person, and they develop a discipline that participates in enhancing the well-being of persons and of the earth. Roy viewed persons and groups as adaptive systems with cognator and regulator subsystems acting to maintain adaptation in the four adaptive modes: physiological–physical, self-concept-group identity, role function, and interdependence.

Application to Vulnerable Populations

Roy used a problem-solving approach for gathering data, identifying the capacities and needs of the human adaptive system, selecting and implementing approaches for nursing care, and evaluation of the outcome of the care provided. The approach includes assessment of behavior and stimuli and is consistent with the nursing process of assessment, diagnosis, planning, implementation, and evaluation.

Example

Hasan is a 35-year-old man who is recently admitted to the oncology nursing unit for evaluation after undergoing surgery for class IV prostate cancer. He has smoked approximately two packs of cigarettes a day for the past nine years. He is married and lives with his wife. He has done well following surgery except for being unable to completely empty his urinary bladder. Hasan is having continued postoperative pain. When he goes home, it will be necessary for him to perform intermittent self-catheterization. His home medications are an antibiotic and an analgesic as needed. In addition, he will be receiving radiation therapy on an outpatient basis. Hasan is extremely tearful. He expresses great concern over his future. He believes that this illness is a punishment for his past life.

Physiological Adaptive Mode

The client's health problems are complex. It is impossible to develop interventions for all of his health problems within this chapter. Therefore, only representative examples are given. Physiological adaptive mode refers to the basic and complex biological processes necessary to maintain life.

Assessment of Behavior

Postoperatively, the patient is unable to completely empty his urinary bladder. He states that he is "numb" and unable to tell when he needs to void. Catheterization for residual urine has revealed that he is retaining 300 ml of urine after voiding. It will be necessary for him to perform intermittent self-catheterization at home. Unsanitary conditions at Hasan's home place him at high risk for developing a urinary tract infection. He states that he is scared about performing self-catheterization.

Assessment of Stimuli

In this phase of the nursing process, the nurse searches for the stimuli responsible for certain observed behaviors. After the stimuli are identified, they are classified as focal, contextual, or residual.

The focal stimulus for the client's urinary retention is the disease process. Contextual stimuli include tissue trauma resulting from surgery and radiation therapy. Anxiety is a residual stimulus.

Infection is a potential problem. The focal stimulus is the need for intermittent self-catheterization. Contextual stimuli include altered skin integrity related to surgical incision, poor understanding of aseptic principles, and unsanitary conditions at Hasan's home.

Nursing Diagnosis

From the assessment of behaviors and the assessment of stimuli, the following nursing diagnoses are made:

1. altered elimination: urinary retention related to surgical trauma, radiation therapy, and anxiety
2. potential for infection related to intermittent self-catheterization, altered skin integrity resulting from surgical incision, poor understanding of aseptic principles, and unsanitary conditions at the client's home

Goal Setting

Goals are set mutually between the nurse and the client for each of the nursing diagnoses. The goals are 1) complete urinary elimination every 4 hours as evidenced by correct demonstration of the procedure for intermittent self-catheterization, and 2) continued absence of signs of infection of the surgical incision and urinary tract.

Implementation

To help the client attain these goals, the following nursing interventions were implemented.

1. To address the issue of incomplete elimination, the client is taught the importance of performing intermittent self-catheterization every 4 hours to prevent damage to the urinary bladder. He is taught to assess his abdomen for bladder distention and the proper procedure for intermittent self-catheterization. He is instructed to keep a record of the exact time and amount of voiding and catheterizations. In addition, the client is taught relaxation techniques to facilitate voiding so that it will not be necessary for him to catheterize himself as often.

2. To address the potential for infection the client is taught the importance of washing hands before touching the surgical incision or doing incision care. The procedure for incision care is demonstrated by the nursing staff, and the client is asked to perform a return demonstration. After the intermittent self-catheterization procedure is explained and demonstrated, the client is asked to perform a return demonstration.

Evaluation

An evaluation of the client's adaptive level is performed each shift.

Self-Concept Adaptive Mode

Assessment of Behavior

The client is extremely tearful. He expresses great concern over his future. Exploration of the client's tearfulness revealed that the client is afraid of dying. Also, the client has not asked the nurse any questions about sexuality. His hesitancy to introduce the subject may be related to his cultural background. In this case, the nurse introduces the topic. Salient findings are 1) the client recently learned of a diagnosis of prostate cancer, 2) he has undergone a recent operation, 3) he is receiving radiation therapy in the hospital and this therapy will continue when he leaves the hospital, and 4) the client has a lack of information about the impact of prostate cancer and chemotherapy on sexuality.

Assessment of Stimuli

The client is an adult, he is married, and has a fifth grade education. He is in an emotionally distant and sometimes abusive relationship. Being diagnosed with prostate cancer at an early age has resulted in a maturational crisis for the client. This is complicated by the fact that several of his relatives have died of cancer. It is important for the nurse to assess coping strategies. One coping strategy that is mentioned is that the client is frequently tearful.

Nursing Diagnosis

The following nursing diagnoses are made:

1. Fear and anxiety of dying related to medical diagnosis and witnessing other family members' deaths as a result of cancer
2. Spiritual distress related to severe life threatening illness and perception of moral-ethical-spiritual self
3. Sexual dysfunction related to the disease process, need for radiation therapy at home, weakness, fatigue, pain, anxiety, and a lack of information about the impact of prostate cancer, and chemotherapy on sexuality
4. Grieving related to body image disturbance, lack of self-ideal, and potential for premature death

Goal Setting

To help the client achieve adaptation in the self-concept adaptive mode, the following goals are set:

1. Decrease fear and anxiety of dying as evidenced by less tearfulness, relaxed facial expression, relaxed body movements, verbalization of new coping strategies, and fewer verbalizations of fear and anxiety
2. Decrease spiritual distress as evidenced by verbalization of positive feelings about self-verbalization about the value and meaning of his life, and less tearfulness
3. Resume sexual relationship that is satisfying to both partners and evidenced by verbalization of self as sexually capable and acceptable, verbalization of alternative methods of sexual expression during the first 10 weeks following surgery
4. Progression through the grieving process as evidenced by verbalization of feelings regarding body image, self-ideal, and potential for premature death

Implementation

The following nursing interventions are implemented to help achieve these goals in the self-concept adaptive mode:

1. *Fear and anxiety of dying related to medical diagnosis and witnessing other family members' deaths as a result of cancer*

Although the client prognosis appeared good, he remained fearful of dying. Time is taken to sit with the client, make eye contact, and actively listen. The client is asked to share an extremely difficult experience he encountered in the past. He is asked how he coped with that experience. Once his present coping strategies are assessed, new coping strategies are suggested.

He is encouraged to express his feelings openly. After allowing the client adequate time to express his feelings, truthful and realistic hope based on the client medical history is offered. A cancer support group will meet each week in the hospital where the client is a patient. The client is given a schedule of the meeting times and topics. He and his partner are encouraged to attend the cancer support group meetings.

2. *Spiritual distress related to severe life threatening illness and perception of moral-ethical-spiritual self*

The client is encouraged to express his feelings openly about his illness. It is suggested that times of illness are good times to renew spiritual ties. The client is supported in positive aspects of his life.

3. *Sexual dysfunction related to the disease process, need for radiation therapy at home, weakness, fatigue, pain, anxiety, and a lack of information about the impact of prostate cancer and chemotherapy on sexuality*

A complete sexual assessment is conducted to evaluate the perceived adequacy of the client's sexual relationship and to elicit concerns or issues about sexuality before his diagnosis with prostate cancer. A private conversation is initiated with the client to gain an understanding of his sexual concerns resulting from his therapy and his beliefs about the effects of prostate in regard to sexual functioning. The client is instructed regarding possible changes in sexual functioning such as a temporary inability to achieve or sustain an erection, for up to several months.

4. *Grieving related to body image disturbance, loss of self-ideal, and potential for premature death*

The client's perceptions regarding the impact of the diagnosis of prostate cancer on his body image, self-ideal, roles, and his future are explored. Hasan is encouraged to verbally acknowledge the losses that he is experiencing. The client is observed to determine which stage of the grief process he currently experiences. The grieving process is explained to the client and to his family, and they are assured that grieving is a normal process. The nursing staff should offer realistic reassurance about the client prognosis. The client is encouraged to attend the cancer support group so that he can talk to others who better understand his grief.

Evaluation
Behavior change is expected.

KING'S THEORY

The focus of King's theory (1971) is on individuals whose interactions in groups within social systems influence behavior within the systems (Gonot, 1989). In other words, the perceptions that people experience as a result of their surroundings influence their own behavior. King's theory is based on three interaction systems. Concepts of self-growth and development, and body image are important (Frey & Norris, 1997; Gonot, 1989). The goal of nursing is to help individuals maintain their health so they can function in their roles.

Application to Vulnerable Populations

It is within this interpersonal system of nurse-client that the traditional steps of the nursing process are carried out. By way of explanation: nurse and client meet in some situation, perceive each other, make judgments about the other, take some mental action, and react to each one's perceptions of the other. Because these behaviors cannot be directly observed, one can only draw inferences from them. The next step in the process is interaction that can be directly observed. When interactions lead to transactions, goal attainment behaviors are exhibited. An assumption underlying the interaction process is that of reciprocally contingent behavior in which the behavior of one person influences the behavior of the other and vice versa (Gonot, 1989).

Example
Elif is 50 years old. She has heart failure. She is married and lives with her husband. She describes him as emotionally distant and abusive at times. She is having continued cardiac pain and palpitation. She will be receiving cardiac therapy on an outpatient basis. Elif is extremely tearful and anxious. She expresses great concern over her future.

From King's framework, Elif is conceptualized as a personal system in interaction with other systems. Many of these interactions influence her health. In addition, her recent diagnosis of heart failure influences her health. Together Elif and the nurse communicate, engage in mutual goal setting, and need to make decisions about the means to achieve goals.

Nursing care for Elif begins with assessment, which includes collection, interpretation, and verification of data. Sources of data are Elif herself, primarily perception, behavior, and past experiences; knowledge of concepts in the systems framework; critical thinking skills; ability to use nursing process; and medical knowledge about the treatment and prognosis of heart failure. Care should well cover the full range of nursing practice: maintenance and restoration of health, care of the sick, and promotion of health. The nurse forms an interpersonal system with Elif. The transaction process includes perception, judgments, mental actions, and reactions of both individuals. The nurse assesses and applies knowledge of concepts and processes. Critical concepts are perception, self-coping, interaction, role, stress, power, and decision making. The nurse's perception serves as a basis for gathering and interpreting information. Elif's perceptions influence her thoughts and actions and are assessed through verbal and nonverbal behaviors. Because perceptual accuracy is important to the interaction process, the nurse analyzes her own perceptions and her interpretation of Elif's perceptions with Elif. It is expected that perceptions might be influenced by her emotional state, stress, or pain.

According to King, self is the conception of who and what one is and includes one's subjective totality of attitudes, values, experiences, commitments, and awareness of individual existence. Elif reveals important information about herself. She is tearful and expresses fear, concern. Her past behavior provides some basis for her present feeling in that Elif has not taken actions to promote and maintain her own health. Clearly, feelings about self and situation are psychological stressors. Elif has physical and interpersonal stressors as well. Physical stressors are a result of the illness. Cardiac function, pain, and palpitation are identified as immediate problems. In the interpersonal system, Elif identifies a distant and abusive relationship with her husband. There is a major lack of emotional support during this very difficult time. Her husband's inability to provide basic emotions is likely to change her own physical status. An additional stressor is the living situation. It is also possible that the lack of personal and perhaps family space contributes to stress. Coping with personal and interpersonal stressors is likely to influence both health and illness outcomes. Elif may need additional resources to help her cope with the immediate situation and the future.

Communication is the key to establishing mutuality and trust between Elif and the nurse and the means to perceptions, establishing patient priorities, and moving the interaction process toward goal setting. Elif is expected to participate in identifying goals. However, direction from the nurse will likely be necessary because of the overwhelming needs and lack of resources. Nurses can find direction for assisting patients to identifying goals based on the assumptions that underlie King's systems framework. Nurses assist patients to adjust to changes in their health status. Decisions about goals must be based on the capabilities, limitations, priorities of the patient, and situation. In this situation, the immediate goals seem to be controlled by cardiac pain and palpitation, although this needs validation by Elif.

The first nursing action will be to obtain psychological assessment and crisis intervention as necessary. Other important goals and actions will be directed toward mobilizing resources, especially husband support. It is possible that professional goals and client goals may be incongruent. Continuous analysis, synthesis, and validation are critical to keep on track.

In addition to decisions about goals, Elif is expected to be involved in decisions about actions to meet goals. Involving Elif in decision making may be a challenge because of her sense of powerlessness over the illness, treatment, and ability to contribute to family functioning. Yet empowering Elif is likely to increase her sense of self, which in turn can reduce stress, improve coping, change perceptions, and lead to changes in her physical state.

Goal attainment needs ongoing evaluation. For Elif, follow-up on pain, palpitation, and cardiac function after discharge will be necessary. An option might be to arrange for in-home nursing services. Having a professional in the home would also contribute to further assessment of the family, validation of progress toward goals, and modifications in plans to achieve goals.

According to King, if transactions are made, goals will be attaine
prove or maintain health, control illness, or lead to a peaceful death
nurse needs to reexamine the nursing process, critical thinking pr

LEININGER'S THEORY OF CULTURE CARE

Leininger's interest in cultural dimensions of human care and caring led to the u.
her theory (Leininger, 1995). She subscribed to the central tenet that "care is the essenc
ing and the central, dominant, and unifying focus of nursing" (Leininger, 1991, p. 35,
unique focus of Leininger's theory is care, which she believes to be inextricably linked with cu.
ture. She defines culture as "the learned, shared, and transmitted values, beliefs, norms, and life
ways of a particular group that guides their thinking, decisions, and actions in patterned ways"
(Leininger, 1991, p. 47). The ultimate purpose of care is to provide culturally congruent care to
people of different or similar cultures in order to maintain or regain their well-being and health
or face death in a culturally appropriate way (Leininger, 1991, p. 39).

Example

A group of Iraqi refugees fled to a city in southeastern Turkey to seek refuge from political
unrest, persecution, and extreme poverty. Providing culturally congruent nursing care to this
group of people is difficult due to differences in language. This leads to difficulty in understanding the lifeways of this group. Children have diarrhea in this group, and it is difficult for
the nurse to observe, interview, and collect data related to cultural practices that might explain
the diarrhea. The nurse helps the group to preserve favorable health and caring life styles about
poverty and diarrhea. The nurse provides help for cultural adaptation, negotiation, or adjustment
to the refugees' health and lifestyles. The nurse can reconstruct or alter designs to help clients
change health or life patterns in ways meaningful to them.

WATSON'S THEORY OF HUMAN CARING

The caring model or theory can also be considered a philosophical and moral/ethical foundation
for professional nursing and part of the central focus for nursing at the disciplinary level. A
model of caring includes a call for both art and science; it offers a framework that embraces and
intersects with art, science, humanities, spirituality, and new dimensions of mind-body-spirit
medicine and nursing evolving openly as central to human phenomena of nursing practice. Concepts of the theory include nursing, person, health, human care, and environment.

Application to Vulnerable Population

Watson emphasizes that it is possible to read, study, learn about, even teach and research the
caring theory; however, to truly "get it," one has to personally experience it; thus the model is
both an invitation and an opportunity to interact with the ideas, experiment with and grow within
the philosophy, and living it out in one's personal/professional life. If one chooses to use the caring perspective as theory, model, philosophy, ethic, or ethos for transforming self and practice,
or self and system, then a variety of questions related to one's view of caring and what it means
to be human might help (McCance et al, 1999; Watson, 1996; Watson & Smith, 2002).

iple

The client, Nesim, is 60 years old, married, and lives with his family. His primary diagnosis hypertension. Under older models of care, the patient might be convinced that he would mply overcome his hypertension—that it would "go away". In the Watson model, however, the nurse should aim to sustain a helping-trusting, authentic caring relationship, and to develop the capacity of the patient to problem solve about his hypertension and to teach him and his family proper care. The nurse educates the patient about hypertension, about improving self-health, thereby enabling and authenticating the deep belief system of the patient. The nurse is support-ive of the expression of positive and negative feelings by the patient. Nesim improves as the nurse creates a healing environment at all levels (physical as well as nonphysical). The patient should be assisted in the creative use of self and all ways of knowing as part of the caring process. The nurse must engage Nesim in the artistry of caring-healing practices that are "human care essentials," which potentate alignment of mind-body-spirit, wholeness, and unity of being in all aspects of care (Watson, 1996, p. 157). The patient should be followed to evaluate the med-ical and dietary treatment of hypertension.

ROGERS' SCIENCE OF UNITARY HUMAN BEINGS

Rogers formulated a theory to describe man and the life process in man (Daily et al, 1994; Rogers, 1990, 1992, 1994). Over the ensuing years, four critical elements emerged that are basic to the proposed system. These are energy fields, open systems, pattern and pandimension-ality (Rogers, 1992). The final concept, pandimensionality, was previously known as multidi-mensionality and prior to that, four-dimensionality.

Application to Vulnerable Populations

Within Roger's model the critical thinking process can be divided into three components: pattern appraisal, mutual patterning, and evaluation. The critical thinking process begins with a comprehensive *pattern appraisal.* The life process possesses its own unity and it is inseparable from the environment. This holistic appraisal requires the identification of patterns that reflect the whole. The pattern appraisal is a comprehensive assessment. Knowledge gained in the ap-praisal process is via cognitive input, sensory input, intuition, and language. The nurse gains a great deal of appraisal knowledge during the interview with the client by using the feeling or sensing level of knowing. Often described as instinctual, intuitive knowledge is best realized through reflection, which assists in appraising patterns. Manifestations of patterns are not static but partial perceptions of the synthesis of the past, present, and future. These perceptions pro-vide the basis for intuitive knowing. Manifestation, patterns, and rhythms are an indication of evolutionary emergence of the human field. Pattern appraisal and rhythm identification, along with reflection, provide the content for appraisal validation with the patient.

Once the client and nurse have consensus with respect to the appraisal, then nursing action is centered on mutual patterning of the client human/environmental field. The goal of the nurs-ing action is to bring and promote symphonic interaction between human and environment. This is done to strengthen the coherence and integrity of the human field and to direct and redirect patterning of the human and environmental fields (Rogers, 1990, p. 122). Patterning activities can be devised with respect to the initial pattern appraisal. The evaluation process is ongoing and fluid as the nurse reflects on his/her intuitive knowing. During the evaluation phase, the nurse repeats the pattern appraisal process to determine the level of dissonance perceived. The perceptions are then shared with the client and family/friends. Further mutual patterning is directed by the perceptions found during the evaluation process. This process continues as long as the nurse–client relationship continues (Bultmeier, 1997).

Example

Ayse is a 32-year-old woman who was recently admitted to the infection-nursing unit for evaluation after experiencing urinary infection and late-stage AIDS. Her weight is 58 kilograms down from her usual weight of about 80 kilograms. She has smoked approximately one pack of cigarettes a day for the past 16 years. She has two children, is married and lives with her husband in conditions she describes as less than sanitary. She describes her husband as emotionally distant and abusive at times. She is having continued pain and nausea. It will be necessary for her to perform intermittent self-catheterization at home. Her home medications are an antibiotic, an analgesic, and an antiemetic. She will soon be receiving radiation therapy on an outpatient basis. Ayse is extremely tearful. She expresses great concern over her future and the future of her two children. She believes that this illness is a punishment for her past life.

Within the Rogerian model, the process of caring for Ayse begins with pattern appraisal, the most important component of the nursing process. The nurse must engage in caring-healing practices which are human care essentials. The purpose is to potentiate alignment followed by mutual patterning and evaluation.

Pattern Appraisal

The history provides a beginning and a major portion of the pattern appraisal. Ayse has a pattern of smoking, which has been associated with poor health. This visible rhythmical pattern is a manifestation of evolution toward dissonance. In addition, Ayse has a pattern manifestation that has been labeled AIDS. This emergent pattern manifests as dissonant. Ayse has a low educational level, which is relevant as patterning activities are introduced. The nurse has reported that Ayse has a manifestation of fear. Ayse reports the fear of dealing with her life after this illness, and the nurse senses this manifestation of fear. Ayse's self-knowledge links the illness to her personal belief of "being punished" for past mistakes. History and focusing on the "relative present" to explore the pattern of punishment is imperative. It is important that the nurse appraise the environment of the hospital and of the others who share her existence. The pain and fear are dissonant manifestations. Dissonance can be perceived in many aspects of Ayse's appraisal: her unsanitary living conditions and her relationship with her husband, the manifestations of AIDS, weight loss, pain, nausea, and tobacco use. Finally, dissonance is also conceptualized as fear and is manifested in the emotional distance that she feels.

On completion of the pattern appraisal, the nurse presents the analysis to the patient. Emphasis can be placed on areas in which dissonance and harmony are noted in the personal and environmental field manifestations. Consensus needs to be reached with Ayse before patterning activities can be suggested and implemented.

Mutual Patterning

Patterning can be approached from many directions. The process is mutual between nurse and patient. Medications are patterning modalities. Ayse is receiving medications. Decisions are made in conjunction with Ayse regarding the use of the medications and the patterning that emerges with the introduction of these modalities. Personal knowledge regarding the medications empowers Ayse to be a vital agent in the selection of modalities. Ayse possesses freedom and involvement in the selection of modalities. Options include therapeutic touch, humor, meditation, visualization, and imagery.

Therapeutic touch can be introduced to Ayse, particularly to reduce her pain. Touch in combination with medications provides patterning that Ayse can direct. The nurse can introduce the process of touch to Ayse's husband and teach him how to incorporate touch into her care. Another option would be to teach Ayse how to center her energy and channel it to the area that is experiencing pain.

Patterning directed at the manifestation of fear is critical. Options include imagery, music, light, and meditation. Fear manifests as her apprehension about self-catheterization. Emphasis needs to be placed on having Ayse direct how, where, when, and with whom the self-catheterization will be taught. Establishing a rhythm to the catheterization schedule that is harmonious with Ayse's life would reduce dissonance. Patterning of nutrition and catheterization based on the pattern appraisal can assist in empowering Ayse to learn self-catheterization. A rhythm will evolve that is harmonious with Ayse and her energy field rhythm and that empower Ayse to direct this phase of her treatment.

Human/environment patterning needs to involve the other individuals who share Ayse's environment, including her husband and children. Options relate to increased communication and sanitation patterns. The nurse talks with the family and Ayse to determine what Ayse would prefer to change in her environment to improve sanitation. Options are introduced that allow pattern evolution integral with her environment that is not perceived as dissonant.

Evaluation

The evaluation process centers on the perceptions of dissonance that exist after the mutual patterning activities are implemented, to determine if they were successful. Specific emphasis is placed on emergent patterns of dissonance that are still evident. Manifestations of pain, fear, and tension with family members are appraised. The nurse continually evaluates the amount of dissonance that is apparent with respect to Ayse as he or she cares for her. A summary of the dissonance and/or harmony that the nurse perceives is then shared with Ayse, and mutual patterning is modified or instituted as indicated based on the evaluation.

ROPER, LOGAN, AND TIERNEY'S MODEL OF NURSING

In the United Kingdom, the Model of Nursing used most predominantly is that of Roper et al. (2002) and bases its principles on a Model of Living. The model is made up of five components: activities of daily living (ADLs); lifespan; dependence/independence continuum; factors influencing ADLs; individuality in living. Roper et al. suggest that these five components are as applicable to a Model of Living as they are to a Model of Nursing.

Example

Hatice is 55-years-old. She has difficult respiration and constipation. She can not do her own cleaning. First, considering 12 activities of daily living and affecting factors, the nurse collects data about the client, and sets nursing diagnoses, goals, and activities.

Diagnosis: Difficult breathing

Goal setting: Effective breathing

Activity: The nurse monitors breathing patterns and respirations and provides clean and normal temperature of the client's room.

Diagnosis: Constipation

Goal setting: Normal defecation

Activity: The nurse provides warm water for the client every morning, and encourages appropriate exercise. After these activities, the nurse should evaluate the results.

PEPLAU'S INTERPERSONAL MODEL

Peplau's interpersonal relations model relates to the meta-paradigm of the discipline of nursing (Forchuk, 1993). These concepts are the view of the person, health, nursing, and environment.

Person. Peplau's model describes the individual as a system with components of the physiological, psychological, and social. The individual is an unstable system where equilibrium is a desirable state, but occurs only through death. This is supported by Peplau's statement that "man is an organism that lives in an unstable equilibrium (i.e., physiological, psychological, and social fluidity) and life is the process of striving in the direction of stable equilibrium (i.e., a fixed pattern that is never reached except in death)" (Peplau, 1992, p. 82).

Application to Vulnerable Populations

The interpersonal relationship between the nurse and the client as described by Peplau (1992) has four clearly discernible phases: orientation, identification, exploitation, and resolution. These phases are interlocking and require overlapping roles and functions as the nurse and the client learn to work together to resolve difficulties in relation to health problems. During the orientation phase of the relationship, the client and nurse come together as strangers meeting for the first time. During this phase, the development of trust and empowerment of the client are primary considerations. This is best achieved by encouraging the client to participate in identifying the problem and allowing the client to be an active participant. By asking for and receiving help, the client will feel more at ease expressing needs, knowing that the nurse will take care of those needs. Once orientation has been accomplished, the relationship is ready to enter the next phase.

During the identification phase of the relationship, the client in partnership with the nurse, identifies problems. Once the client has identified the nurse as a person willing and able to provide the necessary help, the main problem and other related problems can then be worked on, in the context of the nurse–client relationship. Throughout the identification phase, both the nurse and the client must clarify each other's perceptions and expectations. The perceptions and expectations of the nurse and the client will affect the ability of both to identify problems and the necessary solutions. When clarity of perceptions and expectations is achieved, the client will learn how to make use of the nurse–client relationship. In turn, the nurse will establish a trusting relationship. Once identification has occurred, the relationship enters the next phase.

During the phase of exploitation, the client takes full advantage of all available services. The degree to which these services are used is based upon the needs and the interest of the client. During this time, the client begins to feel like an integral part of the helping environment and starts to take control of the situation by using the help available from the services offered. Within this phase, clients begin to develop responsibility and become more independent. From this sense of self-determination, clients develop an inner strength that allows them to face new challenges. This is best described by Peplau who stated that "Exploiting what a situation offers gives rise to new differentiations of the problem and to the development and improvement of skill in inter- personal relations" (Peplau, 1992, pp. 41–42). As the relationship passes through all of the afore- mentioned phases and the needs of the client have been met, the relationship passes to closure or the phase of resolution.

The strength of the model is the focus on the nurse–client relationship. The focus on this re- lationship allows for the nurse and the client to work together as partners in problem solving. The model encourages and supports empowerment of the client by encouraging the client to accept responsibility for well-being. The focus on the partnership of the nurse and the client and the em- phasis on meeting the identified needs of the client, make the model ideal for short-term crisis intervention. The model while focusing on getting sick people well is also applicable to health promotion. The focus of the Peplau model on the nurse–client relationship provides a foundation for many types of interactions between the nurse and the client that enhance health.

Example

Tarkan is a 46-year-old male who is married, and is scheduled for a heart operation next week. The client has had a few hospitalizations and is anxious due to the operation. The first phase of Peplau's model is *orientation*. As the client has previously been cared for at the hospi- tal, he is familiar with the layout of the facility as well as the general rules and regulations of the facility and orientation is quickly established. In the next phase of the relationship, *identifica- tion,* the nurse and Tarkan identify problems that require attention, including the client feelings about the operation and potential to die as a result. The nurse should also identify that the client is experiencing mixed emotions about the operation because he understands it is necessary. Then the nurse also identifies that the client requires additional support because he has been relatively stable for a time and yet requires this operation. In the next phase, *exploitation,* Tarkan quickly begins making use of the available resources and services at his disposal and talks with the nurse about his fears and hopes. He expresses feelings of mixed emotions, and the nurse comforts him by reminding him that his feelings are normal. In turn, he expresses relief.

As the client had been hospitalized twice within a one-year period, the client was provided with information on services that could be accessed to assist him further should the need arise. With the client making full use of the available services, the nurse–client relationship then en- tered the final phase, *resolution.* During resolution, the client becomes less dependent on the nurse for one-on-one interactions and no longer seeks further assistance.

NEUMAN'S HEALTH CARE SYSTEMS MODEL

This section will present the Neuman Health Care Systems Model (Neuman, 1995) as it relates to the meta-paradigm of the discipline of nursing. These concepts are person, health, nursing, and the environment.

Example

Dilek is a 25-year-old woman experiencing violence from her husband and auditory and vi- sual hallucinations. An intrapersonal stressor for Dilek is the limited effect the current medication regime is having on her acute symptoms, including difficulty sleeping. Both interpersonal and extrapersonal stressors exacerbate these intrapersonal stressors. The interpersonal stressors are the strained relationship with her husband related to the charges brought against him for sexual and physical abuse. The extrapersonal stressor is identified as inadequate community resources that could help her stay in her home. Once the stressors have been identified, a determination of the level of prevention required to strengthen the flexible line of defense is made.

In Dilek's situation, the identified stressors have penetrated the line of defense. Therefore, the goal is to prevent further regression. This is a tertiary level of intervention. As tertiary prevention is concerned with maintaining and supporting existing strengths of the client, this is best achieved through intensive conversations of the nurse with the client to emphasize her existing strengths. Dilek is encouraged to express her mixed feelings of relief and sadness about her relationship with husband and her feelings are validated as normal. The alleviation of her psychiatric symptoms is achieved without alteration to her established medication regime.

The primary level of intervention is aimed at health promotion. One of the identified stressors is inadequate community resources. The client attends the local mental health center on a regular basis. However, these appointments with the mental health center occur only once a month. The client should be provided with information related to crisis centers, emergency support, and grief counseling. The nurse follows up to ensure that client makes contact with these resources to strengthen the flexible line of defense.

REFERENCES

Berbiglia, V. A. (1997). Orem's self-care deficit theory in nursing practice. In M. Alligood & A. Marriner-Tomey (Eds.). *Nursing theory utilization & application.* St. Louis, MO: Mosby-Year Book.

Bultmeier, K. (1997). Rogers' science of unitary human being in nursing practice. In M. Alligood & A. Marriner-Tomey (Eds.). *Nursing theory utilization & application.* St. Louis, MO: Mosby-Year Book.

Connerley, K., Ristau, S., Lindberg, C., & McFarland, M. (1999). *The Roy model in nursing practice: The Roy Adaptation Model* (2nd ed., pp. 515–534). Stamford, CT: Appleton & Lange.

Daily, I. S., Maupin, J. S., Murray, C. A., Satterly, M. C., Schnell, D. L., & Wallace, T. L. (1994). Martha E. Roger: Unitary human beings. In A. Marriner-Tomey (Ed.). *Nursing theorists and their work* (3rd ed., pp. 211–230). St. Louis, MO: C. V. Mosby.

Forchuk, C. (1993). *Hildegarde E. Peplau: Interpersonal nursing theory.* Newbury Park, CA: Sage.

Frey, M. A., & Norris, D. (1997). King's system framework and theory in nursing practice. In M. Alligood & A. Marriner-Tomey (Eds.). *Nursing theory utilization & application.* St. Louis, MO: Mosby-Year Book.

Gonot, P. J. (1989). Imogene M. King's conceptual framework of nursing. In J. J. Fitzpatrick & A. L. Whall (Eds.). *Conceptual models of nursing analysis and application* (2nd ed.). Norwalk, CT: Appleton & Lange.

King, I. M. (1971). *Toward a theory for nursing.* New York, NY: John Wiley & Sons.

Leininger, M. M. (1991). *Culture care diversity and universality: A theory of nursing.* New York, NY: National League of Nursing Press.

Leininger, M. M. (1995). *Transcultural nursing: Concepts, theories, research and practice* (2nd ed.). New York, NY: McGraw-Hill.

McCance, T., McKenna, H., & Boore, J. (1999). Caring: Theoretical perspectives of relevance to nursing. *Journal of Advanced Nursing, 30,* 1388–1395.

Neuman, B. (1995). *The Neuman Systems Model* (3rd. ed.). Norwalk, CT: Appleton & Lange.

Orem, D. E. (1995). *Nursing concepts of practice* (5th ed.). St. Louis, MO: Mosby.

Peplau, H. E. (1992). *Interpersonal relations in nursing.* New York, NY: Springer.

Rogers, M. E. (1990). Nursing: Science of unitary, irreducible, human beings: Update 1990. In E. A. M. Barrett (Ed.), *Visions of Rogers' science-based nursing* (pp. 5–11). New York, NY: National League for Nursing.

Rogers, M. E. (1992). Window on science of unitary human beings. In M. O'Toole (Ed.), *Miller-Keane encyclopedia and dictionary of medicine, nursing, and allied health* (p. 1339). Philadelphia, PA: W. B. Saunders.

Rogers, M. E. (1994). The science of unitary human beings: Current perspectives. *Nursing Science Quarterly, 7*(1), 33–35.

Roper, N., Logan, W., Tierney, A., (2002). *The elements of nursing* (4th ed.). Edinburgh: Churchill Livingstone.

Roy, C. (1976). *Introduction to nursing: An adaptation model.* Englewood Cliffs, NJ: Prentice-Hall.

Wadensten, B. B., & Carlsson, M. (2003). Nursing theory and concept development or analysis. *Journal of Advanced Nursing, 42*(2), 118–124.

Watson, J., & Smith, M. (2002). Caring science and the science of unitary human beings: A trans-theoretical discourse for nursing knowledge development. *Journal of Advanced Nursing, 37,* 452.

Watson, J. (1996). Watson's theory of transpersonal caring. In P. H. Walker & B. Neuman (Eds.). *Blueprint for use of nursing models: Education, research, practice, & administration* (pp. 141–184). New York, NY: NLN Press.

CHAPTER 6

Nursing Theories Applied to Vulnerable Populations: Example from Sweden

Barbro Wadensten

An important purpose of theories is to challenge practice, create new approaches to practice, and remodel the structure of rules and principles. Theories should also be used to improve nursing practice. It is therefore interesting to study the content of nursing theories with regard to whether and how they may give guidance in caring for specific groups. This chapter examines definitions of vulnerable people in extant nursing theories and whether these theories can be used in the care of such people. "Vulnerable" is defined here as being in a dangerous position or condition and thereby susceptible to injury.

Different authors have developed various models for the analysis, evaluation, and classification of theories. Fawcett (2000) described the structural hierarchy of contemporary nursing knowledge, making distinctions in terms of the level of abstraction. The first level is the metaparadigm, the second includes conceptual models, and the third, theories. Even within the category of theories, though, types of theories differ in scope, with grand theories being the broadest. Middle-range theories are narrower in scope and are often considered the most useful because they can be empirically tested and applied in practice.

METHOD

Fawcett (2000) examined 10 well-known nursing theories that could be classified as grand-range and middle-range nursing theories according to the structural hierarchy. (Conceptual models have been excluded here because they usually express too little about how care can be structured.) The nursing theories of Henderson (1964, 1966, 1991), Leininger (1978, 1985a, 1985b, 1991, 1995, 1996), Newman (1982, 1990, 1994), Nightingale (1859/1946), Orlando (1961, 1972, 1987), Parse (1981, 1990a, 1990b, 1992, 1997a, 1997b, 1998), Peplau (1952, 1988, 1992, 1997), Travelbee (1966, 1971), Watson (1979, 1987, 1988, 1997, 1999), and Wiedenbach (1964) were selected. The theorists' original works were the point of departure. The content of the theories was analyzed according to Fawcett's (2000) meta-paradigm, which consists of the primary concepts of person, health, environment, and nursing, and the research questions reproduced here were addressed to each theory.

1. Is the concept "human" described and, if so, how?
2. Is human development described and, if so, how?
3. Is the concept "patient" described and, if so, how?

4. Is the concept "vulnerable" used in the theory and, if so, how?
5. With regard to these questions, what consequences do the views expressed by these nursing theories have for how nurses care for vulnerable people?

A content analysis of the theories with respect to questions 1–4 was conducted, and a qualitative analysis of the results was performed. The results are presented here first in terms of four different themes that relate to the concepts listed in the first four questions: human, human development, patient, and vulnerable. Under each theme, the results are reported in alphabetical order by theorist, such that the name is listed if the theme is included in the theory. Thereafter, the results of the qualitative analysis were put together to answer the fifth question, regarding the consequences of the theories (see the Discussion section).

RESULTS

Table 6.1 shows a classification of the theories according to Fawcett's Structural Hierarchy Model. A summary of the concepts (human, descriptions of vulnerable people, and considerations for care of vulnerable people) described by the various theories is presented in Table 6.2.

Descriptions of the Concept "Human"

Henderson (1966) did not describe "human," she only described a person as a patient.

Leininger (1978, 1985) described humans as cultural beings and further (1996) stated that humans are complex beings who wish their holistic view of life, care, culture, and health to remain whole and do not wish to be viewed as fragmented organs or body parts.

Newman (1982, 1990, 1994) described people as dynamic energy patterns that are open and in interaction with the environment. Furthermore, Newman (1994) stated that the human being is unitary and continuous with the undivided wholeness of the universe.

Nightingale (1859/1946) did not describe the concept of human; she described a person as a patient.

TABLE 6.1   Classification of Nursing Theories According to Fawcett's Structural Hierarchy Model

Nursing theorist	Grand- range theory	Middle-range theory
Henderson		X
Leininger	X	
Newman	X	
Nightingale	X	
Orlando		X
Parse	X	
Peplau		X
Travelbee		X
Watson		X
Wiedenbach		X

TABLE 6.2   A Summary of Concepts Described by Theorists

Nursing theorist (Year)	Human	Human development	Vulnerable
		Concept	
Henderson (1964)	only as a patient	no	no
Leininger (1978)	yes	yes	no
Newman (1982)	yes	no	no
Nightingale (1859)	only as a patient	no	no
Orlando (1961)	only as a patient	no	yes
Parse (1981)	yes	yes	no
Peplau (1952)	yes	yes	no
Travelbee (1966)	yes	yes	no
Watson (1979)	yes	yes	no
Wiedenbach (1964)	no	no	yes

Orlando (1961, 1972, 1987) did not describe "human," only a person as a patient.

Parse (1981) described humans as unitary and open, freely choosing meaning *in situ* and bearing responsibility for their decisions. Man coexists while co-constituting patterns with the environment.

Peplau (1952) described "human" as reducible and stated that all human behavior is goal seeking. In subsequent writings, she tended to use the concept of patient (Peplau, 1988, 1992, 1997).

Travelbee (1966, 1971) defined a human being as a unique, irreplaceable individual, in this world only once, unlike any person who has ever lived or ever will live.

Watson (1979, 1988) considered the individual a living, growing entity with three dimensions: spirit, body, and soul.

Wiedenbach (1964) considered humans functioning beings.

Description of Human Development

In the theories of Henderson (1964, 1982, 1991), Nightingale (1946/1859), and Orlando (1961, 1987) there are no descriptions of human development.

Leininger (1985a, 1985b, 1991) claimed that individuals develop and that development is influenced by the cultural environment. Therefore, development during the life span is different across different cultures and in different individuals.

Newman (1982, 1990, 1994) described people as dynamic energy patterns and stated that these patterns are characterized by movement, diversity, and rhythm.

Parse (1981, 1990a, 1990b, 1992) described humans as being able to create and develop their own life patterns. Among the central concepts in Parse's theory are growth and capacity, creativity and transformation. These concepts can be viewed as developmental.

According to Peplau (1952, 1988), human development takes place through interpersonal relations. How individuals experience themselves is a product of socialization, a human function that develops and is revised in a constructive or destructive manner in interpersonal relationships during the life course of the individual.

Travelbee (1966, 1971) pointed out that the capacity and motivation to look for meaning in life experiences is characteristic of human beings. Later life experiences are unique to each individual and are influenced by earlier experiences. Experiences such as illness and suffering can constitute a special opportunity for personal development.

Watson's (1979, 1988) view was that individuals may develop a high degree of consciousness if they can find meaning and harmony in life. Incongruity or disharmony between the self and the ideal self rises increasingly into consciousness, but as an individual matures, he or she becomes more diversified and develops an inner self; the individual also attempts to attain greater spiritual harmony. Watson also said that the individual is influenced and changed by the past, present, and future and that humans have the power to grow and change. This theory thus includes a clear developmental perspective.

Wiedenbach (1964) stated that each human being is endowed with a unique potential to develop but did not describe this development.

None of these 10 theorists actually discussed what the results of human development are expected to be.

Description of the Concept of Patient

Henderson (1964, 1966, 1991) viewed the patient as an individual who requires assistance to achieve health and independence or a peaceful death.

Leininger (1978, 1995) used the concept "client." Her theory is called a transcultural theory, at the heart of which is the notion that the culture influences the need for care.

Newman (1990, 1994) talked about the individual but did not use the concept of patient.

Nightingale (1859/1946) described the patient as a passive person who receives care.

Orlando (1961) stated that people become patients when they submit to medical procedures.

Parse (1981,1990a, 1990b, 1992, 1997a, 1997b, 1998) did not use the concept of patient.

Peplau (1952, 1988) described patients as persons who have problems of one kind or another for which expert services are needed or sought.

Travelbee (1966, 1971) argued that there is a risk in using the concept of patient because it could lead to a stereotyped view of humans. It is important to remember that it is individual human beings who are in need of care.

Watson (1979, 1987, 1988, 1997, 1999) did not use the concept of patient; she instead talked about a person.

Instead of patient, Wiedenbach (1964) used the concept "client" and defined a client as any individual who is receiving help of some kind, be it care, instructions, or advice.

All nursing theorists who described the concept of patient did so in a way that portrays someone who is in need of some help, which indicates that these theorists considered patients vulnerable. Yet even theorists who did not use the concept of patient assumed that the client or person is someone in need of some sort and varying degrees of help or support. Therefore, it is reasonable to conclude that the studied theorists considered these individuals to be in a vulnerable position.

Description of the Concept "Vulnerable"

Orlando (1972) used the concept "vulnerable." She stated that once an individual undergoes medical diagnosis, treatment, or supervision, he or she automatically assumes the status of patient and is vulnerable. That is, patients may not be in a position to control all that happens to them and suffer helplessness as a result. Wiedenbach (1970) also used the concept vulnerable when describing the nursing client. She considered that any person with a perceived need for help is in a vulnerable position.

DISCUSSION

By studying in detail how the concepts "human" and human development are treated in the theories, it is possible to show how the individual is viewed in these theories. Descriptions of the context in which the concept "patient" is used also reveal views on the individual, particularly when the individual is in need of care. Because different theorists use different concepts, it is necessary to study their descriptions of both the individual and the patient.

Only Orlando and Wiedenbach directly used the concept "vulnerable," but it is nevertheless possible to discern in the other theories, through their descriptions of the individual or the patient, that all the theorists studied considered people who are in need of care to be vulnerable and therefore in need of some help or support from nurses. Hence, by studying the views of the theorists on the concepts of human and human development, it is possible to ascertain their beliefs about what attitude the nurse should adopt. Through such an analysis, two groups were identified: theorists who described human development and those who did not.

Views on care of the patient depend on the view of human development. Looking at theorists who considered that human development continues throughout life—Leininger, Parse, Peplau, Travelbee, and Watson, for instance—and thus have a developmental perspective, it is possible to see that vulnerability can lead to growth. According to these theorists, then, when people are vulnerable, they have an opportunity to develop if they can tackle their problems. It is also these theorists who claim that the nurse should support her patients/clients, whereas other theorists are more inclined to view the role of the nurse as one of taking over and helping a passive patient.

This means that two possible approaches to nursing can be perceived, and this has practical consequences for care. The nurse can either take over and do things for the patient or support the patient in the process of tackling the problem. The theorists who did not express a developmental perspective—Henderson, Newman, Nightingale, Orlando, and Wiedenbach—instead had a "take over" perspective and offered nursing actions that could help the patient. The theorists with a developmental perspective—Leininger, Parse, Peplau, Travelbee, and Watson—instead considered that nurses should support the patient in tackling the problem. Theoretically, both approaches to nursing could be valuable, although they do signify two completely different attitudes towards the content of nursing actions.

It may be concluded that the studied theories of Leininger, Parse, Peplau, Travelbee, and Watson convey the notion that the nurse should support patients/clients in their development. The theories of Travelbee and Watson describe human development in terms of a life-cycle perspective. These theories may also provide people with some guidance on possible paths of development. However, they do not discuss the possible desirable outcomes of such development.

Some of the studied nursing theorists have presented descriptions of human development. Leininger, Newman, Peplau, Travelbee, and Watson have all expressed the opinion that early experiences and events influence the way in which the individual experiences and reacts to events later in life. That is, the past influences the manner in which the individual develops, which in turn influences how the individual reacts to different life events and also to the stress experienced during illness and crises. Some, such as Travelbee and Watson, have also stated that crises can present an opportunity for personal development. Therefore these theories give some guidance because they offer the opinion that nurses should support this development. Given this notion, it is possible to construe that it is important to give support and in such a way that allows people to manage the situation. The theorists who consider that humans have the capacity to develop also assume that nurses should believe it is possible and necessary to back up and support the patient. This will have consequences for how the practical care is performed, but the theories do not provide any real guidance on how this practical support can be accomplished.

We can assume that if nurses have adopted the view that humans can develop, they will have a corresponding view with regard to the patient/client. Even if patients are vulnerable, nurses need not consider them totally helpless, and therefore they will support them in tackling their problems, thereby helping them to develop. The nursing actions taken will then reflect a different approach than would those of a nurse who has a take-over perspective.

I consider that we as nurses work on the basis of our individual outlooks on human behavior. I will therefore argue in conclusion that the sort of outlook we have on humans and their ability to manage difficult situations influences how we act. This in turn strongly influences our views on and attitudes toward people we regard as vulnerable. Perhaps we are not always aware of our own outlook or of how to manage our actions and behavior. If we have a theory as our point of departure, we should be aware of it. This would help us clarify for ourselves and for others the standpoint we take and would facilitate cooperation within the staff team as regards how to act.

However, common to all nursing theories is that they fail to specify how support can be provided. The nursing theorists have taken individuality in care into account and mentioned the importance of structuring nursing on the basis of the needs of each individual, but how the nurse should support a vulnerable person is only discussed indirectly. Thus they leave it to each individual nurse to decide what aspects are important in the support he or she provides.

Nursing theories have been analyzed from different viewpoints on different occasions, and their relevance has been discussed (Chinn & Jacobs, 1987; Chinn & Kramer, 1995; Fawcett, 2000; Kirkevold, 1994; Meleis, 1997; Nicoll, 1997). Many authors have analyzed and discussed the applicability of different nursing theories to nursing practice and have arrived at different conclusions. A review of this entire body of literature is not possible here, but it is interesting to point out, in accordance with the intention of this literature review, McCance, McKenna, & Boore (1999), who compared four nursing theories and found that those of Leininger and Watson have great potential for use in practice because they are judged to be less abstract. McCance et al. (1999) posed the important and relevant question of whether busy practitioners can confidently and competently apply a theory if they have limited knowledge and understanding of its underlying philosophies.

With regard to nursing care, the theories could be expected to address more specifically how to care for patients with different needs. Another study (Wadensten & Carlsson, 2003) reviewed 17 nursing theories and found that none of them provided any guidance on how to care for older people. One might expect that nursing theories would more specifically address how to care for persons with different needs, but nursing theories are general and do not provide any precise instructions.

Tierney (1998) critically discussed whether extant nursing theories and models have relevance today and stated that without theory there is no sense of place for new knowledge and no clarity of overall direction for development of the nursing discipline. The nursing theories contain an overall description of the content of care and nursing. It can be said that they define the area of nursing. The theories should of course be seen in a historical perspective, which helps us to understand that part of their purpose was to define nursing, and in this sense they are important. I have often observed that nurses in Sweden feel that theories are unnecessary, probably because they do not understand that theories can guide them in general and specific aspects of care provision. I argue that it is of great value to discuss and develop nursing knowledge; this can be done by developing extant theories or developing new, more concrete nursing theories, because my opinion is that we need theories that can be used in practice. Nursing care needs theories of different scope, and such theories could help the nursing profession in Sweden, as well as in other countries, develop.

A theory is successful if it is efficient and effective in attaining its socially prescribed goals. In the case of nursing, those goals would be the outcomes of patient health and comfort that are fully or partly attributable to nursing care and nursing interventions. The context of what nursing is, has been, and is still, discussed in Sweden. There are different standpoints about the essential nature of nursing care. I turn back to my earlier discussion of how we ought to see the nursing theories in a historical perspective. They have been very important for the development of what nursing care is.

But nurses in Sweden today are not generally familiar with this. Therefore, and also because their opinions about nursing are sometimes not in line with the work of the theorists, I think that many Swedish nurses find the nursing theories unnecessary and uninteresting. Theory should help to provide knowledge to improve practice by describing, explaining, and predicting phenomena. In Sweden, nursing theories are usually perceived as too vague and do not give enough practical guidance. Nurses in Sweden are often trained more directly in practical nursing skills, e.g., how to perform different nursing interventions, without the connection to theory, and they do not understand the value of theory guidance in their work. It is time now in Sweden for nurses to learn more about how theory can improve nursing and the practical work of nursing. It is my strong opinion that nursing needs new theories that can be used in practice, e.g., more specific theories than those that already exist. You cannot assume that busy practitioners can confidently and competently apply a theory if they have limited knowledge and understanding of its philosophies. Therefore nurses in Sweden, and I suppose even nurses in many other countries, need more concrete theories—or guidelines that are derived from theories—to show them how to act in practice.

REFERENCES

Chinn, P. L., & Jacobs, M. K. (1987). *Theory and nursing* (2nd ed.). St. Louis, MO: C. V. Mosby.

Chinn, P. L., & Kramer, M. K. (1995). *Theory and nursing: A systematic approach* (4th ed.). St. Louis, MO: C. V. Mosby.

Fawcett, J. (2000). *Analysis and evaluation of contemporary nursing knowledge: Nursing models and theories.* Philadelphia, PA: F. A. Davis.

Henderson, V. (1964). *Basic principles of nursing care.* Geneva: International Council of Nurses.

Henderson, V. (1966). *The nature of nursing.* New York, NY: Macmillan.

Henderson, V. (1991). *The nature of nursing reflections after 25 years*. New York, NY: National League for Nursing.

Kirkevold, M. (1994). *Omvårdnadsteorier—analys och utv rdering*. Lund: Studentlitteratur.

Leininger, M. (1978). *Transcultural nursing: Concepts, theories, and practices*. New York, NY: John Wiley & Sons.

Leininger, M. (1985a). *Qualitative research methods in nursing*. Orlando, FL: Grune & Stratton.

Leininger, M. (1985b). Transcultural care diversity and universality: A theory of nursing. *Nursing & Health Care, 6*, 209–212.

Leininger, M. (Ed.). (1991). *Culture care diversity and universality: A theory of nursing*. New York, NY: National League for Nursing [NLN].

Leininger, M. (1995). *Transcultural nursing: Concepts, theories, research and practices* (2nd ed.). New York, NY: McGraw-Hill.

Leininger, M. (1996). Culture care theory, research, and practice. *Nursing Science Quarterly, 9*, 71–78.

McCance, T., McKenna, H., & Boore, J. (1999). Caring: Theoretical perspectives of relevance to nursing. *Journal of Advanced Nursing, 30*, 1388–1395.

Meleis, A. I. (1997). *Theoretical Nursing: Development and progress* (3rd ed.). Philadelphia, NY: J. B. Lippincott.

Newman, M. A. (1982). Time as an index of consciousness with age. *Nursing Research, 31*, 290–293.

Newman, M. A. (1990). Newman's theory of health as praxis. *Nursing Science Quarterly, 3*, 37–41.

Newman, M. A. (1994). Theory for nursing practice. *Nursing Science Quarterly, 7*, 153–157.

Nicoll, L. (1997). *Perspectives of nursing theories* (3rd ed.). Philadelphia, PA: J. B. Lippincott.

Nightingale, F. (1957). *Notes on nursing: What it is and is not*. Philadelphia, PA: J. B. Lippincott. (Original work published 1859).

Orlando, I. J. (1961). *The dynamic nurse–patient relationship*. New York, NY: G. P. Putnam's Sons.

Orlando, I. J. (1972). *The discipline and teaching of nursing process*. New York, NY: G. P. Putnam's Sons.

Orlando, I. J. (1987). Nursing in the 21st century: Alternate paths. *Journal of Advanced Nursing, 12*, 405–412.

Parse, R. R. (1981). *Man living—health: A theory of nursing*. New York, NY: Wiley.

Parse, R. R. (1990a). Nursing theory-based practice: A challenge for the 90s. *Nursing Science Quarterly, 3*, 53.

Parse, R. R. (1990b). Health: A personal commitment. *Nursing Science Quarterly, 3*, 136–140.

Parse, R. R. (1992). Human becoming: Parse's theory of nursing. *Nursing Science Quarterly, 5*, 35–42.

Parse, R. R. (1997a). The human becoming theory: The was, is, and will be. *Nursing Science Quarterly, 10*, 32–38.

Parse, R. R. (1997b). The language of nursing knowledge: Saying what we mean. In I. M. King & J. Fawcett (Eds.). *The language of nursing theory* (pp. 73–77). Indianapolis, IN: Sigma Theta Tau International Nursing Press.

Parse, R. R. (1998). *The human becoming school of thought: A perspective for nurses and other health professionals*. Thousand Oaks, CA: Sage.

Peplau, H. E. (1952). *Interpersonal relations in nursing*. New York, NY: G. P. Putnam's Sons.

Peplau, H. E. (1988). The art and science of nursing: Similarities, differences, and relations. *Nursing Science Quarterly, 1*, 8–15.

Peplau, H. E. (1992). Interpersonal relations: A theoretical framework for application in nursing practice. *Nursing Science Quarterly, 5*, 13–18.

Peplau, H. E. (1997). Peplau's theory of interpersonal relations. *Nursing Science Quarterly, 10*, 162–167.

Tierney, A. (1998). Nursing models: Extant or extinct? *Journal of Advanced Nursing, 28*, 77–85.

Travelbee, J. (1966). *Interpersonal aspects of nursing*. Philadelphia, PA: F. A. Davis.

Travelbee, J. (1971). *Interpersonal aspects of nursing* (2nd ed.). Philadelphia, PA: F. A. Davis.

Wadensten, B., & Carlsson, M. (2003). Nursing theory views on how to support the process of ageing. *Journal of Advanced Nursing, 42,* 118–124.

Watson, J. (1979). *Nursing: The philosophy and science of caring.* Boston, MA: Little Brown and Company.

Watson, J. (1987). Nursing on the caring edge: Metaphorical vignettes. *Advances in Nursing Science, 10,* 10–17.

Watson, J. (1988). *Nursing: Human science and human care. A theory of nursing.* New York, NY: National League of Nursing.

Watson, J. (1997). The theory of human caring: Retrospective and prospective. *Nursing Science Quarterly, 10,* 49–52.

Watson, J. (1999). Postmodern nursing and beyond. New York, NY: Churchill Livingstone.

Wiedenbach, E. (1964). *Clinical nursing: A helping art.* New York, NY: Springer.

Wiedenbach, E. (1970). Nurses' wisdom in nursing theory. *American Journal of Nursing, 70,* 1057–1062.

CHAPTER 7

The Ethical Experience of Caring for Vulnerable Populations: The Symphonological Approach

Gladys L. Husted and James H. Husted

As members of mankind, we share with other animals the fact that our nature and relationship to the world makes us vulnerable. We are all prone to encounter, in one way or another, that which blocks our efficient functioning as the kind of being we are. Our vulnerability is an inescapable part of our nature and of the influence of the world in which we live.

This is true not only of animals and humans but of everything that exists. Rocks, rose bushes, and rainbows come into and go out of existence. But to us as humans, and in fact to every animal, there is a noteworthy difference between the alternatives of staying in existence and going out of existence. This is not true of rocks, rose bushes, and rainbows. Animals act to avoid various perils to which they are vulnerable. As rational animals we (sometimes) use our powers of reason to initiate actions to oppose the loss of our well-being.

One of the ways we can do this is through ethical awareness, extending the time frame of our actions and making them more intelligible. Another is by establishing health care systems. The motivation for each of these is a reasoned desire to escape the consequences of various aspects of our vulnerability. Health care systems are far more efficient in achieving this than contemporary ethical systems are. Ethical systems can conflict with the purposes of the health care setting and the objective expectations of patients. When these systems are dominant in a health care setting they expose patients to a virulent form of vulnerability.

Perhaps only in the court system are the benefits of an appropriate[1] ethic, insightfully applied, greater than in the health care system. And only in the court system are the harms of an inappropriate ethic or its inappropriate application greater. At all odds, the health care setting is among the most complex of ethical arenas.

Patients in the health care system suffer a vast multitude of disabilities through injury or illness. This makes the pursuit of a spectrum of individual values, which various patients hold, vulnerable.

AGENCY

For bioethics, one disability defines and sets apart every patient regardless of the nature of his[2] affliction. This is the loss of agency the power of an individual person to initiate and sustain action, the power to act on his purposes. Every patient suffers an impaired ability to take the actions that further his life and his flourishing in that life. This is the overall object of the health care sciences. All of bioethics, properly so-called, is directed against this general disability. There cannot be an ethic for every sort of disability. The onset of disability and loss of well-being and agency sets the standard for the health care setting in terms of ethical awareness in relation to the disabled.

Every patient[3] needs someone to take actions for him. This need is a result of his loss of agency. The vulnerability of a patient is the central concern of bioethics, the concern that he may fail to gain a foreseeable increase in, or even to lose a part of, his agency through the actions of health care professionals. The more acute the potential for loss of agency, the greater the vulnerability. The measure of success for a practice-based bioethic is a patient's vital objective that he shall retain or regain his power to initiate actions. It is here that ethics connects and interweaves with health care and with human life and purposes.

THE NURSE AS A SECOND SELF

According to Aristotle (McKeon, trans. 1941), a friend is, in his famous phrase, "another self" to his friend. Likewise, a nurse is another self to her patients. A nurse who is guided by an ethic based on a professional practice, is "the agent of a patient doing for a patient what he would do for himself if he were able" (Husted & Husted, 2001, p. 53). In filling the defining responsibilities of her profession, such a nurse significantly reduces the vulnerability of a patient.

However, paradoxically, currently fashionable ethical beliefs imparted by her formal education may produce a willingness to aggress against the agency of her patient. The combination of emotivism (ethical actions should be guided by one's beliefs or affective responses) and deontology (ethical actions should not be guided by a sense of professional responsibility but by a strict adherence to rules) can instill an indifference or a blend of resentment and self-righteousness that places a patient in a subsidiary, or even an irrelevant, ethical status.

At the same time, no patient ever came into the health care setting for the purpose of losing his right to self-determination. The great majority of patients assume that a nurse's ethical actions consist in filling her role as nurse. However, a patient may assume a misplaced trust in a health care professional. This simply involves the false assumption that the stable goal of the professional is to help him regain his lost agency. Probably no patient suspects, and none would be comforted by, the knowledge that nurses consider it their ethical responsibility to

- ☐ act on assumed duties whose nature is completely unknown to a patient (the ethic of **deontology**),
- ☐ pursue at every opportunity the greatest good for the greatest number (the ethic of **utilitarianism**),
- ☐ obey an image in her (the nurse's) mind that keeps her informed as to what her culture or society expects of her (the ethic of **social relativism**),
- ☐ follow her emotional state of the moment, however whimsical (the ethic of **emotivism**).

A patient is seldom more imperiled than when he is vulnerable to the misdirected and self-righteous intentions of a nurse.

Being another self, a concerned nurse does not seek to gain dominion over a vulnerable friend but accepts his right to retain his individual identity. She makes it, as far as she can, unnecessary for the patient to defend himself. When appropriate, she defends him. A concerned nurse has no interest in choosing the values or determining the fate of even the most vulnerable patient.

If a nurse were to be shorn of all her out-of-context ethical preconceptions, all that would be left are the ethical demands of her profession. If she is guided by this, her ethical concern is her relation to her patient as an independent ethical equal.

RELATIONSHIP OF NURSE AND PATIENT

"A patient is one who has lost or suffered a decrease in agency; one who is unable to take the actions his survival or well-being requires" (Husted & Husted, 2001, p. 53). Because she is defined as the agent of her patient, it is appropriate that the center of a nurse's professional concern should be her patient. When the center of her attention is not her patient, a nurse is practicing a perverse form of nursing. This perverseness arises through the choice of a flawed and irrelevant standard for nursing. There is nothing in the theory or practice of any health care profession to justify the professional using his or her emotions or preconceptions as inspiration. Nothing other than the well-being of the patient can serve as the standard of professional judgment. Any other standard would not allow an intelligible interweaving of the practice of nursing and the ethic appropriate to that practice.

A patient must exercise the resources of his character that enable him to achieve greater well-being through his power to take independent action. A nurse's standard of success is met when she strengthens these resources and increases the opportunity of her patient to exercise them. For a professional ethic, one defined by a nurse's practice, this is the standard by which she measures her practice. It is the reason-for-being and the ethical guidepost of her profession.

ETHICS OF PROFESSIONAL PRACTICE

The ethic of a concerned nurse must be practice based. An ethic that is not gleaned from practice cannot justifiably be the ethic of a health care professional. It is the ethic of a nurse who is merely going through the motions. Every form of a practice-based bioethic is derived from, and is intended to be appropriate to, the self-determination of a patient, the purposes of a health care setting, and the role of a health care professional. Most nurses eventually adopt some form of a practice-based system. It is a significant benefit to them if they recognize this. An ethic not derived from the practice of the health care professions and the purpose of the health care setting must fail to meet the needs of a patient. Ethical decisions and actions guided by a nurse's feelings or the demands she attributes to her duty often fail. If they succeed, they succeed only by accident. To the extent that a patient is vulnerable, these decisions and actions create a greater vulnerability.

A practice-based ethical system places a nurse in harmony with the nature of the health care system and the trust of her patients. Such a system will produce positive pride in her profession and in herself as a practitioner of this profession. And, as a corollary, it will increase the confidence that each of her patients can appropriately place in her. It will reduce or eliminate the patients' vulnerability, at least in their relation to her.

NATURE OF THE NURSE–PATIENT AGREEMENT

Of necessity, a practice-based system is symphonological, a term derived from *asymphonia*, a Greek word meaning agreement. This is an approach to ethical interaction from professional responsibility, the responsibility encoded in a nurse's professional agreement with her patient. A practice-based bioethic aims to relate professionals and patients internally, to bring them into the same ethical context. It makes human values its focus and ensures that the health care setting is minimally arbitrary and maximally purposeful. This context influences directly or indirectly the way in which a nurse performs (Gastmans, 1998). A practice-based bioethic is based on interaction between a professional and a patient who relate to each other through understanding and agreement. One engages with a nurse assuming that she has agreed to act in her role as a health care professional. In engaging her, one agrees to be a patient, one willing for her to act for him. Logically and ethically there is an inescapable implication that the ethical interactions between nurse and patient will conform to this agreement.

Necessity of the Nurse–Patient Agreement

"How can two walk together lest they agree?" (1 Kings 3:16-28). The simple action of two people walking together is an interaction and is therefore necessarily the product of an agreement. Much more so, the complex and vital actions that take place in a health care system are interactions and are therefore products of a complex and vital agreement.

An agreement is a shared state of awareness established by a decision on the part of each party to the agreement. The agreement between nurse and patient is the foundation of the ethical interaction between them. It is structured by the expectations of each and the commitments that each makes to the other. Each agrees to satisfy these reasonable expectations and to live up to the commitment. The agreement makes their interaction intelligible. It helps each to understand what is expected and what is committed to in their interaction. Whenever a nurse fails to be guided by her professional agreement, her profession becomes, in effect, a hobby. She may feel that ethically she succeeds, but in relation to her patients and her profession, she fails.

NURSING INTERACTIONS

Every action that a nurse takes is an interaction. There are no isolated actions actions without interaction in the health care system. Isolated actions would not be nursing, nor would they be anything of any consequence. A nurse's profession implies that her agreement is to interact. Even in the cases of a patient who cannot actively participate in his care, professional practice remains an interaction. A nurse interacts with the vital functions of her patients. The less a patient can participate in his care, the weaker he is in their interactions, the more vulnerable he is. A concerned nurse does, even for the most vulnerable, precisely what she does for every patient: she acts to overcome his vulnerability, his inability to take action, his patiency. Although with the more vulnerable, her actions may need to be more powerful and more precise. In the context of a practice-based ethic, interaction begins with support for a patient's right to self-determination.

RIGHTS

One evening, strolling across a field in a deserted park, Tom sees Dick approaching from the other side. Tom has recently lost his financial shirt. He is broke and has no bright prospects for the future. Dick is a rich recluse in ill health. He is known to carry large sums of money with him. Tom is aware of this. Tom could rob Dick, solve his financial problems, and no one would be the wiser. Dick, for his part, is unacquainted with Tom. Tom, in common with everyone in town, knows that Dick is subject to hallucinations. On this day, everyone from this small town except Tom and Dick has taken a bus to the county fair. Every circumstance seems to invite Tom to rob Dick. The odds on Tom being caught are minuscule. None of this enters Tom's mind. As they pass, Dick speaks a conventional pleasantry to him and Tom replies in kind. Tom never conceives of robbing Dick. Without thinking about it, Tom has recognized Dick's rights. If you had seen this event, you would have seen the operation of an individual right, Dick's right not to be aggressed against.

Now what is it you have seen?

Rights[4]: the product of a spontaneous and unnoticed agreement. This agreement holds between every noncriminal member of the human species. One instance of this is the agreement existing between Tom and Dick.

Rights: "the product of an implicit agreement among rational beings, formed by virtue of their rationality, not to obtain actions or the product of actions from each other, except through voluntary consent, objectively gained" (Husted & Husted, 2001, p. 4).

Imagine, if you can, a health care setting devoid of this agreement. Without the recognition of individual rights, this system would never have come into being. No one would conceive of something as intricate as a health care system. Human existence would be, in the words of philosopher Thomas Hobbes (1588–1679), "solitary, poore, nastie, brutish, and short" (Oakeshott, 1957, p. 47). To the extent that the recognition of individual rights does not guide interaction, human life must be and is right now solitary, poore, nastie, brutish, and short.

Individual rights belong to each human individual by virtue of his or her membership in the human species. In becoming a patient, an individual does not lose this membership. His rights are not increased—this is not necessary—but neither are his rights decreased because this is not permissible. He is a rational being ethically equal to all other rational beings. The nature of every interpersonal ethical system arises from the attitude of that system toward individual rights. The nature of the ethical practice of every nurse is shaped by her attitude toward the individual rights of her patient.

Ethical practice does not allow a professional to violate the rights of a patient. A dedication to human values is internal to the nature of the health care setting. This dedication presupposes respect for the individual rights of patients. Only when an individual has reason to be confident that he will not be the victim of aggression can he exercise his human virtues in the pursuit of his individual values.

The rights agreement is the ethical foundation for explicit agreements. It is the already-established agreement that explicit agreements will be objective, voluntary, and honored. Harmony is a state wherein each agent can interact without fear of betrayal and aggression. The rights agreement creates a state of harmony among rational beings. Reliance on rights is possible and productive, even though crime is possible in the same way that reliance on health is reasonable despite the possibility of injury or illness. The practice of nursing, ideally, goes beyond respect for rights, but a professional practice-based ethic must begin with a nurse's undaunted pride in her profession and the recognition of the rights of her patients (Hardt, 2001).

THE PARADOX OF GROUP PURPOSE

A bioethical view of rights must be concerned with individual human purposes. How could it be otherwise in view of a patient's individualistic struggles in the health care setting and the defined role of a nurse? It is the view that a patient's pursuit of his purposes should not be aggressed against. Individual purposes are the motivation and precondition of the health care setting and of rights. If people did not act on purposes, rights would have no relevance to ethics, and ethics would have no relevance to human life. Without the protection of rights, human individuals could not act on their purposes. Every moment of their lives would be spent defending themselves. Rights and purposes are intricately interwoven.

Much of the literature about vulnerable patients deals with vulnerable patient populations. As nurses we have to differentiate between vulnerable populations and the vulnerable patient as a unique individual requiring attention to his own specific characteristics. The concept of populations assists our understanding and communication with others; however, it does not create another entity. Populations have no purpose and no rights. No population ever occupied a hospital bed.

Nurses and patients disagree. Patients and patients disagree. Nurses disagree with each other. And it is to the advantage of every individual to accept these differences as relevant, inalienable, and defended by individual rights. The right to different motivations is the reason-for-being of ethics. Any defense of the idea that differences in motivations as such are unjustified would involve an individual in arguing that the motivation of his individual and different point of view is justified; his point being that the motivation behind individual and different points of view are unjustified.

AGREEMENT, BIOETHICAL STANDARDS, AND THE VULNERABLE PATIENT

Virtues are the standards of a practice-based bioethic. Whatever actions a nurse takes to strengthen them are justifiable ethical actions. Whatever actions a nurse takes that weaken virtues are unethical and unjustifiable actions (Husted & Husted, 2001). The rights agreement is the sanction of the virtues. The nurse–patient agreement is an interaction taken in service of the virtues. The virtues, by their nature, are instruments of human purpose, and this nature structures the nature of individual purposes and human persons. Their nature is the inspiration for agreement-making. Bioethical standards, the measuring rods of success, are the virtues of autonomy, freedom, objectivity, self-assertion, beneficence, and fidelity.[5]

Autonomy is the uniqueness of a person, that which makes a person the individual he or she is. It is the right to be who he or she is and act on that basis. If a nurse can strengthen and nurture her patients' autonomy, then she will help them make their purposes and actions their own. She can help them gain a better understanding and acceptance of themselves. This is her ethical means of meeting her agreement.

Freedom is the power (and right) to take long-term action based on one's own evaluation of a situation. A patient who is less able to exercise his ability to take free action is more vulnerable than one who is more able. This is because he is at a greater risk of harm, less able to know, to make known, or to defend what his free action would be. Therefore, nurses or other health care professionals act as the agent through whom patients are able to regain their power to exercise free choice. If she can strengthen and nurture her patients' freedom, she will help them to have a clear vision of what their long-term motivations and values are and what these demand of them in their present situation. She will help them achieve the endurance to take long-term actions toward the pursuit of their values.

Objectivity is the ability to know something and interact with it as it is in itself apart from one's preconceived ideas of it. It is a patient's need to achieve and sustain the exercise of his objective awareness. A patient who is able to contribute information about himself and understand the information given to him in light of available alternatives and his own uniqueness is less vulnerable than one who cannot. All actions that involve the pursuit of benefits and the avoidance of harm occur among the physical realities in which one acts. The loss of objective awareness is a radical form of vulnerability. It makes one vulnerable to the loss of the other virtues.

If the nurse can strengthen and nurture the objectivity of her patient, she will enable a patient to act appropriately on his autonomous and objective awareness of his circumstances. The strength of mind necessary to maintain objective awareness of facts outside of his mind and a stable awareness of items of knowledge that are relevant to his actions are necessary to his endurance and success.

Self-assertion is an agent's self-ownership, the power and right of an agent to control his time and effort, the right to initiate one's own actions. A patient who is able to control his time and effort is less vulnerable than a patient who must rely on others to do this for him. A nurse, as the agent of a patient, assists him in exercising and regaining his power of self-assertion.

Beneficence means competence in acting to acquire what is beneficial in accordance with one's desires and values, the ability to pursue benefits and avoid harms. A patient who is able to define benefit and harm for himself and according to his unique values is less vulnerable than one who cannot. A nurse must exert great care not to view benefit and harm for a patient according to her own idea of benefit and harm. The determination of benefit and harm is very individual. If she can strengthen and nurture his benefit seeking, she will help motivate her patient to retain his values and goals according to his long-term purposes. His courage to accept his own desires for himself, his pursuit of benefit, and his ability to avoid harm will be strengthened.

Fidelity denotes a nurse's commitment to her professional role and a patient's commitment to his life and values.[6] All that a patient endures when he suffers through his vulnerability can be summed up in the fact that he loses his integrity and his power to be faithful to himself and the values he has chosen for his life. A nurse can exert her virtues as codified in the bioethical standards to help a patient regain and/or exert his virtues in order to achieve an active future. If she can strengthen and nurture his fidelity to himself, she can help him to retain a clear understanding of himself in relation to his ambitions. This will assist him in being faithful to his life and flourishing.

JUSTIFIED ETHICAL ACTIVITY

No virtue a nurse can offer a patient is more productive to his life, health, and well-being than her knowledge of who she is both individually and as a health care professional. This is the virtue that enables her to feel and express empathy for her patient. It also is a virtue that enables her to intend to do good, to intend to benefit her patient.

A practice-based bioethic is an outline of the appropriate ways to interpret the health care professional–patient agreement. The bioethical standards, as preconditions of each and every agreement, are the standards of ethical decision making in the health care system. They are the virtues of a person. They are standards because they are the purpose that brings a person into the health care setting to regain or to strengthen his virtues. His agency is constituted by these virtues.

A nurse's standard or measure of ethical justification is the agency of her patient. According to this standard, failing to take action, or acting to frustrate a patient's rightful efforts, undercuts the ability of a nurse to objectively justify her actions. The standards of a patient's success in the health care system are the virtues he seeks to strengthen and regain. If he succeeds in this purpose, his interactions are successful. Insofar as a nurse assists him in this, nurse and patient are equally successful. Insofar as her actions are oriented to this goal, they are justifiable. A committed nurse, through observation and communication, can come to understand how these virtues are expressed (or fail to be expressed) in the actions of her patient. She can discover whether they function and how they function in motivating him. Her understanding can guide and justify her actions.

All of these virtues, by their presence or absence, form the unique character structures of a human individual. The human values that individuals pursue are made possible by these character structures exercised in successful action. They are themselves, human values. The social condition necessary to this pursuit is freedom from aggression. This necessary condition of the achievement of human values is the right of every human individual by virtue of the species wide and unspoken agreement that establishes individual rights. If a nurse maintains respect for her patient's rights, any action she takes will be justifiable.

To the extent that rights can be violated, nothing and no one is secure. Because there are no dependable intelligible sequences to interaction, foresight and predictability are illusory. Under these circumstances, a patient cannot function as a rational being, an individual who possesses purposes and rights. A patient will have a right to do, and to depend on, nothing. The professional will have a right, derived from coercion, to do anything to be unpredictable. To the extent that interactions are guided by unexpected agreements that are secured through deception or force, a patient's rights are violated. The recognition of a patient's rights is the only defense he has in the health care system.

CONCLUSION

When the role of a nurse is not set by a clear and logically comprehensive definition, any action or omission on her part will be allowable. This state of affairs is a violation of her profession. The professional cannot agree to act as the agent of a patient, if something within the profession itself prevents her from acting as the agent of her patient. To the extent that the definition and nature of her role are, actually or potentially, internally contradictory, no agreement is possible.

Rights are not routinely violated in the health care system. If this were the case there would be a revolt and a reformation of the system. When rights are violated, it is usually the rights of the most vulnerable, those who have no voice and cannot defend themselves against the self-righteous irrationality of health care professionals.

Two factors are necessary, and almost sufficient, for a nurse's justifiable ethical interactions: her unwavering recognition of a patient's rights and her unimpeachable adherence to the essence of her profession. In a health care setting that is governed by a practice-based ethic, some patients will be more vulnerable than others but not vulnerable in relation to a nurse. To a great extent, the degree of a patient's vulnerability is a function of a health care professional's character. Sometimes a patient will be completely vulnerable, but the right agreement holds by virtue of his nature and her nature, and ethically, his rights are absolutely invulnerable.

ENDNOTES

[1] "Appropriate" means according to the internal purposes of the setting.

[2] The pronouns she and her are used to designate the health care professional and he and him to designate the patient. This is, in part, for the reader's ease of understanding. More importantly, the singular is preferred to the plural or indeterminate because professionals and patients are individuals, and a practice-based ethic is, necessarily, an individualistic ethic.

[3] The word "patient" is derived from the Greek word *pathos* meaning experiences, suffering, or passivity. Other words with the same root are "pathos" itself (that in experience which evokes empathy or compassion), "pathetic" (evoking tenderness, pity, or sorrow), and "passive" (incapable of action).

[4] "Rights" is used in this chapter as a singular concept denoting an overarching agreement.

[5] "Autonomy" is not used here in its customary dictionary definition of independence. We use autonomy to denote the uniqueness of each individual person. The definition of "freedom" includes everything relevant to a person's independence.

[6] All definitions are taken from Husted & Husted, 2001, and are available from *www.nursing.duq.edu/faculty/husted/index.html.*

REFERENCES

Gastmans, C. (1998). Challenges to nursing values in a changing nursing environment. *Nursing Ethics, 5,* 236–245.

Hardt, M. (2001). Core then care: The nurse leader's role in "caring." *Nursing Administration Quarterly, 25*(3), 37–45.

Husted, G. L., & Husted, J. H. (2001). *Ethical decision making in nursing and health care: The symphonological approach* (3rd ed.). New York, NY: Springer.

McKeon, R. (Ed.). (1941). *The basic works of Aristotle.* New York, NY: Random House.

Oakeshott, M. (Ed.). (1957). *Leviathan.* Oxford: Basil Blackwell.

Leininger's Culture Care Theory: Utility with Vulnerable Populations

Rick Zoucha

In the ever-changing health care environment in the United States, many people have access to services that promote health and well-being and reduce the effects of illness. However, there are also people who are not afforded the same access to health care services as others based on the distinction of vulnerability. According to Campos-Outcalt et al. (1994), vulnerable populations can be defined as groups of people who experience physical disabilities, mental disabilities, cultural differences, geographic separation, and limited economic resources and, because of barriers, might be unable to integrate into the mainstream health services delivery system.

They (Campos-Outcalt et al., 1994) go on to say that "vulnerable populations include, but are not limited to, the urban poor (especially ethnic and racial minorities), Native Americans, rural poor, chronically disabled children and adults, frail elderly, and the homeless." Leininger contends that regardless of economic, political, and even genetic differences, everyone has a culture (Leininger, 1996). This chapter will discuss Leininger's culture care diversity and universality theory and the utility of the theory in working with populations made vulnerable by cultural differences in the research and practice settings.

LEININGER: THEORY OF CULTURE CARE DIVERSITY AND UNIVERSALITY

Leininger (2002) defines cultural care as the "subjectively and objectively learned and transmitted values, beliefs, and patterned lifeways that assist, support, facilitate, or enable another individual or group to maintain health and well-being, improve their human condition and lifeways, or deal with illnesses, handicaps, or death." Leininger (1996) describes culture as the learned values, beliefs, rules of behavior, and lifestyle practices of a particular group of people. Andrews & Boyle (2003) found culture to have four basic characteristics: it is learned, shared, dynamic, and able to adapt to specific conditions. Culture involves all types of behavior that are socially acquired and transmitted by means such as customs, techniques, beliefs, institutions, and material objects (Locke, 1999). According to Leininger (1991) and Andrews & Boyle (1999), humans exist within culture, and culture is viewed as a universal phenomenon. Leininger, in her work and writings, has taken the concepts of culture and an ethical orientation of caring and developed a theory appropriate for nursing practice, research, and education (Zoucha & Husted, 2000).

Leininger's (2002) theory of culture care diversity and universality is the product of over 50 years of research and development in which she studied over 60 cultures and identified

172 care constructs for use by nursing and other health care professionals. The Sunrise Model (Leininger, 2002) depicts Leininger's theory and presents seven cultural and social-structure dimensions: 1) technological, 2) religious and philosophical, 3) kinship and social, 4) political and legal, 5) economic, 6) educational, and 7) cultural values, beliefs, and lifeways (patterns of daily living). The theory describes the diverse health care systems, ranging from folk beliefs and practices to nursing and other health care professional systems used by people around the world. Leininger (1991) describes two systems of caring that exist in every culture she studied.

The first system of caring is generic and is considered the oldest form of caring or nurturing. Generic caring consists of culturally derived interpersonal practices and is considered essential for the health, growth, and survival of humans (Reynolds & Leininger, 1993). Generic caring is often referred to as folk practices and is defined culturally (Leininger, 1996). According to Leininger (1991), the second type of caring is therapeutic, which is cognitively learned, practiced, and transmitted through formal and informal professional education such as schools of nursing, medicine, and dentistry. Professional learning can and does include concepts and techniques to enhance professional practices, interpersonal communication techniques, and holistic aspects of care. Historically, professional care has not always included ideas about folk care because that aspect may not have been valued by nurses and other health care professionals (Leininger, 1995).

In her theory, Leininger (1991) contends that if professional and generic care practices do not fit together, this might affect client/patient recovery, health, and well-being and result in care that is not culturally congruent with the beliefs of the person, his or her family, or community. In order to provide culturally congruent care, Leininger (1995) asserts that professionals must link and synthesize generic and professional care knowledge to benefit the client. This link is a bridge, where a bridge is appropriate, between the professional and folk health care systems (Leininger, 1995).

According to the theory (Leininger, 2002), Leininger contends that there are three predictive modes of care derived from and based on the use of generic (emic) care knowledge and professional (etic) care knowledge obtained from research and experience with the use of the sunrise model. The three modes of action are 1) cultural care preservation/maintenance, 2) cultural care accommodation/negotiation, and 3) cultural care repatterning/restructuring.

Cultural care preservation/maintenance, according to Leininger (1995), refers to professional actions that are assistive, supportive, facilitative, or enabling and to decisions that help individuals, families, and communities from a particular culture retain and preserve care values so that they can maintain well-being, recover from illness, or face possible handicap or death.

Leininger (2002) describes cultural care accommodation/negotiation as creative professional actions that are assistive, facilitative, or enabling and potential decisions that can help individuals, families, and or communities in a particular culture adapt to or negotiate with others for the goal of obtaining satisfying health care outcomes with professional caregivers.

Cultural care repatterning/restructuring is described as the assistive, supportive, facilitative, and enabling actions taken by nurses and other health care professionals to promote actions and decisions that may help the person, family, and or community change or modify behaviors that affect their lifeways to create a new and different health pattern. This repatterning/restructuring (Leininger, 2002) is done while respecting the cultural values and beliefs of the individual, families, and communities while still providing and promoting a healthier lifeway than existed before the changes were co-established with the person, family, and or community. Leininger

(2002) asserts in her theory that the predicted three modes of action serve to guide judgments, decisions, and actions, culminating in the promotion of culturally congruent care.

Leininger (2002) describes culturally congruent care as beneficial, satisfying, and meaningful to the individuals, families, and communities served by nurses. Cultural imposition occurs when nurses and other health care professionals impose their beliefs, practices, and values on another culture because they believe their ideas are superior to those of the other person or group (Leininger, 1995). Leininger uses the concepts of cultural congruence and cultural imposition to focus on acceptable (caring) and unacceptable (noncaring) behavior by nurses in the practice, education, and research arenas.

UTILITY OF THE THEORY IN NURSING RESEARCH AND PRACTICE

In addition to the development of the theory of cultural care, Leininger (1995) developed a research method that is very useful in understanding the phenomenon of culture care for vulnerable populations. As described earlier, vulnerability includes culture differences. Leininger's qualitative ethnonursing research method was created to work in conjunction with her theory (Sunrise Model) and as a guide for research. The ethnonursing research method is described as "the study, documentation, and analysis of the local or emic people's viewpoints, beliefs, and practices about actual or potential nursing care phenomena within a particular culture to generate nursing knowledge." Leininger (2002) suggests the method be used in conjunction with research enablers such as 1) Leininger's observation-participation-reflection enabler, 2) Leininger's stranger-to-trusted-friend enabler, 3) the Sunrise Model enabler, 4) the specific domain of inquiry enabler, and 5) Leininger's acculturation enabler.

The enabler guides can also be used in the clinical setting in an attempt to move the nurse's status in her relationship with her client from that of stranger to that of trusted friend. The notion of being viewed as a friend can promote culturally congruent care in many cultures (Zoucha & Reeves, 1999). This friendlike or personal relationship between the nurse and her client/patient can decrease the cultural difference vulnerability of the person because the culture care needs of the client are known to the nurse. The nurse is then able to promote care that is congruent with the person's culture and promote the health and well-being needs of the person, family, and community.

The connection between the theory and the areas of research and practice is addressed with the use of the identified enablers to promote a deeper understanding of the cultural phenomena of interest regardless of the context (research or clinical practice). This allows for a holistic and comprehensive view of the domain of inquiry and the particular culture being studied. As transcultural nurse researchers and clinicians seek to understand the phenomena of interest for vulnerable populations it is possible to decrease one aspect of vulnerability, that described as cultural differences. If indeed transcultural nurses use the findings of studies in actual clinical practice, then an understanding of the person, family, and community can be viewed from a culture care perspective, thereby increasing the understanding of cultural care needs and exposing the vulnerability that is related to being culturally different.

The problem of personal, family, and community vulnerability with regard to cultural differences is that if nurses pursue an understanding of culture in relation to health and well-being, then there is an ethical motivation to promote care that is culturally congruent. This motivation can possibly decrease the vulnerability for the individual, family, and community. Zoucha &

Husted (2000) contend that cultural caring should consider the person, family, and community in the context of their culture, resulting in the promotion of ethical and culturally congruent care. In agreement with Leininger's theory, Zoucha & Husted (2000) have stated that it is the ethical responsibility and duty of the nurse to promote, provide, and encourage care that is culturally based and congruent with the values, beliefs, and traditions of the individual, family, and community.

Leininger's theory does provide a holistic and emic view of factors that describe culture and those cultural values and beliefs that are meaningful to individuals, families, and communities. However, a critique of Leininger's theory and Sunrise Model reveals that it does not explicitly state, in the context of the Sunrise Model or theory, the related factors of racism, poverty, and history of oppression that commonly affect people other than those in the dominant culture of the United States. Leininger does consider these issues in her writing and presentations but not in the actual explanation of her theory and Sunrise Model in relationship to research and clinical practice. Adding the factors of racism, poverty, and history of oppression to the Sunrise Model as part of the experience for people of different cultures (other than the dominant culture) may assist nurses and other health care professionals in understanding the meaning of vulnerability. Through the use of the theory, nurses and other health care professionals can promote health and well-being while decreasing the experience of vulnerability.

CONCLUSION

Individuals, families, and communities that are identified as vulnerable because of cultural differences can be understood in a manner that seeks to expose that vulnerability and focus on the culture care needs. Leininger's theory of culture care diversity and universality promotes a deep and clear understanding of the individual, family, and community from a unique cultural perspective. Use of the theory and the identified enablers for research and clinical practice allows for the nurse to view the individual, family, and community from the perspective of the seven cultural factors identified in the Sunrise Model: religion, kinship, technology, educational, economic, political and legal, and cultural lifeways. By using this view, nurses and other health care professionals can decrease the vulnerability of the individual, family, and community by uncovering the concern of cultural difference and promoting ethical practice that is congruent with the cultural beliefs of those in the caring relationship with nurses and other health care professionals.

REFERENCES

Andrews, M. M., & Boyle, J. S. (1999). *Transcultural concepts in nursing care*. Philadelphia, PA: Lippincott.

Andrews, M. M., & Boyle, J. S. (2003). *Transcultural concepts in nursing care* (2nd ed.). Philadelphia, PA: Lippincott Williams & Wilkins.

Campos-Outcalt, D., Fernandez, R., Hollow, W., Lundeen, S., Nelson, K., Schuster, B. et al. (1994). Providing quality health care to vulnerable populations. Society of Primary Care Policy Fellows. Retrieved on January 10, 2004, from *http://www.primarycaresociety.org/1994d.htm.*

Leininger, M. (1996). Culture care theory, research, and practice. *Nursing Science Quarterly, 9*(2), 71–78.

Leininger, M. M. (1991). *Culture care diversity and universality: A theory of nursing*. New York, NY: National League for Nursing [NLN].

Leininger, M. M. (1991). *The theory of culture care diversity and universality.* New York, NY: NLN. (Publication No. 15-2402, pp. 5–68).

Leininger, M. M. (1995). *Transcultural nursing: Concepts, theories, research and practice.* New York, NY: McGraw-Hill.

Leininger, M. M., (2002) Culture care theory: A major contribution to advance transcultural nursing knowledge and practices. *Journal of Transcultural Nursing, 13,* 189–192.

Leininger, M. M., & McFarland, M. R. (2002). *Transcultural nursing: Concepts, theories, research and practice* (2nd ed.). New York, NY: McGraw-Hill.

Locke, D. C. (1999). *Increasing multicultural understanding: A comprehensive model.* Newbury Park, CA: Sage.

Reynolds, C. L., & Leininger, M. M. (1993). *Madeline Leininger, culture care diversity and universality theory.* Newbury Park, CA: Sage.

Zoucha, R. D., & Reeves, J. (1999). A view of professional caring as personal for Mexican Americans. *International Journal for Human Caring, 3*(3), 14–20

Zoucha, R. D., & Husted, G. L., (2000). The ethical dimensions of delivering culturally congruent nursing and health care. *Issues in Mental Health Nursing, 21,* 325–340.

CHAPTER 9

Care Giving Beliefs of Parents
of Children with Cancer: Taiwan

Hwey-Fang Liang

Although advanced treatments have increased survival rates, childhood cancer is still a traumatic reality that exists in many Taiwanese families. For children between the ages of 1 and 14 years, cancer is the second leading cause of death (Department of Health, Taiwan, 2002). Approximately 500 to 600 children are diagnosed with cancer each year; approximately 8428 Taiwanese children have been diagnosed with cancer (Childhood Cancer Foundation, R.O.C., 2001).

These children experience countless painful treatments and side effects such as pain, nausea, vomiting, mucosities, anorexia, and weight loss during their illness. Aggressive and lengthy treatments such as chemotherapy, radiation therapy, and surgery, combined with examinations such as blood and bone marrow tests, cause suffering and exhaustion. The diagnosis, treatment, side effects, and examinations affect the child and caregivers both physically and psychologically (Alcoser & Rodgers, 2003), and most caregivers of children with cancer are their parents (Liang, 2002). These parent caregivers are vulnerable because they experience great physical and mental suffering along with their beloved ill children.

Health care and care giving practices are affected by culture. Culture is the learned and shared beliefs, values, and lifeways of a particular group that influence thinking and actions (Leininger, 1995). Parents' beliefs about care giving for children with cancer may affect their care giving behavior. Because of parental decisions to stop treatment for their children, 2.5 % of childhood cancer patients fail to conclude their treatment protocol (Yeh, Lin, Tsai, Lai, & Ku, 1999). Although existing research has shown that Taiwanese caregivers use multiple care practices to provide for their children with cancer (Liang, 2002), it also shows shortcomings in terms of beliefs about care giving, especially within the vulnerable population of parents who are the primary caregivers for their ill children. Therefore, this study reconsidered the beliefs about family care giving among this vulnerable population. The purpose of the research was to learn about the beliefs of Taiwanese parents regarding care giving for children with cancer, applying the ethnographic method.

REVIEW OF LITERATURE

The literature displays an ethnohistory of the Taiwanese that indicates their culture. Named "Formosa" by Portuguese explorers who sailed its waters in 1517 and noted its beauty, Taiwan is an island in the Taiwan Strait in the western Pacific Ocean between the East and South China seas (Unger, 1999). Taiwanese communities do not have a homogeneous population. The population consists mainly of Taiwanese, aborigines, and those of mixed descent, as well as mainlanders from China (Lin, 1993). The largest populations of aborigines, commonly called Taiwanese in the sense of native Taiwanese, are the offspring of the initial immigrants from the provinces of Fukien and Kwangtung in mainland China. In particular, the Hokkien province has the greatest number of immigrants from southern Fukien that speak Min-Nan Hwa, which is the Taiwanese dialect. The Mandarin-speaking Nationalist followers who came to Taiwan from all parts of mainland China in the late 1940s are the most recent additions to Taiwan's population. These people account for about 15% of the population; as a result, Mandarin has become the official and principal language in Taiwan (Taiwan, 1998).

Although many religions have been brought to Taiwan from throughout the world, Taoism and Buddhism are the major religions and prime means of worship. Confucianism influences ethics, morality, and academic thinking enormously for the Chinese people of Taiwan. Supernatural beings such as the spirits of natural objects, ascendants and idolized heroes, and ghosts also inform Taiwanese beliefs (Lin, 1993). The family is the most important organizational unit in Taiwanese society. The family is parent–child dominated, as opposed to the Western family, which is husband–wife dominated. Therefore, Taiwanese parents are almost always available to the growing child (Martinson, Liu-Chiang, & Liang, 1997).

In Taiwan, the primary caregivers for children are their families. Therefore, the participation of the family in caring for the ill child is very common. The mother is the primary caregiver in 52% of families and the father in 19%; in 23% of families, care is shared by both parents (Martinson et al., 1999). Caregivers or families not only participate in caring for ill children, but in many cases also act as the decision makers regarding termination or alteration of treatment. Often these decisions are not discussed with health care professionals, even though the Taiwan Pediatric Oncology Group (TPOG), a team uniting oncology health care providers, recommends and provides biomedicine (chemotherapy, radiology, and surgery) to help children with cancer. Multiple care practices that include Western and folk care practices have commonly been used by family caregivers (Liang, 2002; Liang & Lo, 1999; Yeh et al., 1999; Yeh et al., 2000).

Caring for children with cancer is a lengthy, exhausting, heartrending experience (Davies et al., 1998). Liang (2002) conducted ethnonursing research and found that caregivers promote and expect a care practice of unconditional giving that uses all available cultural knowledge to promote the best and most appropriate methods of health care. This philosophy is influenced by the cultural context of the caregivers. The care beliefs, values, worldviews, social structure factors, environmental contexts, and health care systems of caregivers all influence care giving methods. They need to be closely examined over time in order to understand their influences on human caring, well-being, and issues of health or illness surrounding childhood cancer. This knowledge must then be applied to practical care situations (Leininger, 1991).

METHODOLOGY

Ethnographic methodology (Leininger, 1985; Spradley, 1980) aided in discovering the beliefs about care giving held by the vulnerable population of Taiwanese parents whose children have cancer and by parents who have significantly concerned themselves with their children's health care behaviors and practices. This approach provided an in-depth understanding of research participants' ideas and a means to obtain and access parents' beliefs and care giving practices through a cultural point of view.

Key informants are the most knowledgeable persons about a topic and indicate the values, beliefs, and lifeways of the culture and domain of inquiry; moreover, they are interested and willing to participate in the study (Leininger, 1997). **General informants** commonly do not possess complete knowledge about the domain of inquiry; however, they have broad and general ideas about the domain and are willing to share their knowledge and ideas (Leininger, 1997). Key informants in this study were parents serving as the primary caregivers for their children with cancer who shared specific knowledge pertaining to care giving and beliefs about care giving. They were interviewed in-depth two or three times, each time for 1–2 hours. General informants were interviewed once for 45 to 60 minutes to obtain broad, general reflections about the domain.

As a purposive sample from the vulnerable population parent caregivers the key informants consisted of 15 parents (11 mothers and 4 fathers) of children with cancer, identified as primary caregivers. These informants took care of their children with cancer most of the time, maintained great accountability, and held significant decision-making responsibilities for their children's health. General informants, who numbered 25 and included 18 mothers and 7 fathers, also participated in this study. All informants ranged in age from 27 to 48 years of age and had an educational background ranging from junior high school through college. The religions represented were Buddhism, Taoism, and a combination of the two.

The study's 31 children with cancer ranged in age from 3 to 12 years and had been diagnosed with leukemia, lymphoma, or solid tumors between 1 and 32 months earlier. Two of them were relapse cases. All of them had undergone biomedical treatment protocols in the medical center. The informants, both key and general informants, were enrolled from a pediatric oncology parents club in a medical center located in the central region of Taiwan. All of the informants' children were in the process of oncology treatment during the study. Most of the treatments were suggested by pediatric oncology physicians of the TPOG, which mainly provides Western professional care such as chemotherapy and radiation. In accordance with university research ethics, and with permission from the director of the nursing department at the medical center, the author-researcher was able to conduct the interviews at the pediatric unit in their respective areas for a private and quiet environment. Second or third interviews, if needed, were also conducted in this location.

Instruments used to collect data for this study were the semistructured open inquiry interview guide and the stranger-to-trusted-friend (STF) enabler (Leininger, 1997). The STF enabler assisted the researcher in moving from the position of distrusted researcher to trusted friend in order to gain the parent caregivers' insights regarding their beliefs about care giving practices and the influences of culture on care giving. The enabler applied even if the researcher had previous experiences with children with cancer and spoke the same language. The researcher's transition from stranger to trusted friend was vital to obtaining tape-recorded interviews that possess true, honest, and in-depth data from informants in an initially unfamiliar situation (Leininger, 1997).

Data analysis occurred simultaneously with data collection. Taped interviews were transcribed verbatim. Participation observation was conducted at the pediatric unit in the medical center while the children were hospitalized. Participation observations were written as field notes and then transcribed. All of the data and information from interviews, participation observation, and field notes were coded by the process of examination and comparison with other pieces of data. Domain analysis based on the semantic relationship of the cultural scene assisted in the investigation of a symbolic category consisting of other categories and subcategories

(Spradley, 1980). Taxonomic analysis explored the internal structure of the domain, providing more in-depth analysis. "Componential analysis is the systematic search for the attributes associated with cultural categories" (Spradley, 1980, p. 131). It uses similarities and differences to investigate for contrast, then sorts them out and groups them (Speziale, 2003). Theme analysis determines associations among domains. It is a process used to uncover cultural themes that arise from recurrent patterns. Criteria for the process of systematic analysis include credibility, transferability, dependability, and conformability (Lincoln & Guba, 1985).

FINDINGS

Systematic analysis of the information collected from the vulnerable informants included identification of descriptors, patterns, and, eventually, major themes. Themes that emerged from the data explained the issues surrounding Taiwanese parents' beliefs about care giving for children with cancer. The themes are interpreted below with some verbatim quotes that demonstrate the findings. These themes and patterns emerged from the similarities and differences among these informants.

Theme 1

Theme 1 is integrating supports to assist in the child's fulfillment of his or her treatment protocol. All informants, including key and general informants, concurred in believing that Western care practice, such as a treatment protocol including chemotherapy, radiation, and surgery, could kill or remove evil cells. Also, it is popular to see Western health clinics or hospitals in the environment of context, such as communities in Taiwan. Parents believed the treatment protocols were based on scientific evidence. They trusted Western care practice protocol as well as physicians who were educated with a Western orientation.

Two patterns were abstracted to higher levels of analysis to develop this theme. They are capturing and trusting *guei-zen* (people who can help the children significantly, such as physicians and nurses) and recruiting relatives or friends to maintain the functions of the family. Specific verbatim quotes from the data included, "looking for and capturing *guei-zen* for my child to deal with illness, especially physicians who can make precise diagnoses and treatments and nurses who can give appropriate care and more patience to take care of my child. All of them were my child's *guei-zen*." Another informant said, "My husband has to work, I have to take care of this child. So I asked my mother come to my house to watch the other child. She's only three. So I can accompany with my daughter to do chemotherapy [Sic]."

Friends are other important people who can help. Parents' friends include elder generations, colleagues, or other parents whose children have the same illness and can provide information about the treatment protocol to predict and improve care. Friends can also provide mental support and spiritual comforts for parents during their child's hospitalization.

Theme 2

Parent caregivers believe Western care is effective in treating their children's illnesses. However, side effects and intrusive examinations and treatments are painful and can weaken the child's body. Therefore, parents try to complement the weaknesses of the protocol. Most parents agree to let their children receive folk care, especially food therapy and concoctions of common

Chinese herbs. Two patterns led to the abstract theme: using traditional Chinese medicine to complement the body's deficiencies and using characteristics of food to bolster the body's health. This theme was described by key informants as well as general informants.

"Every time after he took 6MP, his body broke down—nausea, vomiting, bad appetite, does not eat . . . very, very weak. So my mother cooked some herbs with fish and let him drink the broth. And she made juice from organic vegetables and wheat grass. All of that we hoped could reinforce his *yuan-chi* [strength] and nourish his physical strength."

"I cooked chicken with some ordinary traditional Chinese medicine and *s-sen tan* for her to increase her white blood count and complement her *yuan-chi,* even though she seemed not to like that. I also cooked *tang-kuei, huang-chi* [common Chinese herbs] with water to let her drink daily to supplement her physical strength and blood count."

Theme 3

Parents assume many roles in order to help the child. Most Taiwanese parents devote themselves to their ill child. The child is the parents' responsibility for their entire lives. Parents are happy when their child is happy, healthy, and performs well academically. Parents feel sad when a child has poor health. Specific patterns associated with this theme included parents' playing multiple roles for the child. They might change values and attitudes of care giving when they believe it beneficial to the child's health. Most of these parents stated that their daily lives, world views, and values had changed significantly after their child was diagnosed with cancer. They believed that they should stand with their child to conquer the cancer. However, they also described ordinary family affairs that they needed to attend to, such as providing food and supporting the child's health care. They had to play multiple roles to take care of their children in illness and in health, such as doctor, nurse, teacher, friend, guardian, consultant to the health care provider, supervisor, and spouse's inspiration.

Doctor, Nurse, Teacher, Friend, Guardian

Although they support their children's Western treatment protocols, sometimes parents have to be sensitive to their children's reactions and, especially, side effects. One mother said, "I play the roles of doctor and nurse to be very attentive to my child's responses to treatments such as chemotherapy. When he feels better, then I need to act like his teacher to teach him, or like a friend to talk and listen to him." They also act as guardians to protect their children from suffering.

Consultant to Health Care Provider and Supervisor

Parents agreed that most health care providers take good care of their children. However, they still worried that something could happen unexpectedly. They were the people whom the children most trusted and relied on. If parents were busy, they always left at least one or two relatives close to the child who could be consulted by health care providers if necessary. While the child was in the hospital, they acted as supervisors of the work done by the health care providers. As one informant said, "Nurses have to take care of several patients every day. I worry that they might give the wrong medicine to my child. Therefore, I have to be very careful to double check the medicine that they gave my child."

Coordinator and Inspiration for Spouse

Most parents have to change their roles to take care of their ill child. Some of them arrange for relatives, such as sisters and parents, to take care of the other healthy children at home, bring special food for the ill child, or come to the hospital to take care of the child. They have to work as a coordinator to manage time and help for the family and the health care providers. They also cheer up the ill child and the other family members. Parents sometimes have conflicts about their child's health problems. However, they have to support and inspire each other. One father said that "whether husband or wife, they need to work together to inspire and cheer up their families."

Theme 4

Theme 4 involves releasing uncertainties to heaven. Parents understand that even though they provide scientific Western care for their child and catch *guei-zen* to help their children, uncertainties remain. *Guei-zen*'s advanced treatments still may not work well. Therefore, they release all uncertain situations to heaven.

Two recurrent patterns emerged from the data of informants. The first one was negotiating with heaven. Parents or the parents' kin entreat heaven, including their religion's gods, ancestors, and ghosts, to protect their children. Sometimes, some of them worship more sincerely than before. Some of them ask ancestors, ghosts, or gods to change *phone-shui* (known more commonly in the West as *feng shui*), which means the environment of their house, such as the directions of doors, windows, and beds, and even the directions and environment of their ancestor's gravesites. The child's name might also be changed by *ton-gi* (people who can talk and listen to the ghosts) because parents believe the new name from the god could help to protect the child from the devil. Some parents even change their relationship with their child orally, for example, calling the father uncle and calling the mother aunty, or they let the god adopt the child directly so the god can help the child fight the illness. Another method is to change eating habits from a meat diet to a vegetarian diet. "My girl's illness was my fault because of the result of sin, so I couldn't eat meat anymore. I changed to a vegetarian food style." All of these changes were means of negotiating with gods and ghosts.

Another pattern was depending on the child's fate. These parent caregivers do everything they ought to do and leave the rest to fate. One informant said, "I know the doctors and nurses here do everything for my child, and I understand the advanced scientific medicine could help my child, but I know there is something that even the doctor can't control and be sure of. The unsure thing only could depend on the opinion of heaven's opinion. That is my child's fate."

DISCUSSION

The beliefs about care giving that flowed from the data are a fusion of four themes that explain beliefs about care giving among the vulnerable population of Taiwanese parents of children with cancer. Three of these deal with how parent caregivers believe that it is essential to have support from people, including *guei-zen,* friends, and parents themselves, to deal with the child's illness. Beyond this they release uncertain situations, such as the unknown process of a child's illness, old age, sickness, and death, to heaven, and this is the fourth theme. Heaven includes spiritual things that people cannot handle or control. They do everything within their control to negotiate with so-called *guei-zen* and leave the rest to fate. These beliefs about combining people and the great heaven together are methods of providing care giving for children with cancer.

The fact that parents use the efforts of other people to provide advanced treatments for the child (Western medicine), then use non-Western care such as folk care, including traditional Chinese medicine and food function, to make up for the weaknesses of that treatment, reveals a belief about care giving that advanced Western treatment cannot assure a cure for the child's illness. Parents still need to search for other means of care to overcome the shortcomings of Western treatment, even though they provide it without the knowledge of health care providers. Because health care providers were educated in Western-oriented medicine, parents rarely discuss folk care with them publicly. This finding is similar to those of previous studies about using folk or other alternative care for children with cancer (Liang, 2002; Yeh et al., 2000).

Another of the themes involving people, as opposed to heaven, is assuming that many caregivers work hard for the child because they believe this is their responsibility. This is similar to Liang's (2002) study that found that unconditional giving is one of the major themes for Taiwanese caregivers in providing care practices for children with cancer. Even though the participants were different, the concept of unconditional giving was the same.

Conclusions and Recommendations

This study gathered information regarding the beliefs of Taiwanese parents about care giving for children with cancer. Care giving beliefs have powerful meaning and provide direction to care giving practices. Findings from this study support previous work signifying that folk care is an important component of health care for childhood cancer. Parents especially believe in the food function. Health care providers need to understand the value that folk care plays in the care giving beliefs of parents. Health care providers' recognition of and respect for these ideas about integrating *guei-zen* and heaven may earn the parents' trust and help promote culturally sensitive care for parent caregivers. Understanding the love and support associated with families, kinship, and participation in the care giving is essential for the provision of meaningful nursing care. Furthermore, supporting parents as they fill multiple roles for assisting their children or providing a plan to alleviate some of their burden is crucial.

Implications for Nursing

The results of this study afford nurses and other health care providers a culturally sensitive theorem for comprehending beliefs and care giving behaviors of Taiwanese parent caregivers. In professional nursing practice, the participation of families and kinship ties during the child's hospitalization are encouraged and supported. The importance of the social context of care practice for parents of children with cancer has to be identified. Because beliefs about care giving include a combination of Western and folk care practices, *guei-zen,* and heaven, it is essential to integrate scientific, religious, and folk care knowledge into practices to improve competent care for children with cancer and their parent caregivers. In nursing education, knowledge and practices of diverse folk care regarding childhood cancer need to be learned and understood in order that adequate knowledge and advice can be provided to caregivers. Further research needs to probe more deeply into knowledge and experiences regarding care giving after the child has been discharged from the hospital. This will help to promote culturally appropriate health care for children with cancer and their parents within communities.

REFERENCES

Alcoser, P. W., & Rodgers, C. (2003). Treatment strategies in childhood cancer. *Journal of Pediatric Nursing, 18*(2), 103–112.

Childhood Cancer Foundation of R. O. C. (2001, December). *Distribution of childhood cancer in Taiwan.* Retrieved November 10, 2003, from *http://ccf.wingnet.com.tw/people.htm.*

Davies, B., Deveau, E., deVeber, B., Howell, D., Martinson, I., Papadatou, D., et al. (1998). Experiences of mothers in five countries whose child died of cancer. *Cancer Nursing, 21,* 301–311.

Department of Health, Executive Yuan, Taiwan, R. O. C. (2002). *Cause-of-death statistics. Health and national health insurance annual statistics information service.* Retrieved November 9, 2003, from *http://www.doh.gov.tw/statistic/index.htm.*

Leininger, M. (1985). *Qualitative research methods in nursing.* Orlando, FL: Grune & Stratton.

Leininger, M. (1991). *Culture care diversity and universality: A theory of nursing.* New York, NY: National League for Nursing [NLN].

Leininger, M. (1995). *Transcultural nursing: Concepts, theories, research and practices* (2nd ed.). New York, NY: McGraw-Hill.

Leininger, M. (1997). Overview of the theory of culture care with the ethnonursing research method. *Journal of Transcultural Nursing, 8*(2), 32–52.

Liang, H. F. (2002). Understanding culture care practices of caregivers of children with cancer in Taiwan. *Journal of Pediatric Oncology Nursing, 19*(6), 205–217.

Liang, H. F., & Lo, L. H. (1999). From the perspectives of transcultural nursing to view the stressors and coping behaviors of a mother with a cerebral palsy and leukemia girl. *Nursing Image, 9*(4), 10–20 [in Chinese].

Lin, S. S. (1993). *Illness, body and personhood: An anthropological study of women's lives in Taiwan.* Unpublished doctoral dissertation, State University of New York at Buffalo.

Lincoln, Y. S., & Guba, E. G. (1985). *Naturalistic inquiry.* Beverly Hills, CA: Sage.

Martinson, I. M., Leavitt, M., Liu, C. Y., Armstrong, V., Hornberger, L., Zhang, J. Q., & Han, X. P. (1999). Comparison of Chinese and Caucasian families care giving to children with cancer at home: Part I. *Journal of Pediatric Nursing, 14*(2), 99–109.

Martinson, I. M., Liu-Chiang, C. Y., & Liang, Y. H. (1997). Distress symptoms and support systems of Chinese parents of children with cancer. *Cancer Nursing, 20*(2), 94–99.

Speziale, H. J. S. (2003). Ethnography as method. In H. J. S. Speziale & D. R. Carpenter (Eds.). *Qualitative research in nursing: Advancing the humanistic imperative* (3rd ed., pp. 153–180). Philadelphia, PA: Lippincott.

Spradley, J. P. (1980). *Participant observation.* Orlando, FL: Holt, Rinehart & Winston.

Taiwan (1998). In *The new Encyclopaedia Britannica* (Vol. 28, pp. 375–382). Chicago, IL: Encyclopaedia Britannica.

Unger, L. (1999). Taiwan. In *The Encyclopedia Americana* (Vol. 26, pp. 232–238). Danbury, CT: Grolier.

Yeh, C. H., Lin, C. F., Tsai, J. L., Lai, Y. M., & Ku, H. C. (1999). Determinants of parental decisions on "drop out" from cancer treatment for childhood cancer patients. *Journal of Advanced Nursing, 30*(1), 193–199.

Yeh, C. H., Tsai, J. L., Li, W., Chen, H. M., Lee, S. C., Lin, C. F., & Yang, C. P. (2000). Use of alternative therapy among pediatric oncology patients in Taiwan. *Pediatric Hematology and Oncology, 17*(1), 55–65.

C H A P T E R 1 0

Applying Leininger's Culture Care Theory: The Oromo of Seattle

Keesha Morris

To be vulnerable is to be at risk for harm. Harm can take the form of acts of omission or commission by a community, group, or individual. When evaluating the vulnerability of the Oromo people in the United States, there are fundamental precepts that must be taken into account. These are not just factors linked to the Oromo culture but also to the different life experiences that have shaped each individual immigrant or refugee that has arrived on US soil. Madeleine Leininger's theory of transcultural nursing offers a framework for studying this East African population in the form of her Sunrise Model (Leininger, 2001). Chapter 8 of this text, "Leininger's Culture Care Theory: Utility with Vulnerable Populations," was a presentation of the theory. The focus of this chapter is to apply the theory to a specific vulnerable population, the Oromo. Included in this assessment of vulnerability will be a nursing perspective of risk for altered health, along with possible solutions that have been, are being, or need to be implemented.

THE OROMO

Religious and Philosophical Factors

Most of Seattle's Oromo population is located in south Seattle in the communities of Rainier Vista and Holly Park. The total population is thought to be 10,000 or more refugees and immigrants. Some families have also settled in Ballard, West Seattle, Kent, Redmond, and Bellevue (EthnoMed, 2001). In Oromia, located in the horn of Africa (Ethiopia), the population numbers 28 million. Oromians are the third largest nationality in Africa and the single largest nationality in East Africa (Horus, 1995). There are three main religions in Oromia: the traditional Oromo religion, Islam, and Christianity. The traditional belief system advocates one God, or Waaqayoo. Approximately half of the country is Muslim and the other half Christian. Most sources state that a large percentage of practicing Muslims and Christians also practice the traditional Oromo religion (Melbaa, 1998). Most of the Oromo residents at Rainier Vista practice Islam.

Many of the adolescents find it difficult to follow the mandates of their most sacred holiday, Ramadan, which requires the faithful to fast during the daylight hours for an entire month. One of the 13-year-old Oromian residents of Rainier Vista has observed that it is more difficult to follow the precepts of his religion in a country that must separate church and state. "When you're in this country, there are a lot of distractions to Ramadan (eg. cars, making money)." However, some of the teachers in the schools that teach Oromian and other Muslim children are making efforts to accommodate their need to pray five times a day during Ramadan.

"At 1 pm, the time for the midday prayer for devout Muslims, one of the teachers stays in her room with Muslim students so they can pray" (MacDonald, 1999). Other schools allow Muslim girls to attend physical education classes in modest dress and head scarves. The Muslim teens at Seattle's Nathan Hale High School were allowed to start a weekly prayer group on Fridays because they could not arrange transportation to the local Mosque (MacDonald, 1999). These accommodations are scattered throughout different school systems, without any kind of standardization or uniformity. After September 11, 2001, many Muslim Oromians began to fear they would be blamed for the terrorist attacks (Eskenazi, 2001).

Any culturally sensitive actions taken by the community to promote religious freedom will help decrease the vulnerability of the Muslim, Christian, and traditional Oromians. This may be more difficult for the traditional Oromians, who need to sacrifice an animal occasionally for the spirits of deceased ancestors.

Kinship and Social Factors

In Oromo society, members of extended families typically live in the same household. Marriages in rural areas are still prearranged, and girls are eligible to marry at the age of 15. Children are considered full members of the family and the community and are permitted to participate in family discussions that are age appropriate. Children are taught specific tasks. Boys learn to ride horses and throw spears, and girls learn to cook and tend cattle. (EthnoMed, 2001). Girls are expected to be virgins until marriage, and both males and females are circumcised (known in the West as female genital mutilation). A study conducted by Missailidis & Gebre-Medhin (2000) found that women would abandon female genital mutilation if it were not expected by men. The practice is in place to prevent female sexual promiscuity.

The Seattle Oromo community has expressed concern about their children surviving adolescence in the United States without getting involved in violence or drugs. For families from rural Oromia, teenage dating is a new experience because prearranged marriages are the norm. Children are usually disciplined verbally for bad behavior, along with an occasional spanking. An Oromian woman who works for the Refugee Women's Alliance (REWA) reports that the women of Rainier Vista are afraid of Child Protective Services, which renders them unsure of how to manage their children's behavior and teach them respect. Parenting classes offered at the monthly REWA meeting might alleviate some of this anxiety. Two other vulnerability issues she has observed in the Oromo women's community are a lack of health care utilization and depression. Oromo women do not believe in prenatal care. Typically, the Oromo people only seek medical care when they feel sick. If they do go to the doctor, they want a pill to take to make them feel better.

Kibour (2001) found that "during cultural acclimation, psychological disorders, stress, identity diffusion, and identity crisis are most likely experienced by persons who have acculturated in two or more groups" (p. 50). In other words, Oromian immigrants are more vulnerable to depression if they do not get involved in their own racial and cultural group. He also correlated higher levels of education and stable immigration status (the possession of a green card) with lower levels of depression. The Seattle Oromo community has established many outreach and support groups for every age; most hold weekly activities or meetings.

Technological Factors

The high-tech medical approach to childbirth scares the Oromo women of Seattle. They do not understand the need for fetal monitoring and anesthesia. They believe that American doctors "are too quick to perform Cesarean sections for what the women consider normal variations, such as post-term gestational age" (EthnoMed, 2001). This causes them to wait at home until they are in advanced stages of labor before seeking medical attention. This also increases the risk for harm (vulnerability) to the baby and mother during emergency deliveries in inopportune places. In addition, Oromo women are averse to using the technology available to working mothers to pump and store breast milk. Breastfeeding is the traditional method of birth control in the Oromo culture. In the United States, women are returning to work and shortening the traditional 3-year span of breastfeeding, which is contributing to a high fertility rate in Seattle's Oromo community; thereby increasing vulnerability. There are no religious ramifications to contraception. Education in this area for the women by female health care providers would be beneficial. Oromian people like to be given a pill to make them feel better. It is possible oral contraceptives would be effective. Female midwives might also be the answer to the lack of prenatal care. A decrease in technology for childbirth would be seen as an asset in this community.

Educational and Economic Factors

Oromo households in the Seattle area include extended families of up to eight people, nearly half being children under age 10 years. Most of the community members came from rural areas and have had little formal education. Those who came from urban areas are educated and had worked in Ethiopia as health professionals, engineers, teachers, and social workers. Unemployment and underemployment are leading problems for many heads of household (EthnoMed, 2001).

In studying the psychological well-being of Oromian refugees in the United States, McSpadden (1987) found that education played an important role in how well refugees made the transition. Due to the war-torn conditions present in Ethiopia, many Oromians had their education interrupted. An example of a disrupted education is the son of a lawyer, resettled by an agency, who has only a 7th grade education or the son of a large landowner, resettled by a congregation, who left school in the 10th grade to go live in the countryside to escape apprehension by the government (p. 803).

This has far-reaching implications for refugees' perception of self, social status, and expectations. Oromians, who were members of a higher social class in Oromia, find themselves downwardly mobile in the United States in spite of the high expectations they have for themselves. McSpadden (1987) also found that refugees who depend on public welfare or are doing jobs they deem to have no future, rate these factors as the number one contributors to an unhappy life. "Many refugees intertwined going to school or college with getting a job, especially a job of high status" (p. 810). Refugees that were unemployed had strikingly higher levels of stress than those who were employed. In addition, refugees who are resettled by congregational volunteers are more likely to find employment and have opportunities for further education and support than those settled by agencies and caseworkers (p. 812). McSpadden (1987) also reports that in no case have Oromian refugees found their first job without the assistance of an outside source. More private agencies may take the pressure off the overburdened government caseworkers.

Another element that can be evaluated under the education factor is that of language. A refugee's command of the English language has direct impact on employment opportunities and the amount of psychological stress involved in the resettlement process. McSpadden (1987) found that Oromians who had some proficiency with the English language were well educated or had not had their education interrupted in their homeland. In order to decrease vulnerability, English as a second language (ESL) and bilingual programs are imperative for Oromian refugees. Although many school systems have ESL classes for students, there is a shortage of teachers in Washington who are qualified to teach bilingual programs. "Research indicates that students need instruction in both their primary languages and in English in order to best succeed" (Denn, 2001). Using the village model of "helping people to help themselves," assistance could be given to those refugees who have been teachers in Africa to become teachers in the United States. Incentives could include decreased or free tuition for those that wish to work toward giving back to their community, similar to the program already established through the National Health Service Corps.

Political Factors

Oromians structure their government around a democratic system they call the Gada system. "This system organizes Oromo society into groups or sets that assume different responsibilities in society every eight years" (EthnoMed, 1996, p. 1). During the 20th century, Oromo was colonialized by Ethiopia, causing the Oromian citizens to endure political, social, and cultural suppression. However, most Oromians continue to think of themselves as Oromian rather than Ethiopian. The Oromo Liberation Front (OLF) continues to wage a rebellion against the Ethiopians in Africa. The OLF receives financial and public support from many of the Oromian refugees in the United States. In Seattle, there are monthly meetings that only members of the OLF are permitted to attend.

Cultural Values and Lifeways

Prior to the revolution of 1974, which put Ethiopia in power in Oromia, there were three traditional cultural influences. These were the three religious traditions: traditional Oromo thinking, the Coptic Christian church, and the Islamic culture. Merdasa (1991) studied how culture affected the treatment of mental health disorders in Oromia prior to 1974. Traditional Oromo teachings state that each person possesses an *ayana,* which is a special divine agent that can descend upon humans. It is also defined as a person's character or personality. In traditional Oromo culture, the Kallu is the religious leader who investigates the cause of mental disorders and gives advice about treatment. Merdasa (1991) found that mental disorders were generally explained as resulting from disturbances in the relationship between people and divinity. The Coptic church looked upon mental disorders as possession by an evil spirit that could only be treated by priests or monks through prayer, holy water, and exorcism. Muslims believed that mental illness was caused by evil spirits sent by God to punish unfaithful people and treated it with herbal remedies and prayers. Merdasa (1991) found that people attended different healers and religious leaders depending on the reputation of that person, rather than on cultural or religious affiliation. This is thought to be due to the great intermingling of religion and culture among the Oromo people.

Many Oromian refugees are political exiles who fled to avoid death in their own country. The father of one of the Rainier Vista adolescents is an example. He continues to support the OLF's attempts to regain independence from Ethiopia so that he may return home with his family. This is one reason Leininger's Sunrise Model is an effective framework in evaluating the vulnerability of the Oromo people. If a refugee considers himself in a state of indefinite exile, he will resist assimilation into American culture (Sorenson, 1996). This increases vulnerability.

One important aspect of transnationalism is the role that immigrants and refugees play in political activities in both their countries of origin and residence, and their political commitment often has important implications for their sense of self, particularly when those political activities are directed toward the creation of a new homeland for oppressed minorities (Sorenson, 1996, p. 1).

Another factor that can be examined with the Sunrise Model, in conjunction with cultural values and lifeways, is the impact of previous life experience on vulnerability. Many Oromian refugees have had to survive torture and several resettlement attempts in refugee camps in neighboring countries. Robertson (2001) concluded that survivors of government-sponsored torture often experience long-term mental health problems, which can affect future quality of life.

NURSING IMPLICATIONS

For optimal care, with a desired outcome of well-being and decreased vulnerability, the Oromo people benefit greatly when folk medicine and Western medicine are intertwined. An advanced-practice or public health nurse who is using Leininger's culture care theory would plan and make decisions with clients with respect to three modes of action, which are based on the care data obtained from the Sunrise Model. These three modalities are 1) culture care preservation and/or maintenance, 2) cultural care accommodation and/or negotiation, and 3) culture care repatterning or restructuring. These are meant to be "modalities that guide nursing judgments, decisions, or actions in order to provide cultural congruent care that is beneficial, satisfying, and meaningful to people nurses serve" (Leininger, 2001).

Leininger does not use the word intervention in her theory or in her model. Traditionally, the nursing process is based on assessment, planning, intervention, and evaluation. Leininger feels that the term intervention is often "culture bound to Western professional nursing ideologies" (Leininger, 2001). This could convey a position of cultural interference and imposition of value systems. She also believes that the idea of a "nursing problem" does not belong in her theory. A problem prioritized by the nurse may not be given the same relevance by the client of a different culture. The nurse practitioner would use the concepts in the Sunrise Model to guide his or her information gathering. The following is a case study in which the advanced-practice nurse (ARNP) uses Leininger's theory to facilitate her decision-making process.

Case Study: Mrs. S.

Mrs. S. is a 31-year-old Oromo woman who comes into a community family practice clinic complaining of lethargy, headache, and "heart racing" (palpitations). A physical exam reveals pale conjunctiva, koilonychias (thin, concave fingernails with raised ridges), and a smooth tongue with no visible taste buds. The ARNP suspects that Mrs. S. is anemic and knows that this patient must have blood drawn and a stool sample checked for occult blood. The woman is wearing a head covering and is accompanied by her 8-year-old daughter who serves as an interpreter. The ARNP knows enough about the Muslim culture to know that questioning her about gynecological functions will be difficult and that using her daughter as an interpreter would not be wise. The information pertinent to the Oromo culture that the ARNP must gather is outlined in the Sunrise Model.

Technological Factors

The ARNP knows that the optimal solution to overcoming the language barrier is to have an interpreter. The family practice clinic uses an interpretation service that is provided by the telephone service. However, she must first ascertain how comfortable Mrs. S. is with technology. The health care provider is aware that it may be necessary to employ technological diagnostic tools for diagnosis and treatment with this patient and makes it a priority to establish Mrs. S's comfort level. Using her daughter as an interpreter, she asks Mrs. S. what kinds of technology they use in their home. This will begin to give the ARNP an understanding of what Mrs. S. is used to seeing and is comfortable with. Upon discovering that the family is taking computer classes at the local community job resource center, the ARNP feels comfortable in employing the telephone interpretation system.

Religious and Philosophical Factors

The ARNP establishes that Mrs. S. is Muslim and discovers that she is very reticent about answering questions regarding her menstruation. In addition, she does not want to provide a stool sample or undergo a rectal exam to rule out gastrointestinal bleeding. Mrs. S. would like to get a prescription for medication she can take and go home as soon as possible. She is frightened of giving blood and believes that if she is anemic, that will only make it worse.

Kinship and Social Factors

The ARNP finds out that Mrs. S. and her four children live with her sister and her three children in a small house. Mrs. S. and her family moved to the United States 2 years ago, after being in a refugee camp in East Africa for 1 year. Her husband has just found work driving a taxicab. Her children all attend public schools in the Seattle system. Mrs. S. receives social support from the REWA. The ARNP makes a mental note of this information. REWA is probably why Mrs. S. has come to the clinic. They will provide culturally appropriate education to Mrs. S. concerning health care issues and reinforce what the ARNP teaches her.

Cultural Values and Lifeways

The ARNP knows she must find out how Mrs. S. sees herself in her environment and if it is at odds with her culture. In order to provide culturally congruent health care, the health care provider must know how the patient defines health. It is imperative that the health care provider and the patient develop the medical plan together, in accordance with the patient's culture. Does the patient have a traditional healer who is also providing care? Is the patient already taking herbal treatments? What is the patient's diet? Does the patient believe she is sick for spiritual reasons? Mrs. S. has been taking an herbal tea given to her by a local healer. She also believes that prayer would help, along with an increased faith in Allah. She believes her illness could be a punishment.

Political and Legal Factors; Economic Factors

Mrs. S. does not feel it is necessary to respond to questions concerning her political values. Her family fled their homeland to avoid the current regime. They wish to return eventually to their home and extended family. They worry about the safety of those left behind.

Mrs. S. and her family live in subsidized housing and are on Medicaid. The ARNP knows that she can refer Mrs. S. and her children to the Women, Infants, and Children (WIC) program to improve her current diet of *bideenna* (fermented flat bread). Mrs. S. reports eating very few vegetables and little meat due to her economic status.

Educational Factors

It is important to know if Mrs. S. received an education in her homeland. If she is not literate in her own language, then providing her with handouts in Oromiffa will not help her. Mrs. S. comes from an urban area and did receive a 10th grade education. The ARNP feels comfortable providing her with nutritional handouts. She also knows that Mrs. S.'s educational level will help her understand the reasons and importance of the blood the ARBP must draw.

Treatment Plan

Mrs. S. and the health care provider agree on a mutually acceptable plan. The ARNP explains in detail the importance of getting a blood sample, and the patient agrees to have it done. She is found to have iron deficiency anemia. She agrees to monitor her menses and stools over the next month if the ARNP will delay doing a rectal and pelvic exam until it is absolutely necessary. In the meantime, the patient will gladly take an iron supplement and talk to a registered dietician about improving her diet. In addition, she will bring in her tea so the ARNP can see what is in it. The health care provider states her willingness to work with the traditional healer and refers Mrs. S. to the WIC program.

CONCLUSION

Integrated health care is the best approach with the Oromo community in Seattle. Traditional Oromo healers are "skilled at bone-setting, cautery, minor surgical procedures, and treating illnesses using herbal remedies" (EthnoMed, 2001, p. 6). Some of the illnesses (and issues) seen in the Oromo population at the refugee clinic at Harborview Hospital are adolescent violence, anemia, asthma, depression, female circumcision, hepatitis B, parasitic diseases, peripartum problems due to poor prenatal care, and tuberculosis. Many of these illnesses are beyond the scope of traditional medicine in and of itself, and it is necessary to use Western medicine.

Partnerships that have been created in the Seattle area have helped to decrease the vulnerability of the Oromian residents at Rainier Vista. Puget Sound Neighborhood Health Centers, the REWA, and the Job Resource Center are examples of collaborative partnerships that mirror the lower half of the Sunrise Model framework. More solutions for establishing more effective health care delivery to the Oromo population are as follows: 1) provide information for disease prevention, 2) explain diagnostic tests and why treatment might not be given until test results are available, 3) if no medications are given, explain why, 4) take blood from fingers rather than veins, 5) provide same-sex physicians and explain pelvic exams and medical procedures used in childbirth, 6) offer information to new mothers on pumping and storing milk, and 7) offer information on family planning (EthnoMed, 1996).

REFERENCES

Denn, R. (2001, January 3). Growth rate slows for bilingual education enrollment but state still faces a shortage of those teachers, report finds. *Seattle Post-Intelligencer,* p. B4.

Eskenazi, S. (2001, September 21). Aching for peace: Museum film project gives voice to children of Muslim refugees. *Seattle Times,* p. B1.

EthnoMed. (1996). *Voices of the Oromo community.* Retrieved November 16, 2002, from *http://www/ethnomed.org/ethnomed/voices/oromo.html.*

EthnoMed. (2001). *Oromo culture profile.* Retrieved October 10, 2002, from *http://ethnomed.org/ethnomed/cultures/oromo.*

Horus, R. (1995). *Facts about the Oromo of East Africa.* Retrieved October 8, 2002, from *http://www.sas.upenn.edu/African_Studies.*

Kibour, Y. (2001). Ethiopian immigrants' racial identity attitudes and depression symptomatology: An exploratory study. *Cultural Diversity & Ethnic Minority Psychology, 7*(1), 47–58.

Leininger, M. M. (2001). *Culture care diversity and universality: A theory of nursing.* New York, NY: National League for Nursing.

MacDonald, S. (1999, December 4). Schools aiding Muslims, programs target youths from Islamic nations. *Seattle Times,* p. D8.

McSpadden, L. A. (1987). Ethiopian refugee resettlement in the western United States: Social context and psychological well-being. *International Migration Review, 21,* 796–819.

Melbaa, K. (1998). *The Oromian people and Oromia.* Retrieved October 8, 2002, from *http://www.oromo.org/osg/oromo.htm.*

Merdasa, J. L. (1991). Traditional perceptions and treatment of mental disorders in western Ethiopia before the 1974 revolution. *Acta Psychiatrica Scandinavia, 84,* 475–481.

Missailidis, K., & Gebre-Medhin, M. (2000, July 8). Female genital mutilation in eastern Ethiopia. *Lancet, 356,* 137–138.

Robertson, C. L. (2001). *History of government-sponsored torture among Somali and Oromo refugees* [Abstract]. Retrieved October 10, 2002, from *http://apha.confex.com/apha/129am/techprogram/paper_25944.htm.*

Sorenson, J. (1996, October). Learning to be Oromo: Nationalist discourse in the Diaspora. *Social Identities, 2,* 439–468.

CHAPTER 11

Finding Meaning in Death: A Nurse Practitioner's Role

Jennifer Fritz-Millard

Traditional medicine teaches us that illness is something to defeat. The diagnosis of terminal illness is a failure of the clinician's skills and of medicine itself. "In a sense, death must always be defined negatively, for it is the termination of biological life the only mode of existence we know" (Gatch, 1969, p. 4). Nurse practitioners now find themselves in a unique position to assist terminally ill patients by helping them find meaning in their experience, thereby improving their quality of life and potentially easing suffering. In this chapter, I will discuss how nurse practitioners can facilitate the discernment of meaning in terminally ill patients by incorporating Kolcaba's Theory of Comfort, personally encouraging patients to begin their own search for meaning, and referring terminally ill patients to appropriate professionals.

Nurses always have been on the forefront of palliative care and hospice movements. Nurses are taught to holistically care for and treat the vulnerable. We are empowered to critically examine our opinions, biases, and fears in order to give the best possible treatment to our patients. The art of palliative care includes tending to a patient's physical comfort but, more importantly, may include tending to his or her emotional and mental well-being. Tremblay & Breitbart (2001) suggest that since death is an "imminent reality" in palliative care, the role of the mental health professional should be expanded (p. 949). Many times the overtaxed mental health care system is unavailable to dying patients. Nurse practitioners must take the initiative to expand their role and help fill this essential need for the most vulnerable and underserved population the dying.

TERMINALLY ILL PATIENTS AS VULNERABLE

Terminally ill patients are extremely vulnerable on many levels. The loss of strength and control over bodily functions, the pain, and fear are heavy burdens to bear. The terminally ill are vulnerable in that they are losing everything that they have previously known. They experience a profound paradigm shift that puts everything that they have experienced and their hopes for the future in a different perspective. This shift forces patients to view the world through a whole different lens and may change their entire outlook. This shift may lead to suffering.

According to Byock (1997), suffering may occur on any level of a patient's "personhood." People are mind and body combined, and suffering can occur in either realm. Cassel (1991) defines suffering as "the state of severe distress associated with events that threaten the intactness of person" (p. 33). Suffering can take many forms, or it may result in the patient's loss of meaning in life. "Although each person's meaning is different, existence that is merely a burden and lacks a future with any direction or point produces the worst kind of suffering" (Byock, 1997, p. 83).

In today's curative medical climate, clinicians often do not adequately address the needs of this most critically vulnerable population. As a result, the terminally ill are sent unprepared into our health care system, which has both sterilized and desensitized both the end of life and death itself. Terminally ill patients are often sent to medical facilities where they die unseen by the general public. Elaborate funerals are then performed after preparing the deceased for display in a comfortable repose, further helping loved ones to disguise the fact and finality of death. We all, in a sense, alienate the dying by desensitizing the experience for the rest of us. Estranged and vulnerable, the dying person is left to try to make sense of his or her life and impending death.

DEATH IN CLASSICAL LITERATURE

Classic literature has long examined the meaning of life and death. *The Death of Ivan Illyitch*, written by Leo Tolstoy in 1886, portrays a man who struggles to find the meaning of his life and advancing death. He faces his death alone while those around him withdraw as they are unpleasantly reminded of their own mortality and are repulsed by his declining physical condition. Only Gerasim, his butler, gives comfort as he conveys to the dying man that serving him is not only his duty but his privilege as well. This simple man is a caring, straightforward caregiver for the ailing Illyitch and becomes his only real solace. "Gerasim alone did not lie: in every way it was evident that he alone comprehended what the trouble was, and thought it unnecessary to hide it, and simply pitied his sick bairn, who was wasting away" (Tolstoy, 1999, p. 398).

The physician in Tolstoy's story adds a great deal of misery to the plight of Illyitch by focusing on his physical problems and never addressing the obvious fact that the patient is actively dying. Illyitch gradually descends into deep despair as he evaluates his existence and appraises the senselessness, worthlessness, and folly of the life that he has constructed around him. Only when he is able to grasp some meaning in his existence (although bleak) is he able to find peace and release from torment and to die peacefully. Written over 100 years ago, this story still seems starkly appropriate in today's medical and social climate.

DEFINITION OF MEANING

But what is meaning? The *New Merriam-Webster Dictionary* (1989) defines meaning as "purpose," "significance," and "connotation." Circirelli (1998) describes personal meanings as "primarily cognitive interpretations of objects and events in the environment, that occur prior to and stimulate emotional reactions" (p. 714). Gamino, Hogan, & Sewell (2002) suggest that all of us as persons strive to understand and make sense of the world around us, our personal experiences, our relationships with others, and our private thoughts. The meaning of death for each person has a very individual and unique significance that we all must ultimately face alone. Patients' personal meaning of their dying experience can shape the acceptance of their illness and the level of suffering they may endure. Spirituality may be the bridge that enables the patient to move between comfort and meaning.

SPIRITUALITY

There is much in literature concerning spirituality and the meaning of life. Both of these concepts can have very individualistic and unique definitions. When faced with a terminal illness, one's previous experiences and problem-solving schemes are often not enough to make sense of this new reality. Spirituality can help people find meaning in this murky, unfamiliar territory. The consequence of not searching for some meaning or the "why" in a terminal illness can result in resentment or anger. This in turn may lead to suffering.

For some people, spirituality may mean an understanding of or a bond with a higher power. Others may strive to achieve goals that connect them with their spirituality, such as making the world as better place or valuing their life's achievements. Healing any hurts and reaffirming love of family and friends may also have a positive spiritual effect on the terminally ill. Marrone (1999) calls this search for meaning a "psychospiritual transformation, which involves a profound, growth-oriented spiritual/existential transformation that fundamentally changes our central assumptions, beliefs, and attitudes about life, death, love, compassion, or God" (p. 498).

However one chooses to define his or her spirituality, clinicians are obligated to help them explore it in their search for meaning. Nurse practitioners may facilitate this spiritual search themselves or may coordinate spiritual and emotional care with a chaplain, clergy member, grief counselor, or clinical psychologist. Providing support in the grieving process by just listening to the patient's fears and hopes is a valuable way that meaning may be communicated to this vulnerable population.

THEORY OF COMFORT: FRANCES KOLCABA

Frances Kolcaba, a contemporary nursing theorist, has created the Theory of Comfort, which can be a useful tool to help nurse practitioners guide patients on their journey toward meaning. This relatively new and simply applied midrange theory implores nurses to return to their roots and focus on the comfort needs of patients in many areas, including the physiological, social, financial, psychological, spiritual, environmental, and physical. Novak, Kolcaba, Steiner, & Dowd (2001) suggest that terminally ill patients may experience discomfort in any or all of these areas and that the need for comfort must be assessed and addressed on all levels, rather than just in the traditional arena of physical pain management.

Kolcaba defines comfort in nursing as "the satisfaction (actively, passively, or cooperatively) of the basic human needs for relief, ease or transcendence arising from heath care situations that are stressful" (Kolcaba, 1994, p. 1178). This definition is significant because there are few situations that are as stressful, require such global comforting measures, and create as much vulnerability as terminal illness. Kolcaba's theory occurs within an arena composed of three states of being and four contexts within which comfort for the patient can reside. Relief, ease, and transcendence are the three intertwined states of being within which a patient is strengthened. The four contexts in which comfort occurs for a patient are physical, psychospiritual, social, and environmental. The psychospiritual context of comfort is where meaning in life is found.

The theory is built on the premise that all beings react in a holistic manner to complex stimuli and that all beings desire and strive for comfort. Comfort is inherently a multifaceted phenomenon because actions that affect one aspect of a person's comfort indirectly influence other areas as well. Kolcaba proclaims that these direct and indirect results create a greater effect on comfort for the patient than would any action taken individually; thus comfort measures are inherently holistic (Kolcaba, 1994; Kolcaba & Kolcaba, 1991; Novak et al., 2001).

Kolcaba's theory proposes that the interactions among all these aspects of comfort are essential to achieving comfort and are easily assessed and addressed within the field of nursing. Although attaining a state of complete comfort may be an unrealistic goal in palliative care, helping a terminally ill patient find meaning is a small but essential role for nurse practitioners, in addition to the provision of traditional comfort measures and treatments. Kolcaba's theory does not claim that assessing for discord within her seven levels of comfort will take away all of a patient's discomfort. She does maintain, however, that the interactions between comfort measures and the actions themselves may help a patient reach "ease" and "transcendence" (Vendlinski & Kolcaba, 1997).

AGREEMENT IN RESEARCH

The majority of clinical research and literature concerning the end of life suggests that helping or giving patients permission to find meaning in their experience and loss is essential to improving quality of life at the end of life. A 1998 study by Circirelli used a convenience sample of 265 college students compared with older individuals (ages 19–55 years) and attempted to determine a relationship between personal meanings of death in relation to fear of death. Circirelli proposed that those who have positive personal meanings about death experience less distress and more comfort than those who attach negative meanings. Furthermore, "if personal meanings associated with death have negative consequences for the individual, they can generate various death fears" (Circirelli, 1998, p. 714). These fears can affect the way people live their entire lives.

Circirelli (1998) created 30 statements about death and asked participants to rate how each one represented them personally. The Leming Fear of Death Scale was then administered to each participant. He found that those who chose the meaning of death as extinction experienced fear in the greatest quantity, whereas, those who chose the meaning of death as an afterlife experienced less fear, and those who chose the meaning of death as legacy experienced the least fear. This study once again shows that the unknown can generate much fear, distress, and suffering. Those who despair often report greater amounts of uncontrolled pain that those who describe themselves as at peace. Helping patients explore their feelings about death can encourage them to face their fears and conquer them.

Social science has also given emphasis to the importance of finding meaning for the terminally ill. Parker-Oliver (2002) eloquently states, "Hope is entrenched in meaning, and meaning is socially constructed, thus providing the opportunity to assist the dying to find peace and the brightness experienced before a star falls" (p. 115). She maintains that palliative and hospice care allow dying patients to attach meaning to their lives, not in an attempt to continue living, but in order to give value to their unique experience. In this context, hope arises from the search for meaning itself.

Parker-Oliver challenges clinicians working with dying patients to help them discover the meaning in their experience and develop goals despite their grim prognosis. This journey requires that the clinician help the patient transition to a dying role, which creates a paradigm shift for both clinician and patient. This new reality recreates a medical environment where comfort, openness, family, and decision making are emphasized rather that the traditional role of getting well. Dr. Parker-Oliver visualizes a medical model that changes the traditional goal of healing a patient to one of support and comfort

DISAGREEMENT IN THE LITERATURE

Not all the literature agrees that helping the patient find meaning in death is necessary for good end-of-life care. Fulton, Madden, & Minichiello (1996) suggest that participating in the grieving process and finding meaning for the terminally ill is not always necessary. These authors propose that the anticipatory grief theory is flawed and that it is incorrectly embraced on a wide scale by the medical community. They suggest that those individuals who perceive death as a relief to life's suffering and those who maintain optimism about the outcome of their illness may not need to participate in the grieving process at all.

A qualitative analysis of serial interviews with 30 terminally ill patients by Yedidia & Mac-Gragor (2001) set out to find the "narrative context of illness" in order to help physicians more holistically develop individualized treatment plans at the end of life (p. 808). These authors were able to isolate seven motifs from their interviews with patients from varying walks of life, cultures, and ethnicities who were in their last days of life. Only one of these motifs encompassed finding meaning in the experience of dying.

These authors concluded that dying patients tend to view their impending deaths with the same frames of reference that they used consistently to deal with major events and themes throughout their lives. They conclude that some patients do not need to find meaning, and clinicians must assess the whole context of the patient's perspective when constructing an appropriate plan of care.

Furthermore, two separate studies by a research team were analyzed in a paper in which the authors concluded that survivors of a traumatic loss suffered much less distress if they did not attempt to make meaning out of their personal tragedy (Davis et al, 2000). The first study involved interviewing 124 parents 2 weeks, 3 months, and 18 months following the death of their children to sudden infant death syndrome (SIDS). At each interview, the parents were asked whether they had attempted to find meaning or had found meaning in their loss. Then several instruments were used to measure the "psychological adjustment" of the parents. The researchers concluded that the parents who were evaluated as least interested in making sense of their baby's death did significantly better than those who could not find meaning in their loss (Davis et al., 2000; Downey et al, 1990).

The research team undertook another study of 93 people who had lost either a spouse or a child to a motor vehicle accident (Lehman et al., 1987). They interviewed subjects 4–7 years after the incident about their reactions to their loss and their level of psychological distress. They found that about a third of those who had lost a spouse and about a quarter of those who had lost a child did not make sense of or find meaning in their loss (Davis et al, 2000). Furthermore, the percentage of those interviewed who did not try to find meaning in their loss had significantly less psychological distress than the percentage who found meaning in their experience or those who tried to find meaning and were unable to do so.

Although the authors do concede that finding meaning in a tragic loss is important for most people, they suggest that this search is not necessary for everyone. These two studies suggest that the widely held assumption that presumes it is important for everyone to find meaning in loss is incorrect. These authors suggest that not everyone must embark on a painful journey toward meaning to experience peace and come to terms with significant loss.

NURSE PRACTITIONER APPROACHES TO DYING PATIENTS

What techniques and tools can nurse practitioners use to help patients find meaning? Byock (2002) suggests that although finding meaning in the experience of terminal illness is difficult for both caregiver and patient, listening for the common themes of "response to mystery, connection to something larger than oneself which endures into an open-ended future, and experienced source of meaning" helps them move from extreme emotional discomfort to a "seemingly paradoxical sense of personal well-being" (p. 282).

Frances Kolcaba's Theory of Comfort can be used by nurse practitioners to gain a broad perspective on the many dimensions of comfort that a patient requires. Nurse practitioners must help patients find comfort in all four contexts of their lives: the physical, psycho-spiritual, social, and environmental. The psycho-spiritual context is often neglected, and this is where meaning in one's life is found. This relatively new midrange theory is simplistic and solid.

A midrange theory is less abstract than a grand theory and is developed by the theorist to be used easily in a wide range of clinical areas and to be tested by research (Tomey & Alligood, 2002). There is currently no published research on the use of Kolcaba's theory with the terminally ill. Further research on its use in this area would be beneficial to our field. Despite the obvious ethical dilemmas and problems of doing research with the vulnerable population of the terminally ill, more research is required, research that uses the perspectives of the dying themselves rather than retrospective studies concerning the outlook from survivors and treating clinicians.

Our fast-paced medical environment makes it difficult to find time to just sit with a patient and talk about brief and comfortable issues, much less the awkward and disturbing ones. But nurses do make the time. We do it every day in practice and have since our trade began. "Nursing has long been identified as an occupation that offers personalized services and physical ministrations to sick people, including those who are dying" (Feifel, 1977, p. 124). These qualifications make us as nurse practitioners the ideal candidates to take a stand and encourage ourselves and our colleagues to take just a little extra time. Our main concern in practice is the relief of suffering. Suffering for a dying person can come in many forms. Holstein (1997) goes as far to suggest that the search for finding the answer to "what does it all mean?" underlies much of the suffering that the dying person experiences (p. 853).

Gerontologists have long used the tools of life review and reminiscence when working with the elderly. These tools help patients look at their whole lives, both good and bad, in order to make a bigger picture. These techniques have proven to be very therapeutic for the storyteller. What better way to help people celebrate their lives than just sitting and listening for a while to their experience of it? As a clinician, I can think of no better way to honor my patients than by prompting them to find their own unique meaning in their experience and making myself available to them to share these insights.

In order to assess for vulnerability and susceptibility to this kind of suffering, nurse practitioners must ask their patients difficult questions. We must "be" with patients and help them define the "why" of their suffering. Sometimes fear and lack of knowledge may produce anxiety and suffering in themselves. Byock (1997) suggests simply asking the patient, "How are you feeling within yourself?" This open-ended question gives patients permission to describe their suffering and how they feel about it. Simple as this may seem, many medical professionals find it very hard to discuss death with their patients. By discussing death, we inherently must face our personal anxieties about life and death. Many find it difficult to reassure patients when there is no hard clinical proof of existence after life.

CONCLUSION

The majority of research and literature on the subject of terminal illness points to the critical importance of helping the dying patient find meaning in his or her experience and loss. This meaning may encompass spirituality, faith, hope, or even an acceptance of what has happened and what is to come. Despite the recent popularity and expansion of the hospice movement in this country, many clinicians still engage in the traditional medical model of desensitizing the experience of dying for the patient and themselves.

Nurse practitioners must step up to help fill this critical need to assist these alienated and vulnerable patients. Nurse practitioners are particularly skilled in active listening and in treating patients as holistic beings who need care on many levels. Our profession has historically demanded these skills, and we have perfected and taught them to our rising generations. Feifel (1977) suggests that both parties (the clinician and the patient) can mutually benefit from moving from a cure model to a caring model when supporting a patient at the end of his or her life. The holistic and straightforward view of comfort proposed in Kolcaba's Theory of Comfort makes it an easy tool for nurse practitioners to integrate into practice when working with the terminally ill. The time is ripe in our medical climate for nurse practitioners to step up and use and engage our many talents in assisting the most vulnerable of all populations the dying.

REFERENCES

Byock, I. (1997). *Dying well.* New York: Riverhead Books.

Byock, I. (2002). The meaning and value of death. *Journal of Palliative Medicine, 5,* 279–288.

Cassell, E. J. (1991). *The nature of suffering and the goals of medicine.* New York, NY: Oxford University.

Circirelli, V. (1998). Personal meaning of death in relation to fear of death. *Death Studies, 22,* 713–733.

Davis, C. G., Wortman, C. B., Lehman, D. R., & Silver, R. C. (2000). Searching for meaning in loss: Are clinical assumptions correct? *Death Studies, 24,* 497–540.

Downey, G., Silver, R.C., & Wortman, C.B. (1990). Reconsidering the attribution-adjustment relation following a major life event: Coping with the loss of a child. *Journal of Personality and Social Psychology, 59,* 925–940.

Feifel, H. (1977). *New meanings of death.* New York, NY: McGraw-Hill.

Fulton, G., Madden, C., & Minichiello, V. (1996). The social construction of anticipatory grief. *Social Science and Medicine, 43,* 1349–1358.

Gatch, M. M. (1969). *Death: Meaning and mortality in Christian thought and contemporary culture.* Boston, MA: Seabury.

Gamino, L. A., Hogan, N. S., & Sewell, K. W. (2002). Feeling the absence: a content analysis from the Scott and White grief study. *Death Studies, 26,* 793–813.

Holstein, M. (1997). Reflections on death and dying. *Academic Medicine, 72,* 848–855.

Kolcaba, K. Y. (1994). A theory of holistic comfort for nursing. *Journal of Advanced Nursing, 19,* 1178–1184.

Kolcaba, K. Y., & Kolcaba, R. (1991). An analysis of the concept of comfort. *Journal of Advanced Nursing, 16,* 1301–1310.

Lehman, D. R., Wortman, C. B., & Williams, A. F. (1987). Long-term effects of losing a spouse or child in a motor vehicle crash. *Journal of Personality and Social Psychology, 52,* 218–231.

Marrone, R. (1999). Dying, mourning, and spirituality: A psychological perspective. *Death Studies, 23,* 495–519.

Mish, F. C., et al. (Eds.). (1989). *The New Merriam-Webster Dictionary.* Springfield, MA: Merriam-Webster.

Novak, B., Kolcaba, K., Steiner, R., & Dowd, T. (2001). Measuring comfort in caregivers and patients during late end-of-life care. *American Journal of Hospice & Palliative Care, 18*(3), 170–180.

Parker-Oliver, D. (2002). Redefining hope for the terminally ill. *American Journal of Hospice & Palliative Care, 19*(2), 115–120.

Tolstoy, L. (1999). The death of Ivan Illyitch. In C. Neider (Ed.). *Tolstoy: Tales of courage and conflict* (pp. 368–410). New York, NY: Cooper Square.

Tomey, A. M., & Alligood, M. R. (2002). *Nursing theorists and their work* (5th ed.). St. Louis, MO: Mosby.

Tremblay, A., & Breitbart, W. (2001). Psychiatric dimensions of palliative care. *Palliative Care, 19,* 949–967.

Vendlinski, S., & Kolcaba, K. Y. (1997). Comfort care: A framework for hospice nursing. *American Journal of Hospice & Palliative Care, 14*(6), 271–276.

Yedidia, M. J., & MacGragor, B. (2001). Confronting the prospect of dying: Reports of terminally ill patients. *Journal of Pain and Symptom Management, 22,* 807–819.

CHAPTER 12

Giving Voice to Vulnerable Persons: Rogerian Theory

Sarah Hall Gueldner and Geraldine Britton

The human condition of vulnerability is a concept of vital concern to nurses in that a large portion of nursing practice is spent either helping individuals who find themselves in a vulnerable position or helping them avoid vulnerability. However, nursing has been slow in developing theoretical constructs of vulnerability within a nursing perspective (Spiers, 2000). Traditional definitions of vulnerability are framed within an epidemiological approach to identify individuals and groups at risk for harm. Groups most often labeled as vulnerable include the elderly, children, the poor, people with chronic illnesses, people from minority cultures, and captive populations such as prisoners and refugees (Saunders & Valente, 1992). Labels of vulnerability are customarily applied in relation to socioeconomic, minority, or other stigmatizing status (Demi & Warren, 1995) and reflect a tendency to blame the victim rather than prevailing social structures. The generally accepted marker for vulnerability has been the inability to function independently in accord with the values of a particular society. Fortunately, there is growing dialogue about vulnerability from the perspective of the person experiencing it, a view that is more congruent with the philosophical stance of nursing (Morse, 1997; Spiers, 2000).

The Rogerian (Rogers, 1992) conceptual system, which focuses on the person as integral with and inseparable from his or her environment, holds considerable relevance as an innovative nursing framework to use in addressing the problem of vulnerability. Accordingly, the remainder of this discussion will be directed toward application of the theoretical base of Rogerian nursing science to the concept of vulnerability.

A ROGERIAN PERSPECTIVE OF VULNERABILITY

According to Martha Rogers, energy fields are the fundamental unit of everything, both living and nonliving. The fields are boundaryless and dynamic, changing continuously. Two energy fields are identified: the human field and the environmental field. Rogers emphasizes that humans and environments do not have energy fields; rather, they *are* energy fields. Likewise, she insisted that the human field is unitary and cannot be reduced to a biological field, a physical field, or a psychosocial field. As postulated by Rogers, human and environmental fields flow together in a constant mutual process that is unitary rather than separate. Within this worldview, humans are energy fields that exist in constant mutual process with their immediate and extended environmental energy field, which includes, and cannot be separated from, other living and nonliving fields. She also postulated that both human and environmental energy patterns change continually during this process. The inseparability of the human energy field from a person's immediate and extended environmental energy field is perhaps the most central feature of the Rogerian conceptual system.

Phillips & Bramlett (1994) asserted that the mutual human–environmental field process can be harmonious or dissonant. Resonant with Rogers' science, these researchers posit vulnerability as an emergent condition that arises when there is dissonance within the mutual human–environmental field process. This view is consistent with Rogerian scholar Barrett's (1990) theory of power, which associates power with individuals' knowing participation in change within their mutual human–environmental process for the betterment of the whole, including themselves. These authors perceive vulnerability as the opposite condition of power, a condition that may occur when an individual is unable or does not choose to participate in an informed and purposeful way in change. Persons in this situation essentially have no voice and may be intentionally or unintentionally left behind in a compromised position. Within this line of thinking, an individual's sense of dissonance or disharmony within the mutual human–environmental field process would be viewed as a manifestation of vulnerability, placing individuals or groups as risk. Barrett has developed the text-based tool Power as Knowing Participation in Change (PKPC) to measure this concept; a subscale of the tool addresses awareness as an essential feature of knowing participation.

Lack of knowing participation may be associated with a number of scenarios. Individuals may be uninformed or misinformed about situations involved in their unique human–environmental energy field process, or they may be unable to participate due to a specific circumstance such as illness (e.g., stroke) or injury (e.g., hip fracture). Common situations that may limit or prevent knowing participation include compromised vision or hearing, aphasia, difficulty with mobility, and confusion or dementia. Other circumstances that may limit knowing participation include any situation that prevents persons from engaging in sufficient communications within the community, such as lack of transportation or limited language facility. Insufficient means or the inability to move about freely may limit presence, making it more difficult, if not impossible, to be "at the table," so to speak, to achieve representation. Stigmatized individuals or groups such as single mothers, persons who are homeless, and persons perceived as unattractive or different are also at risk for a lack of information or misinformation that may lead to inappropriate participation based on misjudgment. Indeed, information may be intentionally or unintentionally withheld if participation is not welcome.

Parse's (2003) newly published theory of community becoming, which is also an extension of Rogers' nursing science, is particularly applicable to the theoretical tenet of vulnerability. She defines community in terms of the relational experience of being "in community" and describes it as a resource, dynamic and continuously changing to best represent the good of the individual in order to achieve the best for all. According to her definition, community is not a location or a group of people who have similar interests; rather, community is the human connectedness with the universe, including connectedness with yet-to-be possibles. This view represents a paradigm shift, wherein vulnerability is an emergent of the community in process that occurs when an individual or group becomes disconnected from the group and therefore from needed resources. Parse describes a nontraditional model for health service for individuals and families who have become disconnected from resources. The process involves imaging the vision of possibilities and inviting others to capture the vision, thus energizing the community to build partnerships to overcome the disconnect.

Within this perspective/view, vulnerability arises as an emergent when connectedness is compromised by a lack of communication or flawed communication that leads to exclusion from resources. Vulnerability might be seen as an unfortunate estrangement from the process of community. Within this view, persons who are at particular risk for vulnerability are those who for some reason are unable to call enough attention to their needs to garner the support of their community.

Based on Parse's (1997) "human becoming" perspective, her view of nursing practice also differs from traditional nursing practice in that the nurse does not offer standardized professional advice and opinions stemming from the nurse's own value system. Rather, nursing involves what she terms a "true presence with and respect for the other" wherein the nurse dwells with the person or family to enhance their perceived possibles. Parse points out that it is essential to go with vulnerable persons to where they are, rather than to attempt to judge, change, or control them. It is in dwelling with the individual in discussion that meanings emerge, and it is in this process of illuminating meaning that possibilities for transcendence are seen.

In Parse's words, "The nurse in true presence with person or family is not a guide or a beacon, but rather an inspiring attentive presence that calls the other to shed light on the meaning moments of his or her life. It is the person or family in the presence of the nurse that illuminates the meaning, synchronizes the rhythms, and mobilizes transcendence in moving beyond. The person is coauthor of his or her own health . . . choosing rhythmical patterns of relating while reaching for personal hopes and dreams" (Parse, 1997, p.40). She continues, "True presence is a special way of *being with* in which the nurse bears witness to the person's or family's own living of value priorities. True presence is an interpersonal art grounded in a strong knowledge base 'reflecting the belief that each person knows *the way* somewhere within self'" (Parse, 1997, p. 40). Certainly, nowhere is it more important to honor the person as he or she is than when working with those who are vulnerable.

Parse describes a humanitarian model of nursing practice based on true presence and profound respect. Use of this model enables people to find actions that increase their ability to knowingly participate in change to improve their position, thus becoming less vulnerable. Parse refers to this process as the search for the possible beyond the now.

However, in even this overall positive system, some are likely to find themselves in vulnerable circumstances. Some individuals and groups (such as young children) are placed at risk because they cannot speak for themselves and depend on others to advocate for them until they are old enough. Likewise, sick or frail members of the community may be too weak or impaired to participate knowingly in the change process to advance their betterment. They may not be mobile enough, think clearly enough, or be articulate enough to capture community attention and garner the resources they need.

Individuals or families at special risk for vulnerability include those who

- ☐ have energy-draining illnesses or conditions such as stroke, heart attack, cancer, or depression
- ☐ are not included in the dominant culture
- ☐ have compromised language facility, making them at greater risk for being unheard
- ☐ are out of their familiar turf (i.e., new in the community and do not know the "rules" or avenues for help)
- ☐ are unable to comprehend information (i.e., never learned to read, have diminished vision or hearing, are unconscious or have dementia, or are unable to comprehend English)

☐ have illness or injury that limits independence (i.e., broken hips that make it more difficult to stay connected with the community)

☐ lack the ability to access services needed for everyday life (i.e., means for obtaining food, place to live, health services)

☐ are in a position of diminished visibility (i.e., live in a remote area or are homebound, becoming disconnected from community notice)

Viewed from Parse's theory of community becoming, the approach to overcoming vulnerability is a matter of reconnecting the person or group to community. This sometimes happens naturally through family and friends or through social institutions and/or programs such as churches and civic organizations. But it may take the focused attention and time of individuals, such as nurses, to help the person or family as they gain insight about possibles that are available to them.

GIVING VOICE: AN APPLICATION OF ROGERIAN NURSING SCIENCE

Addressing the lack of voice that is so intricately associated with the experience of vulnerability, this section will describe a simple picture tool, the Well-being Picture Scale (WPS) tool, developed within the Rogerian conceptual system to amplify the voice of persons who otherwise might not be heard (Gueldner, Michel, Bramlett, Liu, Johnston, Endo et al., in press).

The WPS is a 10-item non–language-based pictorial scale that measures general sense of well-being as a reflection of the mutual human–environmental field process. It was designed as an easy-to-administer tool for use with the broadest possible range of adult populations, including persons who have limited formal education, do not speak English as their first language, may not be able to see well, or who may be too sick or frail to respond to lengthier or more complex measures. Ten pairs of 1-inch drawings depicting a sense of high or low well-being are arranged at opposite ends of a seven-choice, unnumbered semantic differential scale. The 10 items included are eyes open/closed; shoes sitting still/running; butterfly/turtle; candle lit/not lit; faucet running full/dripping; puzzle pieces together/separated; pencil sharp/dull; sun full/partially cloud covered; balloons inflated/partially deflated; and lion/mouse. Individuals are asked to view each of the 10 picture pairs and mark the point along the scale between the pictures to indicate which they feel most like; for example, a lighted candle or an unlit candle. Psychometric properties were established in a sample of more than 2000 individuals from the United States, Taiwan, Japan, Canada, and Africa.

Conceptual Formulation of Well-Being

Rogers (1992) maintained that "the purpose of nursing is to promote health and well-being for all persons wherever they are" (p. 258). According to Hills (1998), well-being is generally defined as a relative sense of harmony and satisfaction in one's life. Smith (1981) and Todaro-Franceschi (1999) defined health as movement toward self-fulfillment or realization of one's potential, a view that is congruent with Parse's (1997) theory of human becoming. Newman (1994) did not distinguish health from well-being but singularly defined it as a manifestation of expanding consciousness that may occur during, but is not separate from, the experience of illness. This view is supported by the work of Morris (1991) and Hills (1998), who both demonstrated a relationship between well-being and awareness.

Conceptually, the WPS assesses the energy field in regard to four characteristics judged to be associated with well-being: frequency of movement (i.e., intensity) within the energy field, awareness of one's self as energy, action emanating from the energy field, and power as knowing participation in change within the mutual human–environmental energy field process.

Frequency

This term refers to the frequency of innate motion within human and environmental energy fields, described by Capra (1975) as "a ceaseless flow of energy" (p. 226). Frequency specifically describes changes in energy pattern, from lower to higher frequency, denoting the intensity of motion within the energy field. It is postulated that higher frequency is associated with a greater sense of well-being and that it is experienced as a sense of vitality.

Awareness

Awareness refers to the sense an individual has of his or her potential and/or readiness for change within the mutual human–environmental field. It signals readiness for moving toward one's potential and is postulated to be positively associated with a sense of well-being. The concept of awareness is congruent with Newman's (1994) theory of health as expanding consciousness and Parse's (1997) theory of human becoming (unfolding). Barrett (1990) included a subscale of awareness in her PKPC tool, and Hills (1998) discussed enlightenment as a manifestation of expanded awareness, higher-level field motion, and well-being. Ferguson (1980) posited that expanded awareness culminates in a clearer reality and a more integral way of being. Awareness is postulated to be a manifestation of the dynamics of the mutual human–environmental energy field process.

Action

The concept of action is conceptualized as an emergent of the "continuous mutual human field and environmental field process" (Rogers, 1992), reflecting the frequency of the human energy field. Action is viewed as an expression of field energy associated with well-being. Examples of action include activities associated with daily living, such as preparing food, eating, personal grooming, participating in social events, exercising, or doing chores, as well as actively engaging in innovative thinking or the creation of art forms.

Power

As described by Barrett (1990), power is the capacity of an individual to engage knowingly in change. Viewed in this way, Barrett sees it as the degree to which an individual is able to express energy as power to create desired change within his or her human–environmental energy field process. When power is prominent, it is postulated that one would have a sense of confidence; conversely, it is postulated that powerlessness is associated with a sense of vulnerability. Power might also be conceptualized as the capacity of an individual to commute the three aforementioned conditions (energy expressed as frequency, awareness, and action) into an emergent sense of well-being.

WPS Development

More than 10 years of developmental work and field testing of early versions of the WPS has revealed a correlation with several other tools designed to measure aspects of well-being within the Rogerian framework (Gueldner, Bramlett, Johnston, & Guillory, 1996). Johnston (1994), in a sample of nursing home residents and community-dwelling elders, reported a highly significant correlation ($r = 0.6647$) between the WPS tool and her Human Field Image Metaphor Scale, which uses two- or three-word metaphors to measure image. Gueldner et al. (1996) found an even greater correlation ($r = 0.7841$) between the WPS and Barrett's (1990) PKPC tool, which measures an individual's capacity for awareness, choices, freedom to act intentionally, and involvement to bring about harmony in the human–environmental energy field process.

Davis (1989), in a matched sample of 30 males 19–51 years of age who had been hospitalized for traumatic injuries and 30 noninjured males, demonstrated positive significant correlations between the score on the WPS and scores on the PKPC tool ($p = 0.002$) and Rosenberg's self-esteem scale ($p = 0.02$). She also found a difference in the between-group mean scores that approached significance ($p = 0.059$), warranting further consideration in a larger sample.

Hindman (1993), in a sample of 40 nursing home residents and 40 community-dwelling older adults, demonstrated a significant correlation ($p = 0.001$) between the mean score on the WPS and humor as measured by the Situational Humor Response Questionnaire. She also found that the mean score was higher for the community-dwelling group of older adults ($p = 0.001$) than for their counterparts who lived in the nursing home and individuals who perceived their income as adequate ($p = 0.05$). Older participants scored lower ($p = 0.05$) on the WPS.

Hills (1998), in a study of 874 mothers of 6-month-old infants, found that mothers who scored higher on the picture tool also reported higher levels of awareness ($p = 0.001$) as measured by the awareness scale of Barrett's (1990) PKPC tool and well-being ($p < 0.001$) as measured by Cantril's Ladder for Well-Being.

Abbate (1990) used the tool as a pre- and posttest measure of well-being in eight school-aged children (aged 5–16 years) with cerebral palsy who participated in a 10-week therapeutic horsemanship program. The mean of the pretest scores was 82.75, and the posttest mean was 86.38. The scores of four children increased over the 10-week period, one did not change, and the scores of three decreased. All of the children in the study had already been riding horses for several years, leading Abbate to suggest that some of the children may have already achieved the most significant gain from their participation in the riding program prior to the onset of the study. Abbate also noted that even the most impaired children were able to make their own mark on the line (response), some using crayons. This is the only study that has used the WPS tool with children, and the sample was small. However, the findings provide some impetus and direction for developing a children's version of the instrument.

In summary, work by Gueldner et al. (1996), Hills (1998), and Johnston (1994) confirmed a high correlation between scores on the WPS and other measures of well-being developed within the Rogerian conceptual system. Additionally, the work of Davis (1989), Hills (1998), and Hindman (1993) demonstrated a high correlation between the WPS tool and a number of established measures of well-being developed by other disciplines. The work of Abbate (1990), although limited in sample size, demonstrated the potential usability of the tool in younger samples. Given these findings, the WPS is offered as a general measure of well-being mediated through frequency, awareness, action, and power emanating within an individual's mutual human–environmental field process.

The brief instructions for the WPS have been translated into Taiwanese (Mandarin Chinese) and Japanese, producing a tool that can be immediately administered in English, Taiwanese, and

Japanese. The final version of the 10-item tool has been administered to 1027 individuals 18 years of age or older ($x = 35$ years) in the United States, Taiwan, and Japan. The sample was 56% Asian, 34% white, and 10% African American or Hispanic. The overall Cronbach's alpha was 0.8795, and item-to-total analysis revealed that no individual item removal, overall or in the national subgroups, would improve alpha, indicating that each of the 10 items contributed uniquely to the total score. Five of the ten items were completely consistent across countries (puzzle, balloon, sun, eyes, and lion), and all others were consistent across two of the three countries.

CONCLUSION

The WPS is offered as a general index of well-being and for use with international populations and other groups who, for any reason, might have difficulty reading English text. The instrument is seen as having the potential to give research voice to those who are too sick or weak to participate in studies that require lengthy measures of well-being and, perhaps, even to persons with mild to moderate cognitive impairment. A secondary purpose of the tool rests in its potential for use as an easy-to-administer clinical indicator of well-being across a wide sector of clinical settings. Based on the work of Abbate (1990), consideration will also be given to the future development of a children's version of the tool.

REFERENCES

Abbate, M. F. (1990). *The relationship of therapeutic horsemanship and human field motion in children with cerebral palsy.* Unpublished master's thesis, Georgia State University, Atlanta.

Barrett, E. A. M. (1990). A measure of power as knowing participation in change. In O. L. Strickland & C. F. Waltz (Eds.). *The measurement of nursing outcomes: Measuring client self-care and coping skills* (Vol. 4). New York, NY: Springer.

Capra, F. (1975). *The Tao of physics.* Berkeley, CA: Shambala.

Davis, A. E. (1989). *The relationship between the phenomenon of traumatic injury and the patterns of power, human field motion, esteem and risk taking.* Unpublished doctoral dissertation, Georgia State University, Atlanta.

Demi, A. S., & Warren, N. A. (1995). Issues in conducting research with vulnerable families. *Western Journal of Nursing Research, 17,* 188–202.

Gueldner, S. H., Michel, Y., Bramlett, M. H., Liu, C. F., Johnston, L. W., Endo, E., et al. (In press). The Wellbeing Picture Scale: A refined version of the Index of Field Energy. *Nursing Science Quarterly.*

Gueldner, S. H., Bramlett, M. H., Johnston, L. W., & Guillory, J. A. (1996). Index of Field Energy. *Rogerian Nursing Science News, 8*(4), 6.

Hills, R. (1998). *Maternal field patterning of awareness, wakefulness, human field motion and well-being in mothers with 6 month old infants: A Rogerian science perspective.* Unpublished doctoral dissertation, Wayne State University, Detroit, MI (UMI No. 9915666).

Hindman, M. (1993). *Humor and field energy in older adults.* Unpublished doctoral dissertation, Medical College of Georgia, Augusta.

Johnston, L. W. (1994). Psychometric analysis of Johnston's Human Field Image Metaphor Scale. *Visions: Journal of Rogerian Nursing Science, 2,* 7–11.

Newman, M. A. (1994). *Health as expanding consciousness.* New York, NY: National League for Nursing [NLN].

Parse, R. R. (2003). *Community: A human becoming perspective.* Boston, MA: Jones and Bartlett.

Parse, R. R. (1997). The human becoming theory: The was, is, and will be. *Nursing Science Quarterly, 10*(1), 32–38.

Phillips, B. B., & Bramlett, M. H. (1994). Integrated awareness: A key to the pattern of mutual process. *Vision, 2,* 7–12.

Morse, J. M. (1997). Responding to threats to integrity of self. *Advances in Nursing Science, 19*(4), 21–36.

Rogers, M. E. (1992). Nursing science and the space age. *Nursing Science Quarterly, 5,* 27–34.

Saunders, J. M., & Valente, S. M. (1992). Overview. *Western Journal of Nursing Research, 14,* 700–702.

Smith, J. A. (1981) The idea of health: A philosophical inquiry. *Advances in Nursing Science, 4,* 43–49.

Spiers, J. (2000). New perspectives on vulnerability using emic and etic approaches. *Journal of Advanced Nursing, 31,* 715–721.

Todaro-Franceschi, V. (1999). *The enigma of energy.* New York, NY: Crossroad.

UNIT III

RESEARCH

Research is formalized curiosity. It is poking and prying with a purpose. It is a seeking that he who wishes may know the cosmic secrets of the world and that they dwell therein.

Zora Neale Hurston

Source: Bartleby.com, retrieved 2/27/04.

CHAPTER 13

Vulnerable Populations Research: A Center for Excellence

Deborah Koniak-Griffin, Jacquelyn H. Flaskerud, and Adeline Nyamathi

Nursing and interdisciplinary scholars have been conducting research on the health problems of vulnerable populations for about 50 years. According to a recent review of articles published in *Nursing Research* during that period, the number of publications with a major focus on health disparities among vulnerable populations has increased each decade, with a sizable jump since 1990 (Flaskerud et al., 2002). Research efforts, however, have largely been uncoordinated and without a strong theoretical base. Many studies have employed quantitative or qualitative designs that may not be appropriate for vulnerable populations, particularly if the researchers have not coordinated their efforts with a community advisory board or involved members of the target community in the research process. Although race and ethnicity are often used as variables in nursing research, this does not ensure that issues of relevance to vulnerable populations are addressed.

In response to the need for coordinated leadership in building the scientific base for vulnerable populations research and educating scholars on vulnerable populations research methods, the University of California, Los Angeles (UCLA), School of Nursing (SON) proposed development of a Center for Vulnerable Populations Research (CVPR). The CVPR was established in 1999 as a Center for Excellence through a 5-year Research Center Core Grant from the National Institute of Nursing Research (NINR). Initial support for the center was received in a changing political and social environment where government funding opportunities were increasingly directed toward improving health outcomes and eliminating the health disparities of vulnerable populations. Several of the objectives of Healthy People 2000 remained unachieved, and a draft of Healthy People 2010 had been written. The areas of research opportunity established by the NINR for 1999 included identifying ways to adapt prevention interventions to the real-life environment of vulnerable populations and developing community-based approaches to behavior change. The sociodemographic characteristics of Los Angeles County and the nation supported the strong need for establishment of the CVPR; e.g., a growing composition of ethnic/racial minority groups and people living in poverty and/or experiencing stigma. Many diseases were disproportionately affecting these groups.

The CVPR evolved from the UCLA SON's long tradition of building excellence and scholarship through research, clinical facilities, and educational programs (Flaskerud, 2000). The SON's history included development of a nurse-managed clinic at the Union Rescue Mission (URM) in 1983 and affiliations with other clinics serving vulnerable populations. The URM provides primary health care to homeless persons and serves as a site for clinical training of nurse practitioner students and for community-based research by faculty. Knowledge and skills relevant to the care of vulnerable populations are gained and expanded as part of the preparation of students for clinical practice. Faculty research efforts supported by federal, state, and private grants have led to identification of the health problems of vulnerable populations and to descriptions of underlying concepts in vulnerable populations research (lack of resources, increased risks, high morbidity, and early mortality). From the mid-1980s to the early 1990s, faculty conducted vulnerable populations research through individual or small group efforts. Some of the participants included low-income women of color who were infected with or at risk for HIV/AIDS and other infectious diseases or who were abusing drugs (e.g., Flaskerud & Calvillo, 1991; Flaskerud & Nyamathi, 1988, 1999; Nyamathi, 1991, 1992), adolescents in detention (Anderson, 1990) or experiencing unplanned early pregnancies (Koniak-Griffin, 1989; Koniak-Griffin, Lominska, & Brecht, 1993), and homeless adults with chronic mental illness (Wuerker & Keenan, 1997). The methodology employed was innovative, including participatory action approaches and the simultaneous use of qualitative and quantitative methods. As faculty's research trajectories expanded and interdisciplinary teams were forming, there was a heightened need for development of collectivity, collaboration, and core services.

The first effort at creating a focused conceptual area of vulnerable populations research, jointly undertaken by faculty, resulted in a 1994 Institutional National Research Services Award to support pre- and postdoctoral research training in the health-related problems of vulnerable populations. With this award came the creation of a graduate course in the health-related problems of vulnerable populations and monthly seminars for sharing resources and building the knowledge and skills of awardees and faculty in vulnerable populations research and methods. These activities led to further development of the Vulnerable Populations Conceptual Model (VPCM) (Flaskerud & Winslow, 1998), which would serve as a conceptual base for the CVPR.

OVERVIEW OF THE CVPR

The CVPR, an interdisciplinary center within a research-intensive public university system, provides core services to benefit faculty and community partners conducting vulnerable populations research. Its major goal is to build nursing science in the area of the health-related problems of vulnerable populations. To this end, partnerships are established with communities through mutual definition of needs and identification of strengths and resources. Based on this assessment, interdisciplinary scientists, research participants, and community collaborators develop and implement research to eliminate health disparities. Research results are disseminated back to communities of researchers, participants, scholars, ethicists, and policy makers. The center provides consultation and education to interdisciplinary investigators on participatory research methods appropriate for use with vulnerable populations; supports ongoing research; and funds, each year, at least three new pilot/feasibility studies designed to improve the health status of vulnerable populations. Core services assist UCLA faculty and community collaborators to develop research programs, with priority for use of these services given to recipient investigators.

The CVPR infrastructure supports accomplishment of these goals through cores for administration, biolaboratory, participatory research and community partnerships, and research support. These cores facilitate resource sharing and strengthening for research base and pilot studies, partnership building between investigators and communities, and knowledge and skills enhancement for interdisciplinary scholars and community partners to conduct research with vulnerable populations. The team of core leaders is composed of six nurse scholars and three interdisciplinary scholars (representing medicine, public health, sociology, and statistics). Table 13.1 presents the specific aims of the CVPR cores and examples of related activities designed to facilitate collaboration and skills development. The administrative core coordinates activities and projects and facilitates communications among core faculty and affiliated members through a variety of mechanisms, such as written communication, e-mails, the CVPR Web site, and newsletters. Research is disseminated through publications in nursing and interdisciplinary journals; news releases; presentations at regional, national, and international professional meetings; and community events (e.g., forums).

CONCEPTUAL FOUNDATION FOR THE CVPR

Since its establishment, the work of the CVPR has been guided by the VPCM, which was informed by conceptualizations of Aday (1993) on predictors of populations at risk (i.e., social status, human capital, social capital). Other influential writings included the work of Link & Phelan (1996) on determinants of the health of populations and the human rights approach for reducing individual, program-related, and societal vulnerability (Mann & Tarantola, 1996). The VPCM proposes that resource availability, relative risk, and health status are related (see Figure 13.1).

Vulnerable populations are social groups that experience differential patterns of morbidity, mortality, and life expectancy as a result of limited resources and exposure to risks (Flaskerud & Winslow, 1998). Social groups recognized as vulnerable populations include women and children, ethnic people of color, immigrants, gay men and lesbians, homeless persons, the elderly, and those living in poverty. Also included are disabled persons and those subjected to discrimination, intolerance, subordination, and stigma and those who are politically marginalized, disenfranchised, and denied human rights (Amaro, 1995; Carlisle, Leake, Brook, & Shapiro, 1996; Guralnik & Leveille, 1997; Jetter, Orleck, & Taylor, 1995; Link & Phelan, 1996; Mann & Tarantola, 1996). These groups are not mutually exclusive and often overlap. The Health Resources and Services Administration (HRSA, 2000) describes ethnicity, gender, income, and insurance status as among the factors related to poor health. Similarly, the NINR (2000) identifies the poor and members of specific ethnic groups among persons long recognized for suffering health disparities, defined as "differences in the incidence, prevalence, mortality and burden of diseases and other adverse health conditions that exist among specific population groups."

Resource availability refers to human capital; i.e., income, jobs, education, housing, health insurance, social status (power), social connection (integration into society, social networks), and environmental resources (health care access and quality) (Evans, Barer, & Marmor, 1994; Solberg, Brekke, & Kottke, 1997). Relative risk is conceptualized in the VPCM as the ratio of the risk of poor health among groups having fewer resources and exposed to increased risk factors compared with those having more resources and exposed to fewer risk factors (Aday, 1993, 1994; Flaskerud, 1998; Flaskerud & Winslow, 1998). Risk factors may be behavioral (e.g., lifestyle choices; availability, access to, and use or nonuse of screening procedures and health promotion services; exposure to violence and abuse) or biological (e.g., physiological and genetic predisposition). Laboratory assays provide direct measurements at molecular, cellular, and physiological levels that indicate exposures or risk-taking behaviors (Salama, Serrano, & Au,

TABLE **13.1**   Aims and Activities of the CVPR Cores

Core	Specific aims	Examples of activities
Administrative	Continue expanding the scientific knowledge base of health-related problems of vulnerable populations to 1) reduce/eliminate health disparities, focusing on infections, chronic illness, substance use, and environmental quality; 2) facilitate health promotion; and 3) improve outcomes of nursing practice.	Coordination of CVPR activities, monitoring the pilot study program, coordinating monthly colloquium, maintaining communications among vulnerable population researchers and community partners about CVPR activities through written communication, e-mails, the CVPR Web site, and newsletters.
Biolaboratory	Expand the capacity to measure, analyze, and link biological and behavioral markers in vulnerable populations research.	Provide expertise on 1) translation of cutting edge lab technologies to incorporate selected appropriate strategies in participatory research designs, 2) selection of lab technologies/analyses that maximize ability to measure constructs in the CVPR model, and 3) selected in-house and outsourced lab assays or technology-driven strategies.
Participatory Research & Community Partnership	Translate the knowledge, skills, and experience acquired through participatory research methods and community partnerships by university and community investigators into practice/action to	Provide expertise on 1) mentoring new and experienced community and university investigators in use of participatory research methods and establishing community partnerships; 2) strengthening existing community

TABLE 13.1 Aims and Activities of the CVPR Cores (*Continued*)

Core	Specific aims	Examples of activities
	improve the health status of vulnerable populations and to develop science in this area.	partnerships, developing partnerships with a minority-serving university, and seeking new community partners to conduct research addressing health disparities; 3) assisting investigators to develop cultural and linguistically competent programs of community research; 4) developing additional strategies to influence health, social and public policy; and 5) disseminating methods and work/outcomes of the core to participating communities, other investigators, clinicians, ethicists, and policy makers. Conducting a Summer Institute for training in community-based participatory research.
Research Support	Create mechanisms for interdisciplinary preparation of scientists and collaboration of scientists in biobehavioral research with vulnerable populations involving qualitative and quantitative methodology.	Instrumentation, including translation, psychometric testing, developing new culturally sensitive measures, and facilitating Web-based access to research instruments and data on vulnerable populations; biostatistical consultation; data entry management and analysis support; building databases for secondary analyses.

CVPR, Center for Vulnerable Populations Research.

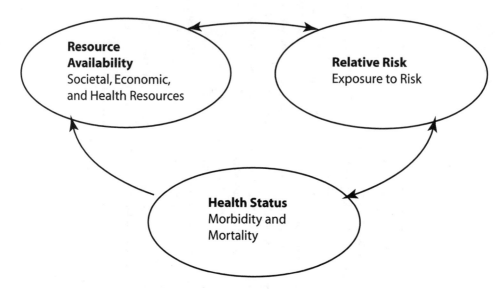

FIGURE 13.1   Vulnerable Populations Conceptual Model
Adapted from Flaskerud and Winslow, 1998, *Nursing Research* 47(2): 69–78.

1999). Disease prevalence and morbidity and mortality rates indicate the health status of a community. There are three proposed relationships among the major constructs: 1) resources and risks, 2) risks and health status, and 3) health status and resources. Lack of resources in a community increases exposure to risk, and increased risk factors can reduce resource availability. Increased exposure to risk factors leads to higher rates of morbidity and mortality, which may exacerbate further exposure to risk factors and affect resource availability by further depleting resources. Nursing research, practice, and ethical and policy analysis are presented in the model as having the potential to affect resources, relative risk, and health status directly as well as indirectly (i.e., intervening in the relationships among these constructs). Research on health-related problems of vulnerable populations can have a behavioral, biological, or health systems focus, or it can have a combination of these.

Extensive research supports the major relationships in the VPCM. A multidisciplinary group of expert scientists and clinicians, convened by the National Heart, Lung and Blood Institute (NHLBI) to review research on risk factors for disparities in asthma health outcomes, emphasized the importance of viewing socioeconomic status and race as fundamental social causative factors that contribute to disparities in access to resources, avoidance of risks, and minimization of the consequences of disease (Strunk, Ford, & Taggart, 2002). The continued widening gap in rates of selected diseases (e.g., diabetes, HIV/AIDS) between ethnic and/or racial groups (e.g., African Americans and whites) suggests that factors other than lifestyle and behaviors, such as availability of social power and economic and health resources, may be influencing the difference. The VPCM has been/is being applied in research conducted by pre- and postdoctoral fellows and faculty at UCLA (Albright, 1999; Conde, 2003; Davis & Curley, 1999; Dixon, Guilliaum, Robinson, & Weathersby, 2000; Flaskerud, 1999; Flaskerud & Kim, 1999; Lesser & Escoto-Lloyd, 1999; Lesser & Koniak-Griffin, 2000; Strehlow & Amos-Jones, 1999; Tullmann & Chang, 1999; Tyson & Fleming, 1999; Winslow & Carter, 1999).

CVPR AND COMMUNITY-BASED PARTICIPATORY RESEARCH

A hallmark of the CVPR is the expertise of its investigators in applying participatory research methods as a framework for many studies and mentoring new investigators in its application. The participatory research model represents a collaborative process in which research questions are developed by the investigators and the "subjects" as full partners in the entire research process (Flaskerud & Anderson, 1999; Reason, 1994). These questions arise in the community, are investigated in the community, and result in research products that belong to and are useful to the community. Community members are acknowledged as both cultural and community experts (McQuiston, Choi-Hevel, & Clawson, 2001). Because of their active involvement, participants also serve as project advocates.

As a systematic approach to inquiry, participatory research incorporates basic principles from formative program evaluation and action research methods (Rogers & Palmer-Erbs, 1994), as well as principles from other fields of inquiry such as feminist theory, cooperative inquiry, and anthropology. Successful employment of participatory research methods leads to the empowerment of participants, organizations, and communities through acquisition of knowledge and skills and the building of community capacity (Israel, Checkoway, Schulz, & Zimmerman, 1994). Community-partnered research projects are increasingly recognized as an effective method to reduce and/or eliminate health disparities. Partnerships may include geographic, ethnic, or university communities and districts served by community-based organizations (CBOs). The North American Primary Care Research Group endorsed participatory research strategies in its policy statement (1998), noting that traditional methods in health research have failed to effect change or to ameliorate social and economic conditions related to health disparities.

Using the participatory research approach, CVPR investigators have conducted several successful studies that have led to empowerment for project participants. Projects vary in the degree of comprehensiveness of the participatory research methods applied, from full use of the VPCM to more limited applications involving participants as members of community advisory boards that provide consultation. HIV/AIDS research with adults and young parents and in studies with adolescents in juvenile detention supports participatory research as a vehicle for facilitating community empowerment and enfranchisement and for engendering a sense of power and control in the lives of participants (Anderson, 1999; Anderson, Nyamathi, McAvoy, Conde, & Casey, 2001; Flaskerud & Anderson, 1999; Flaskerud & Nyamathi, 2000; Lesser, Tello, Koniak-Griffin, Kappos, & Rhys, 2001).

Findings of a recently completed CVPR pilot study showed that lack of availability of resources (income, access to regular medical care) contributed to higher rates of use of emergency/urgent care services and hospitalization among Latino families having young children with asthma (Berg et al., 2004). An ongoing epidemiological study with mine workers in China, led by Dr. Wendie Robbins, incorporates participatory research methods in investigating the relationship between exposure to boron-containing compounds and adverse reproductive effects in men. The following section highlights another CVPR-sponsored, community-based participatory research project.

LAY HEALTH ADVISORS PROJECT

A community-based participatory research project for health promotion within a Latino community was undertaken by the CVPR with support from the NINR (P30 NR05041-02S1,

2000–2002). CVPR investigators formed a collaborative partnership with the Los Angeles County Department of Health Services (LACDHS), CBOs, and community residents to plan, implement, and evaluate this study (Kim, Flaskerud, Koniak-Griffin, & Dixon, unpublished manuscript). In the early planning phase, CVPR investigators approached LACDHS officials to discuss the study, focusing on participatory inquiry and collaborative methods. As ideas were exchanged, LACDHS staff shared information about their experiences conducting outreach programs using community health promoters or lay health advisors (LHAs). A decision was made to apply the LHA model to educate a "target community" about healthy lifestyle behaviors (nutrition, physical activity/exercise, and avoidance of exposure to tobacco smoke) in an attempt to reduce the community's risk for cardiovascular disease.

The use of LHAs (also referred to as lay health advocates, educators, or promoters) for health promotion in underserved communities and with vulnerable populations is a practice that has been reported for over 30 years, particularly in the prevention of sexually transmitted infections (McQuiston et al., 2001; Thomas, Earp, & Eng, 2000) and cervical and breast cancers (Earp et al., 1997; Navarro, Rock, McNicholas, Senn, & Moreno, 2000) and improving maternal–child health (Carrillo, Pust, & Borbon, 1986; Warrick, Wood, Mesiter, & de Zapie, 1992). Surprisingly, few empirical studies have tested its effectiveness. LHAs are ideally suited for active involvement in health promotion efforts. As members of their own community and culture, they are aware of the community's historical roots, strengths, and challenges; have intricate social networks in place; and are well situated to provide culturally competent care in their own communities (Poss, 1999; HRSA, n.d.).

The aims of the study were to 1) conduct a community needs assessment in order to choose a service planning area within Los Angeles County and to determine which community group had the greatest need for health education (healthy nutrition, physical activity/exercise, and smoke-free environment) because of cardiovascular disease risk factors and a lack of health and social resources; 2) develop and implement a LHA training program focusing on the identified community group; and 3) conduct and evaluate an outreach program to reduce cardiovascular disease risk in the target community that would be taught by LHAs using their existing social networks (Kim, Flaskerud et al., unpublished manuscript).

The study had three phases. In phase 1, a community needs assessment was performed by interviewing 33 key informants (RNs, social workers, counselors, teachers, epidemiologists, executives, and health officers from LACDHS primary care and public health clinics, neighborhood clinics, health facilities, school districts, and CBOs). Interview data were supplemented with information from public health reports and statistical data. Two CBOs identified during the data-gathering process provided valuable information that influenced the decision by the research team to select their community (Pacoima, within service planning area 2 of Los Angeles County). Pacoima was found to be 80% Latino, with many residents uninsured and living below the poverty level. Based on poor nutritional status, limited physical activity (evidenced by high rates of overweight and obesity), and high prevalence of smoking, Latinos were chosen as the target vulnerable population for the study. Following recommendations of the LACDHS team (directors, nurses, nutritionists, a program analyst, and health educators), training materials were selected, and the decision was made to offer the training program in Spanish (Kim, Flaskerud et al., unpublished manuscript).

In phase 2, CVPR investigators continued to collaborate closely with CBOs in Pacoima, inviting CBO representatives and residents from the community to join a community advisory board. The community advisory board was instrumental in tailoring the study to the target community; e.g., by suggesting that LHAs be referred to as health promoters (HPs) or *promotoras de salud,* a more meaningful term. The community advisory board also reviewed the training program materials and offered insight into the recruitment of HPs. Twelve HPs participated in the 15-session training, which prepared them to conduct a cardiovascular disease prevention program and to assist with data collection. The sociodemographic characteristics of HPs included a mean age of 39.4 years, time in the United States of 15.11 years, and a mean education of 12.44 years. Several had prior experience in the role of HP. Training was provided by the LACDHS team using *Your Heart, Your Life: A Bilingual Health Promoters' Manual (Su Corazon, Su Vida)* (Alcalay, Alvarado, Balcazar, Newman, & Huerta, 1999). This culturally appropriate, community-based, theory-driven manual was developed and pilot tested by the NHLBI to increase knowledge and awareness of cardiovascular health in the Latino community. Content focuses on prevention of cardiovascular disease through promotion of healthy nutrition and exercise. The CVPR research team provided supplementary information on smoke-free environments, the HP role, class management, principles of protection of human subjects, data collection techniques, and safety issues. Culturally appropriate videotapes, instructional aids (e.g., picture cards, food models), handouts, and opportunities for demonstration and feedback were important training components. During each session, a 10-minute physical activity break was conducted by the facilitators, who used audio- and videotapes to lead the group in practicing low-impact aerobics and stretching, in accord with their individual tolerances.

To assist the HPs in accurately recalling important information from the training program *(Your Heart, Your Life),* a core (shortened) curriculum was provided in addition to the training manual. Each HP practiced teaching using this core curriculum, designed for delivery in three 2-hour sessions, because funding constraints in this pilot study prevented implementation of the entire *Your Heart, Your Life* curriculum. Applying participatory research principles, HPs provided feedback on the intervention program and plans for phase 3, leading to modifications and creative additions to tailor the program to the intended audience. All HPs completed a knowledge questionnaire at baseline and after the training. Satisfactory performance on the posttest was required.

In phase 3, nine HPs implemented the core curriculum and collected baseline, posttest, and 1-month follow-up evaluations (Kim, Flaskerud et al., unpublished manuscript). They successfully recruited participants through use of their social networks at sites such as parent centers, churches, and community organizations. Classes were conducted in Spanish in schools, community centers, homes, and a church. The rate of attrition was extremely low (6%). HPs verbally administered an 11-item health beliefs questionnaire and a 23-item lifestyle behavior questionnaire to assess nutrition, physical activity/exercise, and the presence of smoke-free environments. Additional open-ended questions addressed participants' successes and challenges relating to awareness and motivation issues, incorporating and maintaining specific practices in their daily lives, and cooperation or resistance from family members. The lifestyle behavior measure developed for the pilot study had adequate reliability (Cronbach's alpha = 0.77 for total lifestyle behaviors, $\alpha = 0.71$ for nutrition, $\alpha = 0.68$ for physical activity behaviors, and $\alpha = 0.77$ for smoke-free behaviors). However, reliability for the health beliefs questionnaire was substantially lower.

Complete data are available for the 256 participants who were predominantly women (98%), Catholic (88%), and married (76%). They did not work outside the home (71%), tended to lack health insurance (51%), and had a mean age of 38 years. Most were of Mexican or Mexican-American descent; more than half had lived in the United States less than 14 years (56%) and had less than 9 years of education (60%) (Kim, Koniak-Griffin, Flaskerud, & Guarnero, in press).

Outcome data from participants in the cardiovascular disease prevention program were compared with data collected from a "natural" control group of 122 members of the same community with similar sociodemographic characteristics. The control group completed the baseline and 1-month follow-up questionnaires but did not receive the intervention. Following completion of data collection, they were offered a one-session nutrition class. Results of repeated measures analyses of variance (ANOVAs) revealed a significant interaction between group and time for the total lifestyle behavior questionnaire ($F[1345] = 46.72, p < 0.0001$) and for two subscales: nutrition ($F[1345] = 39.99, p < 0.0001$) and physical activity ($F[1345] = 36.09, p < 0.0001$). Participants in the cardiovascular disease prevention program showed significant improvement over time in these lifestyle behaviors, whereas those in the control group showed no change. On a knowledge measure, group differences over time were not observed; however, data analyses with paired comparison t-tests ($df = 247$) revealed significant increases in scores from baseline to follow-up for overall health knowledge ($t = 2.41, p < 0.05$) and nutrition-related knowledge ($t = 3.16, p < 0.01$) within the treatment group, suggesting a positive knowledge influence of the HPs.

Preliminary themes emerged from the open-ended data on successes and challenges related to behavior changes (Kim, Koniak-Griffin et al., in press). In the area of nutrition, successes included eliminating unhealthy foods from the family diet and incorporating healthier food preparation; challenges were eliciting cooperation of family members and maintaining family interest in healthier foods. For physical activity, successes were expressed as feeling a sense of well-being and weight loss, engaging in daily exercise, and involving family members in an exercise routine. Successes reported for a smoke-free environment were related to discussing and setting up a smoke-free home. The main challenge in this area was setting limits consistently in homes with more than one smoker. Many participants reported at baseline that they could not recall a doctor or nurse ever talking to them about exercising (37.5%), their weight (42.2%), or smoking (50%).

Results from the pilot study demonstrate that HPs can be successfully trained to deliver an education program designed to reduce the risk of cardiovascular disease in underserved Latinos through promotion of healthy nutrition, physical activity/exercise, and decreased exposure to environmental tobacco smoke. This intervention can be delivered at a grassroots level without being attached to sites traditionally used to disseminate health information. Furthermore, HPs can collect data to assist researchers in evaluating intervention effects. The community-based intervention had many promising indicators for sustainability over time, such as a good fit between local providers and the intervention and the use of HPs and members of the community advisory board to advocate for the program. Overall, findings validate the effectiveness of HPs in health promotion and support the need for larger-scale investigations of this alternative health care delivery strategy, particularly in communities with immigrant populations and limited resources (Kim, Koniak-Griffin, et al., in press).

CONCLUSION

Since establishment as a Center for Excellence, the CVPR has advanced knowledge about the health-related problems of vulnerable populations by supporting ongoing research and new pilot/feasibility studies and by providing a variety of educational activities for academics and community members. Investigators are successfully applying community-based participatory research methods rather than traditional research approaches to confront health disparities affecting vulnerable populations. The partnerships established with communities are enhancing the abilities of researchers, participants, and communities to conduct significant research and other activities that appropriately address the needs of vulnerable populations. The contributions of CVPR investigators and affiliates provide strong evidence of how focused efforts can advance science in the area of vulnerable populations. The continued existence of health disparities among vulnerable populations and related national health priorities support the importance of continuing efforts by the CVPR and other academic and community organizations to confront these important issues.

REFERENCES

Aday, L. A. (1993). *At risk in America: The health and health care needs of vulnerable populations in the United States.* San Francisco, CA: Jossey-Bass.

Aday, L. A. (1994). Health status of vulnerable populations. *Annual Review of Public Health, 15,* 487–509.

Albright, A. V. (1999). Vulnerability to depression: Youth at risk. *Nursing Clinics of North America, 34,* 393–408.

Alcalay, R., Alvarado, M., Balcazar, H., Newman, E., & Huerta, E. (1999). Salud para su corazon: A community-based Latino cardiovascular disease prevention and outreach model. *Journal of Community Health, 25,* 359–379.

Amaro, H. (1995). Love, sex and power: Considering women's realities in HIV prevention. *American Psychologist, 50,* 437–447.

Anderson, N. L .R. (1990). Pregnancy resolution decisions in juvenile detention. *Archives of Psychiatric Nursing, 5,* 325–331.

Anderson, N. L. R. (1999). Perceptions about substance use among male adolescents in juvenile detention. *Western Journal of Nursing Research, 21,* 652–672.

Anderson, N. L. R., Nyamathi, A., McAvoy, J. A., Conde, F., & Casey, C. (2001). Perceptions of risk for HIV/AIDS among adolescents in juvenile detention. *Western Journal of Nursing Research, 23,* 336–359.

Berg, J., Wahlgren, D. R., Hofstetter, C. R., Meltzer, S. B., Meltzer, E. O., Matt, G. E., et al. (2004). Latino children with asthma: Rates and risks for medical care utilization. *Journal of Asthma, 41,* 147–157.

Carlisle, D. M., Leake, B. D., Brook, R. H., & Shapiro, M. F. (1996). The effect of race and ethnicity on the rise of selected health care procedures: A comparison of South Central Los Angeles and the remainder of Los Angeles County. *Journal of Health Care for the Poor and Underserved, 7,* 308–322.

Carrillo, J. M., Pust, R. E., & Borbon, J. (1986). Dar a Luz: A perinatal care program for Hispanic women on the U.S.–Mexico border. *American Journal of Preventive Medicine, 2,* 26–29.

Conde, F. (2003). Risk factors for male osteoporosis. *Urologic Oncology: Seminars and Original Investigations, 21,* 380–383.

Davis, C. M., & Curley, C. M. (1999). Disparities of health in African Americans. *Nursing Clinics of North America, 34,* 345–358.

Dixon, E. L., Guilliaum, M. G., Robinson, E. M., & Weathersby, J. H. (2000). Underrepresentation: Minority populations in the health professions. *Journal of Chi Eta Phi Sorority (JOCEPS), 47,* 23–27.

Earp, J. A., Viadro, C. I., Vincus, A. A., Altpeter, M., Flax, V., Mayne, L., et al. (1997). Lay health advisors: A strategy for getting the word out about breast cancer. *Health Education & Behavior, 24,* 432–451.

Evans, R. G., Barer, M., & Marmor, T. R. (1994). *Why are some people healthy and others not? The determinants of the health of populations.* New York, NY: Aldine De Gruyter.

Flaskerud, J. H. (1998). Vulnerable populations. In J. J. Fitzpatrick (Ed.). *Encyclopedia of nursing research.* New York, NY: Springer.

Flaskerud, J. H. (Ed.). (1999). Emerging nursing care of vulnerable populations. *Nursing Clinics of North America, 34,* xv, 261–408.

Flaskerud, J. H. (2000) Developing leadership and excellence with vulnerable populations in research, education, and practice. *Nursing Leadership Forum, 4,* 76–83.

Flaskerud, J. H., & Anderson, N. L. R. (1999). Disseminating the results of participant-focused research. *Journal of Transcultural Nursing, 10,* 340–349.

Flaskerud, J. H., & Calvillo, E. R. (1991). Beliefs about AIDS health, and illness among low income Latina women. *Research in Nursing and Health, 14,* 431–438.

Flaskerud, J. H., & Kim, S. (1999). Health problems of Asian and Latino immigrants. *Nursing Clinics of North America, 34,* 359–380.

Flaskerud, J. H., Lesser, J., Dixon, E., Anderson, N., Conde, F., Kim, S., et al. (2002). Health disparities among vulnerable populations. *Nursing Research, 51,* 74–85.

Flaskerud, J. H., & Nyamathi, A. (1988). An AIDS education program for Vietnamese women. *New York State Journal of Medicine, 88,* 632–737.

Flaskerud, J. H., & Nyamathi, A. (1989). Black and Latina women's AIDS related knowledge, attitudes and practices. *Research in Nursing and Health, 12,* 339–346.

Flaskerud, J. H., & Nyamathi, A. (2000). Collaborative inquiry with low-income Latina women. *Journal of Health Care for the Poor and Underserved, 11,* 326–342.

Flaskerud, J. H., & Winslow, B. (1998). Conceptualizing vulnerable populations health-related research. *Nursing Research, 33,* 69–78.

Guralnik, J. M., & Leveille, S. G. (1997). Race, ethnicity, and health outcomes: Unraveling and mediating the role of socioeconomic status. *American Journal of Public Health, 87,* 728–729.

Health Resources and Services Administration [HRSA]. (2000). *Eliminating health disparities in the U.S.* HRS 00167. Rockville, MD: HRSA.

HRSA. (n.d.) Office of Minority Health. *Overview.* Retrieved July 7, 2003, from *www.hrsa.gov/OMH/overview.htm.*

Israel, B., Checkoway, B., Schulz, A., & Zimmerman, M. (1994). Health education and community empowerment: Conceptualizing and measuring perceptions of individual, organizational, and community control. *Health Education Quarterly, 21,* 149–170.

Jetter, A., Orleck, A., & Taylor, D. (1995). Mothers at risk: The war on poor women and children. In G. J. Demko & M. C. Jackson (Eds.). *Populations at risk in America* (pp. 104–128). Boulder, CO: Westview.

Kim, S., Flaskerud, J. H., Koniak-Griffin, D., & Dixon, E. (2003). Community partnered participatory research for health promotion in Latino community. Unpublished manuscript.

Kim, S., Koniak-Griffin, D., Flaskerud, J. H., & Guarnero, P. (in press). The impact of lay health advisors on cardiovascular health promotion: Using a community-based participatory approach. *Journal of Cardiovascular Nursing.*

Koniak-Griffin, D. (1989). Psychosocial and clinical variables in pregnant adolescents: A survey of maternity home residents. *Journal of Adolescent Health Care, 16,* 23–29.

Koniak-Griffin, D., Lominska, S., & Brecht, M. (1993). Social support during adolescent pregnancy: A comparison of three ethnic groups. *Journal of Adolescence, 16,* 43–56.

Lesser, J., & Escoto-Lloyd, S. (1999). Health-related problems in a vulnerable population: Pregnant teens and adolescent mothers. *Nursing Clinics of North America, 34,* 289–300.

Lesser J., & Koniak-Griffin, D. (2000). The impact of physical or sexual abuse on chronic depression in adolescent mothers. *Journal of Pediatric Nursing, 15,* 378–387.

Lesser, J., Tello, J., Koniak-Griffin, D., Kappos, B., & Rhys, M. (2001). Young Latino fathers' perceptions of paternal role and risk for HIV/AIDS. *Hispanic Journal of Behavioral Sciences, 23,* 327–343.

Link, G. B., & Phelan, J. C. (1996). Understanding sociodemographic differences in health: The role of fundamental social causes. *American Journal of Public Health, 86,* 471–473.

Mann, J. A., & Tarantola, D. (1996). From vulnerability to human rights. In J. A. Mann & D. Tarantola (Eds.). *AIDS in the world, II: Global dimensions, social roots, and responses* (pp. 463–476). New York, NY: Oxford University Press.

McQuiston, C., Choi-Hevel, S., & Clawson, M. (2001). Protegiendo nuestra comunidad: Empowerment participatory education for HIV prevention. *Journal of Transcultural Nursing, 12,* 275–283.

National Institute of Nursing Research [NINR]. (2000). *Strategic plan on reducing health disparities.* Retrieved June 27, 2003, from *www.nih.gov/ninr/researcli/diverstiy/mission.html.*

Navarro, A. M., Rock, C. L., McNicholas, L. .J., Senn, K. L., & Moreno, C. (2000). Community-based education in nutrition and cancer: The Por La Vida Cuidandome curriculum. *Journal of Cancer Education, 15,* 168–172.

North American Primary Care Research Group. (1998, November 6). *Responsible research with communities: Participatory research in primary care. Policy Statement.* Vancouver, BC, Canada: North American Primary Care Research Group.

Nyamathi, A. (1991). Relationship of resources to emotional distress, somatic complaints and high risk behaviors in drug recovery and homeless minority women. *Research in Nursing and Health, 14,* 269–277.

Nyamathi, A. (1992). A comparative study of factors affecting risk level of black homeless women. *Journal of Acquired Immune Deficiency Syndromes, 5,* 222–228.

Poss, J. E. (1999). Providing culturally competent care: Is there a role for health promoters? *Nursing Outlook, 47,* 30–36.

Reason, P. (1994). Three approaches to participative inquiry. In N. K. Denzin & Y. S. Lincoln (Eds.). *Handbook of qualitative research* (pp. 324–329). Thousand Oaks, CA: Sage.

Rogers, E. S., & Palmer-Erbs, V. (1994). Participatory action research: Implications for research and evaluation in psychiatric evaluation. *Psychosocial Rehabilitation Journal, 18,* 3–12.

Salama, S. A., Serrano, M. A., & Au, W. W. (1999). Biomonitoring using accessible human cells for exposure and health risk assessment. *Mutation Research, 436,* 99–122.

Solberg, L. L, Brekke, M. L., & Kottke, T. W. (1997). How important are clinician and nurse attitudes to the delivery of clinical preventive services? *Journal of Family Practice, 44,* 451–461.

Strehlow, A., & Amos-Jones, T. (1999). Emerging nursing care of vulnerable populations. *Nursing Clinics of North America, 34,* 261–274.

Strunk, R. C., Ford, J. G., & Taggart, V. (2002). Reducing disparities in asthma care: Priorities for research: National Heart, Lung, and Blood Institute workshop report. *Journal of Allergy and Clinical Immunology, 109,* 229–237.

Thomas, J. C., Earp, J. A., & Eng, E. (2000). Evaluation and lessons learned from a lay health advisor program to prevent sexually transmitted diseases. *International Journal of STD and AIDS, 11,* 812–818.

Tullmann, D. F., & Chang, B. (1999). Nursing care of the elderly as a vulnerable population. *Nursing Clinics of North America, 34,* 333–344.

Tyson, S., & Fleming, B. (1999). Conceptualizing battered women as a vulnerable population: A case study report. *Nursing Clinics of North America, 34,* 301–312.

Warrick, L. H., Wood, A. H., Mesiter, J. S, & de Zapie, J. G. (1992). Evaluation of a peer health worker prenatal outreach and education program for Hispanic farmworker families. *Journal of Community Health, 17,* 13–26

Winslow, B. W., & Carter, P. (1999). Patterns of burden in wives who care for husbands with dementia. *Nursing Clinics of North America, 34,* 275–288.

Wuerker, A. K., & Keenan, C. K. (1997). Patterns of psychiatric service use by homeless mentally ill clients. *Psychiatric Quarterly, 68,* 101–116.

CHAPTER 14

Client Discourse in the Renal Context: Living on Dialysis

Nick Polaschek

"How can the truth of the sick subject ever be told?" (Foucault, 1990, p. 30).

What do we know about the experience of living on dialysis? Today, several million people around the world with end-stage renal disease (ESRD) continue to live by using various forms of renal replacement therapy. They are a classic example of a group with a chronic condition, untreatable in the past, which can now be managed with modern medical technology. Although there is a large body of literature that objectively assesses the well-being of people with ESRD, there are very few studies that have sought to understand the subjective experience of living on dialysis (Curtin, Mapes, Petillo, & Oberley, 1998; Gregory, Way, Hutchinson, Barrett, & Parfrey, 1998; Nagle, 1998; Faber, 2000).

This absence in the renal literature parallels the obscurity of the renal client experience within the renal setting itself. It is not easy for health professionals to understand the distinctive experiences of people living on dialysis. The professional focus on the complex process of medical management of specific disease entities ("a 43-year-old Caucasian male presenting with mesingio-capillary glomerulonephritis") leaves little time for active consideration of the subjective attitudes of renal clients. It is also difficult for health care professionals, supervising therapies they assume to be valuable and efficacious, to recognize their limitations for clients using them, especially the problems created by the therapies themselves. Instead, there is a focus on the issue of the failure to comply with the therapeutic prescription on the part of people using dialysis.

The prevalent professional viewpoint, an expression of the optimistic ideology of the acute curative paradigm of biomedicine (Morris, 1999), obscures the renal client experience, hiding the vulnerability of this population living with a chronic condition who depend on medical technology to survive. In preventing acute mortality from ESRD, medical science has created a new state of human being, the "renally replaced life." Although this state is defined objectively in medical terms, this is not the only way that it can be understood. The renally replaced life can also be described in terms derived from subjects who are experiencing it (Curtin et al., 1998; Gregory et al., 1998). Articulating their characteristic "concerns" based on the difficulties of living on dialysis may express a dissonance between the client perspective and the dominant professional viewpoint that obscures it (Faber, 2000).

In order to uncover the client perspective on the renally replaced life, appropriate research approaches are needed. Given that the experiences of people living on dialysis are not easily discerned in the renal setting, research that seeks to understand the perspective of renal clients needs to employ methodologies that explicitly take into account the specialized social context of the renal setting (Polaschek, 2003). Because experienced nurses can respond to the concerns of their clients in their practice in the renal setting, nursing researchers are a group who have an orientation and an interest in undertaking the kinds of research necessary to uncover the client experiences of the renally replaced life.

METHODOLOGY: A CRITICAL INTERPRETIVE APPROACH

The research study described in this chapter employed a particular methodology, a critical interpretive approach, in order to understand the experiences of one group of people living on dialysis, white men using hemodialysis in their homes (Polaschek, 2003a). This approach is an expression of the interpretive paradigm in research. It is based on a "radical relativist" stance toward reality that recognizes the interpretive character of all human thought, in contrast to the positivist view prevalent in contemporary scientific study (Schwandt, 1994; Crotty, 1998). It uses a specific synthesis of the hermeneutic and critical social science traditions in research, an alternative to their combination, as critical hermeneutics, used by some nursing researchers (Thompson, 1990; Allen, 1995). In critical hermeneutics, the hermeneutic approach is recognized as foundational but is then included within a definitive critical framework.

By contrast, in the critical interpretive approach developed for this study, the hermeneutic and critical traditions are related in a different way within the interpretive paradigm, reflecting the radical relativist ethos of the postmodern milieu where all "meta-narratives" have lost their absolute authority (Crotty, 1998). In a critical interpretive approach, the hermeneutic is understood as foundational but requiring contextualization in order to become fully meaningful. According to the hermeneutic understanding, the researcher in a study such as this seeks interpretations from participants in a social setting but does so from a distinctive interpretive standpoint, a critical view of the specific context being studied. Within this approach, the critical is a provisional stance rather than a definitive framework.

A critical interpretive approach involves engaging in interpretive work by adopting the critical standpoint that there can be a variety of interpretations reflecting different positions within a specific context and that certain interpretations may be distorted or obscured by the dominant ideology within a social setting. Researchers, when employing a hermeneutic approach with a critical orientation, recognize the character of the specific context in terms of differences in the knowledge and power of various groups within it and do not simply accept the common interpretation at face value. Instead, they attempt to discern a range of interpretations in terms of the different positions of various groups within the social context being studied. By contextualizing the views given by participants, researchers can discern interpretations that may be less visible or even opposed to the dominant viewpoint. Integral to this approach is a recognition that researchers are powerfully positioned in relation to the specific settings they are studying (Lather, 1991).

This research methodology was operationalized in the design for this study of the experience of living on home hemodialysis as a three-phase process. The initial phase involved developing an approach to the research topic. This included both reflection on the positioning of the researcher himself in relation to it and development of a critical standpoint to view the renal setting. This study made use of work about the health care context derived from the French social philosopher Michel Foucault to establish a critical model of the renal setting.

The central phase of information gathering involved an interpretive response to the participants in the study. Six white men were interviewed in their own homes for 1 hour on three separate occasions. From these interviews, written accounts of their experience were produced. In the final phase, the participants' accounts were reinterpreted by contextualizing them in terms of the critical model of the renal setting. By discerning various commonalities across the texts from this critical standpoint, several concerns were described that delineated the common perspective underlying individual views, in contrast to the dominant professional viewpoint in the renal setting.

The application of this methodology involved a dialectic of empathetic engagement and critical reflection in all the phases of the study in order to discern the distinctive features of the experience of participants as renal clients. The outcomes of the study were 1) the critical model of the renal setting and 2) the description of four concerns of the renal client experience.

CREDIBILITY: THE RESEARCHER'S POSITION IN RELATION TO THE STUDY

The credibility of a study employing this type of methodology has two important aspects: the ethical issues involved in the research and the criteria necessary to enable assessment of its quality. The use of the critical interpretive approach raised a number of important ethical issues, which were addressed in the application for ethical approval to conduct the study. These centered on the positioning of the researcher in relation to the study and the renal clients who were participants in it. The powerful location of the nurse researcher in this kind of study provides significant opportunities to misrepresent and even exploit participants while achieving personal professional goals.

Both the methodology developed for the study and the design produced to operationalize it highlighted this relationship between researcher and participants as a key issue for the success of the study. Given the initial recognition that the client perspective is obscured in the renal setting by the dominant professional viewpoint, the methodology itself, including the critical model of the renal setting, sought to delineate the relationship between renal clients and health professionals as a basis to enable the study to uncover the experience of living on dialysis. This approach informed all of the study processes, from the selection of participants, interviews, and production of client accounts to the critical analysis of these to describe the client perspective. In particular, the researcher explicitly addressed the issue of his relationship with each participant before, during, and after the interviews.

In this study, the participants, as clients in the local renal service, knew the nurse researcher who worked within it. This raised specific issues about gaining free consent from potential participants and ensuring privacy of the information that was provided by them for the research. Explicit processes to address these issues were set up. It was decided that these potential problems were manageable and were outweighed by the advantages of working with participants within a common context. "Insider" knowledge of the particular renal setting could enhance full, honest cooperation by participants and enable insight into the client perspective in a way not possible for a more distanced investigator.

Appropriate criteria for assessing the quality of this kind of qualitative study have been summarized as "trustworthiness" (Koch, 1994; Emden & Sandelowski, 1998), meaning that the research is faithful, insightful, and helpful in relation to the particular setting being studied. This is demonstrated first by the transparency of the study, where the methodology, design, and research process are all congruent with one another. It is further demonstrated by its relevance, which means its potential to positively contribute to the setting being studied, in this case the well-being of people living on dialysis. In this study, the congruence of the various aspects of the research project was regularly peer-reviewed throughout the process, and the final report was independently academically reviewed. Since its completion, it has been used locally to critically review aspects of the renal service and has been presented in other professional forums as a contribution to wider reflection on renal service provision. The completed work was fed back to the participants and presented to the local client support group.

Ultimately, the criteria for good qualitative research are relational, reflecting the relational character of the interpretive paradigm in research (Sandelowski, 1997), which specifically involves clear positioning of the researcher in relation to the study and its participants. Crucial to this critical interpretive approach is the clear expression of the dialectic of personal engagement and critical reflection in the study process. The documentation and public presentation of this research project sought to demonstrate that it was true to its aim of describing the experience of people living on dialysis.

A CRITICAL MODEL OF THE RENAL SETTING

In order to establish a standpoint to critically view the renal setting, the study used concepts derived from the work of Michel Foucault (1977, 1980, 1990) as applied in the context of health care (Cheek & Rudge, 1997; Lupton, 1997). The renal setting can be viewed, in Foucauldian terms, as a specialized social context created by a discourse that expresses renal "power/ knowledge" (Foucault, 1977), understood as a single entity. The dominant discourse in the renal context is embodied in the set of diagnostic and therapeutic activities and procedures practiced in nephrology, particularly the technologies of renal replacement therapy. It expresses the optimistic ideology of the acute curative paradigm of biomedicine (Morris, 1999), assuming the value and efficacy of renal replacement therapy.

In Foucauldian terms the renal discourse is one variant of the medical discourses of the body (Cheek & Rudge, 1997). The "clinical gaze" of the medical expert, the nephrologist, defining persons as renal patients through the diagnosis of ESRD and then determining and supervising their renal replacement therapy of dialysis or transplantation, epitomizes the surveillance and normalization of a modern "disciplinary technology," producing the "docile body" that Foucault sees as characterizing contemporary society (Foucault, 1977; Lupton, 1997). In this case, the regimen of treatment, including monitoring both its efficiency and the compliance of the patient with ESRD, produces the "renally replaced" body. The patient's own body is itself modified to accept the technologies of renal replacement therapy. The patient's bodily condition is defined by a range of parameters measured by medical technologies. Bodily activities are altered to accommodate these technologies through dietary restrictions, a medication schedule, and the dialysis regimen (Nagle, 1998). Thus the dominant discourse in the renal context creates the renally replaced life.

All involved in the renal setting participate in the dominant renal discourse; their understandings are created within it and reflect it. The person with a kidney problem becomes a renal patient as, inculcated with the professional viewpoint, they learn to understand their experience in terms of the dominant discourse that shapes renal replacement therapy (Bevan, 2000). However, it is not only the renal patient who is constituted by the renal discourse. The renal physician and the dialysis nurse are also constituted by the renal discourse that gives meaning and authority to their roles. The renal context and all of the various roles within it are all created by the dominant discourse, because it is the therapies generated by this discourse that enable the treatment of ESRD.

There are also several other different discourses, reflecting contrasting perspectives on the renally replaced life, which are based on the different positions of various groups in the renal context. In particular there is also a discourse, fragmentary and little heard, emanating from the recipients of renal therapy themselves. In Foucauldian terms, the dominant discourse, reflected in the professional viewpoint, creates "resistance," a "subjugated knowledge," which could be described as an alternative or counter-discourse reflecting the perspective of the renal client, from his or her position within the renal context (Foucault, 1980).

Over time, individuals with ESRD may find that their experience does not fully accord with the professional viewpoint. Despite the optimism of the dominant discourse they may realize that, for them, living on renal replacement therapy has certain limitations and difficulties, leading them to question or even modify aspects of the interpretation of their situation with which they have been inculcated as renal patients. Their own understanding of their experience will not be easy to discern because it is obscured by the dominant professional ideology. However, their individual interpretations of their renal condition and therapy, although typically framed in the language of the dominant discourse with which they have been socialized since their induction into the renal context, may reflect a dissonance between the professional viewpoint and their own experience. The client discourse, a response to the dominant discourse, reflects the perspective of people living on dialysis.

CONCERNS OF THE CLIENT DISCOURSE

Employing the critical interpretive approach, informed by this critical Foucauldian model of the renal setting, enabled the common client perspective, hidden within individual accounts that naturally tend to use the language and ideas of the dominant discourse, to be uncovered. From the analysis of the set of client accounts, this study described four concerns of the renal client discourse (Polaschek, 2003a). Together, these delineated the shared perspective of people living on home hemodialysis, in contrast to the dominant professional viewpoint.

The first concern is "suffering from continuing symptoms of ESRD and dialysis." According to the dominant discourse, dialysis is an efficacious therapy that removes the symptoms of ESRD. Despite the fact that these men successfully altered their own therapy in order to minimize certain symptoms, their experience showed that some symptoms persist despite renal replacement therapy and also occur as a consequence of the therapy itself. One problem is intermittent painful medical procedures, such as angioplasty, which are necessary to maintain the viability of their treatment.

"The limitations resulting from negotiating dialysis into their lifestyle" is the second concern of the renal client discourse. The dominant discourse indicates that dialysis, in particular self-care treatment, can generally be fitted into a person's usual pattern of activities to allow a reasonably normal lifestyle. Although they tended initially to emphasize continuity in their normal way of life on dialysis, the men's experience revealed the negotiation actually required to fit their treatment into their weekly schedule. Their usual work and leisure activities became more difficult or were curtailed. Their negotiation includes some unauthorized variations in some aspects of their therapeutic prescription, including shortening or missing some treatments.

The third concern is "the ongoingness and uncertainty of life on dialysis." According to the dominant discourse, renal replacement therapy becomes a normal part of life as renal patients become habituated to it over time. Despite these men successfully negotiating dialysis into their lifestyles, their experience suggests rather that renal clients gradually come to realize both the ongoingness of life on dialysis and its inherent uncertainty. The repetitive treatment regimen is intensely boring to them, yet the sense of routinization reduces their anxiety at the uncertainty of life on dialysis. These men cope through hoping that the treatment regimen does not have to be accepted as permanent, because in the future they will be able to escape from dialysis through receiving a kidney transplant.

"An altered interrelationship between autonomy and dependence" is the final concern of the renal client discourse. The dominant discourse indicates that living on dialysis can enable a nearly normal life, and managing their own treatment enhances patients' sense of autonomy. Although acknowledging that performing self-care dialysis does affirm their independence, the experience of these men manifests an altered relationship between autonomy and dependence in various aspects of their lives. These include their personal relationships, their ambiguous relationships with renal staff, and finally their basic reliance on the dialysis machine for continuing life. Renal clients can only achieve autonomy through compliance with the "disciplinary technology" (Lupton, 1997, p. 99) of the dominant discourse itself, but this necessarily involves an underlying contradictory dependence.

CONCLUSION: RESEARCH ON CLIENT EXPERIENCES AND NURSING CLINICAL PRACTICE

The study presented in this chapter sought to understand the experience of one group of people living on dialysis. The obscurity of the client experience in the renal setting exacerbates the vulnerability of the population with ESRD who depend on the technologies of this specialized health care context. The dominant discourse that produces the renally replaced life, expressing the optimistic ideology of the acute curative paradigm of biomedicine, hides the client perspective in the renal setting. In contrast to the dominant discourse expressed in the professional viewpoint, the concerns delineated in this study uncover the difficulties of the renally replaced life from the point of view of the clients.

Describing the shared perspective of people living on dialysis as four concerns of the renal client discourse enables an understanding of individuals' experiences of their renal condition and therapy. As a consequence, it provides the basis for a model of nursing work in the renal setting (Polaschek, 2003b). If the experience of living on dialysis is interpreted in terms of the relationship between the dominant professional viewpoint and client perspective within the renal context, then nursing work can be understood as facilitating renal clients to mediate between these two discourses by responding to their concerns in their own individual situation. While undertaking a range of specific tasks for renal clients, such as supervising their dialysis treatment or educating them about their therapeutic regimen, renal nurses can develop relationships in which they engage with the personal experiences of the client. They can then help individual renal clients to interpret the difficulties they are having in living on dialysis and support them in developing strategies to manage them.

By uncovering the distinctive experiences of people living on dialysis, research can reveal the potential in the service that nurses provide for people with ESRD. The concerns of the client discourse outline the issues that experienced nurses in the renal setting can address with their clients. As a consequence, such research can uncover the nature of nursing work, which is itself obscure in the renal setting. Studies of this kind can also contribute to a revised understanding of issues such as client behavior that is commonly interpreted as noncompliance by renal health professionals.

In general terms, this chapter has offered an example of one type of nursing research into the experience of chronic illness. Positioning themselves in relation to the specialized health care context within which individual clients receive treatment, nursing researchers can study, in terms of their vulnerability as a client population, the experience of living with a chronic condition supported by medical technology. Through enlarging this literature, they can address the obscurity of client experiences within chronic health care settings and provide a resource to enable health care professionals, especially nurses themselves, to humanize the service to people suffering from chronic illness, supporting them to continue to live as fully as possible.

REFERENCES

Allen, D. G. (1995). Hermeneutics: Philosophical traditions and nursing practice research. *Nursing Science Quarterly, 8*(4), 174–182.

Bevan, M. T. (2000). Dialysis as "deus ex machina": A critical analysis of haemodialysis. *Journal of Advanced Nursing, 31*, 437–443.

Cheek, J., & Rudge, T. (1997). The rhetoric of health care? Foucault, health care practices and the docile body 1990s style. In C. O'Farrell (Ed.). *Foucault: The legacy* (pp. 707–713). Brisbane, Australia: Queensland University of Technology.

Crotty, M. (1998). *The foundations of social research: Meaning and perspective in the research process.* St. Leonards, Australia: Allen and Unwin.

Curtin, R., Mapes, D., Petillo, M., & Oberley, E. (1998). Long-term dialysis survivors: a transformational experience. *Qualitative Health Research, 12*, 609–624.

Emden, C., & Sandelowski, M. (1998). The good, the bad and the relative, part one: Conceptions of goodness in qualitative research. *International Journal of Nursing Practice, 4*, 206–212.

Faber, S. (2000). An investigation of life with end stage renal disease: sociocultural case studies analysis. *Canadian Association of Nephrology Nurses and Technicians Journal, 10*(3), Sept, 24–34.

Foucault, M. (1977). *Discipline and punish: The birth of a prison.* New York, NY: Vintage Books.

Foucault, M. (1980). *Power/knowledge: Selected interviews and other writings 1972–1977.* New York, NY: Pantheon.

Foucault, M. (1990). *Politics, philosophy, culture: Interviews and other writings 1977–1984.* New York, NY: Routledge.

Gregory, D., Way, D., Hutchinson, T., Barrett, B., & Parfrey, P. (1998). Patients' perceptions of their experiences with ESRD and hemodialysis treatment. *Qualitative Health Research, 8*, 764–783.

Koch, T. (1994). Establishing rigour in qualitative research: The decision trail. *Journal of Advanced Nursing, 19*, 976–986.

Lather, P. (1991). *Getting smart.* New York, NY: Routledge.

Lupton, D. (1997). Foucault and the medicalization critique. In A. Peterson & R. Bunton (Eds.). *Foucault: Health and medicine* (pp. 84–110). London, England: Routledge.

Morris, D. (1999). *Illness and culture in the postmodern age.* Berkeley, CA: University of California.

Nagle, L. (1998). The meaning of technology for people with chronic renal failure. *Holistic Nursing Practice, 12*(4), 78–92.

Polaschek, N. (2003). The experience of living on dialysis: A literature review. *Nephrology Nursing Journal, 30,* 303–309.

Polaschek, N. (2003a). Living on dialysis: Concerns of clients in a renal setting. *Journal of Advanced Nursing, 41*(1), 44–52.

Polaschek, N. (2003b). Negotiated care: A model for nursing work in the renal setting. *Journal of Advanced Nursing, 42,* 355–363.

Sandelowski, M. (1997). "To be of use": Enhancing the utility of qualitative research. *Nursing Outlook, 45,* 125–131.

Schwandt, T. A. (1994). Constructivist, interpretivist approaches to human inquiry. In N. Denzin & Y. Lincoln (Eds.). *Handbook of qualitative research* (pp. 118–137). Thousand Oaks, CA: Sage.

Thompson, J. L. (1990). Hermeneutic inquiry. In L. Moody (Ed.). *Advancing nursing science through research* (Vol. 2, pp. 223–286). Newbury Park, CA: Sage.

CHAPTER 15

"Growin' Out of It": An Explanation of Childhood Asthma by African American Families

Jane W. Peterson and Yvonne M. Sterling

Asthma is the most common chronic illness in childhood, affecting approximately 5 million children under 18 years in the United States (Centers for Disease Control and Prevention [CDC], 2000; National Institute of Allergy and Infectious Diseases [NIAID], 2001). Asthma is the leading cause of school absenteeism, accounting for an additional 10 million missed school days (NIAID, 2001). Death rates for children with asthma increased by 78% between 1980 and 1993 (Clark, Brown, Parker, Robins, Remick, Philbert et al., 1999; CDC, 1999a). Asthma is more prevalent in African American children than in white children, causing more severe disability, more frequent hospitalizations, and four to six times more death (NIAID, 2000). Thus the burden of the disease falls disproportionately on African American and Hispanic families, particularly those living in the inner city (Clark et al., 1999; CDC, 1999b; Wade, Weil, Holden, Mitchell, Evans, Kruszon-Moran et al., 1997).

We conducted an ethnographic study on a vulnerable population of African American families with chronically ill children. We wanted to better understand how these families respond to the diagnosis of asthma in their children and describe their explanatory models of asthma (Peterson, Sterling, & Stout, 2002). Explanatory models are the beliefs and notions about an episode of sickness (e.g., asthma) and its treatment that are applicable to all those affected by the child's illness (Kleinman, 1980). Explanatory models offer explanations of sickness and treatment to guide choices among available therapies and to shed light on personal and social meaning in the experience of sickness (p.105). Additionally, explanatory models disclose one of the chief mechanisms by which cultural and social structural context affect patient–practitioner and other health care relationships (p.105). Of interest here is how families responded to the questions: Will [the child's] condition have a short or long course and what do you fear most about your child's condition (Kleinman, 1980)? Embedded in many answers was the notion that the child would "grow out of" having asthma.

FAMILY RESPONSES TO CHILDHOOD ASTHMA

The pediatric asthma literature reflects the significant asthma incidence, prevalence, severity, and management challenges in the United States and abroad. This literature is abundant and diverse, describing the impact of asthma on the family (Donnelly, 1994; Horner, 1998; Kurnat & Moore, 1999; Palmer, 2001; Svavarsdottir, McCubbin, & Kane, 2000), quality of life (Erickson, Munzenberger, Plante, Kirking, Hurwitz, & Vanuya, 2002; Sawyer, Spurrier, Kennedy, &

Martin, 2001), and program effectiveness (Capen, Dedlow, Robillard, Fuller, & Fuller, 1994; Yoos et al., 1997). Most of the literature is from the perspective of parents, with a few studies describing the child's view of life with asthma (Ryan-Wenger & Walsh, 1994; Yoos & McMullen, 1996, 1999).

Families of children with asthma face complex experiences and issues and express a variety of needs and concerns. These include time management, financial strain, and family relations (Kurnat & Moore, 1999). Family responsibilities, according to Horner's (1998) findings from a study of 12 families, include learning the ropes and their children's asthma patterns, changing lifestyle and/or environment, and dealing with the asthma itself. Palmer (2001) found a central theme of becoming vigilant in her grounded theory study of 10 caregivers of school-aged children with asthma.

Existing research about the African American family's responses to having and managing a chronically ill child can be found mainly in the literature concerning sickle-cell disease. Published research of the experiences of African American families having a child with other chronic diseases is virtually nonexistent (Sterling et al., 1997).

There is, however, a limited description of ethnically related responses to having a child with asthma. For example, in two studies where 46% of the sample consisted of African American subjects, researchers (Yoos & McMullen, 1996, 1999) found race-related patterns in their study results. In their examination of illness narratives of children with asthma, Yoos & McMullen (1996) found that death was a persistent theme among the African American children. In a later study, they described the accuracy of both parents and children in their perception, interpretation, and evaluation of asthma symptoms; they found that African American parents were more accurate than white parents (Yoos & McMullen, 1999).

Sander (1998) reported that physicians often tell parents that their children will outgrow asthma in an effort to comfort them. The issue of growing out of it was found to be a pertinent theme in the study by Peterson et al. (2002) of African American families of children with asthma. As related to this particular theme, the studies done by Kieckhefer & Ratcliffe (2000) and MacDonald (1996) are of particular note. Findings from these studies suggest that uncertainty is a major concern of parents of children with asthma. Kieckhefer & Ratcliffe found that parents feared that the condition (asthma) would not go away or improve. MacDonald, on the other hand found that the parents expressed the need to master and cope with the uncertainty of the child's asthma.

The notion of whether a child will outgrow asthma has generated much discussion among health care professionals. For example, Altman (1994) believes that outgrowing asthma may be an exception to the rule. Liu, Martinez, & Taussig (2003) conclude that "of all young children who experience recurrent wheezing, only a minority will go on to have persistent asthma in later life" (p. 13). Lui et al. also reported the findings of a study conducted in Australia, consisting of 7-year-old children who were examined for persistence and severity of asthma until they were 35 years of age. At this point, 70–90% of the subjects continued to have asthma symptoms (p. 14). They concluded that asthmatic children may experience remission, but severe asthma persists with age. Roorda (1996) agrees with this premise, stating that the children with severe asthma will more than likely continue to have asthma symptoms into adulthood. Gerritsen (2002) states that there is a transition period from childhood to adulthood where asthma symptoms decrease. However, realistically, more than 50% of children will continue to suffer with asthma in adult life. Others believe that risk factors such as parental cigarette smoking, persistent airway inflammation, pulmonary function, bronchial hyperresponsiveness, and a strong family history contribute to the persistence of asthma into adulthood or to relapse in adulthood (Amdekar, 2001; Panhuysen et al., 1997; Rooda, 1996; Strachan & Gerritsen, 1996).

PARTICIPANTS, SETTINGS, AND METHOD

The ethnographic study presented here (Peterson et al., 2002) was conducted over a 3-year period in two cities in the United States of America: one in the Pacific Northwest and one in the Gulf of Mexico region. The study consisted of 20 African American families (10 from each city) who had a child with asthma. Study participants were recruited from several clinics and by professional referrals in each city. Participants chosen for the study 1) identified themselves as African Americans, 2) had at least one identified caregiver in the family, and 3) had a child who was between 9 and 12 years old with asthma. The child had to have been diagnosed with asthma for at least 1 year and had to be receiving health care monitoring, management, and/or supervision. In addition, the child had to have had at least one emergency department visit, hospitalization, or doctor's office visit for asthma or be using asthma medications in the past 12 months. The child also had to be free from other significant chronic illnesses. Institutional review board approval for the study was obtained in each city before families were contacted. Informed written consent was obtained from each person in the family who participated in the study.

Among the 20 families, 19 (95%) of the adult caregivers were women, and 16 (80%) were mothers of the child with asthma. Furthermore, 8 (40%) were married, and 10 (50%) reported two or more adults living in the household; 17 (85%) of the households included two or more children. Most adult caregivers (17 or 85%) had at least completed high school. As to the employment status of the adult caregivers, 13 were employed for wages outside the home, 5 were not working for wages, and 2 were retired. Of those working for wages, 10 worked full-time and 3 part-time. Family income ranged from $5000 to more than $70,000 per year. Eleven (55%) of the families were below the poverty line.

At the time they enrolled in the study, the children with asthma were 9 to 12 years of age. There were five girls and five boys in each city in grades four through eight. Half of the children rated their asthma as moderately severe, six (30%) said their asthma was not severe, and the remaining four (20%) said their asthma was very severe. Eight children were taking two or more prescribed asthma medications, eight others were taking two prescribed medications, and the remaining four were taking one prescribed medication.

Each family was visited by one of the two African American researchers over the course of 12 months, with an average of 12 contacts per family. Data collection, consisting of participant observation and in-depth semistructured interviews, was conducted in settings in which children and families felt the most comfortable or in which they spent much of their time. These settings included their homes, schools, sports events, churches, and community festivals.

All interviews were recorded on audiotape and transcribed verbatim by a professional transcriptionist. Family genealogies or family networks were also collected. Data were captured on the perceptions of the families "'from the inside,' through a process of deep attentiveness, of empathic understanding (Verstehen), and of suspending or 'bracketing' preconception" about asthma (Miles & Huberman 1994). The observations and reflections of the researchers were recorded as field notes. Data from the field notes were also transcribed. All participants and families were given code numbers and pseudonyms to maintain confidentiality.

The researchers used a qualitative research software program to assist in the organization and coding of data. Data were then analyzed, grouped into clusters, and organized to permit contrast and comparison. Patterns emerged and themes were uncovered. Study findings showed that families have their own explanatory models of asthma. It was also found that these families draw on their cultural context to understand asthma and compared their lived experience with health care providers' explanations of asthma. Specifically, the African American families in this study drew much of their information about asthma from other family members and from personal experience (Peterson et al., 2002). One significant theme that emerged was "growin' out of it." This theme had many facets and is the topic of this chapter.

ETHNOGRAPHY OF "GROWIN' OUT OF IT"

Listening to families, one learns how they understand their child's asthma. A common family response to this diagnosis is to conceptualize asthma in terms of 1) "havin' it," in which families acknowledge that the child has asthma; 2) "growin' out of it," a transition period in which asthma is seen as a temporary condition; and 3) "outgrowin' it," when the child no longer has asthma. Here we use the family's words as they explain their understanding of asthma.

"Havin' It"

When families say their child has asthma, they acknowledge that the child has a health problem that they cannot control. For families, this explains the difference between the child with asthma and other "healthy" children. However, knowing the diagnosis, families anticipate that one day the child will not have it. Family responses to a child having asthma fell into three areas:

1. *In the beginning.* "The first years were rough," one father told us. He remarried during that time. "We were adjusting. During that period, my daughter had a lot of problems with her asthma . . . we [the family] really did not know what to do for her."
2. *Keeps him so wiped out.* "[My son] stays in swimming year round. And that really helps [his asthma]. But when the attack comes on, it's there. Yes, he is wiped out. It takes him the day to feel better. And I think it should not take him that long The treatment also wipes him out when he has to have the asthma treatment. So, I guess that I am just having a harder time with him."
3. *Waitin' an' hopin'.* "Because, you know, just lookin' at him suffering. You know you can't really do nothing about it. Just, make sure he taking his treatments. And looking at him— just lookin' at the suffering I would love for him to grow out of it. I want him to grow out of it."

   "I hope one day she will outgrow it, especially with the way she breathes. I don't know if that's something that can be outgrown, or if it's something that can be corrected. Or is it just a part of her lifelong condition for her at this point?"

   "Because there's nothin' I can really do. You know, I sit there. I watch him with it, and I'm sayin', 'You're gonna grow out of it. You're gonna grow out of it.' I say, 'God will heal you. Now God's gonna heal your asthma. You've just got to wait a little while.'"

Children also voice their hopes saying: "I wish that I could grow out of it [but] it looks like I'm not gonna grow out of it; and I'm just hoping [I will] hurry up and outgrow it."

"Growin' Out of It"

This is a transition period. The child is either said to have asthma but will outgrow it or the pattern of the child's asthma is changing, and this is seen as a sign that the child is outgrowing it. Growing out of it has no specific time frame, although it seems to be tied to both a chronological growing up and emotional maturation. Much of the family time is spent waiting to see if there are symptoms and being cautiously thankful when there are none. This family response can be divided into four areas.

1. *Things are smoothin' out.* "In the past year things have smoothed out and so has my daughter's asthma. Maybe she is growing out of it the way I did," said one parent.

   "At one time when she was very young she had it real bad, and then when she got a little older it sort of faded away."

   "Looks like his asthma is getting better. You know, it look like it's a possibility that he may grow out of it because it's not as frequent as it used to be."
2. *We basically don't have it no more.* This is a conception of asthma based on family experience. "Cuz it seems to me that she's growin' out of it, like kind of all of us have." As one caregiver felt she had grown out of her own asthma, she figured her daughter was growing out of hers. The daughter no longer had symptoms and was feeling well. However, when the girl's peak flow meter readings were low, the mother realized that her daughter still has asthma problems. Because the medication prescribed was not covered by Medicaid, the family was hoping that the child had outgrown her asthma.

   Other families felt that their children were going to outgrow their asthma based on their experiences with other family members.
3. *Lookin' good.* The family set their own criteria for the progress of the illness and when the child has outgrown his/her asthma. One child reported, "I didn't even breathe heavy. And this was an active day today with a lot of exercise and swimming." His mother said, "So, OK that is looking good. If he stays like this between now and 12, then I will figure that he has outgrown it. But I will give it a whole year of not having asthma before I will definitely say that he has outgrown it."
4. *Wait and see.* "He [the doctor] told me that sometime kids outgrow it [asthma] and we'd just have to wait and see if my daughter did or not."

   I asked the doctor, "Will she grow out of it?" And at that time I recall a doctor tellin' me that she will grow out of it. And then I recall also another doctor tellin' me (cuz I always get like a second opinion) that asthma go back and forth. So they don't really know."

"Outgrown It"

When a family can say that their child no longer has asthma, they are definite. Many recite long family histories and name those who have outgrown asthma as evidence that this not only can but does happen. However, families are not foolish. They know of people who had asthma in their old age or died from an asthma attack. This is almost always seen as a certain kind of asthma and not the kind their child has. Therefore, it is hardly talked about and is quickly dismissed from one's mind. "Outgrowing it" responses can be divided into two areas.

1. *I outgrew it, he outgrew it, she outgrew it, they outgrew it.* One mother reminiscing about her father said, "he grew up in Louisiana, he said his asthma was bad when he was down there, but he was OK up here (in Seattle). He smoked cigarettes. He died of cancer they said he had outgrown [his asthma] I guess."

   A mother talking about her own asthma said "I had asthma years ago. But like I grew out of it. And my mom said that she had asthma also when she was a child, and she grew out of it also."

   Mothers also talked about their children. "I have three other children who had asthma. One girl and the other two boys. And they outgrew their asthma. One even had his 10 years."

2. *Some don't outgrow it.* "I don't think she will outgrow her asthma I had a friend whose friend didn't outgrow it. I just hope, it's just better controlled. And then I also knew a lady that I work with. I mean, she was like in her 50s, 60s, and she had it. I don't know whether she had asthma or bronchitis, but she used to have the inhaler."

   A mother expressing ambivalence said "on top of my mind, he gonna grow out of it. In the back of my mind, I know that he's not gonna grow out of it, you know."

   "I hope she's outgrowin' it. And I still wonder sometimes because I know it has to do like with their lungs I don't know if you can ever outgrow it. Because I remember talkin' with someone at work because she thought her son had outgrown it, and when he went into the service he couldn't stay in the service because he started having asthma attacks and she thought he had outgrown it I was a child and I outgrew it, and I just got it back cuz I done got old, you know."

DISCUSSION

Families have previously described (Peterson, Sterling, & Weekes, 1997) their feelings about asthma, likening it to an unwelcome visitor or an intruder. Faced with the reality of a child's diagnosis of asthma, families have a need to "contain the intrusion," a phrase used by Blueblood-Langer (1996) when describing families who had a child with cystic fibrosis. The need to contain the intrusion means accepting change on the families' own terms. The shock that their child has a serious illness forces families to look for ways to help ease the child's hurt. With asthma, this means finding a way to help the child breathe with ease. The plethora of medications and the advances in acute medical care for children with asthma has made this possible. However, the models held by the families differ significantly from those held by health care providers.

   Families see age as the single most important indicator of managing asthma and see the ultimate outcome as not having asthma. Health care providers see adherence as the most important indicator of asthma management, with the outcome being to live normally with asthma. The two models are shown in Figure 15.1.

   Although families and health care providers agree, eventually, on the "havin' it" stage or the diagnosis and immediate treatment, the chronic character or nature of asthma is not shared. Families watch as the child gets older for changes that indicate the asthma is fading out. Health care providers, on the other hand watch for adherence to the asthma management plan to ensure that

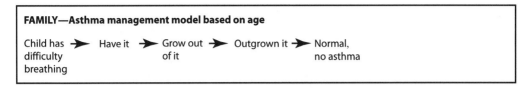

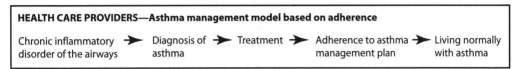

FIGURE 15.1   Asthma Management Models

the child participates in his or her desired activities. Families are missing an understanding of the chronic nature of asthma; the cases they cite of older people with asthma are in the minority and viewed as atypical. Therefore families' view of "havin' it" often fits with the diagnosis of the health care providers, and both parties work well together.

However, the families' concept of "outgrowin' it" does not fit with the health care providers' concept of a chronic disease to be managed over one's lifetime. Sander (1998) makes the cogent remark that failure to outgrow asthma is discouraging for children and their families. However, promoting and supporting the belief of permanent remission of the asthma symptoms can be misleading, harmful, and lead to false hope. Furthermore, families usually reframe advice from health care providers to fit their own concept. At the point when the family says the child no longer has asthma, health care providers want to continue to treat this chronic disease. As a result, families tend to ignore their advice. When this attitude persists, health care providers need to be clear about what they want to convey to families with children who have asthma. If families hear, understand, and accept health care providers' explanations of asthma, then the use of scientific language and detailed physiological descriptions may be appropriate. However, asthma management plans should be individualized. It is imperative that health care providers modify their language and understand the family's conception and explanatory model of asthma. This is not a matter of giving incorrect scientific information or embarrassing people who have different beliefs and language about a condition. It is about using the languages and concepts of both the health care providers and the family to bring about the best health outcomes for a child.

Most of the children in this study classified their asthma as moderate to severe. Furthermore, most of the families had a strong history of asthma. Their beliefs with regard to growing out of asthma were significant, based on the absence or change in pattern of asthma symptoms. Yet, the belief of a permanent remission of asthma was dispelled when they learned of a recurrence of asthma symptoms in their children, adult friends, or relatives.

There is clear and consistent evidence that remission of asthma symptoms during childhood may not preclude the possibility of relapse during the adult years (Amdekar, 2001; Gerritsen, 2002; Lui et al., 2003; Warke et al., 2002). As noted earlier by Sander (1998), physicians sometimes tell parents that their child will outgrow asthma as a measure to comfort them. Health care professionals, particularly nurses, must be familiar with accurate, evidence-based asthma information, particularly those factors that may place children and adolescents at risk for recurrent asthma. They must seek and confirm this information during all health care visits and use assessment data, including the family's explanations, as a basis for family asthma education.

In conclusion, the notion that the adult caregivers in this study believe and hope that their children will outgrow asthma could make them vulnerable for negative or poor health outcomes. These beliefs can significantly affect the management of their children's asthma. Asthma, like any chronic illness, is a family affair. Therefore, those beliefs (whether accurate or not) may also be imparted to other family members. Successful asthma management involves multidisciplinary and family collaboration and ongoing education.

REFERENCES

Altman, L. K. (1994, January 4). Childhood asthma seldom outgrown. *New York Times*. Retrieved November 4, 2003, from *http://web.lexis-nexis.com/universe*.

Amdekar, K. (2001). Natural history of asthma in children. *Indian Journal of Pediatrics, 68*(Suppl. 4), S3–S6.

Blueblood-Langer, M. (1996). *In the shadow of illness*. Princeton, NJ: Princeton University Press.

Capen, C., Dedlow, E., Robillard, R., Fuller, B., & Fuller, C. (1994). The team approach to pediatric asthma education. *Pediatric Nursing, 20,* 231–237.

Centers for Disease Control (CDC). (1999a). *Facts about asthma*. Retrieved 7/15/01, from *http://www.cdc.gov.od/oc/media/facts/astha.htm*.

Centers for Disease Control (CDC). (1999b). *Asthma Prevention Program of the National Center for Environmental Health: At-A-Glance* Retrieved 4/19/04, from *http://www.cdc.gov/nceh/airpollution/asthma/ataglance/ataglanceprint.htm*.

Centers for Disease Control (CDC). (2000). Measuring childhood asthma prevalence before and after the 1997 redesign of the National Health Interview Survey United States. *Morbidity and Mortality Weekly Report, 49*(4), 908–911.

Clark, N. M., Brown, R. W., Parker, E., Robins, T. G., Remick, D. G., Philbert, M. A., et al. (1999). Childhood asthma. *Environmental Health Perspectives, 107*(Suppl. 3), 421–429.

Donnelly, E. (1994). Parents of children with asthma: An examination of family hardiness, family stressors and family functioning. *Journal of Pediatric Nursing, 9,* 398–408.

Erickson, S., Munzenberger, P., Plante, M., Kirking, D., Hurwitz, M., & Vanuya, R. (2002). Influence of sociodemographics on the health-related quality of life of pediatric patients with asthma and their caregivers. *Journal of Asthma, 39*(2), 107–117.

Gerritsen, J. (2002). Follow-up studies of asthma from childhood to adulthood. *Pediatric Respiratory Reviews, 3*(3), 184–192

Horner, S. (1998). Catching the asthma: Family care for school-aged children with asthma. *Journal of Pediatric Nursing, 13,* 356–366.

Kieckhefer, G., & Ratcliffe, M. (2000). What parents of children with asthma tell us. *Journal of Pediatric Health Care, 14,* 122–126.

Kleinman, A. (1980). *Patients and healers in the context of culture*. Berkeley, CA: University of California.

Kurnat, E., & Moore, C. (1999). The impact of a chronic condition on the families of children with asthma. *Pediatric Nursing, 25,* 288–292.

Lui, A., Martinez, F. & Taussig, L. (2003). Natural history of allergic diseases and asthma. In D. Leung, H. Sampson, R. Geha, & S. Szefler (Eds.). *Pediatric allergy. Principles and practice*. St. Louis, MO: Mosby.

MacDonald, H. (1996). "Mastering uncertainty:" Mothering the child with asthma. *Pediatric Nursing, 22*(1), 55–59.

Miles, M. B., & Huberman, A. M. (1994). *Qualitative data analysis* (2nd ed.) Thousand Oaks, CA: Sage.

National Heart, Lung and Blood Institute. (1997). *Expert panel report 2. Guidelines for the diagnosis and management of asthma* (NIH Publication No. 97-4051).

National Institute of Allergy and Infectious Diseases (NIAID). (2001). *NIAID fact sheet. Asthma: A concern for minority populations.* Retrieved November 6, 2003, from *http://www.niaid.nih.gov/factsheets/asthma.htm.*

National Institute of Allergy and Infectious Disease (NIAID). (2000). *NIAID fact sheet.* Retrieved May 8, 2001, from *http://www.niaid.nih.gov/factsheets/allergystat.htm.*

Palmer, E. (2001). Family caregiver experiences with asthma in school age children. *Pediatric Nursing, 27*(1), 75–81.

Panhuysen, C., Vonk, J., Koeter, G, Schouten, J. vanAlterna, R., Bleeker, E., et al. (1997). Adult patients may outgrow their asthma. A 25 year follow-up study. *American Journal of Respiratory & Critical Care Medicine, 155,* 1267–1272.

Peterson, J., Sterling, Y., & Stout, J. (2002). Explanatory models of asthma. *Journal of Asthma, 39,* 577–590.

Peterson, J. W., Sterling, Y. M., & Weekes, D. P. (1997). Access to health care: perspectives of African American families with chronically ill children. *Family & Community Health, 19*(4), 64–77.

Ryan-Wenger, N., & Walsh, M. (1994). Children's perspectives on coping with asthma. *Pediatric Nursing, 20*(3), 224–228.

Rooda, R. J. (1996) Prognostic factors for the outcome of childhood asthma in adolescence. *Thorax, 51*(Suppl. 1), S7–S12

Sander, N. (1998). Belief systems that affect the management of childhood asthma. *Immunology and Allergy Clinics of North America, 18*(1), 99–113.

Sawyer, M., Spurrier, N., Kennedy, D., & Martin, J. (2001). The relationship between the quality of life of children with asthma and family functioning. *Journal of Asthma, 38*(3), 279–284.

Strachan, D., & Gerritsen, J. (1996) Long-term outcome of early childhood wheezing: Population data. *European Respiratory Journal,* (Suppl. 21), 42s–47s.

Sterling, Y. M., Peterson, J. W., & Weekes, D. P. (1997) African-American families with chronically ill children: Oversights and insights. *Journal of Pediatric Nursing 12(5),* 292–300.

Svavarsdottir, E., McCubbin, M., & Kane, J. (2000). Well-being of parents of young children with asthma. *Research in Nursing & Health, 23,* 346–358.

Taylor, W. R., & Newacheck, P. W. (1992). Impact of childhood asthma on health. *Pediatrics, 90,* 657–662.

Wade, S., Weil, C., Holden, G., Mitchell, H., Evans, E., Kruszon-Moran, D., et al. (1997). Psychosocial characteristics of inner-city children with asthma: A description of the NCICAS psychosocial protocol. *Pediatric Pulmonology, 24,* 263–276.

Warke, T., Fitch, P., Brown, V. Taylor, R. Lyons, J., Ennis, M., & Shields, M. (2002). Outgrown asthma does not mean no airways inflammation. *European Respiratory Journal, 19,* 284–287

Yoos, H., L., McMullen, A., Bezek, S., Hondorf, C., Berry, S., et al. (1997). An asthma management program for urban minority children. *Journal of Pediatric Health Care, 11,* 66–74.

Yoos, H., L., & McMullen, A. (1999). Symptom perception and evaluation in childhood asthma. *Nursing Research, 48*(1), 2–7.

Yoos, H., L., & McMullen, A. (1996). Illness narratives of children with asthma. *Pediatric Nursing, 22*(4), 285–290.

CHAPTER 16

Immigrant Vulnerability: Does Capitalism in the United States Matter?

Jenny Hsin-Chun Tsai

International migration (or immigration) is an ancient phenomenon. With globalization, this old phenomenon is happening faster and becoming more diversified than ever before. In 1997 in the United States alone, 25.8 million persons or 9.7% of the total US population were immigrants (Schmidley & Gibson, 1999). In 2000, immigrants increased to 28.4 million, representing 10.4% of the nation's total population (Lollock, 2001). Schmidley & Gibson's (1999) projection indicates that from 1995 to 2050, 40% of the total immigrant population will be Hispanic, 30% will be from Asia and the Pacific Islands, 20% will be non-Hispanic whites, and 10% will be African American (p. 1). As a result, demand for culturally competent care is knocking on the doors of clinicians, educators, researchers, and health care administrators harder than ever before.

Scientists believe that as a result of the extensive changes involved in immigration, the health of immigrants is threatened and their risk for poor health is increased after resettlement. In other words, changes experienced during transition add to the vulnerability of immigrants (Meleis, 1996). With regard to mental health, Ödegaard's (1932) investigation in the United States regarding mental illness in adult immigrants, Rutter, Yule, Berger, Yule, Morton, & Bagley's (1974) survey of children in the United Kingdom; Munroe-Blum, Boyle, Offord, & Kates' (1989) study of children in Canada; Barnes' (2001) screening of recent refugees in the United States; and many other works show various kinds and degrees of adverse mental health consequences for immigrants and refugees.

Studies from other scholars further show factors that are associated with the health status and vulnerability of immigrants. For example, Anderson's study (1985) with Indo-Canadian and Greek women in Canada found that the women's help-seeking experiences were affected by their own perceptions of health, inability on the part of health professionals to grasp the circumstances of their lives, and their experiences of discrimination. Studies with Polish immigrants (Aroian, 1990), Iranian immigrants (Lipson, 1992), and Korean immigrants (Nah, 1993) in the United States showed that language and occupational accommodation were two key factors for successful resettlement. The existence of ethnocultural communication in the area where immigrants move was also found to be important for immigrants' health (Baker, Arseneault, & Gallant, 1994). Weitzman & Berry's work with poor immigrant women in New York (1992) indicated that being poor and being an immigrant contributed to these women's limited use of US medical care and poor health status. These women faced even greater barriers to health care than poor and uninsured Americans did.

Transition during immigration and resettlement adds to the vulnerability of immigrants. Nevertheless, this vulnerability is not a static, self-contained entity. Immigrant vulnerability is produced in ongoing interaction with social, economic, political, and cultural structures of the receiving country. Chopoorian (1986) reminded the nursing profession that a lack of consciousness about social, political, economic, and cultural factors prevents nursing from arriving at a comprehensive view of human health. Such a lack of consciousness about these issues keeps the profession in a peripheral role in the larger arena of social, economic, and political affairs of the United States. In order to promote the health of immigrant, as Anderson (1991) suggests, health professionals need to "acquire, through their education, a theoretical base that allows them to analyze the socioeconomic and political factors that influence health care delivery" (p. 716) and other aspects of everyday life. Partial findings of a critical ethnographic study (Tsai, 2001) will be presented in this chapter to show the effects that the receiving country's economic structure has on the vulnerability of immigrants. This will be illustrated through events of their daily lives, their psychosocial reactions, and the adaptive strategies they used during resettlement in the receiving country. Implications for US health professionals will be discussed thereafter.

DESCRIPTION OF THE STUDY

This critical ethnographic study took place in a metropolitan area in the northwest region of the United States between 1998 and 2000. The study was designed to explore how immigrant families' lives are shaped by the larger societal context of the receiving country. Data were collected from nine Taiwanese immigrant families recruited through community snowball referrals. Participants were protected through compliance with the university-approved procedures for human subjects.

Sample

A total of 29 participants, representing these 9 families, contributed to the overall data. Of the 29 participants, 16 were parents with a mean age of 45.3 years [standard deviation (SD) = 2.4). Nine completed college (16 years) in Taiwan, and four had advanced education (3 master's degrees and 1 doctorate) in North America. As for the 13 children, they were between 8 and 21 years of age, with a mean of 16.1 years (SD = 3.7). Their education ranged from second grade to first year of college. These families arrived in the United States as immigrants between January 1989 and August 1998 through three mechanisms: own employment ($n = 3$), sponsored by siblings who were naturalized US citizens ($n = 4$), and returning to the United States ($n = 2$) (in which case, one of the key family members already had permanent resident status or citizenship in the United States). Most families ($n = 8$) lived in middle-class areas.

Data Collection

Participants were interviewed one to three times, alone or with other family members. All interviews were semistructured and were conducted primarily in Chinese. English was occasionally used with children who were limited in Chinese proficiency or to convey certain ideas. All of the interviews were conducted at home, with the exception of one participant who chose to meet at a restaurant because his parents and sibling did not participate. The length of visit for each interview ranged from 1.5 to 10 hours. Interviews were recorded on audiotape with the consent of the participants. During the interview visits, observations were undertaken to learn about family dynamics, family structure, family affect, daily family activities, the physical home environment, network contacts, and opinions about extrafamilial environments.

In addition to interviews and observations, each participant completed a demographic and immigration questionnaire at the end of the first interview. The children's version had 21 items and collected each child's demographic information. The adult version had 41 items that gathered each adult participant's individual information and his or her family information. Both Chinese and English versions were available. Assistance was available at the scene to help them complete the questionnaires.

Data Analysis and Scientific Rigor

Descriptive statistics (frequency, mean, and SD) were used to analyze the questionnaire data. Narrative analytical technique (Riessman, 1993) guided the analysis of the interview data. In the first step, interviews were transcribed from audiotapes to paper (in Chinese). Both verbal and nonverbal communications were preserved in the Chinese transcripts. After close examination of the Chinese transcripts, portions of the Chinese language transcripts (i.e., narrative segments) were selected, translated, and preserved in the English language transcripts for in-depth analysis.

Substantive and methodological codes were written next to the highlighted narrative segments. Other analytical notes were also written next to the related narrative segments. Ongoing comparisons of stories across different family members in the same family and across families were made during the analysis process. Ongoing consultation with senior researchers and colleagues with diverse backgrounds, as well as confirmation with participants, refined the analysis. Fewer and fewer new codes were generated with each newly analyzed interview after half of the interviews were analyzed. Codes gradually merged and became more abstract and analytical. HyperRESEARCH (1999), a computer-assisted qualitative software, was used to manage the data and emerging codes.

FINDINGS

The in-depth analysis revealed that four aspects of US societal context shaped the everyday lives of immigrants. One of these was economic: the norms, values, and practices defined by US capitalism (the others being immigration policy, western imperialism, and social class). Marketing culture, insurance, and credit were the three themes of the economic context identified in the data related to US capitalism.

Marketing Culture

Marketing culture refers to "the degree with which the norms and practices of business for selling products and making profits for business owners influence immigrants" (Tsai, 2001, p. 168). Similar to what occurs in the rest of the US population, families in this study received multiple phone calls, mailings, or in-person visits for various product sales and donations. Taiwan is a capitalist country, yet the economic structure and culture differ from those of the United States. The United States emphasizes individualism and the free market. Taiwan emphasizes collectivism and tighter government control.

Participant families had different cultural knowledge about and conceptions of telecommunications and product sales. Many of them complained about their contacts with sales representatives in the United States. "Ordering magazines is the same [problem]. They knock on your door all the time. Ask you to order, ask you for donation. Many of this type of problem," said one family (Tsai, 2001, pp. 168–169). They were distressed, bothered, and frustrated by these practices and the hassles derived from these practices. As one participant said, "We only called Taiwan for a few minutes. Why it cost so much?! We later knew the reason [because we did not sign up for any long-distance promotion plan]. There is only one phone company in Taiwan. You just need a phone and then you have everything" (mother of two, living in the United States for 18 months at the time of the interview) (Tsai, 2001, p. 168).

Some families were concerned and worried about being cheated or having financial or even legal complications because "there are charges against some wrongdoing all the time in America. Lawsuits are everywhere" (Tsai, 2001, p. 169). The levels of frustration and worry were found to be higher in the participant families who were less proficient in English or who did not have friends or relatives in the area to which they moved.

Families usually thought of strategic solutions to decrease their stress level and protect themselves after a few bad experiences with sales people. For instance, some families chose to say no to everything and stick with whatever (telephone company, magazine subscription) they had at the time. After learning from friends or relatives with knowledge about the US marketing culture, another strategy was sometimes adopted by the immigrants: speaking with a strange foreign accent or improper grammar in hopes that this would stop salespersons from further explaining their products. Some families adapted to the US marketing culture by adjusting their personal perceptions. They treated the money lost to purchasing products they regretted as the "tuition" they had to spend as part of their immigration journey. "Be careful" was the phrase used by some participants throughout the interviews.

Insurance

Insurance is "the types and amounts of insurance necessary to adequately protect the families" (Tsai, 2001, p. 171). Health and life insurance were exported from the United States to Taiwan decades ago. Thus Taiwanese are familiar with the concepts of health and life insurance. Because of the increasing use of cars in Taiwan, car insurance was adopted in Taiwan in the mid-1990s. After participant families immigrated, they began to realize that there are many more types of insurance in the United States and, as one participant said, "everything needs to be insured." The expense of insurance was much higher than they had expected.

The participant families' greatest concern was the cost of health insurance. Taiwan has a universal health care system. Having to purchase one's own health insurance when not employed was a new concept to families who were new to the United States. For one family that immigrated as an investment, they did not know that they needed to purchase individual health insurance until they were involved in the local Taiwanese community. Families felt helpless with the high cost of health insurance; at the same time, they could not go without insurance. Unfortunately, the road to finding a health insurance plan was not straightforward either. There are many insurance plans offered by different companies. Before participant families could even make a decision, they had to learn about copayments, deductibles, preferred doctors, prevention, and so forth. For participant families who spoke limited English, choosing an insurance plan was challenging. They had to rely on relatives or friends in the area (more so than did those who were comfortable with English) to resolve the insurance issues.

To overcome the problems with insurance, the first step was staying as healthy as possible to avoid health care expenses while the family was looking for jobs that offered benefits. One family said, "When we just got here, we had no insurance. Could not get sick! We bore with it for half a year. Took some over-the-counter drugs [when we're sick]" (Tsai, 2001, p. 173). Some families flew back to Taiwan for their health care needs, usually the nonemergency kind, because as one participant said, "add a round trip ticket on top of [the treatment cost], I still have plenty left. It's still cost-effective" (Tsai, 2001, p. 172). A few families would just pay for the insurance regardless of the cost because they knew the importance of having insurance in the United States.

Credit

Credit refers to "the degree of which the value of credit affects immigrant families in the U.S." (Tsai, 2001, p. 174). In capitalism, credit means money and profits (Weber, 1992). Credit history, a widely used concept in the United States, is employed to assess a prospective customer's potential for profit making for the business owner. A good credit history means a potential for making profits from this prospective customer. However, credit history is not a concept that exists in Taiwan. Thus families living in the United States for the first time were surprised and confused when apartment managers asked about credit history and requested investigation fees. Although families in the study were lucky enough to have the investigation waived, some of them had friends who could not even rent a place because they had no credit history at the time. One family said that a friend had to pay 6 months rent in advance in cash in order to secure the place.

The lack of credit history not only presented problems for immigrants' access to housing, it also hampered their ability to get loans and credit cards and, ironically, chances to build up their credit history. In the area of loan and credit card applications, no family was lucky with these services. As one unhappy family described their experience: "American banks were not willing to loan to us because he wants you to use credit as deposit, right? Chinese use properties as deposit for loans. That's the difference" (Tsai, 2001, p. 128). Families eventually turned to Chinese-owned banks for help. Regardless of the fact that the process with Chinese-owned banks was not completely smooth, families at least got the loan or credit card from the bank as a start.

DISCUSSION

Decades of studies of immigrant experiences have informed us of the resettlement experience and the threats to immigrant health in countries such as Canada, the United Kingdom, and the United States. Analysis of the stories of nine Taiwanese immigrant families reveals that immigrants' everyday life is inseparable from the economic structure of the receiving country. Three capitalist practices—the marketing culture, insurance, and credit—create a living context that increases immigrants' vulnerability in the United States.

The financial burden, potential legal ramifications, and limited access to housing, loans, and health care are not the kinds of experiences that immigrants to the United States anticipate before their immigration. Literature has shown that when people move into a new country they have to adapt, to varying extents, with regard to the language used by the receiving country, the physical environment, the culture, the systems, the loss of social support, and economic survival (Aroian, 1990; Baker et al., 1994; Lipson, 1992; Sam & Berry, 1995; Tsai, 2001). The adaptive processes can last from years to a lifetime. These unexpected experiences are additional stressors that place immigrants in the United States at risk while they are attempting to manage the other demands they must face as immigrants. Moreover, as part of the capitalist environment or economic structure, people in the United States are always bombarded with sales promotions for new products, business changes, new insurance coverage, and increases in health care costs. Even Americans who were born and raised in the United States struggle to understand the changes and choices available to them and to deal with these economic practices. Immigrants, particularly new immigrants, easily get lost in the massive amount of information thrown at them. Making an informed decision is a much more challenging and stressful process for new immigrants than for native-born Americans and established early-wave immigrants. In other words, immigrants' vulnerability exists on a continuum. The degree of the vulnerability increases when the receiving country's economic structure intersects with immigrants' language challenges, unfamiliarity with the systems, and/or limited access to local social networks for support. In this study, the participant families (who had been in the United States no more than 10 years) discussed their self-doubt about the decisions they made; they revealed their worries and frustration about the financial and legal consequences of their decisions. Unlike those citizens born in the United States, immigrants can face deportation for numerous legal issues (e.g., not reporting an address change to the immigration authority, speeding tickets, credit problems, or crime). Thus not only are immigrants concerned about the same financial and legal consequences as the people of the receiving country, but they also need to worry about the legal consequences specifically tied to their immigration status.

Navarro (1993) argues that the problems of the US health care system can not be understood without including capitalism—the moving force behind the financing and delivery of health services in the United States—in the discussion. Health insurance companies are controlled by corporate owners and have a tremendous power over how services are provided by health care providers. Profit and efficiency are the bases for their decision. Insurance premiums are raised to cover growing medical costs and ensure profits. As a result, employers shift the cost of insurance premiums to their employees and/or provide limited choices of insurance plans or no insurance at all. More people become uninsured and seek help in the emergency department only when their conditions are too severe to be ignored (Himmelstein, Woolhandler, & Hellander, 2001; Kleinke, 2001). Because capitalism in the United States has such an intimate relationship with immigrants' everyday experience, I would further argue that this economic framework has not only shaped the nation's health care system, it also has driven the production of goods and marketing, the creation of insurance policies, and access to those things which fill basic needs. To decrease immigrants' vulnerability and promote their health, it is absolutely essential to include capitalism in the discussion.

IMPLICATIONS FOR HEALTH PROFESSIONALS

Health professionals have ample opportunities to work with immigrants: in acute care settings, primary care settings, long-term care facilities, community clinics, workplaces, home settings, and schools. In fact, health professionals are in a valuable position to ensure health equity for immigrants. Presented here are some ways for health professionals to be true health advocates.

As a micro-level approach, during visits health professionals should include questions that can help them better understand the effects of the US capitalist economic structure and practices on the stress levels and well-being of immigrant clients. Because immigrant clients are already using their individual resources (e.g., personal intelligence and knowledge, social networks) to develop sufficient strategies to overcome those stressors, health professionals can (should) serve as another resource for these clients. If immigrant clients do not have enough individual resources to develop effective adaptive strategies, health professionals should then initiate the discussion and collaborate with the clients to formulate some potentially practical and successful strategies.

In addition to changing their own practices, health professionals have to share their knowledge with their colleagues and policy makers to heighten their awareness of the effects of the receiving country's economic structure on immigrants' vulnerability and health status. Thus fewer health professionals and policy makers will use culture or language barrier as a catch-all category to explain all immigrant experiences (McGrath, 1998; Tsai, 2003). Instead, more will have a more comprehensive understanding of immigrants' experiences and health care needs. As a result, more health professionals and policy makers will provide relevant interventions for the immigrant population and engage in the reconstruction of social and health policies that are driven by US capitalism—a system that goes beyond immigrants' control yet has a tremendous effect on their everyday life.

CLOSING THOUGHTS

Immigrants are at a higher risk for poor health. Nevertheless, their risk is not solely a result of language skills, education, levels of assimilation to the receiving country, or knowledge about the systems of the receiving country. The historical, sociocultural, economic, and political structures play significant roles in shaping immigrants' everyday experiences and health status. This chapter provides some preliminary insights into the effects of the US economic structure on immigrant vulnerability. To provide culturally competent care to the immigrant population, further investigation into each of these structural effects and their interactions with immigrants' vulnerability is crucial. Cross-national comparison is needed as well. Of course, it is also necessary to have more health professionals and policy makers who can recognize that the health experiences and stresses immigrants identify are indeed products of complex social processes. Immigrants then will not be blamed for their problems while the "causes" of the problems lie in the larger societal context.

ACKNOWLEDGMENTS

This chapter is based on the author's dissertation study. The study was supported in part by the American Nurses Foundation, the Psi-Chapter-at-Large of the Sigma Theta Tau International, the Robert Gilbert Foundation of the Association of Child and Adolescent Psychiatric Nurses, and the Hester McLaws Nursing Scholarship Fund of the University of Washington School of Nursing. An earlier version of this chapter was presented at the 2nd State of Science Congress in Washington, DC, in September 2002.

REFERENCES

Anderson, J. M. (1985). Perspectives on the health of immigrant women: A feminist analysis. *Advances in Nursing Science, 8*(1), 61–76.

Anderson, J. M. (1991). Immigrant women speak of chronic illness: The social construction of the devalued self. *Journal of Advanced Nursing, 16,* 710–717.

Aroian, K. J. (1990). A model of psychological adaptation to migration and resettlement. *Nursing Research, 39*(1), 5–10.

Baker, C., Arseneault, A. M., & Gallant, G. (1994). Resettlement without the support of an ethnocultural community. *Journal of Advanced Nursing, 20*(6), 1064–1072.

Barnes, D. M. (2001). Mental health screening in a refugee population: A program report. *Journal of Immigrant Health, 3*(3), 141–149.

Chopoorian, T. J. (1986). Reconceptualization the environment. In P. Moccia (Ed.). *New approaches to theory development* (pp. 39–54). New York, NY: National League for Nursing.

Himmelstein, D., Woolhandler, S., & Hellander, I. (2001). *Bleeding the patient: The consequences of corporate health care.* Monroe, ME: Common Courage.

HyperRESEARCH (Version 2.03). (1999). Thousand Oaks, CA: ResearchWare.

Kleinke, J. D. (2001). *Oxymorons: The myth of a US health care system.* San Francisco, CA: Jossey-Bass.

Lipson, J. G. (1992). The health and adjustment of Iranian immigrants. *Western Journal of Nursing Research, 14*(1), 10–29.

Lollock, L. (2001). *The foreign-born population in the United States: March 2000, current population reports* (US Census Bureau, Current Population Reports P20–534). Washington, DC: US Census Bureau.

McGrath, B. B. (1998). Illness as a problem of meaning: Moving culture from the classroom to the clinic. *Advances in Nursing Science, 21*(2), 17–29.

Meleis, A. I. (1996). Culturally competent scholarship: Substance and rigor. *Advances in Nursing Science, 19*(2), 1–16.

Munroe-Blum, H., Boyle, M. H., Offord, D. R., & Kates, N. (1989). Immigrant children: Psychiatric disorder, school performance, and service utilization. *American Journal of Orthopsychiatry, 59*(4), 510–519.

Nah, K. (1993). Perceived problems and service delivery for Korean immigrants. *Social Work, 38*(3), 289–296.

Navarro, V. (1993). *Dangerous to your health: Capitalism in health care.* New York, NY: Monthly Review Press.

Ödegaard, O. (1932). Emigration and insanity. *Acta Psychiatrica et Neurologia,* Supplement 4, Copenhagen, 11–206.

Riessman, C. K. (1993). *Narrative analysis: Vol. 30.* P. Manning, J. Van Maanen, & M. Miller (Eds.). Newbury Park, CA: Sage.

Rutter, M., Yule, W., Berger, M., Yule, B., Morton, J., & Bagley, C. (1974). Children of West Indian immigrants—I: Rates of behavioral deviance and of psychiatric disorder. *Journal of Child Psychology and Psychiatry, 15,* 241–262.

Sam, D. L., & Berry, J. W. (1995). Acculturative stress among young immigrants in Norway. *Scandinavian Journal of Psychology, 36*(1), 10–24.

Schmidley, A. D., & Gibson, C. (1999). *Profile of the foreign–born population in the United States: 1997* (US Census Bureau, Current Population Reports P23–195). Washington, DC: US Government Printing Office.

Tsai, J. H. C. (2001). *One story, two interpretations: The lived experiences of Taiwanese immigrant families in the United States.* Unpublished doctoral dissertation, University of Washington, Seattle.

Tsai, J. H. C. (2003). Contextualizing immigrants' lived experience: Story of Taiwanese immigrants in the United States. *Journal of Cultural Diversity, 10,* 76–83.

Weber, M. (1930/1992). *The protestant ethic and the spirit of capitalism* (A. Giddens, Trans.). London, UK: Routeledge.

Weitzman, B. C., & Berry, C. A. (1992). Health status and health care utilization among New York City home attendants: An illustration of the needs of working poor, immigrant women. *Women and Health, 19*(2/3), 87–105.

CHAPTER 17

Child Health in a Barrio of Managua

Susan P. Colvin, Mary de Chesnay,
Teodora Mercado, and Carmen Benavides

The purpose of this study was to identify some characteristics that enhance or limit the ability of mothers and community health workers to meet the health needs of children in a selected barrio of Managua, Nicaragua. The study was a joint United States–Nicaraguan study that was conducted within the framework of participatory action research (PAR) in order to provide information requested by the community health workers in the barrio. The interview questions were designed by the Nicaraguan nurses and a community leader who served an important function: accessing the mothers who were interviewed.

PAR is a methodology that enables people to transform their communities by developing plans for action toward specific purposes that they define in concert with the investigators. PAR is similar to ethnography in that the design entails detailed descriptions of the problem from the point of view of the subjects, rather than that of the researchers. PAR is a respectful way of conducting research because the design is implemented with the cooperation of the community and enables the community to use the data immediately. As such, PAR is particularly useful as a research method for studying vulnerable populations because the techniques are somewhat owned by the community being studied.

For this study, a team of nurse researchers from two universities (in Nicaragua and the United States) collaborated on a broader study to explore how to improve the health of the children who live there. Reported here is the outcome of a project that addressed some dimensions of the broader issues of health care for children in Nicaragua. The broad research question was: What are the community's primary concerns about health care of the children in this barrio (neighborhood)?

Faculty from the Nicaraguan school developed a model for nurses to use in assisting the community and later involved their sister school in the United States in a variety of projects designed to improve the health status of people who reside in this barrio. Every year since 1993, students and faculty from the United States school have traveled to Nicaragua to work with the Nicaraguan faculty and the families of the barrio on community assessment, clinical interventions, and health teaching. Because about 60% of the population is younger than 17 (MINSA, 2000), the team decided to focus this particular study on children. The study elicited concerns of mothers in the barrio and included feedback to the *brigadistas,* a group of community health workers who live in the barrio, so that they can develop an action plan in concert with the Nicaraguan nurses.

LITERATURE

There are few studies on the health of children in Nicaragua, and those found in the literature center around the most basic problem, infant mortality, and its leading cause, diarrhea. Inextricably linked to poverty, childhood diarrhea and the resulting dehydration have been the subjects of epidemiological studies in the developing world. In one of the few studies available, an optimistic picture for Nicaragua was provided by Sandiford, Morales, Gorter, Coyle, & Smith (1991) who concluded that infant mortality rates dropped sharply—an average of 4.7 deaths per 1000 live births each year from 1974 to 1986—with a low of 63 deaths per live births in 1986. Sandiford's team attributed these results to several factors, including income, nutrition, breastfeeding, maternal education, access to health services, provision of water, and antimalarial programs.

Peña, Wall, & Persson (2000) performed a cohort analysis of infant survival in León (Nicaragua) from 1988 to 1993 in which they found that the infant mortality rate was 50 per 1000 live births. They concluded that poverty and social inequity increased the risk but that infant mortality risks were lower among families with educated mothers. Though the study was conducted in one city, the demographics of this city are similar to other parts of the Pacific coastal region. Notably lacking is information from the Atlantic coastal region.

Several studies were conducted in Nicaragua on diarrhea and its medical treatment, oral rehydration and antibiotics (Hudelson, 1993; Jacobs, Jiménez, Gloyd, Gale, & Crothers, 1994; Paniagua, Espinoza, Ringman, Reizenstein, Svennerholm, & Halander, 1997; Smith et.al. 1993). These studies indicated that although antibiotics and oral rehydration solutions are provided to families, many mothers tend to favor home remedies. In a randomized double-blind study by Jacobs et al. (1994), statistically significant results indicated that homeopathic remedies were often used instead of the prescribed medical treatment.

All of the studies found in the literature are highly quantitative and have a narrow focus. No studies were found from the point of view of the people affected, nor were there any studies that produced results that could be used by the people to improve their health care outcomes.

METHODS

The study was conducted in two phases: the interview phase and the community feedback phase. In the first phase, interviews were conducted with mothers who reside in the barrio. After the interviews were analyzed, a community meeting was arranged in order for the researchers to share the data and discuss how the findings might be used by the *brigadistas*. (*Brigadistas* are community residents who have received some first-aid training and function as health resources for the people in the community. *Brigadistas* range in age from early adolescents to adults.) More than simply a means to share the results of the interviews, the community meeting is central to the idea of action research (discussed more fully in Chapter 19) in that it is here that the results are turned over to the community to use.

Additional interviews were conducted with nurses in Bluefields on the Atlantic coast, a region isolated geographically from Managua, for the purpose of gaining a sense of the commonalities of child health issues across the country. The findings were also validated by nurses who work in a northern community near Jinotega.

Sample

The sampling method was purposive, and the sample of 10 mothers residing in the barrio was drawn from a total population in the barrio of about 10,000 people. In addition, interviews were conducted with nurses who are familiar with the barrio and data from the health ministry Ministerio de Salud (MINSA) were used for background. The study was approved by the American university's institutional review board. Procedures to protect the rights of subjects were instituted, consistent with US federal policies regarding research with human subjects. However, it is important to note that the usual connotation of "subjects" does not apply in PAR because the community members are active participants, not recipients of experimental treatments. The mothers' age range was between the high teens and 20s, and there was a mix of single and married women.

Setting

Description of the Barrio

This barrio was (and is) a marginal urban community, settled primarily by people who lost their homes during natural disasters or who were displaced from the countryside by civil war and relocated to southeast Managua. About 10,000 people live there, and 52.6% are women, many of whom are single mothers. The rate of unemployment in 1999 was 45%; in addition, many people functioned in low-level jobs (15%) such as street vending and housekeeping (11%) (Guevara, 1999). A system of informal health care was instituted by community leaders who recruited older, responsible children and adolescents called *brigadistas* to assist in identifying health problems and referring people to the Centro de Salud (health center.)

According to Guevara (1999), there are 1310 houses in the barrio and 1.2 families per house (extended families). Sixteen percent of the homes have dirt floors, and the others are mostly cement (UPOLI, 2000). Of the homes, 66.7% have latrines, and 34.2% use open air; 51% throw or burn garbage in empty places near the house. There are no lighted streets. In terms of education, 14.8% of the children in the barrio finish primary school, and 7% finish secondary school, but 14.7% of the population is illiterate (Guevara, 1999). Of the total population in the barrio under study, 40.7% completed elementary school, and 35.3% completed secondary school (UPOLI, 2000). Education was generally valued by members of the community, and there was a school in the barrio.

Approximately 50% of children under age 5 years are vaccinated against the usual childhood diseases and polio. Fifty percent of the population has pediculosis (lice). Food establishments tend to operate without health licenses (Guevara, 1999). Attempts to grow food in gardens meet with varying degrees of success but are hindered by the scarcity of water.

Research Team

Nursing faculty from two schools (Nicaraguan and American) worked together to conduct this study. The schools are described briefly here in order to emphasize the close collaboration of the research team.

Nicaraguan School

The Nicaraguan school of nursing, Universidad Politécnica de Nicaragua (UPOLI) in Managua, Nicaragua, with about 230 students, is administered within a small private university of about 6000 students and is operated under the auspices of the Baptists. Founded in 1943, the school of nursing was the first in the country and was originally operated by the Baptist Hospital. In 1978, the school began to offer the baccalaureate degree in nursing, and 2600 graduates have earned that degree. The school established a nursing center in the barrio, and funds were obtained in partnership with Canadian nurses to build a community center, which includes rooms for clinical services. The faculty and students conduct health assessments, teach residents about health, and refer residents to the formal health care delivery system (the Centro de Salud). Most of the faculty are nurses with master's degrees. They are committed to teaching students professional principles and are experts in community health nursing. Proud of their work in the barrio, the faculty are modest about their many accomplishments. Beginning with a community diagnostic assessment in 1992, the school has integrated theory into practice by addressing real health needs.

American School

The American school of nursing at Duquesne University in Pittsburgh offers three degrees: baccalaureate, master's degree, and doctorate. The school is operated under the auspices of a Catholic university. In 1992, the Center for International Nursing invited 20 Nicaraguan nurses to the American city for a course on management and leadership. The group included faculty from the Nicaraguan school, and they expressed an interest in partnering with the faculty at the American school. A sister school relationship (*hermanamiento*) was signed in 1995 by the two deans of nursing, and many student–faculty exchanges and research projects have been completed or are in progress.

Instrumentation

In PAR, the instrument consists of both the interview questions and the ability of the researcher to elicit rich emic data, i.e., data from the viewpoint of the participant. For this study, the American pediatric nurse (first author Colvin) worked with Nicaraguan faculty members (Mercado and Benavides) and a community leader to develop the questions, conduct pilot interviews, and recruit the sample. The second author (de Chesnay) served as facilitator and methodologist. The American nurses had worked for many years with the Nicaraguans and, through participant observation, were familiar with the barrio. A semistructured interview guide was translated into Spanish to answer questions of concern to the Nicaraguans and was used as a starting point for the interviews with mothers. Questions were designed to elicit information about the following general areas of concern: health status of children, sources of information and support to families, and access to the health care delivery system. The interview questions were

1. Do you think the boys and girls of this generation are healthier than the past generation?
2. How do the children in your community find out about good health?
3. Who are the best sources of information about good health?
4. Where is the best place to go to get help if you or your children are sick?
5. How far do you have to go to get help if you or your children are sick?
6. In your community, who are the best people at helping those who are sick?
7. Have you ever been to the hospital? If so, what did you like and dislike about the hospital?

8. Have you ever been to the Centro de Salud (or another health center)? If so, what did you like and dislike?
9. What is the best thing about living in your community?
10. What are the three most serious health problems of children in your community?

Procedures

The first activity was a meeting of the research team and the community leader, an adult woman who served as the primary *brigadista* and whose guidance was essential to the project. Interviews were conducted with her and one other mother to pilot the interview guide and plan. Data were translated into English for analysis and then content analyzed to identify key themes that could form the basis for action strategies. Several discussions were held among the members of the research team as to the meaning of the data. Finally, a meeting was held with the community *brigadistas* in order to share data and develop an action plan.

RESULTS

Health Status of Children

Most of the participants indicated that children of the current generation were not as healthy as children of their own generation and they cited as a primary cause the deteriorating status of the economy as expressed in poor water quality, food shortages, and sanitation problems. The children's health problems most identified by the mothers were diarrhea, fever, grippe (influenza), respiratory disease, skin rashes, malnutrition, mosquito-born malaria and dengue fever, and parasites. Wanting to keep their children fed and homes clean emerged as a strong value of these mothers.

"Children's health was better before, when I was growing up. There were better jobs . . . parents could give their children more and better foods. I think this affected our health."

"The children are less healthy. There is not good water. If the children want to be clean they can't."

"There was not much garbage (in my time), and the garbage was picked up. The water was better."

"Children's health is worse now. Now there are too many parasites, and people cough too much."

"The drinking water is dirty, and the street is full of trash."

"Rashes are caused by all the dust in the barrio."

Sources of Information and Support

The mothers indicated that children's best sources of knowledge about health are their families and the schools but also commented on the success of billboard campaigns, a prominent government-sponsored source of information for the people who do not have access to radio or television.

"Always the parents. They get the information from their parents. Neighbors are important, too—good neighbors are important—they help."

"Parents, teachers, and health workers [*brigadistas*] in the barrio and sometimes the church."

"Parents and teachers tell children to keep their house and hands clean . . . and teach good nutrition—like eating fruit and hand washing."

For themselves, mothers identified the nurses in the health center as their best source of knowledge and their primary resource in the event of illness or injury, saying: "[We go to] the Centro de Salud or hospital if it's an emergency." Others indicated that "some neighbors are nurses."

Almost all the mothers indicated that their primary source of medical support was the Ministry of Health center located just outside the barrio (Centro de Salud). However, two mothers reported that the Catholic church was a resource. This is not surprising because even during the Sandinista times under a Communist system of government, the Catholic church was respected by the people. There have been many other religious groups prominent in Nicaragua over the years, and they too have had a major impact on communities by doing social service work and providing medical care. To quote the study participants: "[We go] to church for spiritual health. I would go there."

Accessing the Health Care Delivery System

When asked about modes of travel, all respondents indicated that they walked. Most stated that they could walk to the Centro de Salud in about 15 minutes. Transportation is limited, and there is a complicated process mothers need to go through to accomplish even the most mundane chores. "We don't have a car, so we walk, and it's hard if it's an emergency. Sometimes a neighbor will drive us in an emergency."

The mothers reported that there is a strong informal network of resources they use prior to accessing the formal health care delivery system. Mothers indicated that they use the *brigadistas,* their family members who live with them (mothers or in-laws), and neighbors (some of whom are nurses).

"First I get help from the *brigadistas.*"

"Neighbors—they help us, we help them."

Experiencing the Health Care Delivery System

We asked the mothers about their experiences with the hospitals and the Centro de Salud. In general their perceptions of both places were positive, but common criticisms were long waiting periods to be seen by a nurse or doctor and dirty conditions. All the mothers had been to a hospital at least once, particularly the maternity hospital. A majority commented that they liked the attention they received.

"I was in the hospital to have a baby—it was too crowded."

"I was in the hospital to have a c-section (caesarian delivery). There was good attention to the mothers."

"I went to the maternity hospital for babies. The attention was OK but there was not enough attention to the mother. I had to wait outside while I was in labor and could only go in to deliver the baby and then stay for 12 hours after I had the baby."

"When I was working I had insurance so I went to the hospital when I didn't feel good for gyn[ecological] care. The attention was good, but I did not like how long you must wait—sometimes 3–4 hours, and there are too many sick people."

"Only for the delivery of children . . . I did not like it. There was bad care. It's the worst hospital."

"Only to one hospital. Everything was OK, but the nurses are not well behaved and don't give attention to people."

"To the Children's Hospital. The baby had vomiting and diarrhea. We went in the morning and stayed the next day. He had good attention, everything was good. He was 1 year old."

All mothers had visited the free Centro de Salud. Most had favorable comments.

"For general health care . . . I also went to the Centro in the barrio of El where I lived before for prenatal care. There were less people there, but sometimes the clinic had to close because there were no doctors."

"Today I went for a PAP test. I got quick attention."

"To Centro here . . . the care for the baby is good. The bad thing is that the wait is too long. I wait very long with the baby."

"There was nothing good. I did not get good attention. I took my son to see the psychiatrist there; he needed to see a psychiatrist. They kept sending him to one doctor then another. He could not see the right doctor. This is the only clinic I have been to . . ."

"I get good attention but I can't get medicine. I got better attention at another clinic but it cost lots of money."

"Some of the ladies [nurses] are not polite and the doctors don't tell you anything unless you ask, but I got good attention. I took my oldest child to a private clinic near the new Centro. It was private and I had to pay and wait a long time, but it's closer. He has a kidney infection. If the children have a fever, I take them to the Centro."

Living in the Barrio

The Nicaraguan nurses had a long-term relationship with the barrio and many active projects. They were particularly interested in what people liked best about living in this barrio and were gratified to hear from the mothers that the mothers appreciated the efforts of the two schools of nursing in working with the community.

"It's stable and well-organized. A good place to raise children. And it also has organized health care at the Centro."

"It's pretty—everyone works together to keep it clean, everyone gets along."

"We can own our houses. I moved here 10 years ago from León. The bad thing is the water. There's no water."

"Electricity is good but the water is bad."

"I was able to buy a house here. We can live here with the whole family."

"It's a nice, tranquil barrio. People don't intrude."

DISCUSSION

The findings revealed a consensus among residents on some aspects of health needs. For example, parents and other family members emerged as the primary source of health information for children. Schools and churches play a lesser role as sources of information. A majority of mothers perceived the health of their children as somewhat poorer compared with their own generation.

What is apparent in the interviews is the prominent role that the new Centro de Salud plays in the lives of the residents of the barrio. All respondents had visited the Centro, and most had favorable impressions of the care they received. If prevention of disease is the focus, the residents overwhelmingly rely on the nurses at the Centro for information about good health. In addition, the Centro is by far the first choice for barrio residents to go to when they are acutely ill. Mothers, by and large, see the Centro as accessible—it is located on the outer perimeter of the barrio. Although access to transportation is difficult, they do not complain about having to walk 15 minutes to get to the Centro.

The country continues to be plagued with environmental problems, and barrio residents are particularly affected by problems of sanitation, clean water, and the associated problems of mosquitoes and other pests. Respiratory and gastrointestinal diseases continue to adversely affect the population. Many middle-income houses in Managua have rain-collection tanks on the roof, but there is no such device in the barrio, although the nurses have identified installing a tank on the community building/clinic as a priority.

The last phase of the study involved presenting the findings to the community. The meeting was held in the community center, an informal setting in which the *brigadistas* sat in a circle with the two pediatric nurses and the community leader. Once the formalities concluded, the meeting began with a review of the project and the information gathered from mothers. Information was prepared in Spanish and distributed to the *brigadistas,* who were then encouraged to comment. Their concerns centered around issues of sanitation and water storage. Related concerns were the prevention of dehydration and diarrhea in children. The handout included the symptoms of dehydration and methods and treatment with oral rehydration solution.

Because respiratory diseases emerged as a major problem, information was also presented about ways to reduce local environmental pollution such as the smoke from cooking fires in homes and secondhand smoke. These homes are one-room buildings with a center fire pit for cooking, and the fire is left burning all day. There is poor ventilation, so the smoke inside the homes becomes intense and creates a variety of respiratory conditions. Methods to treat respiratory distress that were taught included postural drainage, breathing exercises, and chest percussion.

Malnutrition was the third major problem, and this topic was addressed by presenting information about the best diets for small children, taking into account which foods provide nutrients and are available within the community. Breastfeeding is supported through a national program, and the presentation to the *brigadistas* included encouragement to breastfeed.

An example of a unique concern of the *brigadistas* was the practical problem of gangs roaming the streets at night. This led to the question of what to do at night if a child is having difficulty breathing. The prescribed intervention would be immediate transport to the hospital. However, the gangs make it is unsafe for barrio residents to leave their homes. Because of this, principles of rescue breathing (in contrast to CPR, which can be dangerous) were explained with the proviso that the child should be transported as soon as possible. It would be interesting to see whether the barrio could negotiate with the gangs for a truce for emergency purposes.

The MINSA nurses in Bluefields (a port city on the Atlantic coast) verified that the same problems identified in Managua were also concerns along the Atlantic coast. However, with the unemployment rate of 95% in the Atlantic coast versus 80% in Managua (as reported by the nurses in Bluefields), these nurses thought that the problems of child health were exacerbated by the despair of the people.

The findings were independently validated by a second Nicaraguan–American team of nurses providing services in a rural community near Jinotega in the northern part of the country, near the border with Honduras. Although data were not collected systematically through the same methods, it is clear that the barrio represents a microcosm of the country in terms of the questions studied.

The desperation of the people in the barrio is tempered by hope and persistence. The residents of this particular barrio receive support from the two schools of nursing, who have made a long-term commitment to the community. The study generated information about specific health factors and problems that can be addressed by the Nicaraguan nurses in the development of future projects. The relevance of the projects is validated by the collaboration of the nurses with the *brigadistas* and the community leader.

Based on the findings from this project, further studies are planned. First, it became obvious during this study that children's health and mental health are related, so the team is currently working on a follow-up study dealing with violence against women and children. Second, the data need to be compared with new statistical information gathered by MINSA to analyze trends. Third, interventions that are specific to the problems in this barrio will be developed and tested. For example, the problem of night transportation to the hospital needs to be solved in light of the information about gang activity.

ACKNOWLEDGMENT

The authors thank the barrio residents for their participation and the schools of nursing at Universidad Politécnica de Nicaragua and Duquesne University for partial funding of the study.

REFERENCES

Guevara, M. (1999). *Synthesis of the community project: Anexo Villa Libertad.* Managua: UPOLI.

Hudelson, P. (1993). ORS and the treatment of childhood diarrhea in Managua, Nicaragua. *Social Science Medicine, 37,* 97–103.

Jacobs, J., Jiménez, L. M., Gloyd, S., Gale, J., & Crothers, D. (1994). Treatment of childhood diarrhea with homeopathic medicine: A randomized clinical trial in Nicaragua. *Pediatrics, 93,* 719–725.

Figueroa de Robles, E. (2000). Handout prepared by Chief Nurse and given to S. Colvin as personal communication. Ministerio de Salud (MINSA).

Paniagua, M., Espinoza, F., Ringman, M., Reizenstein, E., Svennerholm, M. M., & Halander, H. (1997). Analysis of incidence of infection with enterotoxigenic *Escheria coli* in a prospective cohort study of infant diarrhea in Nicaragua. *Journal of Clinical Microbiology, 35,* 1404–1410.

Peña, R., Wall, S., & Persson, L. (2000). The effect of poverty, social inequity and maternal education on infant mortality in Nicaragua, 1988–1993. *American Journal of Public Health, 90,* 64–69.

Sandiford, P., Morales, P., Gorter, A., Coyle, E., & Smith, G. (1991). Why do child mortality rates fall? An analysis of the Nicaraguan experience. *American Journal of Public Health, 81,* 30–37.

Smith, G., Gorter, A., Hoppenbrouwer, J., Sweep, A., Perez, R., Gonzalez, C., et al. (1993). The cultural construction of childhood diarrhea in rural Nicaragua: Relevance for epidemiology and health promotion. *Social Science Medicine, 36,* 1613–1624.

UPOLI Escuela de Enfermería. (2000). *Diagnostico comunitario en el Anexo Villa Libertad como linea de base del Centro de Atención de Enfermería: 1999.* Managua: UPOLI Escuela de Enfermería.

CHAPTER 18

Medication Practices of African American Seniors

Lenore K. Resick, Mary de Chesnay,
Debra Kubinski, Roberta Zolkoski

As the population of the United States shifts to that of an older population, the topic of medication use among aging Americans must be viewed as an emerging health issue by the nursing profession. The urgency of investigating this topic was underscored by a group of African American inner-city community leaders, who noted that older adults living in residences within their community seemed to be experiencing problems with medication use. These leaders noted that older community members appeared to be prescribed many medications and were not sure how to take them and whether to mix them. The leaders asked this university-based research team to investigate the ways in which these seniors take their medications and to use the vehicle of the nurse-managed center operated by the school of nursing to intervene and assist residents who were experiencing problems. The leaders also requested the dissemination of more information about medication administration in "lay terms."

This study was a form of action research (discussed more fully in Chapter 19) in which community residents took an active role in conducting research relating to their health. This study was initiated by the community, and most data were collected by a member of the community. The family nurse practitioner and manager of the nursing center operated by the school was the leader of the research team. Action research elicits data from the emic point of view or the point of view of the community residents affected by the policies and practices of nurses providing community-based care. The significance of the study is that the question posed by the community was answered, and the data were used by the nursing center's staff to increase their understanding of the culture of the community they serve.

The importance of the topic of medication use by older African Americans is supported by population projections provided by the United States Bureau of the Census. According to estimated census figures, the growth rate of the population of African American seniors is expected to increase by 50% between the years 2000 and 2025; that is, the percentage of African Americans in this age bracket is expected to rise from 8.2% of the total population in the year 2000 to 12.3% of the total population in the year 2025 (US Bureau of the Census, 1995). Furthermore, research indicates that the prevalence of disease varies by race and ethnicity, with older African Americans generally having more health problems than their elderly white counterparts (Cooper, 1993).

The long-term objective of the study was to educate the community about medication administration so that older adults could take control over their own health. The purpose of the study was to elicit information about types of medications and the participants' knowledge of their use.

LITERATURE

The literature dealing with medication use among the elderly reveals studies of inappropriate drug prescribing (McVeigh, 2001; Psaty et al., 1993; Schmader et al., 1994; Willcox, Himmelstein, & Woolhandler, 1994) as well as studies on pharmacodynamics and pharmacogeriatrics (Craig, 1994; Katz, 1993; Paolisso et al., 1994; Piraino, 1995). Additional studies revealed that older persons are twice as likely to receive prescription medications and are more likely to take more than one medication compared with the rest of the population (Piraino, 1995; Sternberg et al., 2003).

Variations in pharmacokinetics resulting from changes in the physiological processes related to aging affect clearance, metabolism, and bioavailability of drugs in the elderly (Craig, 1994; Katz, 1993; Paolisso et al., 1994; Piraino, 1995). Therefore, as health problems increase with aging and more therapeutic agents are added to the medication regime, there is the increased likelihood of drug interactions, adverse reactions, and drug-related side effects (Bjerrum, Andersen, Petersen, & Kragstrup, 2003; Stone, 1991).

It is well documented that the elderly account for an increase in the prevalence of drug-related hospitalizations (Colt & Shapiro, 1989; Grymonpre et al., 1988; Ives, et al, 1987). Lamy (1990) reported that adverse drug reactions account for 10–30% of hospital admissions in the geriatric population. Stone (1991) explained that combinations of medications greatly increase the probability of a drug interaction, specific drug adverse effects, and iatrogenic problems in the elderly. Furthermore, polypharmacy in the elderly is a significant factor in falls and contributes to difficulties in screening geriatric patients for vulnerabilities to a variety of health problems (Kinn & Clawson, 2002; Miller et al., 2000).

The literature supports the finding that little information is currently available on drug utilization patterns and the management of adverse drug reactions in older adults in the community setting (LeSage, 1991; Pollow et al., 1994). Also, the literature is scarce with regard to medication-taking behaviors among high-functioning and low-functioning seniors living in the community, including older African Americans (Wallsten et al., 1995), and there are limited reports addressing the perceptions of older African Americans from the emic (person's point of view) perspective.

METHODOLOGY

The design of this study was ethnographic, and data collection took place over a 1-year period, beginning with a series of participant observation activities (Resick, Taylor, Carroll, D'Antonio, & de Chesnay, 1997). Observations about medication interactions and patterns of medication administration were initially made at the nursing center by the nurse practitioner/primary researcher while she was in the process of establishing rapport within the community. Interviews with elderly African American participants followed, although the cultural informants were not necessarily clients at the center.

After institutional review board approval was obtained, pilot interviews were conducted to aid in the development of a semistructured interview guide. Initially, interviews were conducted in the neighborhood in which the nursing center was located; later interviews included African American seniors living in a different area of the state. Once the interview guide was refined, interviews were conducted with 22 residents of the community (primary setting) and 3 residents from a distant site (secondary setting), resulting in a total sample size of 25. All cultural informants were African Americans over the age of 65 years because they were the community of interest and because the concern about medication was initially expressed on behalf of these citizens by African American leaders. Results are presented collectively because no differences between these two sample populations were noted.

Setting

The primary setting was an urban neighborhood of a large western Pennsylvania city. The secondary setting, urban but smaller in size, was also in Pennsylvania and was located approximately 100 miles from the first. The demographic composition of both settings was similar, consisting primarily of white Americans with clusters of African American neighborhoods. The wellness center was located in the primary setting and was operated by the research team's school of nursing and funded (originally) by the Department of Housing and Urban Development (HUD). This center was established at the request of community leaders, who expressed concern that the residents constituted a medically underserved population (Resick et al., 1997).

Data Collection and Analysis

Data were collected through interviews in the homes of the cultural informants with a semi-structured interview guide designed by the team to obtain data regarding medication knowledge, beliefs, and patterns of use. Conducting the interview in the homes of the participant was a convenience to the participants, but it also enabled the interviewer to record specific drug names as printed on the drug labels. All interviews were audiotaped, and transcriptions were typed to permit review by the team and to ensure accuracy.

Accuracy was maximized by intensive review of the tapes and discussions within the team. Data from the participant observation experiences in the first phase of the study were discussed by the research team, as were preliminary interview data, in order to determine areas of agreement and disagreement and aid in the refinement of the semistructured interview guide. Further team discussion led to the decision to include a similar but less urban secondary site for the expressed purpose of comparative data analysis. Following the completion of the 25 interviews, team discussions focused on audiotape review, accuracy of transcription, and analysis of data. Data analysis resulted in the identification of an emerging typology of themes that related to the research questions regarding medications and their use. A culminating strategy included the submission of data for review by individuals not originally associated with the team, including a nursing master's degree student and nursing doctoral students, as a way of validating the decision trail of conclusions. The final stage involved review of results by all members of the research team, with an emphasis on evidence to support conclusions in order to ultimately come to consensus about meanings.

RESULTS

Sample

The sample consisted of 25 African American seniors, including 5 men and 20 women. There were many areas of consistency among participants, and no striking gender, demographic, or environmental differences were noted. One of the first steps in data analysis was to identify and categorize the medications taken by this sample and to identify their most common health problems, but these data were secondary to the main focus. The most frequent medications were antihypertensives, calcium channel blockers, anticoagulents, and diuretics. The medications seemed to be consistent with the most common chronic disease problems, which were hypertension, coronary artery disease and history of myocardial infarction, stroke, and congestive heart disease.

Responses

The following section highlights informant responses using pseudonyms selected by the informants to maintain confidentiality. Responses were organized according to the typology of the 16 themes (the sections that follow) that emerged during data analysis.

System and/or Routine for Self-Medication

Participants described using a daily pill dispenser, keeping medications on a designated table or tray, or placing nighttime medications next to the bed. Participants said they kept medications in one place to be a visible reminder. Referring to medications by name indicated incorporation into daily routines or patterns of living, so pills became known as pills "in the morning," "after breakfast," "with meals," or "at night." Practices for taking medications were linked to daily activities so medications would be taken at mealtime, after coming downstairs, after going upstairs, after bathing, or before sleeping. Participants referred to support and/or assistance from spouses, children, friends, and neighbors to prepare medications, remind them to take medications, or maintain a calendar and/or chart to help keep track of medications due and when taken. For example, Ms. Carolyn relied on her friend to remind her and check on her evening medications.

Accountability and Responsibility

Most participants took medications as prescribed without question unless problems arose with side effects, at which time they would exercise independent decision making and then notify the doctor. Ms. Ruth recalled that once she was taking many medications and they were making her sick, so she stopped taking them and then called and told the doctor she had stopped taking them. He gave his approval. Ms. Liz explained that she altered her potassium chloride dose depending on her dietary intake of potassium. Ms. Carolyn independently decided to take her evening pills at bedtime because she took her morning pills late; she explained that the visiting nurse often placed the pills in the evening slot, but she always took them at bedtime because that was "the right way."

Two male informants stated they did not take their water pill (diuretic) on days they had to leave the house but took the pill when they returned home, if it was not too late. Ms. Beverly said she quit medications "years ago" and has not returned to her doctor for between 1 and 2 years; her concerns included cost, smoking (she smoked and was told to quit), and fear of a diagnosis of another blocked coronary artery.

Ms. Jessy said she took pills "when I feel like it," took one pill at a time to monitor effects, did not like to take medications, was dissatisfied with the health care delivery system, and said "I spend a lot of time alone because I just don't trust people." Mr. Lloyd said he used garlic and cranberry as substitutes for prescription medications because of cost, and he demonstrated inaccurate knowledge of medication actions. Ms. Ruth explained an approach that was symptom-oriented, leading her to conclude that she didn't need Zantac or potassium chloride at times. She also said that she skipped a dose of insulin once in awhile.

Knowledge of Medications

Participants very rarely knew drug names. Medications were referred to by appearance, size, color, what they were taken for, or what they did: "for my heart," "for blood pressure," or "for breathing." Participants were able to explain how to take medications, such as "with food," "wait between puffs," or "rinse mouth after puffs." The participants demonstrated a very pragmatic, practical approach that focused on what medication knowledge was really needed in most cases.

Response to Taking Medications

Almost all participants stated they did not like to take pills unless absolutely necessary and that they would stay away from medication if able. Mr. Harry said he never took his prescribed sedative, explaining that "I read in my pill book that it would be detrimental to my body." Ms. Ruth explained that if her "arthritis is real bad . . . will take pain pill . . . not too often, only when I have to . . . I can endure pain." Ms. Ruth stated she had a lot of pain because of her arthritis, and the doctor wouldn't order a pain pill for her. (Ms. Ruth presented contradictory information.)

Over-the-counter (OTC) drugs were not used by most participants; a few took OTC medications for colds, arthritis, upset stomach, and headache. They stated that the doctor knew of the use of these medications. Many commented that they were concerned about interactions with prescribed medications or that the OTC medications could create health problems because of chronic disease.

Response to Medication Side Effects

Participants identified pain in the stomach, nausea, and increased blood sugar as associated with medication use. Participants reported side effects to the doctor, which resulted in a change in therapy, such as discontinuing the medication, decreasing the dose, or trying a different medication. Participants expressed being in touch with physical feelings and changes, especially when taking new medications. Most participants commonly and readily called the doctor with medication problems. Ms. Rose stated she knew she should not take aspirin with a nonsteroidal anti-inflammatory drug (NSAID), but the same doctor ordered both of these medications and she thought "he should know what he's doing." However, she started bleeding from her colostomy and was unsure what to do, so she took the aspirin just once in a while, not daily as prescribed. She had not talked with the doctor about this, although she said she "can call the doctor," but in the meantime is waiting to see what happens.

Interaction with the Health Care Delivery System

Negative comments about the doctors or health care services were rare, but they were expressed. Ms. Jessy stated she felt "too rushed," and in reference to her health maintenance organization, she stated it was "run by a corporation and they are out for just the profit; they don't care whether you're sick or well, and they don't care if you get well." Ms. Beverly and Ms. Jessy recalled doctors questioning their ability to pay, so they did not return to those doctors, although there were other contributing factors in these situations.

Positive comments were expressed by the majority of the participants, including "Doctors work well together as a team," "Doctors explain things," "Can ask the doctors questions," "Nurses call and check on them," and "Pharmacists are very good." Comments usually indicated that participants felt the doctors and nurses cared about them.

Response to Missing a Dose

Participants expressed that they were not overly concerned if they forgot a medication, explaining that they would take the medication when they remembered, and, if late, would wait until the next dose was due. Most favored waiting until the next scheduled dose, and most identified problems with doubling up doses to make up for missed medications, registering greater concern about taking too much medication than taking too little. In the words of Mr. Harry, he would "use good common sense" if a medication was missed.

On the whole, participants rarely acknowledged forgetting. Ms. Mary stated that she "can't recall the last missed dose." Ms. Jeannie explained that she never forgets, said it is "automatic." Ms. Alice described having a pill box dispenser that keeps her from forgetting. Ms. Liz replied that she "don't miss too many . . . ready for breakfast, I have everything right there." Ms. Eulah emphasized "no, that's part of what I got to do to keep me goin' for the day . . . I want to get better so bad."

Attention to Prescription Refills

Participants explained that they sometimes ran out of a medication for "a day" or "a while" because there was no refill prescription, there was a problem with insurance coverage, or they were unable to pick up the medication because they had no transportation. Mr. Ooch explained that he had a bag of extra medication as "back-up."

Response to Expiration Dates

Participants were not generally aware of the expiration date when asked. Many participants had a bag or box of "old medications," but this didn't seem to confuse them or lead to a problem.

Sharing of Medications

All participants responded strongly with "no" and "never" in response to questions about routinely sharing, lending, or borrowing prescription medications. Ms. Mary said "I think that would be the worst thing in the world; me borrowing somebody's medicine or give somebody something that I'm taking." Ms. Ruth recalled borrowing a prescription medication once because she was out of town without her medication and someone had her "exact same medication." She explained that she did not use this person's patch, however, because it was the "wrong strength," and the pharmacy sent some of hers down.

Reaction to the Cost of Medications

Almost all participants had insurance coverage. Only one participant had to self-pay, and that person incurred a cost of $103 per month. Ms. Ruth stated that insulin needles are expensive, so she uses them twice, explaining that a doctor told her this was "okay." Mr. Lloyd mentioned cost as one factor for substituting garlic pills and cranberry capsules for prescription medication. Some participants explained that with insurance coverage paying for refills on a monthly basis, it is difficult to get prescriptions refilled as soon as they run out and before the new prescription is needed.

Use of Home or Folk Remedies

In response to this question, participants explained healthy eating practices, which included fruits, vegetables, bran, and a decrease in red meat and fat in their diets. Some participants mentioned hot water applications and hot baths as treatments for pain. Some participants explained using mustard, vinegar and water, and garlic and water for stomach upset, sore throat, or "phlegm." Ms. Millie discussed many "medicinal herbs" she used but not in place of prescription medications. She stated that both herbs and medications were important but said she could "replace medicines if she could talk with her friend." There was no evidence supporting the practice of using folk or home remedies in place of prescription medications, except for Mr. Lloyd, who did use garlic pills and cranberry capsules. This was related to inaccurate knowledge and concern for costs.

Male to Female Ratio or Gender Influence

The 20 women and 5 men demonstrated no apparent cohort differences in their approach to taking medications or in their health care practices.

Religious Influence

Many participants referred to church and the Lord, but religious beliefs were not raised as an issue that affected their ability to take prescription medications. Ms. Emma indicated a slight conflict between her religious beliefs and her use of medications but concluded that "He [God] sent the medications."

Environmental and Demographic Effects

There was a sense that informants at the primary site were neighbors or resided together, which may have reflected an environmental, demographic, or geographical connection or effect, although informants in the secondary site resided in separate communities within this city.

References to Future Plans

Participants' responses with regard to future plans indicated they planned to learn from the interaction with the researcher. They had "plans to do something," if their initial answers in the interview did not seem sensible or "right" to them, or if the interviewer persisted in this line of questioning, leading them to question their decisions. Plans included taking a list of all medications to the pharmacist for evaluation, getting a notebook to record blood glucose values, buying groceries, and not relying on the wheelchair but to start using the walker. Contradictory responses were noted, suggesting that maybe participants had become confused or were looking for the "right" response because of concerns that their behaviors or plans were not acceptable, i.e. stemming from concern that they were expected to have future plans.

DISCUSSION

The study did not identify a significant health need, but new insights were gained about medication practices of the community served by the nursing center. Results reflect that these African American seniors tended to be knowledgeable about their medications and followed the prescribed regimen. These individuals tied medication practices to daily routines, such as mealtimes, bathing, and getting up or going to bed, and referred to their routines as strategies for helping them remember to take their medications. If routines were disrupted, however, medications were sometimes forgotten, but most participants had developed a method for dealing with forgotten meds, using a conservative approach to avoid overmedication. Consequently, medication times were readjusted or the participants would wait until the next dose was due.

These participants had, in fact, developed creative problem-solving strategies by which to incorporate medications into their lifestyles, including the use of calendars and charts and the establishment of support and backup systems, relying on family members, friends, and neighbors. Further evidence was provided by the men, who elected to delay taking their diuretic until they had completed errands and returned home for the day. Most participants understood primary drug actions, stating this one was for "my heart," "my blood pressure," or "my breathing" and knew if they needed to take medications with food or wait between puffs, although they generally did not know expiration dates. These African American elders took an active role in the technique of self-administration and were involved, for the most part, in making decisions about their drug therapy. Although they expressed trust in their nurses and physicians, commenting "he should know what he's doing," and would usually take prescribed medications without question, there were times when problems arose, and participants exercised independent decision making first and then notified health care providers. Participants, for the most part, were sensitive to physical feelings and changes, especially when taking new medications, and would stop taking a medication and notify the doctor or nurse if side effects developed.

With regard to sharing medication, these individuals responded with a strong "no," indicating that they "never" routinely shared or borrowed medications. Almost all of the participants stated they did not like to take pills unless absolutely needed, and none relied on the use of narcotics or sedatives. Some participants expressed concern about the cost of their drug therapy, but this posed a problem for only one individual, who stated that cost was one reason why he substituted for prescription medication.

Prescription refills were delayed at times because of insurance coverage and transportation, but this was not identified as a significant problem. Some participants used folk remedies along with their prescribed medicines, which they identified primarily as eating practices, especially the use of garlic, along with hot water applications and baths. Religious beliefs did not create an area of conflict with regard to medication use or practices. No gender influences or environmental and demographic effects were detected in this sample, although some could have been neighbors and friends. There were rare negative comments and only a few mixed reactions regarding health care providers and the health care delivery system. For the most part, comments were positive, indicating that these individuals felt the doctors and nurses cared about them and were available to answer questions and provide explanations.

CONCLUSIONS

African Americans in this sample population exercised control over their medication practices and developed routines and procedures to help them remember medication schedules and instructions. Prescribed medications were generally taken without question, but if problems were experienced, these individuals exercised independent decision making until health care providers could be notified and consulted. Although in-depth knowledge of drug actions was limited, there was a general sense and understanding of desired drug effects, side effects, and the potential for drug interactions. Data did not support an increased use of over-the-counter medications, especially sleeping medications, as reported in the literature, nor did the data support literature reports that claim elders tend to share their medications.

The study has significant implications for nursing practice. Although these results identified no major health concerns in this sample population, they underscore the important role of the health care provider and the health care system in maintaining a high level of wellness among our aging citizens. Nurses working with older adults living in the community must individually assess these clients with specific emphasis on medication knowledge and self-administration practices. Strengths must be identified and built upon in order to empower the individual through knowledge and a supportive and collaborative health care culture. Aging adults must be assisted in self-care activities to ensure the correct use of prescribed medications as well as to aid in the development and maintenance of their active roles as health care consumers. Failure to achieve optimal outcomes with regard to medication therapy in the home setting may be linked to the health care system's failure to assess individual needs and beliefs specific to medication administration, as well as the lived experience of the aging adult within a community and cultural context. It is the vital role of professional nursing to bridge this gap.

Precise recommendations followed from this study and included integration of these findings into the treatment plan by nursing faculty who practiced in the university-affiliated health center located within this urban Pennsylvania community. Furthermore, study results, along with recommendations and ongoing health care plans, were shared with the community leaders who requested this investigation. Additionally, a lay guide for medication administration in the home setting was recommended as a collaborative effort in conjunction with the school of pharmacy located within this university setting.

As a limited ethnography, this study stands alone and no further research is planned at this time. However, it would be valuable to replicate this study in other communities with diverse samples in order to add to this growing body of nursing knowledge. Specific areas of research dealing with medication administration, the aging population, and the health needs of African Americans would contribute essential information by which to guide evidence-based nursing practice and aid in the attainment of optimal health care outcomes. Limited nursing research in these areas, coupled with inconsistent research findings, adds additional support to warrant further investigation. Also, collaborative research projects involving representatives from other cultural and ethnic groups are strongly recommended in order to develop a sense of universal patterns and concerns.

ACKNOWLEDGMENT

This study was funded through a provost office faculty research grant.

REFERENCES

Bjerrum, L., Andersen, M., Petersen, G., & Kragstrup, J. (2003). Exposure to potential drug interactions in primary health care. *Scandinavian Journal of Primary Health Care, 21*(3), 153–158.

Colt, H., & Shapiro, A. (1989). Drug-induced illness as a cause for admission to a community hospital. *Journal of the American Geriatric Society, 37,* 323–326.

Cooper, R. S. (1993). Health and the social status of blacks in the United States. *Annals of Epidemiology, 3*(1), 137–144.

Craig, G. M. (1994). Clinical presentation of orthostatic hypotension in the elderly. *Postgraduate Medicine Journal, 70*(827), 638–642.

Grymonpre, R. E., Mitenko, P. A., Sita, D. S., Aoki, F.Y., & Montgomery, P.R. (1988). Drug-associated hospital admissions in older medical patients. *Journal of the American Geriatric Society, 36,* 1092–1098.

Ives, T. J., Bentz E. J., & Gwyther R. E. (1987). Drug-related admissions to a family medicine inpatient service. *Archives of Internal Medicine, 147,* 1117–1120.

Katz, M. D. (1993). Anticholinergics increase risk of adverse drug reactions in elderly. *Provider, 19*(4), 53.

Kinn, S., & Clawson, D. (2002). Health visitor risk assessment for preventing falls in elderly people. *British Journal of Nursing, 11*(5), 316–321.

Lamy, P. P. (1990). Adverse drug effects. *Clinics in Geriatric Medicine, 6*(2), 293–307.

LeSage, J. (1991). Polypharmacy in geriatric patients. *Nursing Clinics of North America, 26*(2), 273–290.

McVeigh, D. M. (2001. Polypharmacy in the older population: Recommendations for improved clinical practice. *Topics in Emergency Medicine, 23*(3), 68–75.

Miller, K., Zylstra, R., & Standridge, J. (2000). The geriatric patient: A systematic approach to maintaining health. *American Family Physician, 61,* 1089–1111.

Paolisso, G., Gambardella, A., & Galzerano, D., (1994). Insulin resistance and hypertension in the elderly optimal drug therapy. *Drugs and Aging, 4,* 403–409.

Piraino, A. (1995).Managing medication in the elderly. *Hospital Practice, 30,* 59–64.

Pollow, R. L., Stoller, E. P., Forster, L. E., & Duniho, T.S. (1994). Drug combinations and potential for risk of adverse drug reaction among community-dwelling elderly. *Nursing Research, 43*(1), 44–49.

Psaty, B. M., Savage, P. J., Tell, G. S., Polak, J. F., Hirsch, C. H., Gardin, J. M., & McDonald, R. H.(1993). Temporal patterns of antihypertensive medication use among elderly patients. *Journal of the American Medical Association, 270*(15), 1837–1841.

Resick, L., Taylor, C., Carroll, T., D'Antonio, J., & de Chesnay, M. (1997). Establishing a nurse-managed wellness clinic in a predominantly older African American inner city high-rise: An advanced practice nursing project. *Nursing Administration Quarterly, 21*(4), 47–54.

Schmader, K., Hanlon, J. T., Weinberger, M., Landsman, P. B., Samsa, G. P., Lewis, I., Uttech, K., Cohen, H. J. & Feussner, J. R. (1994). Appropriateness of medication prescribing in ambulatory elderly patients. *Journal of the American Geriatric Society, 42,* 1241–1247.

Sternberg, S., Chandran, A., & Sikka, M. (2003). Alternative therapy use by elderly African Americans attending a community clinic. *Journal of the American Geriatrics Society, 51*(12), 1768–1772.

Stone, J. (1991). Preventing physical iatrogenic problems. In W. Chenitz, J. Stone, & S. Salisbury (Eds). *Clinical gerontological nursing: A guide to advanced practice* (pp. 359–375). Philadelphia, PA: W. B. Saunders.

Wallsten, S. M., Sullivan, R. J., Hanlon, J. T., et al. (1995). Medication taking behaviors in the high- and low-functioning elderly: MacArthur field studies of successful aging. *Annals of Pharmacotherapy, 29,* 359–363.

Willcox , S. M., Himmelstein, D. U., & Woolhandler, S. (1994). Inappropriate drug prescribing for the community-dwelling elderly. *Journal of the American Medical Association, 272*(40), 292–296.

United States Bureau of the Census. (1995). *Statistical abstract of the United States* (115th ed.). Washington, DC: Government Printing Office.

CHAPTER 19

Women with Dissociative Identity Disorder: Solution-Focused Nursing

Margaret McAllister

Queensland, Australia, has a major childhood sexual abuse and neglect problem. With a population of almost 3.5 million, Queensland has about 780,000 (21%) children. According to the Australian Institute of Health and Welfare, a total of 22,069 notifications of abuse and 18,122 investigations (56% finalized) were reported in 2000–2001 (Johnstone & Kelly, 2001). This equates to 7.4 in 1000 children in Queensland investigated, which is marginally lower than the rates in the United States and Canada (National Child Abuse and Neglect Data System, 2002). Although they account for only 3% or the child population, the rates of abuse and neglect for Aboriginal and Torres Strait Islander children was 15.2 per 1000 children, double the rate for other children (Angus & Woodward, 1995).

Although most children go on to recover from these experiences, especially if the environment becomes more nurturing, many will suffer serious consequences. Sheldrick (1991) has claimed that 20% of childhood sexual abuse victims display serious mental health problems, such as dissociative identity disorder, in adult life.

Many effective services, staffed by dedicated clinicians, community workers, and volunteers, exist in Queensland to help women overcome traumatic childhood experiences. These include health services such as hospitals, general practice physicians, counseling services, psychologists, psychiatrists, and other mental health professionals. They also include services such as housing, legal centers, courts, neighborhood centers, and community services such as migrant and domestic violence resource centers and services specific to Aboriginal people (Dimopoulos et al., 1999). Although these services are staffed by a variety of professionals, each of whom is guided by his or her own disciplinary discourse, the predominant approach is a problem orientation.

PROBLEM ORIENTATION

The problem orientation remains the dominant and preferred approach in health care, and it has a number of strengths. Problem solving has been described as scientific because it involves deductive reasoning, and this kind of thinking helps clinicians be more dispassionate, rational, and logical in their approach to resolving issues. However, the problem orientation also has a number of weaknesses because it tends to set up a dichotomy between the problem solver and the problem so that the client is seen as the one with the problem that needs to be fixed. In this way of thinking, the clinician does not need to look within or around the self for possible contributors or solutions to the problem. This in part explains why disorders and illnesses are most commonly conceptualized as located and best treated individually (or biologically), rather than socially and culturally. A problem orientation, with its emphasis on detachment and impartiality, also tends to dismiss the adoption of a passionate stance in relation to particular issues, but sometimes passionate engagement is what stimulates compassion, involvement, and quality care.

SOLUTION ORIENTATION

A solution orientation is not positioned against or in opposition to the problem orientation. Rather, emphasis is placed on a different part of the problem-solving continuum, solution searching and solution generation. This means that instead of nurses assessing and exploring problems as their primary activity, they will now spend more time on the positive and creative challenge of solution generation. This activity uses all of the cognitive skills required for problem solving but does not privilege rationality over creativity. Thus a solution orientation involves logic and creativity, deductive and inductive thinking, imagination and reason, problem solving, and solution searching. A solution orientation also works with what is going right with an individual or group and seeks to maximize those potentials by building on strengths, achievements, and capacity.

In order to link theory to practice, this solution orientation will be explained in relation to the results of a recent study. (Table 19.1) From August 1997 to February 1999, at the invitation of staff at the only Queensland private mental health facility dedicated to the provision of care for people diagnosed with dissociative identity disorder or trauma, I led an action research study to explore, describe, and develop acute care for women who dissociate (McAllister et al., 2003).

TABLE 19.1   A Solution Orientation

Asks what the client wants to change and how
Opens space for future possibilities through a focus on exceptions and resources
Invites client to clarify main issues and priorities for health service
Continuously channels client and caregiver toward goals or desired actions
Assumes client is competent, resilient, and resourceful
Views client as unique and maintains a position of curiosity
Views nursing as interaction that opens new possibilities
Focuses on a process of collaborative inquiry
Privileges the voice and expertise of the client
Builds on client's ideas and language
Seeks to be open, collaborative, and respectful
Asks: Have we achieved enough to end?

McAllister, M. (2003)

ACTION RESEARCH METHOD

Action research was chosen because of its capacity to engage participants, raise consciousness about nursing, accumulate and share understanding of phenomena, and enact change (Clifford & Gough, 1990; Elliott, 1991; Lovat, 1988). Action research is a spiraling process of data collection and analysis, and in this case it involved two main data sources: focus interviews with nurses and postacute clients. The study was approved by the researcher's university Human Research Ethics Committee, a formal committee charged with ensuring that the rights of subjects are protected. The university and the health service gave ethical clearance, and each participant gave informed consent. Data were collected, stored, and presented according to the requirements of both committees. The risk that mild emotional distress could be inadvertently elicited during data collection and analysis was minimized by continual reassurance that participants need not divulge anything they did not want to, that pseudonyms would be used to protect privacy, and that information revealed would be kept confidential by the researcher and only shared in documents that had the participants' approval. Fourteen nurses and ten postacute clients participated in the study. Only those patients who had been discharged from acute care were invited to participate. At the request of the patients, nurse and patient data were gathered separately.

Focus Interviews and Workshops

An initial letter briefly outlining the study was distributed to all participants. Focus interviews with a group of two to three nurses were organized within working hours so that participants were not burdened to give of their free time. Interviews explored typical daily activities. Later, the principal researcher facilitated a series of workshops. The first workshop provided information on action research and data collection, and another workshop provided a summary of the literature review on the therapeutic relationship between nurse and patient. Participants formed small groups to review their interview transcripts and to critically reflect on the completeness of this data. Themes were collated and categorized by a process of directed cue sorting. This process resulted in the generation of many concepts, which were subsequently distilled into 30 subthemes. These subthemes were subsequently sorted into three main themes through a process of directed cue sorting. Groups then constructed patient–nurse narratives that they felt encapsulated the elements of a therapeutic relationship. The narratives were taped and transcribed by the principal researcher.

Storytelling gave participants the opportunity to speak and to have their feelings and views heard. It also developed a level of cohesion and commitment that enabled the study to progress smoothly. A final 2-hour workshop involving nurse and patient participants was held to present and discuss the findings.

PHASES OF CARE

An important outcome of the study was the design of a framework that sees acute care as comprising three main phases: joining, building, and extending (see Figure 19.1).

A NURSING MODEL FOR ACUTE CARE PEOPLE WHO DISSOCIATE

The Joining Phase: Getting to Know the Person	The Building Phase: Processing and Coping Skills	The Extending Phase: Using Skills for Life
• **Knowledge:** impaired knowledge of self, fragmented memories, fragmented identity, perception of self as a victim • **Attributes:** fearful, lonely, angry, numb, despairing, ashamed, vigilant, on edge, tired • **Skill deficits:** in trust, coping mechanisms, in disclosing secrets • **Excesses:** keeps secrets, excessive use of dissociation, self harm, testing, and avoiding others	A milieu which facilitates patients' ability to: • **Recover from trauma:** explore their own fragmented memories; disclose, feel, and grieve; resolve and store memories safely • **Make connections:** within self and within community; trust self and others • **Build resilience:** problem solve, find safety, use supports, value self, avoid trauma	• **Knowledge:** self-knowledge is deeper, identity is coherent and stable, accepts self, knows how to avoid and minimize trauma response • **Attributes:** positive self-regard, able to ventilate strong emotions safely, feels appropriately • **Skills:** uses coping mechanisms such as the support of others and self-talk; able to relax, unwind, debrief; can build and maintain relationships; has connections, avoids tests, able to trust and disclose

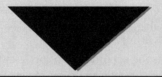

SOLUTION-FOCUSED NURSING
• Improves flexibility • Develops creative problem solving
• Reminds of the need for time-out, of opportunities to revitalize self
and develop coping abilities

FIGURE 19.1   Nursing Model for Acute Care of People Who Dissociate

Joining Phase

The joining phase is when the client meets the acute care team. It involves assessment, goal setting, and planning of care. The study revealed some important insights for working in this phase, which subtly yet powerfully shifted the focus from a problem to a solution orientation.

First, in assessing clients, it is important to identify not just their presenting problems but also their strengths because these attributes can be harnessed in the building phase when creative approaches to coping and developing resilience are the focus. Second, problems may be seen not only as deficits in knowledge, skills, or attributes but as excesses. For example, clients could be assessed as having a knowledge deficit when what they really have is memory gaps or repression, rendering them unable to recall the origin of their trauma and, therefore, unable to process past events. At the same time, clients may be assessed as having a coping skill excess if they use dissociation so frequently that they cannot participate in meaningful work or leisure because they are numb and depersonalized. In keeping with a solution orientation, the framework considers the client to be affected by both problems and strengths. Thus the aim is to achieve a balanced level of self-knowledge, social skills, and personal attributes.

Building Phase: Recovering from Trauma

Throughout acute care, the aim for nurses is to facilitate growth in their clients so that they are more likely to engage in the work that will help them recover from past traumas, make connections within the self system and in the social system, and build resilience so that they are less vulnerable to future stressors.

Clients requiring acute admission to the trauma unit often present in crisis and are at risk of harming themselves and others. Frequently, they have self-harmed or attempted suicide, or they may be experiencing emotional dysregulation (e.g., depression, numbness, or irritability). It is important to understand that the urge to act, rather than feel, may be irresistible for some clients. After all, the psychological effects of abuse and the experience of affective pain are possibly far more damaging and frightening than the time-limited physical acts of harm. Furthermore, self injury may also represent a way of taking control of one's past victimization. In this act, a person becomes a subject not an object, an aggressor not a victim. But this kind of way of being is not a positive connection with the world and does not facilitate healing. For the client to be able to process the trauma, the feeling needs to be linked to the memory, and acting out needs to be replaced with something less dangerous such as thinking, feeling, or talking.

Sometimes if clients dissociate, there are internal personalities who fight amongst each other, and the body is the place where that fight takes place (Goodman, 1995). For the dissociated client, the body is the one thing that all the identity states (also known as parts or alters) share. Thus it is not surprising that parts will fight over the body as this excerpt from a story told by a nurse illustrates.

"Over the past month Ellen was cutting herself—usually on her arms, legs, and abdomen. Sometimes she burned her ankles with a cigarette lighter. The part that cuts is 'Nell,' a persecutory alter, who is very angry and wants the 'little ones' to die."

Nell is in battle with the little ones, who she thinks cannot keep secrets. Because of their inability to keep secrets, the whole self-system is in danger because if one identity learns of the abuse, the perpetrator might be discovered, and Ellen and her identities would be punished. This fear of punishment is what motivates Nell to keep the little ones quiet and to feel so aggressive toward them. Thus the story reveals that the part who is self-harming is actually trying to keep the body safe from a bigger hurt, but Nell's behavior, although understandable, has serious consequences because it is Ellen and her body that ultimately suffer.

From this story, one is sensitized to the knowledge that self-harm, struggle, and defensive battles are strategies that the identity states have used to keep the body safe. Childlike, inadequate, desperate solutions have been chosen. It is the nurse's opportunity here to communicate understanding of the motivation but also to offer feedback that such solutions are inadequate. In the long term, the nurse can work with Ellen and her parts to find safer solutions and learn ways to communicate with each identity in order to resolve the conflict.

When the client recovers from the new trauma induced by self-harm, it may also be useful to find alternative places for this urge to self-harm to be carried out, a place other than the body. For example, the client can be helped to act the conflict out on a doll by drawing or making cuts on the doll, or by cutting paper, tearing phone books, punching pillows, or throwing plastic bottles. In other words, nurses can help to move the battleground from the body to a safer place, a site for healing.

Within this acute-care unit a range of services is provided, from individual supportive therapy, group support to art expression, leisure groups, crisis intervention, and telephone counseling. In this way, hospitalization becomes a time for intensive therapeutic work. It is not simply a place of asylum from life's troubles but a place for restoration and repair. The aim is to provide a milieu that carefully balances work, play, and rest so that individuals do not become exhausted but also do not waste valuable opportunities to practice finding safety, problem solving, feeling, and relating.

Building Phase: Making Connections

Connections have deep significance in therapeutic work with women who are dissociated. First, women with dissociative identity disorder have many identities who may not be known to one another. Thus a very important part of individual therapy is to help clients come to know their many identities and to map out the sometimes complicated communication pathways within the self-system.

Encouraging the client to keep a journal is an important way to encourage inward exploration and raise self-knowledge. It also acts as a shared communication medium for the client's identities, offering them each a way to be heard without having to resort to extremes. In this setting, nurses also use the journal as a starting point for daily discussions about progress. In this way, clients are reminded that acute care is not just a place of asylum but an opportunity to develop self-awareness, resilience, and adaptive coping skills.

Within the ward environment, nurses also focus on facilitating social connections for clients. Many women who have survived trauma remain vulnerable to further abuse and exploitation, perhaps because they have long felt disconnected and lack the faith and capacity to make enduring, meaningful, and mutually satisfying close relationships. It may also be helpful to discuss that it is not just vulnerable women who experience disconnection. Over the last 50 years, we as a society have become less connected with our neighbors, church, community, and families, and now all people can benefit from making a concerted attempt at establishing deeper social connections.

Group psychoeducation, art expression, games, and informal gatherings take place regularly. Not only do groups help people see they are not the only person to have suffered such terrible trauma, but they can also see others risking disclosure and learn that punishment does not follow. The group work helps to build trust and facilitate connections between people. It also builds the individual's resilience to future stress or trauma.

Extending Phase: Building Resilience

Resilience is a process of overcoming and defending against adversity. And, as has been explained, the client group represented in this study remains vulnerable to future trauma. Whether they will succumb to that trauma in the same ways may well depend on how resourceful and strong they have become in the recovery experience.

Resilience in a client can be promoted, even during times of crisis, by conveying optimism and faith in the person's ongoing capacity to cope. Interactions with the client in the emergency setting or during any brief intervention can incorporate resilience work. For example, one can simply show the client another way to think about the issue or gently reframe negative self-talk so that he or she can see the self in new and more positive ways.

People who dissociate tend to lack the social support that can help build resilience and resistance to future stress and trauma (Van der Kolk, 1996). This story illustrates the resilience that is facilitated in a group.

> Every day we find ourselves helping each other out in some way. Because we know what it feels like to be zoning out, afraid, or switching we can see it in others. So, we help each other get through it. We might kick a ball, or make them a drink, or join them in throwing plastic bottles against a wall. We might pace in circles with them, draw, or sit and hold hands. We're like a sounding board. We're always giving reassurance.

In these encounters, peers are encouraged to see themselves as supporters, not rescuers. It may be useful to encourage clients to focus on supporting general concerns and to leave the specifics of the traumatic experience alone because, as clients, they may be very susceptible to vicarious trauma.

Moving On

The overall goal for acute care is to achieve a place of safety that is sustainable. Thus when the individual feels and can demonstrate increased self-control and is no longer at risk of harm to self or others, then that person may be ready for community-based psychotherapy. It is important to note that the end of acute care does not signal termination of therapy. Rather, the context of care changes to offer clients the opportunity to apply newly learned coping mechanisms, problem-solving strategies, social skills, and trauma responses in a less controlled setting and in relationships with friends, work colleagues, and family.

A STRONGER IDENTITY FOR NURSES AND NURSING

Throughout this therapeutic relationship, it is not only the client who grows; ideal caring is reciprocal. In this study, nurses tended to see their role as one of facilitating solutions rather than solving problems, as sharing control rather than taking it away, as teaching rather than parenting, and as supporting rather than curing. These are some reasons why they find this role rewarding. Because each client who dissociates has unique fears, problems, and resources, skilled helping requires conversation, flexibility, and creativity. Every new strategy that nurses and clients devise and which leads to positive experiences adds to the nurse's tool kit.

The idea that caring is reciprocal; that nursing work can be proactive and solution oriented—focused on joining, building, and extending—is relevant for nurses working in a range of practice settings. For example, nursing care for the aged can be extended when nurses approach aged clients by assessing their strengths as well as problems and develop a milieu that treats illnesses, facilitates social connections, and builds resilience, place, meaning, and contentment.

Insights for changes in practice that emerge from a solution orientation also have clear cross-cultural relevance. Groups that may be disadvantaged by their cultural differences from the mainstream know only too well that constantly searching for, and noticing problems in, their person or their group tends to keep them from appreciating things that are going right. It may also be that some problems may never be resolved completely, and a focus on the negative is inherently pessimistic. A solution orientation, however, with its emphasis on creativity and novel approaches, invites cultural groups to do things differently and to be proud of their innovative approach to solving local and distinct health issues.

REFERENCES

Angus, G., & Woodward, S. (1995). *Child abuse and neglect Australia, 1993–94: Australian Institute of Health and Welfare: Child welfare series No. 13.* Canberra: AGPS.

Clifford, C., & Gough, S. (1990). *Nursing research: A skills-based introduction.* New York, NY: Prentice Hall.

Dimopoulos, M., Baker, R., Sheridan, M., Elix, J., & Lambert, J. (1999). *Consultancy report: Mapping pathways of service provision: Enhancement of family violence protocols and interagency linkages. Canberra, Australia:* Partnerships Against Domestic Violence, Commonwealth Government.

Elliott, J. (1991). *Action research for educational change.* Philadelphia, PA: Open University.

Goodman, L. (1995). Persecutory alters and ego states: Protectors, friends, and allies. *Dissociation, 8*(2), 91–99.

Johnstone, H., & Kelly, S. (2001). *Child protection Australia 2001–02. Australian Institute of Health and Welfare: Child Welfare Series No. 32.* Canberra: AGPS.

Lovat, T. (1988). Action research and the praxis model of religious education: A critique. *British Journal of Religious Education, 11*(1), 30–37.

McAllister, M., Higson, D., McIntosh, W., O'Leary, S., Hargreaves, L., Murrell, L., et al. (2001). Dissociative identity disorder and the nurse–client relationship in the acute care setting: An action research project *Australian and New Zealand Journal of Mental Health Nursing, 10,* 20–32.

McAllister, M. (2003). Doing practice differently: Solution-focused nursing. *Journal of Advanced Nursing, 41,* 528–535.

Sheldrick, C. (1991). Adult sequelae of child sexual abuse. *British Journal of Psychiatry, 158*(Suppl. 10), 55–62.

CHAPTER 20

Interaction Between Caregivers and Families Expecting an Impaired Child: Finnish Health Care

Hanna Maijala

Major fetal malformations are diagnosed in 1200–1800 newborn children in Finland every year, a rate of 2–3% (Ritvanen & Peippo, 1998). The incidence of fetal impairments and malformations discovered during the last trimester of pregnancy is 3–5%, and in pregnancies terminated by a miscarriage, the frequency is even higher (Ämmälä, 1992).

The life situation of a family expecting an impaired child is challenging because these families have to face not only the normal pregnancy-related developmental changes but also a traumatic crisis (Allen & Mulhauser, 1995; Driscoll, 1993; Heiskanen, 1994; Hunfeld, Wladimiroff, Passchier, Venema-Van Uden, Frets, & Verhage, 1993; Leon, 1990; Matthews, 1990; McNeil & Nimby, 1998; Shiloh, 1996; VanPutte, 1988; Wheeler & Pike, 1993). In most cases, the fetal impairment comes as a surprise, and the situation is generally experienced as unclear, partly due to the uncertain prognosis concerning the unborn child. The family has to live with uncertainty in regard to the child's survival and the severity of impairment, and the parents may have to make a decision about the continuation or termination of the pregnancy (Bourguignon et al., 1999; Chitayat & Babul-Hirji, 2000; Gevers, 1999; Lorenzen & Holzgreve, 1955; Zuskar, 1987).

Each family member reacts to the situation in an individual way, and these reactions have an impact on the family as a whole (Anderson, 1996; Boyd, 1996; Hanson et al., 1998; Mercer et al., 1988; Wright & Leahey, 1994). Individual methods of coping with the stress are drawn on and used by the family for adjusting their internal actions with the external reality so as to reach a state of balance. However, the appropriate means of handling the stress are not always available (Bomar & Cooper, 1996; Hanson et al., 1998; Mealey et al., 1996). According to earlier research, there are also some inadequacies in the manner and means of helping these families as well as in the training of their caregivers (Chitty et al., 1996; Leon 1995; Loenzen & Holzgreve, 1995; Posa et al., 1997; Posa, 1998).

This chapter deals with the interaction between caregivers and families expecting an impaired child as perceived within the framework of the Finnish health care system. The discussion is based on research undertaken by the author for her doctoral thesis published in 2004. The thesis comprises five articles and a concluding summary based on the articles.

The purpose of the research was to develop a practical nursing theory to describe caregivers' interactions with families expecting a child diagnosed with a fetal impairment. The goal was to generate data that would enhance the interaction between families and the caregivers and contribute to the well-being of the families. The research was conducted at the Department of

189

Nursing Science of the University of Tampere, in cooperation with Tampere University Hospital in Finland. The study used grounded theory methodology.

The mothers and fathers ($n = 29$) of families expecting an impaired child and the nurses and doctors ($n = 22$) who worked with these families participated in the research as informants. The data were gathered with the use of semistructured interviews that were audiotaped. The supplementary data consisted of essays ($n = 5$) written by each parent. The data were analyzed with the method of constant comparison based on the approach of grounded theory. The conclusion consisted of defining the content of interaction, giving titles to the focal concepts that describe the interaction, and defining their interrelations as well as the overall structure of the interaction process. The present chapter is focused in part on the findings that describe the perceptions of the parents and families with regard to their own actions and those of other family members during interactions that occur within the care system. It also focuses on the families' reported experiences of receiving and giving help.

ACTIONS OF CAREGIVERS THAT ENHANCE FAMILY SURVIVAL

According to the parents, when the initial information about impairment in their unborn child was received, the shock and concern were often manifested as crying. It was quite usual that parents were shocked at first, which often kept them from remembering to ask questions or participating in an active discussion with the caregivers. This initial information sometimes also created such a perplexing experience that the parents felt discouraged from asking questions or hearing what the answers might be. Some parents were shy in expressing their wishes, not wanting to be difficult or of any trouble to the caregivers. Other parents did express their need for information to the caregivers, both immediately and by writing down questions before appointments. The questions were often practical and related to the child, the nursing procedures, and what to expect in the future. The parents found it important to make a stand for their own cause and to be able to make their own decisions. Sometimes their wishes were expressed purposefully because an active patient was thought to receive better care.

In relating their experiences, parents indicated that a matter-of-fact, realistic, and calm attitude on the part of caregivers was helpful. Parents indicated they felt a need to cry undisturbed, without any interference that might further upset them. The parents viewed a partnership with the health care providers as needing to be characterized by an attitude on the part of the health care providers that reflects the dimensions of speaking the same language, discussing questions together, listening, and answering. Parents were better able to cope if the health care providers gave thorough, well-informed explanations. Parents thought that both positive and worrying aspects of the child's impairment and potential treatment could be concretely presented, for example, by illustrating a point with a drawing or by relating the experiences of children with similar impairments. Parents were also told what could and could not be known for certain.

It is essential to respect the decisions of the family regarding the continuation or termination of the pregnancy. Parents appreciated it when personnel expressed understanding and acceptance of the family's decision, regardless of what that decision was. Also, parents considered it important that the caregivers continue to offer the choice of terminating and not terminating, right up to the time of the operation. Parents also expressed that not being left alone after making their decision made them feel that the caregivers were on their side and that they appreciated their wishes about practical aspects of care being taken into account in those cases in which they decided to have abortions.

Regardless of the family's choice about abortion or not, examinations and nursing procedures are not the only way to help. Results of this study show that the healthy coping of the family can be strengthened by caregivers' arranging sick leave and taking care of pain medication.
Active nursing care shows the parents that the family's experience is being taken seriously by the
caregivers. Active caring can manifest through telephoning the parents at home, making frequent
visits while they are on the ward, and encouraging them to contact their health care providers.

According to the parents, the medical personnel strengthened the family by responding to
the presence of the father in a manner that enabled him to feel included in the care. Parents liked
it when the father was greeted and asked about how he was feeling. Caregivers could also
strengthen the family by allowing the father to be present on the in-patient ward at all times, independent of hospital schedules, possibly by reserving a separate patient room for the parents.

As experienced by the parents, showing kindness meant a smile, warm-hearted cheerfulness,
correct behavior, and a positive interest in their experience. A free atmosphere occasionally light-
ened with humor was valued. Sometimes psychological support was offered directly by providing opportunities for discussion and sometimes indirectly by guiding the parents to use the
resources designed to help in situations of crisis. The informative and human dimensions that
support the survival of the family run in a close parallel relationship to each other.

ACTIONS OF CAREGIVERS THAT COMPLICATE FAMILY SURVIVAL

This study has shown that parents perceive it as a threat to family survival when caregivers are
involved in examinations that they do not explain. Ignoring the parents' need for information was
often manifested by leaving the parents without answers, presenting only general information, or
not explaining the details clearly. Sometimes parents felt that caregivers were reluctant to disclose information and that they avoided certain issues or conveyed information only to each
other.

Caregivers' verbal undermining of a mother's fears or a lack of reaction to her tears was experienced as negative by the parents. Parents also considered it insensitive when no advance
warning was given about probable pain in connection with medical procedures to be performed
on mothers or when the warning was given too bluntly. Sometimes parents perceived that their
fears would not be heard; therefore, they sometimes tried to reach out for the caregiver's understanding by crying.

Further communication problems were perceived during examinations in which caregivers
discussed the child's situation with each other or with students while the parents are present but
did not give any explanation to them. A tone of astonishment (implying surprise at the parents'
thoughts or feelings) in the caregivers' voices during their discussion was experienced as particularly upsetting to the family. Talking past the parents also occured during telephone conversations
with outsiders in the presence of the parents. Another form of breaking the family's internal support system was questioning the father's presence when the parents both preferred to be involved.

The use of heavy medical terminology by the caregiver also made it harder for the family to
cope because of misunderstandings and confusion. On the other hand, colloquial expressions
such as "water on the brain" or "abnormal shape of the skull" could seem so appalling that the
rest remained unheard. In the case of twin pregnancies, parents found it confusing if the names
used for the fetuses, A and B, changed evey time the caregivers did. Inappropriate words used to
describe the parts of the mother's body and also the use of words other than those in the parent's
native language could be experienced as offensive.

Unnecessary expressions of shock, excessive politeness, exaggerated expressions of sympathy, empty words of comfort, or showing pity were manifestations of the kind of compassion that weakened the parents' survival mechanisms. Occasionally a caregiver assumed the mother had emotions that did not correspond to her actual experience.

All waiting and delay was stressful for the parents. They found it difficult, for instance, if following the receipt of serious information they had to wait several weeks for their next appointment. Waiting for test results in a state of uncertainty or a delay of further examinations was often found to be difficult. Sitting in a waiting room waiting for a caregiver who is late for the appointment was also perceived as negative. Waiting for admittance to the ward or, when already there, waiting for access to one's own patient room was also stressful. Sometimes it was perceived as distressing to wait for an ultrasound examination to be over.

Parents found it offensive if caregivers, who were outsiders from the family's point of view, interfered in their affairs by expressing personal opinions. For instance, talking about birth and a child to a mother whose own perception is that she will be undergoing a miscarriage may be upsetting. Similarly, expressions of a caregiver's opinion with regard to termination of the pregnancy or instructions from the caregiver for the parents to think about the decision together sometimes complicated decision making. In the same way that the caregivers' actions could enhance the coping ability of the family, the parallel dimensions of informative and human factors could also be found in the actions that weakened the coping process.

EXPERIENCES OF CAREGIVERS: HELPING THE PARENTS COPE

Ideally, caregivers prepared to meet with the parents by doing background work if any earlier data were available. This entailed getting acquainted with the case history and literature as well as planning for the practical arrangements. To be prepared also meant getting ready psychologically, thinking of one's own participation and taking the unexpected into account.

At the initial stage of interaction, the approach was tentative and open, and the parents' need for support was assessed. The caregiver's actions were situation specific and family centered. Sometimes talking was the natural choice, and sometimes it was good to remain silent. Actions were adjusted according to the severity of the impairment and in proportion to the reactions of the family. If the abnormality was mild, the seriousness of the situation could be undercut, and any strong reactions from the parents could be calmed. However, if the situation was grave, the caregiver sometimes found him- or herself shocked.

Caregivers who associate themselves with the family's situation experience it as if living side by side with the parents. The caregiver may grieve with them and wait anxiously for further information on the impairment. Sometimes the parents' emotions may be strongly transferred to the caregiver as a sense of panic or an impulse to scream, even though those emotions are kept under control. Particularly when the situation is serious, compassion may be expressed in words, by silence, or through touch, taking the parent by the hand or hugging. A caregiver may even cry with the parents. Sometimes it is difficult to express compassion in a supportive way, and even though the commitment to the interaction is genuine, a real interaction does not occur.

The parents' questions are paid proper attention by responding as well as possible, asking for clarifications, and making notes. Often the caregiver is not able to give explicit and exact answers because it is the lack of certainty that is generally at the core of the question. To make it easier for the parents to cope with uncertainty, caregivers may make new appointments for consultation or offer the parents an opportunity to contact them. During the discussions they can explain further what has been diagnosed, what it means, and what choices are available.

Like the parents, the caregivers also experience the fact that concentrating on the examination of the child may cause the parents to be ignored. For instance, during an examination, caregivers may focus their attention on the ultrasound monitor. Wondering about the fetal impairment, they may talk only to each other or remain silent. Supporting a family in a matter-of-fact manner means limiting the conversation to issues pertinent to the moment, such as the child's current condition or what will be done next; this should especially be done in acute situations. Caregivers also express a practical approach by defining situations, like explaining the reason for an examination at the very beginning. Asking actively about the parents' feelings should be avoided in order to ease the parents' distress. Aggression can be responded to by neutrally justifying the parents' decisions. In some cases, an official approach can be emphasized as an expression of respect. Honest, positive support can be expressed by avoiding empty promises, admitting that nothing is guaranteed where childbirth is concerned, and bringing up issues that may be unpredictable. However, at the same time, hope can be given by pointing out the options of helping.

When caregivers act as negotiating partners, they discuss the issues important to the family with the parents in an atmosphere of equality. The caregivers may express their personal opinions, e.g., that it is usually beneficial to see the lost child. She/he may also say that it is wise to tell something about the expected child's situation to the other children in the family, or that it is good for parents who have lost a child to go through a mourning period before a new pregnancy.

Respect for the family's decisions is expressed by paying attention to the parents' wishes and conveying them to the rest of the personnel when planning the practical arrangements. The personnel also present the options available for the parents and provide them with the information necessary for decision making.

Giving practical support to the parents often means helping with simple things, like meals and clothing, arranging a peaceful patient room, and seeing that the father gets some rest, too. Support may be expressed by offering to remain on the ward, administering pain relief without delay, giving sleeping medication, or suggesting an ultrasonic investigation. According to caregivers, one form of practical support may be arranging someone to accompany the mother or guiding the parents to visit the neonatal unit before the birth of their child.

Providing active care is a maternal attitude that helps the parents experience their situation in a tolerable way. Attention is focused on contributing to parents' coping, being available in connection with issues important to the family, and doing all that is necessary for them like making sure they are visited frequently enough on the ward, telephoning them at home, and telling them who to contact at night.

Caregivers contribute to the strengthening of the family's internal support by encouraging the father to participate in care along with the mother and also by paying attention to his need for support, and his questions and opinions. Interaction between the parents should be paid attention to and ideas and thoughts should be discussed with them. A caregiver may ask the mother how the father experiences the situation if it is difficult to establish a direct contact with him. In some cases, interaction with the father is more intense than with the mother. Also, the parents need to be given an opportunity to be alone and the presence of their other children be allowed if the parents wish.

A caregiver may also feel as if she/he were positioned in between the parents' interaction. This is the case when the caregiver asks one parent questions that the other hastens to answer.

Sometimes, it is difficult to approach a withdrawn father or manage to pay attention to him successfully. A female caregiver may experience that it is easier to attend to a woman than to a man.

Securing the continuity of a care relationship is accomplished by telling the parents about one's work schedules, giving the parents necessary details for making contact, encouraging the parents to make contact, and keeping appointments and schedules. If necessary, parents are guided to see others, like a pediatrician, social worker, hospital clergy, or psychiatric nurse. The caregiver may inform the personnel of a postnatal clinic about the mother's discharge and arrange with them to make a home call. The parents are encouraged to share their experience with people who are or have been in a similar situation by writing them, and by attending peer support groups.

Caregivers perceive that they receive relatively scarce feedback directly from families, and in most cases no information is obtained after the care is concluded. Some feedback may be obtained in connection with checkup appointments, via medical colleagues, and through the mothers' written recollections of her experience. A family's ability to cope occupies the caregivers' thoughts even after the conclusion of the cooperation. This is especially true when the shocking situations that led to a child's unexpected death and the parents' strong reactions to what happened are remembered. The situation may be discussed over a long period of time and some parents may never be forgotten.

PARENTS' EXPERIENCES IN OBTAINING HELP OR NOT BEING HELPED

Successful interaction produces an experience of obtaining good care and of being in reliable hands, as well as an awareness of being helped. The parents' perception is that a caregiver is careful and does her/his best while focusing on the situation of the family carefully and earnestly. Consequently, the parents trust her/his words based on her/his professional skills and they are able to maintain a peaceful attitude toward future events. Obtaining appropriate mental support can give the parents a sense of having hope, of having been approached and cared for by a professional on a personal level, and an experience of not feeling left alone. The caregiver has contributed to their moving forward and there has been no experience of being undermined.

One of the ways to obtain help is by gaining a clearer understanding of the information received. Naturally, receiving some positive information about the child's situation is pacifying. Comprehending the overall situation with its various alternative factors decreases, among other things, the need for psychological support and increases the trust in one's survival. Information obtained in appropriate amounts enables the parents to comprehend and process it. Consequently, preparing for the future, letting go of feelings of guilt, and eliminating frightful prospects have become possible for the parents.

A highly personal psychological strengthening seems to knit together the family's own coping strategies and to enhance their mutual interaction. The strengthening includes an experience of having grown as a human being through the process of questioning the matter of course expectations of having a healthy child and through the change of one's priorities and values. Going through the experiences associated with fetal impairment may have produced the thought that life could hold nothing worse in the future. Psychological strengthening also involves an experience of learning and sharpening one's ability of perception as well as an outlook that there is a meaning in the experience.

Parents' disappointment and distrust is directed toward their experience of health care as a whole: caregivers' professional skills, obtaining information, and practical arrangements. The parents may suspect that the time used for examinations has been insufficient and the tests have been carried out by uninformed personnel. They may also be bitter because the abnormality was not detected earlier. An experience of not being heard or defended, or being left to provide for one's own care are some of the reasons that cause distrust.

Parents may feel that responsibility for the flow of information lies solely with them. They may also feel that the care given to the mother is insufficient. For instance, she may not have been given any health instructions on how to take care of her basic physical condition. An experience of not having been helped often contains a perception of a thin connection with the care personnel. Interactions between the parents and the personnel may have been minimal or nonexistent. In pressed situations of investigation, conversation often remains superficial and if the only words exchanged are limited to a short greeting at arrival the contact may be experienced as disturbing. Parents do not always think to ask caregivers about questions that bother them. A child's specific impairment is an issue rarely discussed within the course of basic health care while in specialized nursing questions connected with the family's overall situation can easily be left out.

The father may sometimes remain an outsider in the family's situation. He is not always given attention and the fact that it is possible for him to be present may not be actively expressed by the caregivers. He may cope with the situation without expecting any attention, satisfied with the fact that he is not asked to leave the hospital. He may perceive the ward as a women's realm, where the father is an outsider. The parents experience the lack of emotional support as being left alone, without an opportunity to contact a caregiver, and as an absence of expressions of compassion from the personnel.

The perception of not being helped may come from the parents' experience of feeling crushed by unexpected or shocking information delivered to them bluntly or indiscreetly. Parents may also feel that their participation has been somehow restricted. They may feel that they have become an object of bidding and hostility, for instance, when they express an opinion different from that of the caregiver's. The end result is an experience of fear, anger, shock, and a withdrawal from contact.

CAREGIVERS' PERCEPTIONS OF SUCCESSFUL AND UNSUCCESSFUL HELPING

From the caregiver's point of view, successful helping typically includes an experience that the family has received the help offered. The caregiver experiences that she/he has fulfilled the parents' expectations and the relationship with them is confidential. The atmosphere between them is warm and contains intimacy. The caregiver feels that issues important to the family have been handled and she/he trusts in the survival of the family.

In the caregiver's estimation, giving information has eased the family's apprehension and feelings of guilt, and sometimes the information in and of itself has been hopeful. When the caregiver has the experience of being able to help the family, she/he gains a sense of having succeeded in her/his work, and appreciation received is experienced as rewarding. The experience of having been able to contribute something to the family's survival decreases the strain of working and increases job satisfaction. The caregiver's collaboration with the parents can be rewarding and the results may give joy to all involved.

Along with the increase in professional experience, the caregiver's fears diminish, and confidence in the adequacy of her/his professional skills is enhanced. The caregiver experiences she/he is working with the parents in her/his personal way, trusting her/his intuition. Her/his calmness is enhanced by the realization that every situation can be handled. A leniency with regard to her/himself and the other personnel grows and unreasonable demands are not made. The caregiver is capable of admitting her/his ignorance and perceives that she/he has learned something that has changed her/his own values.

Parents may turn down opportunities the caregiver offers for discussion, which may appear to the caregiver that the parents do not wish to talk about their feelings, be asked about their situation, or listen to the caregiver. One of the outcomes of such an interaction is that information is not comprehended by the parents. There may be misunderstandings, or it may appear that the information was not received. This can happen even if the caregiver's own assessment is that everything has been explained appropriately, perhaps several times, to the parents. In some cases, the father remains a bystander.

Occasionally parents accuse caregivers of causing their child's serious situation and this may be manifested in a long complaint processes. While the caregivers understand that often the accusations are not directed against them personally, becoming a target may be experienced as frustrating and unfair. When the tone of interaction is negative, caregivers often have a sense of inadequacy and failure.

Seeing both the challenging situations of fetuses and parents' distress may make working with a family emotionally taxing for caregivers, and they may feel that they will never get used to the most serious situations. Not being able to show one's feelings, or if mothers do not seem to react in an appropriate way, may also be experienced as stressful by caregivers.

The interactions experienced by a caregiver and the family of a child with fetal impairment and the experiences of help given and help obtained are presented in a compact form in Figure 20.1.

CONCLUSIONS

On the basis of the previous research results, it can be stated that caregivers acting within the Finnish care system understand well the shock a fetal impairment causes to a family, the demanding decision making needed to choose termination or continuation of a pregnancy, the importance of the family's internal relationships, and how to be sensitive to the family's social background. In this respect, the informative starting point of the caregivers is good.

The study also concludes that when successful, the interaction between parents and caregivers is an inter-professional collaboration that contributes to the survival of families and brings satisfaction to caregivers. As to the developmental point of view, however, a significant finding is that according to the parents' perception, the caregivers' actions, both in the dimension of information and that of humanity, contain a number of elements that complicate the families' survival.

From the point of view of the whole family, the fact that fathers are not always included in the care calls for attention. Usually it is not experienced as a problem that the children of the family are not included in the active care. Still, caregivers would be able to help them too, e.g., to better understand the parents' grief, and to help process any feelings of guilt, grief, or fears (Leon 1986, 1990, 1995).

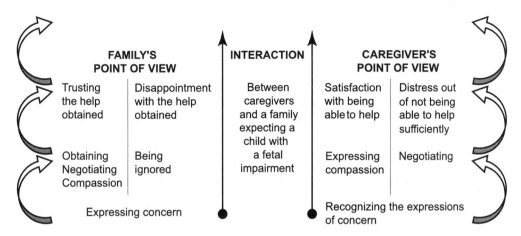

FIGURE 20.1 Interaction Between Caregivers and a Family Expecting a Child with a Fetal Impairment

In conclusion, the following propositions, partly included also in previous international research, are made for developing family nursing practices, caregivers' education, and health care administration (see Jorgensen et al. 1985; Langer & Ringler, 1989; Lemons & Brock, 1990; Bewley, 1993; Holzgreve & Miny, 1993; Seller & Barnes, 1993; Allen & Mulhauser, 1995; Dallaire et al. 1995; Leon, 1995; Lorenzen & Holzgrave, 1995; Chitty et al. 1996; Bryar, 1997; Pearson, 1997; Posa, 1998; Statham et al. 2000):

1. Instructions for securing psychological support for a family expecting an impaired child should be devised in the units of basic health care services and specialized nursing, covering the practical activities from the issuing of the first information during pregnancy to the follow-up appointment after the delivery or termination of pregnancy. The goal is to assign for each family a doctor–nurse team in charge of ensuring that the family obtains support as part of the overall care and, when necessary, makes sure that services such as a person with psychiatric education or a hospital clergy are available for the family.
2. The education of health care personnel should be developed by paying more attention to enhancing interaction skills, particularly a conscious utilization of the experiential dimension of interaction, which means that the caregiver understands her/his counteremotions and performs systematic self-evaluations.
3. The education of health care personnel should be developed by paying more attention to the sociopsychological processes that are associated with fetal impairment, the course of pregnancy when expecting a child with abnormality, and the loss of a child caused by a fetal impairment, either through termination of pregnancy or the death of the fetus.
4. The education of the personnel in basic health care should be increased in regard to fetal impairment.
5. The care of a family expecting a child with a fetal impairment should be improved by paying more attention to the needs of the father and the siblings.

6. The health care organizations should increase their resources of personnel, time, and space to accommodate the work with the families and the associated internal cooperation of the personnel.

REFERENCES

Allen, J. S. F., & Mulhauser, L. C. (1995). Genetic counseling after abnormal prenatal diagnosis: Facilitating coping in families who continue their pregnancies. *Journal of Genetic Counseling, 4,* 251–265.

Ämmälä, P. (1992). Sikiödiagnostiikka. In M. Haukkamaa (Ed.), *Obstetriikka* (pp. 223–237). Helsinki: Recallmed Oy.

Anderson, E (1996). Family roles. In P. J. Bomar (Ed.), *Nurses and family health promotion: Concepts, assessment, and interventions* (2nd ed., pp.70–82). Philadelphia, PA: W. B. Saunders Company.

Bewley, C. (1993). The midwife's role in pregnancy termination. *Nursing Standard, 8,* 25–28.

Bomar, P. J., & Cooper, S. (1996). Family stress. In P .J. Bomar (Ed.), *Nurses and family health promotion: Concepts, assessment, and interventions* (2nd ed., pp. 121–138). Philadelphia, PA: W. B. Saunders Company.

Bourguignon, A., Briscoe, B., & Nemzer, L. (1999). Genetic abortion: Considerations for patient care. *Journal of Perinatal and Neonatal Nursing, 13,* 47–58.

Boyd, S. T. (1996). Theoretical and research foundations of family nursing. In S. M. H. Hanson & S. T. Boyd (Eds.), *Family health care nursing: Theory, practice, and research* (pp. 41–54). Philadelphia, PA: F. A. Davis Company.

Bryar, S. H. (1997). One day you're pregnant and one day you're not: Pregnancy interruption for fetal anomalies. *Journal of Obstetric Gynecologic and Neonatal Nursing, 26,* 559–566.

Chitayat, D., & Babul-Hirji, R. (2000). Genetic counselling in prenatally diagnosed non-chromosomal fetal abnormalities. *Current Opinion in Obstetrics and Gynecology, 12,* 77–80.

Chitty, L. S., Barnes, C. A., & Berry, C. (1996). Continuing with pregnancy after a diagnosis of lethal abnormality: Experience of five couples and recommendations for management. *British Medical Journal, 313,* 478–480.

Dallaire, L., Lortie, G., Des Rochers, M., Clermont, R., & Vachon, C. (1995). Parental reaction and adaptability to the prenatal diagnosis of fetal defect or genetic disease leading to pregnancy interruption. *Prenatal Diagnosis, 15,* 249–259.

Driscoll, J. W. (1993). The transition to parenthood. In C. S. Fawcett (Ed.), *Family psychiatric nursing* (pp. 97–108). St. Louis, MO: Mosby-Year Book.

Gevers, S. (1999). Third trimester abortion for fetal abnormality. *Bioethics, 13,* 306–313.

Hanson, S. M., Kaakinen, J. R., & Friedman, M. M. (1998). Theoretical approaches to family nursing. In M. M. Friedman (Ed.), *Family nursing: Research, theory & practice* (pp. 75–96). Stamford, CT: Appleton & Lange.

Heiskanen, T. (Ed.). (1994). *Henkinen tuki ja onnettomuudet: Takaisin elämään.* Porvoo: SMS-Tuotanto OY.

Holzgreve, W., & Miny, P. (1993). Genetic counselling in prenatal diagnosis. *European Journal of Obstetrics, Gynecology and Reproductive Biology, 49,* 125–129.

Hunfeld, J. A. M., Wladimiroff, J. W., Passchier, J., Venema-Van Uden, M. U., Frets, P. G., & Verhage, F. (1993). Emotional reactions in women in late pregnancy (24 weeks or longer) following the ultrasound diagnosis of severe or lethal fetal malformation. *Prenatal Diagnosis, 13,* 603–612.

Jörgensen, C., Uddenberg, N., & Ursing, I. (1985). Diagnosis of fetal malformation in the 32nd week of gestation: A psychological challenge to the woman and the doctor. *Journal of Psychosomatic Obstetrics and Gynecology, 4,* 73–83.

Langer, M., & Ringler, M. (1989). Prospective counselling after prenatal diagnosis of fetal malformations: Interventions and parental reactions. *Acta Obstetricia et Gynecologia Scandinavica, 68,* 323–329.

Lemons, P. K., & Brock, M. J. (1990). Prenatal diagnosis and congenital disease: Role of the clinical nurse specialist. *Neonatal Network, 9,* 15–22.

Leon, I. G. (1986). Intrapsychic and family dynamics in perinatal sibling loss. *Infant Mental Health Journal, 7,* 200–213.

Leon, I. G. (1990). *When a baby dies: Psychotherapy for pregnancy and newborn loss.* Binghamton, NY: Yale University.

Leon, I. G. (1995). Pregnancy termination due to fetal anomaly: Clinical considerations. *Infant Mental Health Journal, 16,* 112–126.

Lorenzen, J., & Holzgreve, W. (1995). Helping parents to grieve after second trimester termination of pregnancy for fetopathic reasons. *Fetal Diagnosis and Therapy, 10,* 147–156.

Matthews, A. L. (1990). Known fetal malformations during pregnancy: A human experience of loss. *Birth Defects, 26,* 168–175.

McNeil, T. F., & Nimby, G. T. (1998). Anomalies and the mental health professional. *Annals New York Academy of Science, 18,* 10–20.

Mealey, A. R., Richardson, H., & Dimico, G. (1996). Family stress management. In P. J. Bomar (Ed.), *Nurses and family health promotion: Concepts, assessment, and interventions* (2nd ed., pp. 227–244). Philadelphia, PA: W. B. Saunders Company.

Mercer, R. T., Ferketich, S. L., DeJoseph, J., May, K. A., & Sollid, D. (1988). Effect of stress on family functioning during pregnancy. *Nursing Research, 37,* 268–275.

Pearson, L. (1997). Family-centered care and the anticipated death of a newborn. *Pediatric Nursing, 23,* 178–182.

Posa, T., Väisänen, L., & Väisänen, E. (1997). *Ultrasonographically detected fetal defect need more support.* Kiawah Island: Annual Family in Family Medicine Conference 1997.

Posa, T. (1998). *Ultraäänitutkimuksella todettu sikiöpoikkeavuus vanhempien kriisinä.* [Abstract in English: Ultrasonographically detected fetal defect as a parental crisis]. Doctoral dissertation, Oulu: Acta Universitatis Ouluensis D, 457.

Ritvanen, A., & Peippo, M. (1998). Synnynnäiset epämuodostumat. In P. Aula, H. Kääriäinen, & J. Leisti (Eds.), *Perinnöllisyyslääketiede* (pp.153–167). Helsinki: Duodecim.

Seller, M., Barnes, C., Ross, S., Barby, T., & Cowmeadow, P. (1993). Grief and mid-trimester fetal loss. *Prenatal Diagnosis, 13,* 341–348.

Shiloh, S. (1996). Genetic counseling: A developing area of interest for psychologists. *Professional Psychology: Research and Practice, 27,* 457–486.

Statham, H., Solomou, W., & Chitty, L. (2000). Prenatal diagnosis of fetal abnormality: Psychological effects on women in low-risk pregnancies. *Baillière's Clinical Obstetrics and Gynaecology, 14,* 731–747.

VanPutte, A. W. (1988). Perinatal bereavement crisis: Coping with negative outcomes from prenatal diagnosis. *Journal of Perinatal and Neonatal Nursing, 2,* 12–22.

Wheeler, S. R., & Pike, M. M. (1993). Families' responses to the loss of a child. In C. S. Fawcett (Ed.), *Family psychiatric nursing* (pp. 140–161). St. Louis, MO: Mosby-Year Book.

Wright, L. M., & Leahey, M. (1994). *Nurses and families: A guide to family assessment and intervention.* Philadelphia, PA: F. A. Davis Company.

Zuskar, D. M. (1987). The psychological impact of prenatal diagnosis of fetal abnormality: Strategies for investigation and intervention. *Women & Health, 12,* 91–103.

A Phenomenological Inquiry of Hope in Illness: Gays and Lesbians with HIV/AIDS

Kevin C. Krycka

HIV/AIDS continues to devastate individual lives, families, and communities across the globe. Its staggering dimensions are well documented by the World Health Organization and other agencies (United Nations Programme on HIV/AIDS, 2004). HIV/AIDS makes our will to live problematic as well as our need to understand the human condition in broader medical, social, and psychological terms. It confounds our best efforts at cure and continues to reveal glaring shortcomings in public attitudes and health policy toward gays and lesbians in particular. Undoubtedly, the persistence of heterosexism (the belief that only heterosexual relationships are normal and are therefore privileged) and homophobia will further confound the long-term care needs of gays and lesbians with HIV/AIDS. The two forces, a lack of cure on the horizon and the magnifying scope of fear, even hatred, against those with HIV/AIDS, stifle the development of a psychologically healthy self-image in those infected.

The phenomenological study reported here examines the experience of hope for those living with HIV/AIDS. It reveals that human beings who are able to access an embodied (level of immediate experience as it is directly known) understanding of their lived experience of hope in illness freely develop new strategies for living with a life-threatening disease. They are able to follow emergent experiences from within that contradict old patterns of prejudice, fear, and hopelessness—be they rooted in personal, institutional, or cultural sources. They find new words for the unimaginable that once structured the experience itself, which paradoxically creates fresh personal understanding and opens the door for a deeper exploration of the meanings their lives hold.

Language and languaging (the act of making words out of experiences) are key components in establishing, strengthening, and maintaining individual, institutional, and cultural identities and inequalities, both positive and negative (O'Brien & Howard, 1998). In this study, the power of language is seen in the words the participants chose to describe actual experiences. Logically, language and languaging choices by the participants are key indicators of changes in their negative or positive identities and inequalities.

It has long been established that gays and lesbians experience firsthand the power of unequal treatment as individuals. It is O'Brien & Howard's (1998) contention that institutions (e.g., medical and psychiatric) and cultures are likewise equal opportunity purveyors of these negative identities and inequalities. Thus when we seek to help gays and lesbians who are ill with HIV/AIDS, we must realize that many forms (individual, institutional, and cultural) of bias and negative valuation come along with them. Experiences of hatred, fear, and suspicion are common and may remain at levels hidden to the individuals at whom they are directed, only emerging through the words they choose when describing their experiences.

THE ILLNESS CONTEXT

It is important to note the broader philosophical context for understanding the psychology of hope in illness. Existential–phenomenological philosophers and psychologists believe individual experience takes place within a context, which contains multiple sources of knowledge (Gadamer, 1975; Polka, 1986). Valle & Halling (1989) note that this tradition (existential phenomenology) sees the individual as neither at the whim of a forever-constructing culture nor locked in self-referential isolation. This philosophical perspective sees realities as reciprocal.

For those suffering HIV-related limitations or disability, a dynamic of reciprocation is evident. As pointed out so eloquently in Toombs' (1993) examination of the experience of illness and the meanings generated by it, meanings derived from life-threatening illness begin and end with the hermeneutic of patient and doctor. Toombs rightly contends that both doctor and patient actively co-create the illness experience itself. Likewise, thinking and, by extension, saying are always situated and perspectival. Furthermore, thinking and saying transcend human mental life in that they imply more than what is known and said (Gendlin, 1997; Merleau-Ponty, 1955/1964).

Most research on hope in illness (Hall, 1994; Klenow, 1992; Perakyla, 1991; Rabkin, Williams, Neugebauer, Remien, & Goetz, 1990; Snyder et al., 1991) has relied on observation, surveys, experimentation, and interviews. Each of these methods is subject to the researcher's interpretation and the biases of the natural scientific method. They limit the scope of the world of everyday life to measurable data. A human life with its unique understandings and meanings cannot be so limited.

The phenomenological method described by Giorgi (1970, 1971, 1975, 1985, 1988) and used here safeguards against these limitations by returning to the experience as it is lived (Husserl, 1931/1962). The unique feature of this method is its articulation of the essences of experience, rather than generalizations. These essences, or themes, provide an in-depth look at the experience itself, revealing the lived experience in its most naked form. The use of Focusing (Gendlin, 1982), which was learned by the participants, enhances the felt-quality of the description of hope in illness, thereby giving the research a more proximal or grounded and embodied foundation.

RESEARCH SITUATION, PROCEDURES, AND PARTICIPANTS

Existential–phenomenological theory (see overview in Valle & Halling, 1989), pioneered in the last century, has developed its own method of analysis (Giorgi) that seeks to illuminate the basic dimensions of the experience under study and to report these dimensions in understandable terms. It allows us access to the participants' world and reveals the meaning of the situation, as it exists for them.

In this study, the basic dimensions of the experience of hope in persons living with HIV/AIDS were sought. It was determined that continuing with the methodology employed in previous studies by the author (Krycka, 1997, 1999) of this chapter (who is hereafter referred to as "I") would be best for this kind of investigation; therefore, it has been employed here.

The experiences shared and analyzed here come from five gay and/or lesbian individuals whom I (the author and researcher) had trained in Focusing (Gendlin, 1982) prior to their participation in this study. Focusing is a mind–body awareness technique taught in six steps. The six steps are clearing a space, finding the felt-sense, getting a handle, resonating, asking, and receiving. The process is well developed and researched in medical settings (Focusing Institute, 2004). The process is noted for its ability to help develop "direct access to embodied knowledge and the new steps of change and resolution that come from it" (Focusing Institute, 2004).

Individual interview sessions were audiotaped and transcribed. The participants, briefly described in Table 21.1, were each asked in an interview to "describe how you experience hope in relation to your illness." After transcription, the interviews were given to the participants for review and clarification during a second interview. To ensure validity, participants were allowed to review their interviews and check back with their own recollections to see if there was still a match between word and experience. These revised interview transcripts were then brought to phenomenological analysis.

The initial analysis involved searching for content dimensions and themes and listing them for each participant. These themes, at first highly individual and idiosyncratic, were brought together in the second stage of analysis. The results obtained by merging the thematic representations of individuals form the underlying dimensions of the experience of hope in illness. In keeping with an emphasis on returning to the experience as it is directly known (Husserl, 1931/1962; 1954/1970), the analysis uses little jargon, relying instead on the words of the participants to give flesh to their experience of hope while living closely with their own mortality.

The dimensions or themes structuring the experience under investigation are co-constituted out of the researchers' experiences and from the experiences of those who participated in this study. It is important to keep in mind that it was the participant's willingness to speak candidly about being ill and being gay or lesbian that enabled us to see deeply into the human process of dying (and living while dying).

What was seen was the eventual letting go of embattled strategies for fighting to live, fighting for a cure. When this happened, what emerged was something unique to the experience of being a gay or lesbian person with HIV/AIDS, although it may also be seen as a basic constituent of the experience for others as well. It is believed that the Focusing attitude of nonjudgment, the acceptance of what is and of welcoming new experiences has helped significantly in the achievements of the study.

For those unfamiliar with analysis of this type, let me say one thing further. This kind of qualitative work relies on the psychological openness of the researcher to the experience being

TABLE 21.1   Demographic Information

Identifier	Age	Relationship status	Education	Occupation
Becky	34	Partnered	Master's	Psychotherapist
David	48	Partner deceased	Community college	Unemployed
Joshua	28	Partnered	High school	Unemployed
Sarah	42	Single	Master's	Educator
Tim	45	Single	Master's	Mechanic

studied (Halling, Kunz, & Rowe, 1994). The analysis proceeds from the standpoint that there is little distinction between the observer and the observed.

ANALYSIS AND COMMENTARY

What follows are themes of hope in illness that emerged from analysis of the interviews. The themes presented here are technology, captivity, polarization, and consent. Themes are in some way an abstraction of the reported experiences of hope, yet they are true to the experiences themselves. The themes are presented in the order in which they arose from the analysis. This is an important aspect of the findings in that the first three themes may appear unrelated to hope at first glance. However, in the process of analysis it became clear that technology, captivity, and polarization were nested within the larger picture of hope that needed to be expressed. Said another way, these three themes were actually part of the hope in the illness experience.

Theme of Fascination

The first theme noted in the descriptions of hope was the participants' fascination with aspects of their medical conditions. A particular interest in the technological facts was noted, be it a newly placed Hyckman tube for intravenous feeding or mountains of data on various medical conditions. Participants expressed being drawn into their various new psychological or physical symptoms. There was no end to the trails we could follow in unraveling the mystery of their illnesses.

Becky, one of the participants, 34 years old and living with a brain infection brought on by later-stage AIDS, can help illustrate this. Below is a brief narrative summary of two interviews with her.

I sat with Becky in her living room one sunny Sunday afternoon. She had spread out in front of her a stack of new test results. She stated she had a "brain tumor," an inoperable one. With studied intensity she explained to me what each test meant, with a wide eyed expectation that I would also be enthralled with her telling. She said excitedly, "Look at this. This indicates it's probably not spreading. Although without another MRI [Magnetic Resonance Imaging] they don't know for sure. My brain is responding, though, to treatment my doctor says." She used clinically significant but distant wording. Her excitement was indeed genuine; it captured for the moment what it meant for her MRI to change since her last visit with her physician.

It has been said that the brain is like a computer and that the body is like a machine. Becky and another female participant, Sarah, spoke of "my brain." Surely they owned "brain" in some fashion, but it was not wholly theirs, either. Their charts were attended to, focused on, the facts made explicit to us. Becky's brain would die taking her along with it. These moments of intensity always ushered in a distance for Becky and Sarah, a distance that they slowly became aware of as we shared time together.

During a second interview with Becky, Tim, and Sarah, their fascination with one objective fact or another of their conditions gradually revealed inability to hold much of the depth of the meaning. Talking of the brute facts eventually slowed to a pace where a more gracious welcoming could come. The once psychologically necessary fracturing of experience faded into an awareness characterized by less distance and greater proximity to the very thing they sought to describe.

Toombs (1993) often notes that patients refer to illness as a psychic object, as an "it," when attempting to communicate about illness. This is an attempt to go around the limits of the technologically bound language with which we have become familiar. In some very important way, the employment of such language, distant though it may be, helps alleviate the anxiety that is, perhaps, brought out by the interview situation itself.

In a culture, an era, fascinated with medical and technological facts and focused on the parts of things, it should be of no surprise that a prime way of interacting with illness would come through an objectified perception. What is important to note is that the participants needed to wade through what was most psychologically familiar to them before they could fully describe their experience of hope. This description came in the second interview, where clarity and revision were sought.

Theme of Captivity

Another theme that emerged was the theme of captivity. David, 48 years old, spoke of how at first HIV infection was not merely an unwanted fact in his life but a hindrance to many daily activities. David became ill quickly after HIV exposure and was hospitalized many times in the proceeding 4 years. He spoke of his "real life" and his "real-now life with AIDS." For him, his real life, the life he wished he still had, appeared to be forever lost.

The participants expressed that when they became ill, even with a cold, they experienced a shift in the usual way they experienced their bodies and lives. Most of us can surely relate to this theme. Typically, we see illness as an unwelcome visitor, and the adjustments we need to make to accommodate it are done so be grudgingly (Marcel, 1942). Being ill signals to us that we are now different than we were before. Common to the experience of severe or life threatening illness is the experience of fragmentation between "my real, healthy self" and the "self I now find myself with." As with David there is sadness, regret, anger, bargaining, and even despair.

We are painfully reminded of the loose grip we have on life. Our physicians and caregivers deliver an increasingly complete set of descriptions of what will come to us in the course of our illness. "I think I'll probably eventually lose control of bodily function and slip into a coma," said David. Such prediction brings with it more uncertainty. The uncertainty of the body and the uncertainty of the wisdom of our attachment to it extend the experience of anxiety.

Marcel (1942) writes of a metaphysic of hope in which he states that hope's mission is to respond to the signal of distress piqued by our anxiety over the captivity our illness represents and to lift us up, as it were, to a broader view of life and what remains of it. He maintains that real hope, although borne of distress for some, is not in fact limited or ultimately fashioned by it.

Another male participant, Joshua, 28 years old, said, "You know, the worst thing of this is that I can't play with my dog anymore and that I've had to give the cats away; that and being chained to this machine now so I can't even go to the bathroom without major assistance."

Captivity is a typical experience of illness. It speaks of the forcible removal of those things we are attached to: sunlight, driving a car, petting a cat; and the fate to which we have been assigned. Throughout this study, participants spoke of the sense of captivity their illness brought before they spoke about their experience of hope. It became clear in the analysis that the themes common to this group of people represented a way into something much more interior and private, such as hope.

Theme of Polarization

A third theme revealed the deeper character of this softening from a stance of only experiencing illness-as-loss to experiencing illness-as-more-than-loss and captivity. These moments came for two participants as a clear, lucid recognition of being both body and more. For others it gave way to what can only be called a flight into wellness.

Three participants reported traveling to bookstore after bookstore, workshop after workshop to sit at the knees of an endless stream of gurus and saints in a desperate attempt to get back to health, to become whole and young, untouched by disease or infirmity. Such reactions take form around issues buried deep within their psyche.

The narrative that follows exemplifies a subtle aspect of illness-as-more. Joshua tells us of times when he was struggling against his potential death as he substituted one kind of hoping for another. His story elucidates the pitfall of continuing to live life as if all is the same when it clearly is not the same.

Joshua, a young man with advanced AIDS, said, upon reflecting on this time of frantic hopefulness, "I was seesawing back and forth between two worlds, almost. On the one hand was the leukemia creeping up in my body and the pain in that for me. On the other hand, I seemed to leap at any chance for a cure. You name it, I tried it. I went to church again with my mother . . . the first time in years. I hit the bookstores for the latest vitamin therapy." Joshua saw in his "seesawing" an attempt to regain something and push something else away simultaneously. He relied on a hoped-for outcome, a proof that such faith was indeed real. But this kind of faith, probably not a true kind of faith according to Joshua, is caught up in the having of more things, a healthy body, a clear mind, a reestablishment with the activities and loves of old.

If we stay in the awareness of multiple losses associated with illness and the frantic attempt to reclaim those losses, we are likely to experience a further inner tightening as many in this study did. Such tightening can lead to meaninglessness and despair as it did with Tim.

"At one point after my first OI (opportunistic infection) I thought I was going to be dead in a couple of weeks. Then when I didn't die, I thought 'What's the point? I'm just going to go through this crap again and again. Hell no. I'm not going to feel this bad again.'"

In each of these cases, as in helplessness and loneliness, we miss what we have had. Like the man in sorrow for having to give away his cherished pets, we are let down and see this so clearly. Actually feeling these losses helped alleviate the grip of such loss. During the interviews, the participants' feelings were freed up so that they then could speak more directly of their experiences of hope. A similar dynamic was reported in a previous study on the recovery of hope and will (Krycka, 1997).

Theme of Consent

The final theme in the experience of hope in illness involved consent. It began to reveal itself during our interviews, most often when a participant made a statement such as "I do not feel like this (HIV/AIDS) is all of me." Not necessarily said in those words, a force emerged that contests the inevitable outcome of the disease while owning the brute facts. Consent, as a theme of hope in illness, did not mean giving up, as one might assume. Instead, it formed the nexus of where hope resided for these people.

This last theme itself reveals many levels of potential paradox. It was not until the final stage of the analysis that the paradoxical nature of the embodied self-understanding of hope in illness came clear and the proximal language of the deep experience of hope was revealed. The final analysis put the flesh on the bones of the previously mentioned themes. From Tim:

> I hated to think about this second interview. It made me have nightmares again. The kind I had when I first was diagnosed. But then I took a breath, like we do, and could feel I had already changed. I didn't really feel dread anymore. I'm not that good with words, but I don't know; it's like I'm just now feeling hopeful. Going through all that stuff . . . and none of it was good in my book . . . it feels okay. I guess my "experience of hope" [motioned with quotation marks] isn't that religious kind of thing. **I'M** hopeful. **ME.** Not because of this or that. It's just me that's feeling hopeful.

Marcel (1942, p. 38) conveys the same in more philosophical terms.

> Because I am condemned never to recover from this illness, or not to come out of this prison, I do not mean to give up, I do not consent, from this very moment, to be the useless creature which my illness or my captivity may finally make of me; I will counter the fascination which the idea of this creature might have for me with the firm determination to remain what I am.

All of the participants clearly came to this position while in the study. It appears that as the participants learned better how to employ Focusing in their daily lives, they came to understand that they were more than their illness. To say "I am not my diagnosis" was no mere rallying point for denial of illness. Rather, what needs to be stressed is the very real embodied perception that, as David put it, "I am more than this illness believes me to be."

As a psychologist, it is alternately invigorating and challenging for me to hear such language come so clearly from an embodied place. All my training has told me to disbelieve such language or at least regard it cautiously. Yet these participants firmly showed me that my opinion of their words meant very little to them. In fact, as they described their experience of hope, it was obvious that I became the witness to their often-startling recognition of being more-than-ill, of being more-than-body.

CONCLUSIONS

The persons I have sat with over this last year have taught me that having a terminal illness does not necessarily mean being "trapped as in a sea of ice." In listening and in the analysis, I discerned what I believe to be an evolution of hope that involved negotiation with other lived aspects of the illness such as fascination, captivity, and polarization. This negotiated hope became evident through listening to the shifts experienced while we sat with each other during the interviews. It started first by fully understanding, or as nearly as possible understanding, the nature of the experience of illness itself and then opened up to a more readily recognizable theme associated with hope.

During the interviews we would, at moments, simply sit with each other, saying nothing, perhaps watching out the window to see the leaves turn up, silvery edged, against the wind. Except that we would keep dipping down into silences, drinking in a long stretch of quiet or laughing over our creaking and snapping joints. Our conversation did not appear remarkable although it was focused on the question at hand.

Any person with a life-threatening condition such as HIV/AIDS lives in uncertainty. The lives of those dying can remind all of us of a basic uncertainty about the ground on which we stand. But the lives of these participants reveal something more of the human spirit. They reveal a tacit knowledge that all is not what it seems, that we are more than our skin and dying cells, more than what appears at first glance or at the surface of our conversations.

The participants in this small study may be unusual in some respects. First, the sample contains two lesbian women with HIV/AIDS, which is an atypical occurrence epidemiologically. There may be gender differences unexplored in the analysis because they did not appear in the texts. This is one aspect of the research that could be explored further using narrative methods.

In spite of the unusual burdens placed on the ill, especially those with HIV/AIDS (Carson, Soeken, Shanty, & Terry, 1990), some persons so affected come to employ this embodied dialogue in their own lives and what remains of them with great positive effect.

The evidence for the presence of hope in illness is not refuted; rather it is extended by this study because the charge of this study was to describe as faithfully as possible the embodied experience of hope in illness. Connecting with the language of the body had the noticeable effect of taking us further into the life slipping away. It appears that the use of embodied experience—advanced by techniques such as Focusing—and the formation of a dialogue with such experience, forms the basis of a lived authenticity wherein hope resides.

This study examined what happens when gay and lesbian individuals explore the experience of hope in a time of life-threatening illness. It revealed psychological movement at the individual level and furthered a deeper understanding of the psychology of hope. It is through examination of the embodied experience of illness that patients and caregivers alike are offered a strategy to regain a sense of themselves in their experience that is linked to the development of positive self-ideals and images of the future. The results of this research indicate that looking to our embodied experience of illness will, in fact, supply us with a basic understanding of the experience of hope in illness and an embodied sense of hope that is neither otherworldly nor simplistic.

Finally, this chapter has suggested that hope, as seen through an analysis of the struggles of gays and lesbians with HIV/AIDS, appears as a negotiation at the horizon of death. Its emergence foreshadows a new but more complicated direction of promise for mental and physical health in times of uncertainty and change brought on by the nearness of mortality.

REFERENCES

Carson, V., Soeken, K., Shanty, J., & Terry, L. (1990). Hope and spiritual well-being: Essentials for living with AIDS. *Perspectives in Psychiatric Care, 26*(2), 28–34.

Focusing Institute. (2004). Retrieved January 4, 2004, from *http://www.focusing.org/research.*

Gadamer, H. G. (1975). *Truth and method.* New York, NY: Seabury.

Gendlin, E. T. (1982). *Focusing.* New York, NY: Bantam.

Gendlin, E. T. (1997). How philosophy cannot appeal to experience, and how it can. In J. McCumber & D. M. Levin (Series Eds.) & D. M. Levin (Vol. Ed.). *Northwestern University studies in phenomenology and existential philosophy: Vol. 2, Language beyond postmodernism: Saying and thinking in Gendlin's philosophy* (pp. 3–41). Evanston, IL: Northwestern University.

Giorgi, A. (1970). *Psychology as a human science.* New York, NY: Harper & Row.

Giorgi, A. (1971). Phenomenology and experimental psychology. In A. Giorgi, W. F. Fischer, & R. Von

Eckartsberg (Eds.). *Duquesne studies in phenomenological psychology.* (Vol. 1, pp. 6–16). Pittsburgh, PA: Duquesne University.

Giorgi, A. (1975). Convergences and divergences between phenomenological psychology and behaviorism. *Behaviorism, 3,* 200–212.

Giorgi, A. (1985). *Phenomenology and psychological research.* Pittsburgh, PA: Duquesne University.

Giorgi, A. (1988). Validity and reliability from a phenomenological perspective. In W. J. Baker, L. P. Moss, H. V. Rappard, & H. J. Stamm (Eds.). *Recent trends in theoretical psychology* (pp. 167–176). New York, NY: Springer-Verlag.

Hall, B. (1994). Ways of maintaining hope in HIV disease. *Research in Nursing & Health, 17,* 283–293.

Halling, S., Kunz, G., & Rowe, J. (1994). Contributions of dialogal psychology to phenomenological research. *Journal of Humanistic Psychology, 34*(1), 109–131.

Husserl, E. (1962). *Ideas: General introduction to pure phenomenology.* New York, NY: Collier. (Original work published 1931.)

Husserl, E. (1970). *The crisis of European sciences and transcendental phenomenology.* Evanston, IL: Northwestern University. (Original work published 1954.)

Joint United Nations Programme on HIV/AIDS. (2003). Retrieved January 4, 2004, from *http://www. unaids.org/Unaids/EN/Resources/Publications/Corporate+publications/AIDS+epidemic+update+-+ December+2003.asp.*

Klenow, D. J. (1992). Emotion and life threatening illness: A typology of hope sources. *Omega, 24*(1), 49–60.

Krycka, K. (1997). The recovery of will in persons with AIDS. *Journal of Humanistic Psychology, 37(2),* 9–30.

Krycka, K. (1999). The lost language of hope: Explorations of the lived-experience of life-threatening illness through focusing. *Focusing Folio, 18(1),* 93.

Marcel, G. (1942). Sketch of a phenomenology and metaphysic of hope. In G. Marcel (Ed.) *Homo Viator: Introduction to a metaphysics of hope.* New York, NY: Harper and Row, 29-67.

Merleau-Ponty, M. (1955/1964). *The primacy of perception* (J. M. Edie, Trans.). Evanston, IL: Northwestern University.

O'Brien, J., & Howard, J. (Eds.). (1998). *Everyday inequalities: Critical inquiries.* Malden, MA: Blackwell.

Perakyla, A. (1991). Hope work in the care of seriously ill patients. *Qualitative Health Research, 1*(4), 407–433.

Polka, B. (1986). *The dialectic of Biblical critique: Interpretation and existence.* New York, NY: St. Martin's.

Rabkin, J. G., Williams, J. B., Neugebauer, R., Remien, R. H., & Goetz, R. (1990). Maintenance of hope in HIV-spectrum homosexual men. *American Journal of Psychiatry, 147*(10), 1322–1326.

Snyder, C. R., Harris, C., Anderson, J. R., Holleran, S. A., Irving, L. M., Sigmon, S. T., et al. (1991). The will and the ways: Development and validation of an individual-differences measure of hope. *Journal of Personality and Social Psychology, 60*(4), 570–585.

Toombs, K. (1993). *The meaning of illness: A phenomenological account of the different perspectives of physician and patient.* The Netherlands: Kluwer.

Valle, R. S., & Halling, S. (Eds.). (1989). *Existential-phenomenological perspectives in psychology: Exploring the breadth of human experience.* New York, NY: Plenum.

CHAPTER 22

Nontraditional Vulnerable Populations: The Case of International Students

Leehu Zysberg

When vulnerable populations are discussed in nearly any context, and especially in health-related settings, certain groups come to mind almost automatically. It seems that certain social categories draw most of our attention when considering the terms "at risk" or "vulnerable." A search for the key word "vulnerable populations" in popular search engines (e.g., the National Library of Medicine's PubMed, Yahoo) showed the following recurring categories: certain age groups (e.g., the elderly, minors), ethnic backgrounds (e.g., African American, Hispanic), socioeconomic status (e.g., the poor), cognitive impairment (e.g., the mentally challenged), and physical location characteristics (e.g., prisoners, the homeless). More recently, issues such as cultural diversity, sexual preference, and gender have also become the focus of attention in this field as per guidelines for institutional review boards (IRBs) for conducting research with human subjects (IRB, 2004).

When dealing with definitions of populations it becomes obvious how arbitrary such classifications are, given the nature of social categories. By definition, social categories pertaining to populations, social groups, and so on are endless. Each and every individual belongs in many of them at any given moment (Dubrin, 2004; Myers, 2002). Hence, there may be an added value in eyeing social groups that do not usually fall into the traditional view of vulnerable populations as such.

The purpose of this chapter is to present an exploratory qualitative study focusing on one such potential vulnerable population. Based on the preliminary results, drawing on theoretical frames (e.g., the theory of reasoned action, the health belief model, and reversal theory) to discuss some directions and conclusions that may shed light on what makes a vulnerable population in this current social context may be useful.

INTERNATIONAL STUDENTS AS A VULNERABLE POPULATION

By the end of the year 2002, there were over 586,000 international students in college-level academic institutions across the United States (Institute of International Education, 2004). These students, before they even arrive in the United States, must be accepted for specific programs of study, show that they have a minimum amount of funds as required for their studies and relevant expenses, and acquire health insurance. They are not US citizens, and they are usually not required to pay taxes. With the exception of chronic conditions contracted while in the United States, they are not covered by Medicare or its equivalents. This is a group that is highly educated, financially stable, and health insured. In what way, then, are international students a vulnerable population?

FRAMEWORK OF THE STUDY

The study was aimed at exploring the international students' perceptions of their health-related welfare and their perceived level of comfort with the health care systems in the United States. The study followed a descriptive–qualitative design (Isaac & Michael, 1997) to allow for an exploratory approach because literature reviews revealed that the existing empirical work in this field was meager. The results revealed a pattern of decision-making processes and behaviors that suggest that international students may meet the criteria for a vulnerable population.

Sample

Twenty-five international students volunteered to participate in a study entitled "International Students' Relationships with Health Delivery Systems in the United States." The author approached potential participants on two campuses. One was a prominent university in a large metropolitan area, and the second, a community college serving a mix of rural and urban communities, was located in the northwestern United States. Except for one participant who declined, all the students approached showed willingness to participate. The participants were students at all academic levels from freshmen students in an AA program to advanced doctoral candidates. The age of the participants ranged from 25 to 46, and 22 (88%) were married. Of the participants 20 (80%) were women and 5 (20%) were men, and they were generally healthy. Although a few reported chronic health conditions, none were terminal or disabling. The participants were staying in the United States for a period ranging from 4 months to 3 years at the time of the study. Participants came from the following countries of origin: Gambia, Israel, Korea, Russia, Sweden, Taiwan, and the Ukraine.

Instruments

Data were collected by means of interviews. The purpose of the interview was to get the participants' general impressions and perceptions of their interactions with the health care system in the United States. A few guiding questions were used.

1. Do you have health insurance?
2. What do you usually do when you or someone in your immediate family does not feel very well?
3. Have you ever looked for professional health care? If so, how? Where did you go? How did you arrange for it? Could you describe the interaction with the health care agency to which you turned?
4. Based on your experience, what is your general opinion of the health care delivery system in the United States?

Prior to the interview procedure, approval from each academic institution and oral consent from each participant were obtained. The interviews were conducted individually in a private room and lasted between 20 and 35 minutes. The interviewer documented the sessions in writing.

Procedure and Analysis of Data

Interviews were conducted on campus at the convenience of the participants. The data were collected as interview transcripts. The data analysis followed the principles of content analysis. The transcripts were reviewed to extract content units into which interview material was assigned. A new content category was created whenever a new issue was encountered that could not be accounted for by the existing content categories. The assignment of content into categories was conducted independently by two judges to minimize bias on the part of the experimenter. Issues that were not agreed upon between the judges were either discussed until agreement was achieved or excluded from the results if agreement could not be achieved.

RESULTS

Contact of Participants with Health Care Agencies

It is interesting to note that the participants seemed eager to talk about their experiences with the health care system. The preliminary impression was that most of them had "a full belly" and that discussing their experience allowed them to "let some steam out."

All the participants had health insurance (as mandated by the US State Department). All of them had at least some interaction with health providers, and it is interesting to note that the overwhelming majority of them (22 or 88%) had been to a hospital emergency department. Approximately half of the participants (12 or 48%) had contacted health agencies for a condition they experienced themselves; the rest did so for a family member (typically a child).

Responses of Participants to Altered Health Conditions

The purpose of this analysis was to assess how easy or difficult it was for the participants to turn to health professionals; in other words, the perceived accessibility of health services in the eyes of the participants. The overwhelming majority of the participants (20 or 80%) reported postponing seeking professional help. Of those who delayed treatment, some reported waiting a while for a health problem to go away (50%). Others reported using traditional/folk remedies (15%), consulting informally with a family member and or friend who was a health professional (30%), and self-care practices (5%).

Patterns of Usage of Health Services and Agencies

What happened when professional health services were clearly required? What was the typical pattern of interface or interaction the participants showed when it came to health provision agencies? The overwhelming majority (22 or 88%) went to the emergency department when a clear need for professional health care arose, even when the need was not acute (e.g., headaches that would not respond to over-the-counter pain medication, sleep disturbances, and signs of mild depression). A minority (3 or 12%) scheduled appointments with family health and/or other specialty health professionals, predominantly physicians. Only a minority of the participants reported being under the regular care of a family health professional who managed the care program for them or their family members (5 or 20%).

An additional intriguing pattern emerged from the participants' stories. A few mentioned returning to their homeland for short visits for medical care. This was especially popular with dental care. Others reported postponing care for existing conditions until their scheduled return to their homeland. The reasons for this behavior were twofold. The leading one was cost-effectiveness. Participants reported that the estimated cost of travel plus the cost of care in the homeland was significantly lower than the cost of care alone in the United States (this taking into account their coverage under local insurance!). The second reason, mentioned mainly when it came to dental care, was that they felt they could trust the dental professionals in their home country better than they could the local professionals.

General Perceptions of the US Health System

The general impressions and perceptions provided by the participants fell into the following categories.

1. *Overly expensive or unaffordable.* Although insured, all the participants, without exception, reported perceiving the services and medications offered as "ridiculously expensive," "unbelievably priced," and "totally unaffordable for me." Most of the participants reported deep resentment of the co-pay that was often required, and although many American citizens may share this sentiment with the sample in this study, it is interesting to note the different basis for it.

   Most of the participants were from welfare states in which health services were provided free of charge or for very small payments by the patients. Many of the participants noted that, for example, "compared to what I had to pay at home, what's required here is absurdly expensive." Although these lower health expenses in the countries of origin are, of course, enabled by a heavier tax burden, the perception of direct payment for health services and products seems to have a negative effect on the participants.

2. *Administratively convoluted and/or inaccessible.* Participants reported avoiding the health service providers, mainly because they perceived them as inaccessible. Based on previous experience, 60% reported being unable to schedule an appointment within what they perceived as a reasonable timeframe for their health needs. Another complaint was what the participants perceived as limited or inadequate availability of doctors and other health professionals. As a result, they tended to withdraw and avoid contact with the system as much as possible, and most of them were not under the care of a primary health professional or a case manager (e.g., family health professional). The pattern that arose from the content analysis was one of unplanned "emergency" appointments, even when the complaint was not acute. Hence, the main resource that seemed accessible enough on short notice was the emergency department.

3. *Ambiguity, vaguenes, and hostility.* Most of the participants found it difficult to manage their interactions with the health services providers. They perceived them as impersonal. Therefore, they felt ambiguous about their rights as patients, and 60% reported perceiving the system as hostile toward patients, making such statements as "They don't really care about my health at all, just about proper payment," "How do they expect me to know when I'll be ill a month or more in advance?" and "There's no one to talk to when I need real help." It is important to note that these statements and the content they represent do not relate to the insurance companies but to the health care providers themselves.

4. *Dealing with insurance companies, claims, and payments.* The last major content category raised by the participants was the perceived complexity and misunderstanding of the insurance system and how to handle it. Some expressed fear of rising premiums and

payments if they filed too many claims, so they avoided the system as much as possible. However, all have mentioned in one way or another a sense of awkwardness and discomfort regarding the insurance management. This in turn seemed to deter them from approaching the system. "I just don't want all the headache of filing claims and filling all those papers and waiting and waiting" and "I wouldn't know what to do if I had to fill out all the papers" were two opinions that were heard.

Other Experiences with the Health System

Despite the obvious struggles and problems reported, students also reported successful, positive experiences. Two students gave birth while in the United States. Both reported very positive experiences with the care they got and the way the process was professionally managed (although they did mention struggling with the administrative aspects of the process). Another student, who was under the care of a primary health professional, reported a very smooth process. Students who were in health-related study programs (e.g., nursing, dental assisting) reported going through the needed vaccination and health-screening processes (usually managed by the school they attend) in a satisfactory manner.

All in all it seemed that the health conditions of most participants were eventually treated, but in many cases treatment was postponed or accompanied by adverse emotions as described in the previous section. None of the students interviewed was, at the time of the interview, in an extremely deteriorated or neglected health condition, although some reported medical conditions that had gone untreated.

DISCUSSION

International Students as a Vulnerable Population

Campos-Outcult et al. (1994) have offered three criteria for the definition of vulnerability in a social group: lack of access to care, fragmentation of care/lack of continuity, and lack of cultural competence (in other words, understanding the way the system works). International students, based on the preliminary results reported here, meet these criteria. Although insured and theoretically eligible for full health care, most of them perceived care as inaccessible, especially because of cost (which, again, is more of a perceived than an actual barrier) and the availability of health professionals when needed. Because of these perceptions, the students interviewed seemed to demonstrate an exaggerated use of emergency department services. As a result, treatment was fragmented because the clients did not have a professional available to them who was possessed of the whole picture to ensure continuity of care and proper follow-up. A lack of cultural competence was partly evident through the perception of ambiguity or vagueness in the system. This perception may have occurred because the students seemed to draw on the models of health care they knew from their countries of origin when trying to cope with the local health care system in the United States.

Understanding the Dynamics of a Nontraditional Vulnerable Population

The population discussed here, if considered vulnerable, requires a slightly different frame of reference for understanding. Unlike most traditional vulnerable groups, this one, at least theoretically, has adequate resources, both financially and cognitively. A cultural model would also be hard to apply here, because it seems that students with different cultures, backgrounds, and lengths of stay in the United States demonstrate similar patterns. What seems to be the problem, then? One of the most popular approaches to paradoxical behavior is the one dealing with the cognitive roots of behavior. A few models will be reviewed here and used to better understand the phenomenon at hand.

Theory of Reasoned Action

Fishbein & Ajzen (1975) presented a model linking attitudes and behavior, trying to answer another kind of paradoxical question: Why don't people always actually do what they think and believe in? In a series of theoretical and empirical works, they asserted that the link between attitudes and behavior is moderated by behavioral intent. Behavioral intent, in turn, is moderated by factors such as perceived self-efficacy, perceived obstacles, and the overall expected benefit of the behavior (Ajzen, 1991).

Health Belief Model (HBM)

Drawing on the theory of reasoned action, the Health Belief Model attempts to understand and even predict health-related behavior based on intrinsic and extrinsic factors. Intrinsic factors may be the value a person attaches to a given action (e.g., consulting with a health professional). This may be influenced by a combination of the perceived benefits of action and the perceived threats of inaction. A combination of intrinsic and extrinsic factors may account for perceived barriers to action (e.g., cost–extrinsic; fear of bad news–intrinsic). Additional extrinsic factors involved in understanding action are the behavioral cues, which usually come from the immediate environment, sending covert messages of action or inaction (e.g., a friend who used a certain health service successfully may be a positive cue). Additional factors related to self-perception and self-efficacy have also been linked to the model (Rosenstock, Strecher, & Becker, 1994).

Reversal Theory

A model originally created to account for self-defeating behavior in children is beginning to be applied in various health-related contexts (Finfgeld, Wongvatunyu, Conn, Grando, & Russel, 2003). This model views behavior as aimed at meeting goals determined by physiological and emotional factors. Motivations to behave may vary, focusing on intrinsic and/or extrinsic goals. Self-defeating or maladaptive behavior may result from the need to manage frustration, satiation, or environmental pressures (Apter, 1981, 2001). The model suggests a mechanism of behavior that may allow the reversal of counterproductive behaviors by reversing the goals toward which behavior is aimed.

Integration of Models to Understand Vulnerability in International Students

The three theoretical models (the theory of reasoned action, the Health Belief Model, and reversal theory) may help explain the paradox of the vulnerability of international students. The three models have a few key elements in common.

1. All of the models assume that motivations to behave are multilayered and are influenced by different factors.
2. All assume that people follow a relatively consistent pattern with regard to attitudes, emotions, or physiological factors.
3. All assume that behaviors are expressed or suppressed by a combination of cues (representing the value of behavior and the barriers to the behavior) and a perception of self-efficacy.
4. All models agree on the importance of environmental factors and cues in triggering behaviors or creating inhibition.

Based on the content raised in the study, international students seem to apply patterns of knowledge they bring from the health systems they know in their countries of origin to coping with the local health systems. Naturally, this may lead to maladaptive perceptions because the systems, by definition, are not the same, and therefore attitudes, or any other theoretically consistent pattern, will discourage prompt use of the system. Previous experiences and environmental cues in the form of experiences of other family members or friends (that have a high chance of being similar to their own) may even worsen the tendency for maladaptive behaviors. Lack of understanding of the system or a clash of values and attitudes (e.g., "one shouldn't pay for health care out-of-pocket") may pose perceived barriers to seeking professional health care. The process may account for the paradoxical conditions that can turn a knowledgeable, financially stable, and insured group into a vulnerable group. Figure 22.1 presents an integrated model for nontraditional vulnerable populations based on the models reviewed here.

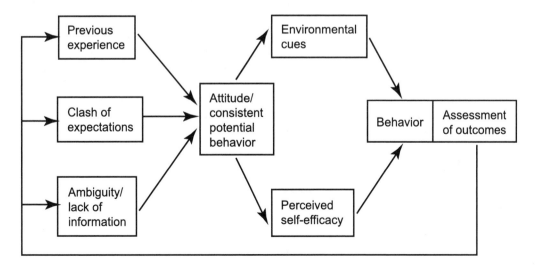

Figure 22.1   Nontraditional Vulnerable Populations: Integrated Model

Implications for Future Study and Practice and Limitations

This preliminary and exploratory study focused on what seemed an unlikely vulnerable population and probed the ways in which it may actually be classified as one. The assumed processes underlying the phenomenon involve biases in decision-making processes, based on a clash of attitudes and environmental cues.

One of the major roles of nursing in the promotion of wellness and health is education. Education also seems to be one of the most efficient strategies for dealing with vulnerable populations (Campos-Outcult et al., 1994). Education seems to increase perceived control, empower patients, and inform them of the options available to them (Myers, 2002). None of the students who participated in this study reported getting instruction from a health professional as to how to use the system. Could that be a direction for action for nursing and other health professionals in coping with the vulnerability of international students?

A similar process can be used to assess other nontraditional vulnerable populations and help encourage a body of research allowing better provision of health care to diverse populations, regardless of specific culture. Understanding paradoxical perception processes better will enhance the ability to educate target populations to use health services more efficiently, with the hope of promoting good health rather than treating deteriorated acute health conditions. Education aside, other structural adjustments in health care provision may, in the future, help reach more diverse populations and even cost less than they do now. How could these interventions cut down costs? A more efficient use of health care, less use of emergency department services, and an increased sense of continuity of care will help increase the quality of care and decrease its cost to all parties involved.

On the more general level, examining nontraditional at-risk or vulnerable groups is good for us as researchers. It forces professionals and researchers to take a fresh look at our current reality in which social categories and social groups abound. It will potentially help us avoid the entrapment of viewing social dynamics and their implications as "given" or "scientific constants" and keep on promoting evidence-based knowledge by simply doubting what we know.

This study, although it may point in a few interesting directions, is limited in scope and power. It was based on a relatively small sample that is not fully representative in terms of countries of origin and geographic dispersion in the United States. Being exploratory and descriptive in nature, cause and effect relationships were not fully established but rather were postulated from existing theories. Based on the preliminary results, model-driven hypotheses may be generated and tested on wider-scope samples, examining the general model for nontraditional vulnerable populations in a more specific manner.

ACKNOWLEDGMENTS

The author thanks Betsy Davidson and Anna Zisberg for their comments and help in the preparation of this chapter.

REFERENCES

Ajzen, I. (1991). The theory of planned behavior. *Organizational Behavior and Human Decision-Making Processes, 50*, 179–211.

Apter, M. J. (1981). The possibility of structural phenomenology: The case of reversal theory. *Journal of Phenomenological Psychology, 12,* 173–187.

Apter, M. J. (2001). *Motivational styles in everyday life: A guide to reversal theory.* Washington, DC: American Psychological Association.

Campos-Outcult, D., Fernandez, R., Hollow, W., Lundeen, S., Nelson, K., Schuster, B., et al. (1994). *Providing quality care to vulnerable populations.* Retrieved December 10, 2003, from *http://www.primarycaresociety.org.*

Dubrin, A. J. (2004). *Applying psychology: Individual and organizational effectiveness* (6th ed.). Upper Saddle River, NJ: Prentice Hall.

Finfgeld, D. L., Wongvatunyu, S., Conn, V. S., Grando, V. T., & Russel, C. L. (2003). Health belief model and reversal theory: A comparative analysis. *Journal of Advanced Nursing, 43*(3), 288–297.

Fishbein, M., & Ajzen, I. (1975). *Belief, attitude, intention and behavior: An introduction to theory and research.* Reading, MA: Addison-Wesley.

Institute of International Education. (2004). *Open doors project.* Retrieved December 10, 2003, from *http://www.opendoors.iienetwork.org/?p=36523.*

I. R. B. (2004). *Investigator handbook.* Champaign, IL: IRB.

Isaac, S., & Michael, W. B. (1997). *Handbook in research and evaluation* (3rd ed.). San Diego, CA: EdiTS.

Myers, D. G. (2002). *Exploring psychology.* New York, NY: Worth.

Rosenstock, I. M., Strecher, V. J., & Becker, M. H. (1994). The health belief model and HIV risk behavior change. In R. J. Diclemente & J. I. Peterson (Eds.). *AIDS: Theories and methods of behavioral interventions.* New York, NY: Plenum.

CHAPTER 23

"Can't Keep Me Down": Life Histories of Successful African Americans

Mary de Chesnay

The purpose of the study presented here is to document success stories of African Americans, with the ultimate aim of developing clinical interventions based on data from successful adults that would be culturally appropriate in helping children. The investigator developed the life history methods described here in the early 1990s for a study in the southeastern United States. Although data were collected, the research team did not reach consensus on the conclusions and interpretation, and that study was not published. The study was reproduced in the Northeast and Midwest and is being extended to the Pacific Northwest, and some of those data are presented here. Because of the volume of material generated in life histories, only data relevant to the purpose of this book are presented here.

The initial literature review revealed many examples of dysfunction in African American families, yet many adults are highly successful members of society-at-large as well as their own subculture. A new literature review was conducted in preparation for this book, and it is evidence of progress that investigators have started to focus their attention on the strengths of African American families, although there continues to be research on the most vulnerable of African Americans.

African Americans are significantly at risk for health disparities (Institute of Medicine, 2003). Themes of dysfunction and risk are apparent in the literature in terms of depression (Fuller-Thomson & Minkler, 2000), child protection for child abuse victims (Brissett-Chapman, 1997), HIV/AIDS (Carten & Fennoy, 1997; Mitrani, Prado, Feaster, Robinson-Batista, & Szapocznik, 2003), delinquency (Cross, 2003; Paschall, Ringwalt, & Flewelling, 2003), substance abuse (Ensminger, Hee, & Fothergill, 2002), foster care (Kemp & Bodonyi, 2000), early pregnancy (Yampolskaya, Brown, & Greenbaum, 2002), and nutritional problems (Basiotis, Lino, & Anand, 1998; Hargreaves, Schlundt, & Buchowski, 2002; Lee, Murray, Brody, & Parker, 2000).

METHODOLOGY

The life history is a technique derived from anthropology, and it is useful when the ethnographer wishes to tell the story of individuals who are particularly representative of their culture or subculture as a way of further describing that culture beyond the ethnographic material. Life history differs from autobiography in that the agent of interpretation is the researcher, not the one whose life is being described. The informant tells his or her story to the researcher who then interprets the story in light of the research questions and the cultural context in which the person lives.

There are many examples of detailed life histories in the anthropological literature (Davison, 1989; Early, 1993; Gmelch, 1986; James, 2000; Levy, 1988; Scheub et al., 1988; Sexton, 1981).

In the study reported here, the life histories are abbreviated stories told by people who have something to teach others through the recounting of their path to success. Success for the study was both self-defined and defined by members of the communities in which informants lived or were raised. For the purposes of this study, success means a sense of prosperity and general satisfaction with accomplishments in terms not limited to the attainment of material possessions but that include such factors as sense of satisfaction at his or her state in life.

It is important to note that the data derived from this study are emic data (from the person's viewpoint) rather than etic (from the researcher's viewpoint). Emic data are more powerful for the purpose of developing culturally appropriate interventions because of the increased likelihood of relevance to the target audience.

The author (hereafter referred to as "I") developed the methodology as a set of techniques that included interviewing, genograms, and time lines in order to focus on the research question: How does one become successful despite the potential obstacles of growing up African American? Although life histories traditionally are part of ethnographies and the researcher lives with the persons being interviewed, in this study, the researcher lived within the community but was not conducting a broader ethnography. A similar method of focusing life history material for briefer reports was developed by Hagemaster (1992), who presented a clear outline for interviews conducted solely as life histories. The usefulness of narratives was described by Mattingly & Lawlor (2000). Beery, Sommers, & Hall (2002) used an adaptation of Hall's (1996) methodology of focused life stories to explore women's experience with pacemakers.

Sample

Key informants were recruited purposively so that responses could be obtained from an adult sample diverse in age, gender, and socioeconomic status. Genograms and specific demographic data about the sample are not presented here in order to protect participants' privacy. The small number increases the risk of recognition of key informants, who, in some cases were prominent members of the community.

In all, 14 people were interviewed until it was determined that data saturation was reached. Although data saturation across informants is not an important consideration in life histories because these stories traditionally stand alone, it was decided to develop a typology from the data, which required a sense of consistency of results. Of the 14 people interviewed, 9 were men and 5 were women. Ages ranged from 29 to 82 years. Most of the older people were not college educated and had worked in factories, retail, or service jobs. Of the younger people, most were college educated, and four were professionals (an attorney, a physician, and two college professors).

Key informants were either approached by the researcher or referred by people within the community known to both the referring person and the researcher. The researcher spent much time in participant observation within the community and had developed relationships with people who either agreed to be interviewed or who referred others.

Setting

Key informants were interviewed in their homes, the office of the investigator, or in a private place convenient to the informant. Every attempt was made to maintain privacy. In one case, the interview needed to be rescheduled because of interruptions. In another case, small children were present, creating several interruptions, but the informant chose to continue, and an additional shorter interview was scheduled later.

Instrumentation

There were three instruments: a semistructured interview guide, a genogram, and a time line. Generally, we began with the genogram, a family tree in which patterns of family relationships and health status can readily be seen. The genogram was developed as a clinical tool in family therapy and is now widely used as an assessment tool in nursing and medicine. The genogram model developed for family therapy (McGoldrick & Gerson, 1986; McGoldrick, Gerson, & Shellenberger, 1999) was adapted by me for use in my own clinical practice as a family therapist and as an instrument of research in an earlier study (de Chesnay, Marshall, & Clements, 1988). The purpose of the genogram was to shortcut the analysis of family data.

Genogram questions involved gathering information about the family of origin and successful role models within the family. Interviews included broad questions about the definition of success, facilitators and barriers, and stories from the informants' youth. Generally three or four interviews lasting about 2 hours were necessary. Interviews were audiotaped for accuracy.

The timeline data collection tool is simply a horizontal line on a blank page with "birth" at the left end and "present age" at the right end. Informants were asked to indicate on the line the critical events in their lives and the ages at which the events occurred. The time line helped to clarify the sequence of events important to the person. Informants were given copies of the genograms and time lines and were encouraged to change them as needed during the intervals between interview sessions. Several informants also requested copies of the audiotapes.

In life history research, the researcher is an instrument, and the interaction between ethnographer and key informant can affect the accuracy and believability of results. Because the interviewer in this study was not African American, special attention was given to establishing rapport during the consent process as well as during the interviews. For enhancing accuracy and replicability, the data were subjected to external review by an African American nurse researcher familiar with the method. She validated the decision trail. These discussions were extremely helpful to the interviewer and increased confidence in the interpretation of results. After the institutional review board gave approval, the informants were recruited, the consent forms were explained and signed, and the interviews were scheduled, conducted, and analyzed.

RESULTS

The vast amount of data generated from these 14 life histories is too much to report in a single chapter. Rather, the results reported here include the commonalities that emerged from the data to generate a typology of success among African Americans. In order to give the reader an appreciation for the richness of the data collected in life histories, abbreviated biographical material is included for one of the informants, disguised to protect his privacy.

Mr. Sweet (he chose this pseudonym because "my wife says I am the sweetest man she ever met") was a 74-year-old factory worker who had spent most of his life working for the same company. He had retired twice, once from his regular full-time job and once from a part-time job as a handyman. He was active in his church and was seen as generous to others and a leader within his circle of friends and acquaintances. Referred by an acquaintance, Mr. Sweet agreed to participate even though he did not quite see why I would want to interview him. He chuckled: "but if you want to ask me questions, well go on, my wife says I have a lot to say about stuff I don't know anything about!"

He had been married to the same woman for 50 years and had four grown children, eight grandchildren, and two great-grandchildren. He defined his life as "service to my family and my God." As a blue-collar worker, he earned a steady salary sufficient to put his children through college, a fact of which he was extremely proud. The decisions he made in life were satisfactory to him, and he expressed that he had few regrets. He defined his success in terms of raising a family of children "who really have something to contribute to black folk and their church."

Mr. Sweet was modest about being referred to the study as an example of a successful man, but, on reflection, he acknowledged that he "must have done some things right" because the pressures "on black men as I was growing up" were intense and led to the downfall of many of the friends of his youth, who "ended up in jail or died young." He tended to minimize his experiences with racism and discrimination as he was growing up during segregation by interpreting racism as a problem of others. "It took me awhile but I finally figured out that if folks don't like me cuz of the color of my skin, well then, that's saying something about them, not me."

Mr. Sweet's genogram showed a family of origin that was intact and nuclear in both his and previous generations, with some divorces and nonmarried relationships in his wife's family and among his children. He was the only surviving member of his family of origin with the exception of a younger unmarried sister. His genogram also showed some of the health problems prevalent among African American families: diabetes and heart disease. He was in good health but reported he had "high [blood] pressure" for which he took medication.

On the time line, he indicated the following ages at which significant events occurred: age 4, when his mother died (he was raised by his grandmother and aunts); age 12, when he quit school to work in order to help his family; age 17, when he met his wife; age 19, when they married; age 28, when he earned a GED and a job promotion; age 35, when he was honored by his church; and age 69, when he retired comfortably enough for his wife to quit work.

Concepts

Transcending Racism

Racism was a universal in that all informants talked about the effects of racism on their lives, but it was striking that they tended to frame their reaction to racism as a problem of "the other" (the racist), and they made a clear distinction between their own feelings and behavior and those of the other. There was a philosophical sense underlying the anger about racism that made clear that these people were determined to transcend it. They tended to acknowledge their own anger about ongoing discrimination but without bitterness. Rather, they described how they had decided to channel their anger into activism. Examples of statements they made in response to questions about racism they had experienced follow.

"I know I didn't do anything besides sit in the diner and try to eat my lunch, but when the men around me started on about being with a, you know, the 'n' word, I got pretty mad, but I thought about what my mama told me, and she always said they [racist people] was ignorant and I should just pretend like I didn't hear."

"Yeah, well, you have to understand; I grew up in the segregation days and that was just the way it was. It was hurtful to have white folk looking down on us and it was a struggle to get a good job, but today things are so different and my children have it some easier. I always had the hope that my children wouldn't have to go through all that—and they still do—racism is still very much with us, but my children got to have advantages I didn't have, and that makes it all worthwhile."

"I still get mad every time I see it [racism], but, you know, it isn't really my problem. Racism is about the person being a racist, not about me."

"Oh, I guess, sure, racism was a barrier, there's no telling what I could of been if I grew up white, but I tried not to let it get me . . . I just knew the day would come when color don't matter—and I still believe that—even though that day hasn't come yet. Meanwhile I do what I can to help my people."

"Don't take offense now, but I really don't like to be around white people . . . some of them are honest folk trying to make a living for their families just like me, and some of them want to step over everybody else to get ahead . . . to make themselves powerful . . . but I figure we all God's children, and I can't allow myself to sink to their level."

Valuing Education

Although not all the key informants were well educated, they all valued education and saw it as a good way to have a better life. Their stories indicated hard work on the part of parents to provide a college education for their children and respect by children for the better-educated members of their families. In some cases, the person interviewed was the only one in the family who had earned a college degree, and these people discussed their education as "a blessing." They perceived that their less fortunate family members who had not earned a degree were proud of them.

"I never had much schoolin'—had to work the farm when I was growin' up and didn't even finish the 8th grade, but I was determined that I would send my children to college."

"My aunt had a college degree—she was a teacher—and we all [brothers and sisters] looked up to her because she just knew about everything! I would sit with her for hours and just to try to get her to talk to me about everything she knew. I used to pretend I was a teacher, too. I wanted to be just like her, except she didn't have children and I wanted to have kids, and I was gonna send them all to school, too. At my graduation [from college] my aunt was right there in the front row smiling up at me and I thought 'isn't it great—I made it—I'm gonna be just like her.' "

"I was the first [in my family] to go to college and my parents were so proud of me. I have a doctoral degree now and my daddy still brags about me as if I were a little girl . . . my brother wasn't so lucky—he would've liked to have been a doctor, but Mama got sick and [my brother] quit school to work because they didn't have insurance and my daddy didn't make much—he was a farmer. . . . I always felt bad about my brother. He would have made a wonderful doctor, but he never complained, and when I graduated he told me 'you done good little sister—you done me proud.' "

Family Support

A surprising result was that the people interviewed for this study tended to come from intact nuclear families. That is not to say that successful people do not come from single-parent families. No attempt was made to stratify the sample; the sampling was purposive and it just happened that all but one of the people interviewed came from intact nuclear families. All the informants talked about family support in some way, including the one from a single-parent home whose genogram showed a large extended family.

"My parents were extremely self-sacrificing . . . to make sure we all had a college educa-tion. Neither of them finished high school—they had to work—but they made sure we could [go to college]."

"I was raised by three parents—my mom and dad but also my mother's mother who lived with us. If one of them couldn't help me with a problem, there were two more I could go to . . . of course, sometimes they all got involved and I had more help than I wanted . . . but I always felt their love."

"Probably more was expected of me because my father had high expectations of me, and my mother made me sit down and do my homework before anything, even my chores. I remember once when I had a tough exam coming up and I really couldn't get into the subject, I actually volunteered to do the laundry, and my mother caught me out and told me she could do laundry but she couldn't take my exam and I just better get to work."

"My aunts lived next door and my parents had to work, so when I came home from school I went to my aunts' house and did chores for them till my parents came home . . . they [aunts] were always on me to study hard and get good grades so I could get into college."

Church as Extended Family

A strong theme was spirituality, which was closely linked to growing up in the black churches. Even though some of the informants were no longer associated with their churches, they talked about their early childhood experiences as giving them and their families spiritual strength. They tended to define their spirituality in terms of their connectedness, not just to God, but also to their community and their people.

"Church was the center of our world. We sang in the choir, went to Sunday school, spent most of our free time with people from the church—often marrying within the church. Of course, it was natural because in segregation, we couldn't have white friends."

"Church was a safe haven . . . we could be ourselves and feel safe."

"Pastor was a good spy for my parents. When I was doing something I shouldn't and it got back to my parents, almost always it was our minister who told on me. Not a bad thing, although I thought so then, but he was just looking out for us—trying to protect us."

"I'm not a particularly religious person now, but when I was growing up I went to church and made some lifelong friends . . . there's something special about friends you've had for a long time . . . and my church friends I knew I could always count on."

Perseverance

There was great consistency in the informants' statements regarding the dominant concept that emerged from the data: perseverance. Informants told many stories of "sticking with it" and refusing to give up. Perseverance seemed to be both an attribute of the individual and a child-rearing strategy. As an attribute, perseverance was seen as strength in that these people knew they had to depend on themselves and could not count on the mentoring and support by their super-visors that their white counterparts could expect. The informants made many statements about their families' encouragement to persevere, and they talked about how their family love and sup-port inspired them to find the strength to work hard to achieve their goals.

"No matter what they do to me, they can't keep me down—I always come back."

"I hear white people criticizing affirmative action, but if it weren't for that I couldn't have gone to college. I'm convinced that, without affirmative action, I would've ended up like so many of my friends—dead or in jail . . . so I just made up my mind to ignore the criticism."

"I just made up my mind that no one was going to stop me."

"I didn't care how much it took, I was going to make it . . . and make my parents proud."

"Every time I thought about quitting, I said to myself, 'no one is going to do for me except me.'"

"There were some nights I thought I just didn't want to wake up in the morning, but then, somehow, when I prayed for strength, God always answered my prayers . . . sure enough . . . it didn't take courage so much as will . . . I just decided if God would do his part, I had to do mine."

"My parents sacrificed so much for me . . . for all of us kids . . . that I just couldn't let them down. So every time I would hear some snide comment or hit a discrimination barrier, I would look at my [family photographs] pictures and say to myself, 'this is for you, Mama, or for you, Daddy.'"

"I was too stubborn to quit . . . you hit me down and I just bounce right back up."

DISCUSSION

Although transcending racism was a dominant theme in the study, it seems reasonable to conclude that perseverance was the key factor in the success of the people interviewed. The ability to persevere enabled the informants to overcome the effects of racism while working toward their goals and to make use of resources such as family support, education, spirituality, and connectedness within the church. There seemed to be a sense of strong self-image in these people, a self-esteem that a lifetime of racism could not erode.

The approach of social support was used in a program, Healthy Men in Healthy Families (pseudonym), designed to serve low-income urban African American men. Detailed analysis of the data showed that men continue to experience the effects of racism. It is an external factor in matters such as obtaining a job, but it is also an internal factor in that it strongly affects self-esteem (Aronson, Whitehead, & Baber, 2003).

In a study comparing the way that Hispanic, African American, and white children cope with disabilities, Hanline & Daley (1992) suggested that the ability to "reframe" helps African Americans rise to meet challenges and is a factor in their ability to integrate a child with disabilities into the family. Reframing a negative aspect as a successful problem-solving strategy is consistent with earlier findings on creative problem solving (de Chesnay, 1983, 1983, 1986) and might be an area for further research and for family therapy interventions as suggested by Stevenson & Renard (1993). For example, participants in the study reported here often reframed their experience of racism in terms of how tough yet compassionate they believed the experience made them.

The concept of family support is gaining attention in the literature on African American families, with a noticeable switch in focus from weaknesses (Myers, 1982) to strengths and resilience (Boyd-Franklin, 1989; Hill, 1999; Kaslow, Thompson, & Twomey, 2000; Kruzich, Friesen, Williams-Murphy, & Longley, 2002; Mandara & Murray, 2000, 2002; Owens, 2003; Scannapieco & Jackson, 1996). The results of the study presented here indicate a strong family network as a key factor in success, which is consistent with the findings of a study on coping with disability in which authors used a family strength model to emphasize that, although African Americans experience disability more often than whites, they are insulated by strong family ties that enable them to adapt over time (Alston & McCowan, 1994). In their family strength model, Alston & Turner (1994) describe strong religious and community ties as sources of support for families who have prevailed over time despite disruptive influences. Many other authors report similar findings about the relationship of family functioning and positive outcomes, whether in one-or two-parent homes (Conger, Ebbert, Sun, Simons, McLoyd, & Brody, 2002; Cosey & Bechtel, 2001; Fuller-Thomson & Minkler, 2000; Gorman-Smith, Tolan, Henry, & Florsheim, 2000; Taylor, Casten, & Flickinger, 1993; Timberlake & Chipunga, 1992; Wiley, Buur, & Montanelli, 2002; Winter, 2000).

In a study of vocational rehabilitation outcomes of African Americans, Dunham, Holliday, Douget, Koller, Presberry, & Wooderson (1998) found that college was a strong predictor of success in overcoming disabilities. It is not surprising that education was seen as a key strategy in success because education usually means an income sufficient to meet one's own needs as well as the needs of families. Education can also be an indicator of prestige, particularly in families in which few members are well educated.

The finding of spirituality in the life history study was closely linked with connectedness to family and community. There is support for this relationship in the literature. In their model of parental religiosity, family processes, and youth competence in two-parent African American families, Brody, Stoneman, & Flor (1996) depict linkages that explain the interactions of achievement, educational attainment, family cohesion, and marital stability. The development of resilience within spirituality was the guiding theme of Haight's (1998) ethnographic study on the socialization of African American children.

African American caregivers benefit from spirituality and support from the church. In three studies on the difficulties of coping with mental illness (Pickett-Schenk, 2002), stroke (Pierce, 2001), and HIV (Poindexter, Linsk, & Warner, 1999), a strong theme of spirituality linked with caring emerged and resulted in positive outcomes for patients.

The results of the study are consistent with the literature on all of the emergent themes and suggest specific interventions and recommendations for further research. First, implications for nursing and family therapy seem to call for an emphasis on strength rather than weakness or dysfunction resilience rather than hopelessness. As nurses and therapists, people come to us when in a state of stress, illness, or dysfunction, but we can choose to emphasize how they can mobilize resources to overcome their presenting problems. Racism is an ongoing factor in the lives of African Americans, and the addressing of institutionalized racism is a social problem beyond the scope of this research. However, there are clearly things that successful African Americans do that can be taught to children to help them transcend racism. Providing multicultural experiences, educational assistance, and social and family support helps children develop a strong self-image that is not impervious to racism but mitigates its demeaning effects. Helping children to reframe racism from being a problem "within the self" to a problem "of the other" places experience within a context the child can understand.

Further research is underway to validate and extend the findings. Currently, the study is being replicated in the Pacific Northwest with African American interviewers. Additional life histories with successful adults will provide a picture of commonalities of experience around the country. Clinical interventions need to be refined and tested. Finally, the study is being expanded to examine success in other contexts, such as coping with bereavement and becoming an advocate for social justice.

ACKNOWLEDGMENTS

The author is grateful to Dr. Ora Strickland for her help in validating the decision trail and to Dr. Jane Peterson for her critical review of the manuscript.

REFERENCES

Alston, R,. & McCowan, C. (1994). Family functioning as a correlate of disability adjustment for African Americans. *Rehabilitation Counseling Bulletin, 3*(4), 277–290.

Alston, R., & Turner, W. (1994). A Family Strengths Model of adjustment to disability for African American clients. *Journal of Counseling and Development, 4,* 378–384.

Aronson, R., Whitehead, T., & Baber, W. (2003). Challenges to masculine transformation among urban low-income African American men. *American Journal of Public Health, 93*(5), 732–742.

Basiotis, P., Lino, M., & Anand, R. (1998). Report card on the diet quality of African Americans. *Family Economics and Nutrition Review, 11*(3), 61–64.

Beery, T., Sommers, M., & Hall, J. (2002). Focused life stories of women with cardiac pacemakers. *Western Journal of Nursing Research, 24*(1), 7–27.

Brissett-Chapman, S. (1997). Child protection risk assessment and African American children: Cultural ramifications for families and communities. *Child Welfare, 76*(1), 45–64.

Brody, G., Stoneman, Z., & Flor, D. (1996). Parental religiosity, family processes and youth competence in rural, two-parent African American families. *Developmental Psychology, 32*(4), 696–706.

Carten, A., & Fennoy, I. (1997). African American families and HIV/AIDS: Caring for surviving children. *Child Welfare, 76*(1), 107–126.

Conger, R., Ebbert, W., Sun, Y., Simons, R., McLoyd, V., & Brody, G. (2002). Economic pressure in African American families: A replication and extension of the family stress model. *Developmental Psychology, 38*(2), 179–193.

Cosey, E., & Bechtel, G. (2001). Family social support and prenatal care among unmarried African American teenage primiparas. *Journal of Community Health Nursing, 18*(2), 107–115.

Cross, W. (2003). Tracing the historical origins of youth delinquency & violence: Myths and realities about black culture. *Journal of Social Issues, 59*(1), 67–82.

Davison, J. (1989). *Voices from Mutira: Change in the lives of rural Gikuyu women.* Boulder, CO: Lynne Reinner.

de Chesnay, M. (1983). The creation and dissolution of paradoxes in nursing practice. *Topics in Clinical Nursing, 5*(3), 71–83.

de Chesnay, M. (1983). Problem solving in nursing. Image. *Journal of Nursing Scholarship,15*(1), 8–11.

de Chesnay, M. (1986). Jamaican family structure: The paradox of normalcy. *Family Process, 25*(2), 293–300.

de Chesnay, M., Marshall, E., & Clements, C. (1988). Family structure, marital power, maternal distance, and paternal alcohol consumption in father-daughter incest. *Family Systems Medicine, 6*(4), 453–462.

Dunham, M., Holliday, G., Douget, R., Koller, J., Presberry, R., & Wooderson, S. (1998). Vocational rehabilitation outcomes of African American adults with specific learning disabilities. *Journal of Rehabilitation, 64*(3), 36–42.

Early, E. (1993). *Baladi women: Playing with an egg and a stone.* Boulder, CO: Lynne Reinner.

Ensminger, M., Hee, S. J., & Fothergill, K. (2002). Childhood and adolescent antecedents of substance abuse in adulthood. *Addiction, 97,* 838–844.

Fuller-Thomson, E., & Minkler, M. (2000). African American grandparents raising grandchildren: A national profile of demographic and health characteristics. *Health and Social Work, 25*(2), 109–119.

Gmelch, S. (1986). *Nan: The life of an Irish traveling woman.* Prospect Heights, IL: Waveland.

Gorman-Smith, E., Tolan, P., Henry, D., & Florsheim, P. (2000). Patterns of family functioning and adolescent outcomes among urban African American and Mexican American families. *Journal of Family Psychology, 14*(3), 436–457.

Hagemaster, J. (1992). Life history: A qualitative method of research. *Journal of Advanced Nursing, 17,* 1122–1128.

Haight, W. (1998). "Gathering the spirit" at First Baptist Church: Spirituality as a protective factor in the lives of African American children. *Social Work, 43*(3), 213–222.

Hall, J. (1996). Geography of childhood sexual abuse: Women's narratives of their childhood environment. *Advances in Nursing Science, 18*(4), 29–47.

Hanline, M., & Daley, S. (1992). Family coping strategies and strengths in Hispanic, African American and Caucasian families of young children. *Topics in Early Childhood Special Education, 12*(3), 351–367.

Hargreaves, M., Schlundt, D., & Buchowski, M. (2002). Contextual factors influencing the eating behaviours of African American women: A focus group investigation. *Ethnicity and Health, 7*(3), 133–147.

Hill, R. B. (1999). *The strengths of African American families: 25 years later.* Lanham, MD: University Press of America.

Institute of Medicine. (2003). *Unequal treatment: Confronting racial and ethnic disparities in health care (2003).* Washington, DC: National Academy of Sciences.

James, D. (2000). *Doña María's story.* Durham, NC: Duke University.

Kaslow, N., Thompson, M., & Twomey, H. (2000). Ratings of family functioning of suicidal and nonsuicidal African American women. *Journal of Family Psychology, 14*(4), 585–599.

Kemp, S., & Bodonyi, J. (2000). Infants who stay in foster care: Child characteristics and permanency outcomes of legally free children placed as infants. *Child and Family Social Work, 5,* 95–106.

Kruzich, J., Friesen, B., Williams-Murphy, T., & Longley, M. (2002). Voices of African American families: Perspectives on residential treatment. *Social Work, 47*(4), 461–470.

Lee, E. J., Murray, V., Brody, G., & Parker, V. (2002). Maternal resources, parenting and dietary patterns among rural African American children in single-parent families. *Public Health Nursing, 19*(2), 104–111.

Levy, M. (1988). *Each in her own way: Five women leaders of the developing world.* Boulder, CO: Lynne Reinner.

Mandara, J., & Murray, C. (2000). Effects of parental marital status, income and family functioning on African American adolescent self-esteem. *Journal of Family Psychology, 14*(3), 475–490.

Mandara, J., & Murray, C. (2002). Development of an empirical typology of African American family functioning. *Journal of Family Psychology, 16*(3), 318–337.

Mattingly, C., & Lawlor, M. (2000). Learning from stories: Narrative interviewing in cross-cultural research. *Scandinavian Journal of Occupational Therapy, 7,* 4–14.

McGoldrick, M., & Gerson, R. (1986). *Genograms in family assessment.* New York, NY: W. W. Norton.

McGoldrick, M., Gerson, R., & Shellenberger, S. (1999). *Genograms: Assessment and intervention.* New York, NY: W. W. Norton.

Mitrani, V., Prado, G., Feaster, D., Robinson-Batista, C., & Szapocznik, J. (2003). Relational factors and family treatment engagement among low-income HIV-positive African American mothers. *Family Process, 42*(1), 31–45.

Owens, S. (2003). African American women living with HIV/AIDS: Families as sources of support and of stress. *Social Work, 48*(2), 163–172.

Paschall, M., Ringwalt, C., & Flewelling, R. (2003). Effects of parenting, father absence, and affiliation with delinquent peers on delinquent behavior among African American male adolescents. *Adolescence, 38*(149), 15–35.

Pierce, L. (2001). Caring and expressions of spirituality by urban caregivers of people with stroke in African American families. *Qualitative Health Research, 11*(3), 339–352.

Poindexter, C., Linsk, N., & Warner, S. (1999). "He listens and never gossips:" Spiritual coping without church support among older, predominantly African American caregivers of persons with HIV. *Review of Religious Research, 40*(3), 230–243.

Pickett-Schenk, S. (2002). Church-based support for African American families coping with mental illness: Outreach and outcomes. *Psychiatric Rehabilitation Journal, 26*(2), 173–180.

Scannapieco, M., & Jackson, S. (1996). Kinship care: The African American response to family preservation. *Social Work, 41*(2), 190–197.

Scheub, H., Mack, B., Schildkrout, E., Obbo, C., Wilks, I., Romero, P., et al. (1988). *Life histories of African women*. London: Ashfield.

Sexton, J. D. (1981). *Son of Tecún Umán: A Maya Indian tells his life story*. Prospect Heights, IL: Waveland.

Stevenson, H., & Renard, G. (1993). Trusting ole' wise owls: Therapeutic use of cultural strengths in African American families. *Professional Psychology: Research and Practice, 24*(4), 433–442.

Taylor, R., Casten. R., & Flickinger, S. (1993). Influence of kinship social support on the parenting experiences and psychosocial adjustment of African American adolescents. *Developmental Psychology, 29*(2), 382–388.

Timberlake, E., & Chipunga, S. (1992). Grandmotherhood: Contemporary meaning among African American middle-class grandmothers. *Social Work, 37*(3), 216–223.

Unequal Treatment: Confronting Racial and Ethnic Disparities in Health Care (2003). Washington, DC: National Academy of Sciences-Institute of Medicine.

Wiley, A., Buur, H., & Montanelli, D. (2002). Shelter in a time of storm: Parenting in poor rural African American communities. *Family Relations, 51*(3), 265–283.

Winter, M. (2000). Culture counts. *Human Ecology, 28*(1), 12–17.

Yampolskaya, S., Brown, E., & Greenbaum, P. (2002). Early pregnancy among adolescent females with serious emotional disturbances: Risk factors and outcomes. *Journal of Emotional and Behavioral Disorders, 10*(2), 108–115.

UNIT IV

PRACTICE

When working with others during times of despair, vulnerability and unknowns, we are challenged to learn again, to reexamine our own meeting of life and death. As we do so, we engage in a more authentic process to cultivate and sustain caring, healing practices for self and others.

Jean Watson

Source: Watson, J. (2003). Love and caring: Ethics of face and hand—An invitation to return to the heart and soul of nursing and our deep humanity. *Nursing Administration Quarterly, 27*(3), 197–202.

CHAPTER 24

Cultural Traits and Nursing Care Particular to Japan

Yukie Takemura

According to Leininger (1985), the real meaning and quality of life, health, and nursing care are best understood from a holistic frame of reference that takes into account the social structure of the person. Nurses must see the meaning of events from the viewpoint of those they care for in order to understand their health care needs (called the emic view). This is especially important when a nurse cares for a person from a different culture or subculture. Care is established when a patient has accepted an action of care. Care arising from the one-sided understanding of the caregiver (from the nurse's own cultural perspective) may not be accepted as care by the patient. This chapter presents some information about Japanese culture that might enable nurses to improve caring for Japanese patients.

JAPANESE PERSONAL PERSPECTIVES AND INTERPERSONAL PERSPECTIVES

Japanese culture has been compared, inappropriately, with Western culture. For example, a dichotomy often used to understand and compare cultures is individualism–collectivism. Hamaguchi (1998) pointed out that the concept of the "individual" is not universal and that the distinctions in the dichotomy of individualism and collectivism are "culture-bound." That is, when using the Western concept of individualism (consisting of autonomous individuals), Japan is characterized as a nonindividualistic and collectivistic culture. Thus Japanese are portrayed as soldier ants or worker bees that sacrifice their interests as individuals to contribute to the group. To understand Japanese cultural traits, a uniquely Japanese view (an emic framework from the point of view of the Japanese person) must be developed and used.

According to Hamaguchi (1998), in Japan a person is structurally defined in relation to nature and other persons. The group or organization is considered a network system that shares among its members an interpersonal context that includes relationships, situations, and shared values. Therefore, Japanese culture can be considered to be an example of relationalism (all things are related) (Kumon, 1982) or contextualism (behavior takes place within a context) (Hamaguchi, 1998), rather than collectivism (individuals not an end to themselves). Although Western societies promote the realization of the individual self as the goal of life, the Japanese ideal of life is to exist among others harmoniously (Nonaka & Takeuchi, 1995).

Japanese Relationships and Communication Style

Japanese culture is characterized by respect for relationships with others. However, compared to Americans, who seem to express their thoughts and feelings readily, Japanese are less likely to disclose their inner experience (Barnlund, 1975). Barnlund explained this phenomenon in terms of the public self and the private self. The private self indicates aspects of the person that are not often shared with others. The public self identifies aspects of the person that are easily shared with others. Barnlund (1975) explained that Japanese have a narrow range of public self and a wide range of private self. Americans have the reverse. In Japan, the inner experience is often communicated nonverbally when the listener carefully guesses at it and not by the speaker's disclosure of self. Japanese verbal communication is characterized by an indirect, localized, self-controlled, situation-oriented, chain of monologues (Nishida, 1996), which avoids outright opposition between one person and another and preserves harmony.

In contrast, Americans communicate fast in a manner that is direct and to the point. Americans may perceive that conversation with the Japanese is endless, pointless, and strained, and made up of numerous evasive sentences. They may also perceive that it involves a great deal of wasted time because there are long silences (Barnlund, 1975). Sekiguchi (1999) stated that, if Western communication is seen as a rally in tennis, Japanese communication is like just hitting the ball. That is, one side hits a slow ball to a place where the other party cannot return it; the other party sees the rolling ball, guesses the intent, and this time takes a new ball from his or her own pocket and hits it similarly the other way. The topic itself is often not important. Thus a subtle understanding is born between the two people while the sequence is repeated.

Cross-Cultural Communication and Value Transformation

In the modern age, vast amounts of information are exchanged rapidly and go beyond national borders. Although Japanese traditional culture and values are influenced by Western culture and values to a degree, traditional Japanese personal perspectives and communication styles are still the basis of the behavior and thought of people in Japan today. When doing work that is closely related to a person's way of life and values, such as nursing, the cultural traits of Japan cannot be ignored. Western nurses should understand the fundamental differences in communication style and act accordingly, and Japanese nurses must understand that Western patients will behave very differently from Japanese patients.

A NURSING CARE MODEL APPROPRIATE FOR JAPAN

Modern Japanese nursing was born after World War II when Western nursing models were incorporated into nursing education and practice in Japan. More recently, Western values and beliefs about nursing have been fused with Japan's traditional values, culture, and nursing models, which have been modified to be useful in Japan. Takemura & Kanda (2001, 2003) interviewed and observed nurses at hospitals in Japan and attempted to identify the process of nursing care. Their findings are useful for those nurses caring for Japanese patients and probably also for East Asians who have cultures that resemble Japanese culture. Following are the major themes identified in their studies.

Realizing Meanings and Values and Changing for the Better

Takemura & Kanda (2001) found that Japanese nurses do not simply aim to solve patients' problems but also to help them explore meanings and values of their experiences with illness, hospitalization, and treatment in order to be satisfied with their lives during their illness and health care. Making a change for the better (resolution of nursing problems) in the patient's internal and external environment (physical, psychological, and social conditions) is an important element in nursing care. However, regardless of how good the patient's condition becomes, when patients cannot find value or meaning in their improvement, Japanese nurses do not feel they have performed good nursing. In order to perform better nursing (i.e., for the patient to realize meanings and values), knowing the patient and attending to the patient are recognized as critical nursing actions. Moreover, gaining the patient's trust, helping the patient participate in medical care, and working with the family while preserving harmony are also recognized as important elements of nursing care both in Japan and in the West. These aspects of nursing care probably reflect the universal mission of nursing. However, approaches to these elements by Japanese nurses are uniquely Japanese.

Knowing the Patient

To help patients explore the meanings and values of their experiences with illness, Japanese nurses get to know the patient; then they identify the target, direction, and conditions of nursing care. For the duration of nursing care, the nurses implement care with the aim of changing patients' internal and external environments for the better. Getting to know the patient is an especially important process and becomes the basis of all decision making.

Distinguishing Between the Patient's Perspective and One's Own

Tanner et al. (1993) indicated that knowing the patient means two things: knowing the patient's typical pattern of responses and knowing the patient as a person. Takemura & Kanda (2003) stated that knowledge of the patient as a person includes both the patient's subjective world (patient's perspective of world) and the holistic patient (nurse's perspective of the patient). They found the importance of ascertaining the former while distinguishing it from the latter to be particularly evident in Japan. Of course, the importance of understanding the patient's perspective was pointed out in the West as well, as in Benner and Wrubel's (1989) observation that, while taking the history, nurses attended to the patient's story of the illness. For the nurse to understand the context and meaning of the symptoms is central to curing and healing. The reason why this is important in Japan is that in traditional Japanese society, people had vague boundaries between self and others and did not distinguish between an individual's perspective and that of others in a strict sense.

Nonaka & Takeuchi (1995) pointed out that oneness of the self and the other, oneness of humanity and nature, and oneness of body and mind represent Japanese intellectual tradition. Japanese philosophy integrates the teachings of Buddhism, Confucianism, and major Western philosophical thought. Although a typical Western individual conceptualizes things from an objective vantage point, a Japanese person does so by relating himself or herself to other things or persons. Therefore, the Japanese perspective is tactile and interpersonal. The structure of the Japanese language also facilitates the sympathetic unity of self with other people. In the Japanese language, omission of the subject is frequent and verbs do not agree with the subject of the sentence. A message is often communicated through the use of context, not by the grammatical code as in English. The present and past are also expressed without strictly differentiating between them. The perspective of a Japanese speaker can be shared naturally and smoothly by others (Nonaka & Takeuchi, 1995). On the other hand, conveying one's thoughts and emotions as one's own is difficult, and this causes a general tendency among Japanese to mix the thoughts and feelings of others with one's own. Nurses in Japan require special awareness and effort to distinguish and ascertain the world experienced by the patient and the world experienced by the patient as surmised by the nurse.

Three Modes to Know the Patient

Takemura & Kanda (2001) further discovered that Japanese nurses use three modes to get to know a patient: the considerate mode, professional mode, and narrative listener mode. Which mode was primarily used and the differentiation of the use of modes depending upon the context differed depending on the nurse.

The considerate mode is the manner normally used when a Japanese person wants to know another person and is guessing, in a nonverbal manner, the other's thoughts and emotions. The Japanese traditionally place more value on silence than on speech. They tend to keep words to a minimum and leave much of what they wish to communicate implied rather than stated (Nishida, 1996). Japanese patients expect their nonverbalized needs and emotions to be understood by nurses, and they tend not to explain or elaborate by putting them into words. Nurses must surmise the world experienced by the patient based on observation of the patient's facial expression, eye movements, body movements, pauses or silences, and the patient's condition and context. They can avoid making the patient feel uncomfortable by being mindful of the world experienced by the patient that the nurse has conjectured. When using the considerate mode, words or actions of the patient that would be superficially rude, incomprehensible, or troublesome change to understandable ones. The considerate mode allows nurses to provide care without having uneasiness towards the patient. However, when the nurse forgets that the patient's world as surmised by the nurse is not the world actually experienced by the patient, slight discrepancies may occur between the nurse's assumptions regarding care needs and the patient's actual needs. This may cause the nurse to feel that his or her own effort and expectations ended in failure.

The professional mode is what can be called a rational method of knowing a patient, and Japanese nurses learn this through specific training given during nursing education programs. In this mode, the nurse's aim is to provide appropriate nursing care for a patient who is a completely independent being. Therefore, the nurse wants to know the patient. The nurse wants to know necessary and important information in order to assess a patient's problems or to evaluate whether problems are resolved. However, in Japan there is little disclosure and little clear indication of intent from a patient. The nurse must first listen to the patient's conversation through a filter of inference and judgment as a professional, then provide appropriate care. Sometimes, information obtained from the patient is used by the nurse to perform nursing care that satisfies the nurse and not the patient. In this mode, generally the nurse has difficulty accepting what a patient means. One nurse related that, looking back on herself in the past while primarily using this mode: "I thought I listened to the patient, but I've realized I didn't. I thought I had an interest in the patient, but I've realized I didn't. I didn't take advantage of the patient's thoughts and only my thoughts instead."

In the professional mode, the nurse uses patient responses regarding care to evaluate nursing care. The patient's responses are also linked to the evaluation of the nurse's competency. When problems are resolved with the patient acting as the nurse expected, the nurse feels competent as a nurse and feels happy. When encountering an unexpected patient response, the nurse feels as if his or her own ability as a nurse has been questioned. This also somewhat complicates the nurse's acceptance of the patient's message for what it means.

In principle, the patient's perspective can be conveyed through verbalization of the patient's own experience and cannot be ascertained by either the considerate mode (the traditional method of knowing a person in Japan) or the professional mode, which is learned in nursing education. However, nurses in Japan might need to go beyond these communication styles and employ the narrative listener mode. The narrative listener mode is not intended to be directly linked to aims such as selection of nursing care. The narrative listener has an interest in the patient and the patient's life and wants to know the patient and understand his or her lived experience. This mode is used by some nurses who are considered excellent by patients and colleagues. It is an important mode that holds the key to knowing a patient's perspective. When using this mode, the nurse temporarily reserves his or her point of view in order to distinguish it from the patient's point of view. In this way, the nurse listens to the patient's conversation without filtering it as a nurse. One nurse indicated differentiation with the professional mode in the following way: "First, listen to conversations to know the patient. Afterwards, do this again, but this time, listen as a nurse for assessment." The narrative listener mode helps make the perspective of the patient known and minimizes the chance of the unpleasant betrayal of nurses' one-sided expectations when the care provided depends primarily on the nurse's conjecture. Additionally, the nurse does not feel threatened, because unexpected patient responses can also be readily accepted.

Strategies to Know a Patient's Perspective

For the Japanese, even if the nurse wants to hear the patient's perspective directly from the patient, emotions and other related perceptions are difficult to express verbally. Takemura & Kanda (2003) clarified the strategies Japanese nurses use to encourage patients to talk about themselves, their feelings, perceptions, and hopes.

The most important is gaining the patient's trust. When a nurse attends to a patient and indicates a strong interest in that patient, the patient recognizes the special existence of that nurse and comes to trust him or her. The patient displays signs such as relating rarely expressed true feelings to that specific, trusted nurse. As in the tennis example, there are times when a ball with a slightly different trajectory than normal is hit or a ball flies to a slightly different place than normal. One nurse stated that when she caught a sign like this, even if other work was planned, she would postpone it so that the chance to develop trust would not be missed. Overlooking the signs often shown by the patient is linked to a loss of confidence in the nurse; the chance to hear the patient's true feelings may not come around again. It is important to note that when a patient selects a specific nurse to divulge what is in his or her heart, sharing that information without the patient's permission with other members of the medical care team can also be perceived as a betrayal of trust by the patient.

Besides preparing conditions in which the patient can confide, such as conversing in a place where privacy is protected to encourage the patient to talk about his or her true feelings, letting the patient know times when the nurse is available is also an important method. The skilled nurse takes the opportunity during normal communication to lead the discussion around to the concerns of the patient.

Emotional messages often are communicated through nonverbal signals. With respect to patients who are reluctant to verbalize their true feelings, the nurse must use a communication style in the considerate mode, i.e., closely observing the patient, immersing himself or herself in the patient's context, imagining the world experienced by the patient, and conveying this interpretation to the patient and confirming it with the patient.

If the patient does not provide self-disclosure even when these methods are used, family members, such as the spouse, can also be asked how they feel about the concerns of the patient. A spouse can help express the patient's concerns, because they often share feelings and experiences with the patient.

Patient's Participation in Decision Making in Japan

In the findings of Takemura & Kanda (2001), the nurse recognizes participation in medical treatment and care as the patient's own problem and reflection of the patient's thoughts, hopes, and values as important elements of better care. Up until at least the 1980s, for many Japanese, the notion of patients' rights, sharing information, and shared decision making between patients and physicians had been quite radical (Kimura, 1987). Recent increasing pressures to emphasize patients' rights, patients' autonomy, and informed consent are illustrated by the burgeoning patients' rights movement, recent legal cases, and newly issued guidelines on informed consent; however, patient autonomy coexists with physician paternalism and family autonomy in Japan (Fetters, 1998).

The tendency in Japan to restrict the assertion of one's own wishes, accept surrounding opinions, and to try to preserve harmony are not limited to medical treatment. The influence of Buddhist thought encourages detachment from earthly desires and passion as well as suppression of the egoistic self (Fetters, 1998). In Japan medicine has been known as *jin-jutsu* (benevolent art) since ancient times and was seen as the performance of *jin,* a Confucian concept, by a physician. Therefore physicians had a paternalistic and authoritarian position relative to the patient. In addition, the respect for knowledge and status became standard with the influence of Confucian thought; entrusting a physician to make decisions was definitely not seen as a childlike attitude but rather as an exemplary attitude (Fetters, 1998). Thus, even today, for many patients, asserting their own wishes to physicians as a customer or contracting party is extremely difficult.

In recent times, because of improvement in cure rates, changing options, and respect for the patient's right of self-determination and quality of life, disclosure to the patient by the medical staff and encouragement of decision making by the patient are increasing. However, in Japan, even if competent, a patient generally needs to share decision making with relatives. In instances of serious illnesses in particular, facts—and even the diagnosis—may not be revealed to the patient, and having the family make decisions in the patient's place is not unusual (Fetters, 1998). According to Confucian thought, in East Asia every individual is born to a family, possessing special relations to other family members. To this end, the injury, disease, or disability of one family member must be handled as a problem by the entire family (Fan, 1997). Fan (1997) also pointed out that, while the Western principle of autonomy is a self-determination-oriented principle, the East Asian principle of autonomy can be labeled as a family determination-oriented principle. Family can be viewed as an autonomous social unit by the physician, and it is not the patient alone but the entire family that has real authority in clinical decision making.

Concluding that the Japanese patient is willingly taken out of control of his or her own care is a biased view. Rather, the sense of directly controlling one's situation is not emphasized in Asian cultures. Even if controlled by someone else, if one is in accord with one's environment as a result of external control, one feels good (Yamaguchi, 2003). Consignment of one's decisions to family and physicians is supported by the Japanese craving for amae (dependence), which appears as a characteristic of interdependence. This means that the person desires to depend on particular persons in good relationships and has the capacity to accept dependence in a relationship and receive special interests and consideration from others (Doi, 1971; Fan, 1997; Fetter, 1998). It is seen as important for nurses to provide care in hopes that the patient will find true meaning and greater satisfaction in life by the nurse's ability to ascertain the patient's unexpressed perspective. A Japanese nurse, through the narrative listener mode, uses strategies to work with the patient to relate his or her emotions, hopes, and values with respect to the illness and treatment and life in the future. Difficulty in expressing opposition to the decisions made by the physician and family must be considered by the nurse, and an easy-to-express environment must be provided. A nurse should also keep in mind that the patient is receiving a benefit with the concession of his or her own personal wishes. Preserving the relationship with the physician and family is also a priority.

Considering the Patient's Family in Japan

In the research of Takemura & Kanda (2001), working with the family while preserving harmony and making use of all resources are important elements of better nursing. In Japan, a family caregiver may not want to use formal nursing services despite obvious need. In order to understand this behavior, one must understand the concepts of shame and guilt in Japan. As early as 1946, Benedict pointed out that in contrast to the guilt culture in the United States, Japan has a shame culture, and Japanese behave in certain ways because of their fear of shame (Benedict, 1946). Japanese do, in fact, tend to act while heeding *sekentei* (appearances to the public). Hamaguchi (1982) asserted that a person in Japan exists as a *relatum* (one who values harmony, interdependence, and mutual reliance with others). Balance between oneself and others and suitable behavior for the social position that a person occupies become important. The Japanese feel shame when their behaviors do not suit their formal and informal social position or when they seem inferior to other persons in a similar position; they feel guilt when they do not adequately fill their role and when the balance is disturbed (Hamaguchi, 1982; Makabe and Hull, 2000). When seeking to avoid shame beforehand, Japanese can be seen as actively striving not to damage relations with people.

With the influence of Confucianism in Japan, care of the aged has been traditionally considered to be the fixed responsibility of the succeeding generation. If this social norm is not followed, the older person feels shame and guilt with respect to the family, relatives, and *seken* (the public). The family as a whole also come to feel shame and guilt with respect to relatives and *seken*. Of course, this social norm is being disrupted by changes in society such as declining birth rates, a trend toward the nuclear family, an increase in the number of working women, the introduction of a public long-term care insurance system, and the spread of service-provision systems.

However, regardless of social changes, roles assigned to the family over a long period of time and a sense of expectation of these roles exist in the individual as well as in Japanese society, and family roles have a great deal of influence on the use of services. Yamamoto & Wallhagen (1998) clarified the fact that Japanese home caregivers carefully monitor the situations that surround them and find the way that is safest for them while maintaining harmony with the family and society. In their research, the decision to use formal services is made when the caregivers can justify their tolerance limit to themselves, negotiate successfully with other family members at their given level of authority, and perceive a service as available to them. Careful assessment of the social issues might give new insight for future care plans in situations where the caregiver chooses not to use professional services despite obvious need.

BEYOND CULTURAL DIFFERENCES

In this chapter, the uniqueness of Japanese culture has been introduced with a focus on its differences from the West, although there are some commonalities. Knowledge of Japanese traditional culture and respect for cultural differences is critical in order to capitalize on these commonalities. Humans live meaningful lives supported by the values of the culture to which they belong. Behavior seen as incomprehensible and paradoxical to others is produced as a natural offshoot of that culture. When a nurse deeply understands a patient's culture or subculture, the nursing care provided can more profoundly meet patients' needs.

REFERENCES

Barnlund, D. C. (1975). *Public and private self in Japan and the United States: Communicative styles of two cultures.* Tokyo: Simul Press.

Benedict, R. (1946). *The chrysanthemum and the sword: Patterns of Japanese culture.* Boston, MA: Houghton Mifflin.

Benner, P., & Wrubel, J. (1989) *The primacy of caring: Stress and coping in health and illness.* Boston, MA: Addison-Wesley.

Doi, T. (1971/1981). *The anatomy of dependence* (J. Bester, Trans.). Tokyo: Kodansha International.

Fan, R. (1997). Self-determination vs. family-determination: Two incommensurable principles of autonomy. *Bioethics, 11,* 309–322.

Fetters, M. D. (1998). The family in medical decision making: Japanese perspectives. *Journal of Clinical Ethics, 9,* 132–146.

Hamaguchi, E. (1998). *The principles of Japan research.* Tokyo: Yuhikaku.

Kimura, R. (1987). Bioethics as a prescription for civic action: The Japanese interpretation. *Journal of Medicine and Philosophy, 12,* 267–277.

Kumon, S. (1982). Organizing principles in Japanese society. In E. Hamaguchi & S. Kumon (Eds.). *Japanese groupism.* Tokyo: Yuhikaku.

Leininger, M. M. (1985). Nature, rationale, and importance of qualitative research methods in nursing. In M. M Leininger (Ed.). *Qualitative research methods in nursing.* Philadelphia, PA: W. B. Saunders.

Makabe, R., & Hull, M. M. (2000). Components of social support among Japanese women with breast cancer. *Oncology Nursing Forum, 27,* 1381–1390.

Nishida, T. (1996). Communication in personal relationships in Japan. In W. B. Gudykunst, S. Ting-Toomey, & T. Nishida (Eds.). *Communication in personal relationships across cultures* (pp. 102–121). Thousand Oaks, CA: Sage.

Nonaka, I., & Takeuchi, H. (1995). *The knowledge-creating company: How Japanese companies create the dynamics of innovation.* New York, NY: Oxford University.

Sekiguchi, I. (1999). Issues of Japanese verbal communication. In I. Sekiguchi (Ed.). *Modern Japanese communication environments* (pp. 147–174). Tokyo: Taishukan.

Takemura, Y., & Kanda, K. (2001). The elements and the process of "good nursing practice" perceived by nurses. *Japanese Journal of Nursing Research, 34*(4), 329–339.

Takemura, Y., & Kanda, K. (2003). How Japanese nurses provide care: A practice based on continuously knowing the patient. *Journal of Advanced Nursing, 42,* 252–259.

Tanner, C. A., Benner, P., Chesla, C., & Gordon, D. R. (1993). The phenomenology of knowing the patient. *Image: Journal of Nursing Scholarship, 25,* 273–280.

Yamaguchi, S. (2003). Culture and control orientations. In S. Yamaguchi (Ed.). *Social psychology: An Asian approach* (pp.115–130). Tokyo: University of Tokyo.

Yamamoto, N., & Wallhagen, M. I. (1998). Service use by family caregivers in Japan. *Social Science and Medicine, 47,* 677–691.

CHAPTER 25

Predisposition to Non-Insulin-Dependent Diabetes Mellitus Among Immigrants from the Former Soviet Union

Nataly Pasumansky

Scientific articles and media report a worldwide epidemic of diabetes. Surveys about the prevalence of diabetes in the United States report that diabetes has increased 33% between 1990 and 1998 and is steadily increasing (Levetan, 2001). According to a report from the Centers for Disease Control (CDC), diabetes is currently the sixth leading cause of death in the United States. Prevention and treatment of diabetes is a difficult task and requires both a cultural and an individual approach. The National Diabetes Information Clearinghouse emphasizes that certain ethnic groups have an increased incidence of diabetes among adults 20 years and older. Many cultural groups, new immigrants among them, are known to have an increased incidence of diabetes. With the stress of immigration and the changes in lifestyle and diet, new immigrants are more prone to diabetes. One such group, immigrants from the former Soviet Union, needs special attention because among them are many elderly and chronically ill persons. This chapter addresses the predisposition to non-insulin-dependent diabetes mellitus (NIDDM) among immigrants from the former Soviet Union (hereafter referred to as immigrants).

Immigrants from the former Soviet Union often have poor dietary habits and sedentary lifestyles that put them at risk of developing obesity, a major risk factor for diabetes. With the collapse of the Soviet Union, many people became poor and resorted to a diet they could afford, a diet that was usually high in calories and carbohydrates with few fresh fruits and vegetables. In addition, with little emphasis on prevention of health problems, these immigrants have little awareness of healthy diet and lifestyle options. Therefore, diabetes is often diagnosed late, when the disease is already in progress. After immigration, persons with diabetes and pre-diabetes have a difficult time learning a new language and finding a job, causing them to pay less attention to their health. In addition, these immigrants often are poor and have no access to basic health care.

Health care access is also complicated because of diversity. They come to the United States from different republics of the former Soviet Union. The majority come from Russia and the Ukraine. Most of them know the Russian language; however, some immigrants from other places, such as Latvia or Uzbekistan, do not know or are not fluent in Russian. In addition, they have different customs and religions. Even though interpreter services may be helpful, it is still not easy to accommodate the diverse cultural groups in this vulnerable population.

Nurse practitioners who manage these patients must understand their specific cultural behaviors and dietary habits. Advanced-practice nurses may be particularly appropriate to provide care for these immigrants because they usually spend more time with patients than physicians do. In addition, advanced-practice nurses provide individualized treatment plans that are cost-effective. Nurse practitioners may have more expertise at gaining patients' trust because of the additional time they spend with patients and their focus on health promotion, such as lifestyle modifications. With an increased knowledge of health practices and an awareness of the historical background of immigrants, nurse practitioners may have patients with higher adherence/compliance rates.

A culturally sensitive approach to diabetes education and treatment would seem to be particularly helpful when caring for immigrants not only due to differences in culture but also with regard to the stress of immigration. Diabetes treatment depends on factors such as stress, diet, and lifestyle; therefore, cultural aspects and trends are building blocks for understanding how to treat diabetes in these immigrants. However, little is known about this population and diabetes. Nurse practitioners need to assess risk factors and develop plans for the prevention of diabetes and diabetic complications in these immigrants.

LITERATURE REVIEW

Taking a cultural approach to diabetes treatment and prevention is important for nurse practitioners and other health care providers. The literature currently addresses diabetes in different ethnic groups such as the Chinese, Vietnamese, Cambodians, and Latinos (Adams, 2003; Mull, Nguyen, & Dennis, 2001; Rankin, Galbraith, & Huang, 1997). Increased mortality from chronic diseases, including diabetes, among the immigrants was a major concern for Israel and has been studied from a variety of perspectives (Ben-Noun, 1994; Rennet, Luz, Tamir, & Peterburg, 2002). Chronic diseases are reported as significantly higher in immigrants than in native Israeli veterans (Brodov, Mandelzweig, Boyko, & Behar, 2002; Rennet et al., 2002). This problem of chronic diseases among immigrants significantly influenced Israeli mortality statistics and necessitated changes in the Israeli medical system. However, little is known about diabetes among the community of these immigrants in the United States.

Preventive Care Practices Among Immigrants from the Former Soviet Union

There are indications in the literature that in the former Soviet states, health promotion is poor and people go to their provider only if they have health problems, especially in the middle-age group (Aroian et al. 2001; Mehler, 2001). Female immigrants tend not to use health screening resources such as blood pressure and cholesterol checks, Pap smears, mammography, and breast self-exams. According to Ivanov & Buck (2002) and Duncan & Simmons (1996), these immigrants do not believe in health promotion and usually do not visit a clinic for screening exams. In addition, women do not receive information about the need for such screening measures. Heavy cigarette smoking, high alcohol consumption, poor nutrition, and little attention to physical fitness have contributed to chronic health problems in this population (Duncan & Simmons, 1996; Mehler, 2001). The authors did not mention, however, the importance of glucose screening for this population with multiple risk factors.

Russian articles about diabetes say that people are aware of healthy lifestyles and health promotion, but they pay more attention to these things when they already have some health problem. According to the Ministry of Health of the Russian Federation, there is no appropriate preventive care for diabetes. When, in 2003, the Ministry of Health did an investigation in Tumen (a medium-sized city in Russia), millions of patients were diagnosed with diabetes. These patients already had serious cardiac problems as a result of hidden diabetes (Ministry of Health, 2003). In one article Manvelov (1999), a Russian physician, wrote that 50% of patients who suffered a cerebrovascular accident (CVA) may have had diabetes as a risk factor before the CVA occurred. He also stated that the diabetes rate in Russia is between 4 and 5%, but in some populations it may be as high as 20%. This high prevalence of diabetes among Russians discloses as well the genetic component of diabetes that makes it a unique problem for Russian immigrants in the United States or elsewhere in the world.

The adverse effects of diabetes can be minimized with appropriate care that doesn't involve medication, as is the case with some other chronic conditions, such as cardiovascular disease. "Medical nutritional therapy, exercises and diabetes education" can treat diabetes and prevent complications (Levetan, 2001). Even though these immigrants are usually highly educated, they have little knowledge of disease prevention. The CDC task force has recommended diabetes education information in communities (CDC, 2003). However, because of the language and cultural barriers, they do not attend community education meetings. Education one-on-one by nurse practitioners may be more beneficial for them.

Diet and Obesity Among Immigrants from the Former Soviet Union

Dietary habits vary within different cultural groups. Immigrants are a diverse group, and they have different eating patterns. However, knowing the most common diet pattern is important for nurse practitioners so that they can discuss dietary changes if needed. Brown (2003) emphasized that more studies are needed to examine nutritional habits among ethnic groups and how important it is for health care providers to understand the patient's specific cultural diet in order to help people adjust for a healthier lifestyle.

Diet habits depend on cultural differences and vary from country to country within the former Soviet Union. Diets in Russia are typically high in carbohydrates and fat and low in vegetables. Oystragh (1980), a Russian-speaking physician in Australia, conducted a study on Russian Jewish immigrants in Australia. In his practice he performed routine urine and serum glucose tests on new patients and found that, in his caseload, 15 of 158 (9.49%) patients were diabetic. This was compared with the average Australian incidence of 3%. Oystragh attributed the increased diabetes rate to two main factors: the high-stress period of immigration and a diet "extremely high in starches, where potatoes, bread, cakes, biscuits are eaten in almost every meal" (Oystragh, 1980, p. 270). The author observed only a small group of immigrants, but he believed that this small group provided an accurate picture of the dietary habits of many Russian immigrants.

Obesity as a result of poor dietary habits is a major risk factor for developing NIDDM. Nikitin (1989) found that people who migrate to the east region, Siberia, increase their risk of developing diabetes. He found obesity to be an important risk factor. In his study, more than half of the women who migrated to Siberia experienced a rapid weight gain during the first years of migration (Nikitin, 1989). One recent study of 644 Russian immigrants in New York found that they were "invisible minorities" at increased risk of developing diabetes and its major predisposing factor, obesity (Hosler, 2003). In Popkin's study (1998), data were collected from a Russian longitudinal monitoring survey, and a consistent increase in adult, and particularly elderly, obesity was found. In his research, Popkin (1998) found the overall increase in total obesity was more than 5 percentage points per 10-year period in Russia. Popkin (1998) also emphasized that NIDDM and many cardiovascular conditions related to NIDDM, such as hypertension, dislipidemia, and atherosclerosis, are increasing rapidly in poor countries.

Another study conducted in Russia by Zabina et al. (2001) said that in Russia, as in the United States, the causes of chronic disease are typically related to lifestyle risk factors such as poor diet and inadequate physical activity. According to their survey of 542 men and 1151 women living in Moscow, more than half of the men were current smokers, and more than half of both men and women had a body mass index more than 25, signifying the obesity problem (Zabina et al., 2001). This study is consistent with the findings of Duncan & Simmons (1996) in which physical assessment data of 30 immigrants showed that 65% of participants were overweight, but only 14% of them were advised to lose weight. Duncan & Simmons (1996) questioned whether immigrants are aware of obesity as a health problem. To the contrary, studies from the Ministry of Health of the Russian Federation showed that Russian immigrants who have been diagnosed with diabetes are aware of the importance of diet in its treatment because many studies published in Russian are about a healthy diet in diabetes (Sharafertdinov, Mesheryakoba, & Plotnikova, 1997). However, a review of the Russian-language literature did not show the presence of encouraging information about diabetes prevention and suggestions for diet change prior to disease onset.

Medication Versus Natural Remedies

In the former Soviet Union, as in other countries including the United States, there are various medication treatments for diabetes. However, the use of natural remedies in eastern European cultures remains open to discussion. Wheat, Brownstein, & Kvitash (1983) found that former Soviet Jewish patients were found to consider all drugs as poison and believed more in natural remedies. Today, the use of natural remedies for diabetes treatment in the former Soviet community is relatively unknown because of varying levels of knowledge about natural remedies among the population. As in many other countries, urban and highly educated people may not even be aware of their culture's traditional natural remedies; but the rural population may believe in natural remedies as the best treatment. Nurse practitioners as primary care providers need to know the risks and benefits associated with these natural remedies.

Multiple studies in Russia have shown an increased interest in the use of natural remedies. One of those studies about green coffee was done at the Moscow Center for Modern Medicine, Russian Ministry of National Defense. Green coffee contains 55% chlorogenic acid, which is an antioxidant. Volunteers for the study received 90 mg/dl of chlorogenic acid or placebo. Results showed that blood glucose levels dropped 15 to 20% for those who received chlorogenic acid. The researchers concluded that chlorogenic acid has a potential role in the management of diabetes (Fields, 2003).

Another study used tea from blueberry leaves (known as *chai cherniki* in Russian) for gastric colic and diabetes. Blueberry leaves extract contains caffeoylquinic acid and hydroxicinnamic acid (Jimenez del Rio, 2003). A study conducted in the Moscow Center for Modern Medicine, the same center that did research on green coffee, showed that blueberry leaves extract "possesses physiologically significant glucose-reducing potencies" (Jimenez del Rio, 2003).

The literature does not reveal if these remedies are used often by Russian-speaking patients in the former Soviet Union or by immigrants. More studies are needed in the United States for detecting the risks and benefits of those natural remedies because in the United States, these remedies are not widely found.

Stress and NIDDM

Immigrants from the former Soviet Union experience high psychological stress. Smith (1996) noted that they leave to escape very poor living conditions and joblessness but often face the same problems after entering the United States. They tend to end up in inner-city apartments and experience crime problems, low status, and low-paying jobs. With the stress of adapting to these multiple factors, they pay little attention to their own health. Brodov et al. (2002), studying 13,742 patients from two cohorts (Soviet Union and Israeli born), found a statistically significant difference in mortality between the two groups (14.7 and 18.5%, $p < 0.001$, respectively). The main causes of mortality in this study were a high number of chronic diseases (especially coronary artery disease). However, the authors suggested that the cause of these chronic diseases is psychological stress. Stress has an adverse effect on many chronic diseases, and NIDDM is among them.

Many immigrants may consider stress a major risk factor for NIDDM onset (Meyerovich, 2003; Sidorov, 2001). Multiple studies have shown how stress affects glycemic control negatively in clients that already have type I or type II diabetes. On the other side, little research exists on the correlation of stress and the onset of diabetes. In their research, Peyrot, McMurry, & Kruger (1999) found that stress affected glycemic control mostly because stress caused poor compliance with health regimens. These authors suggested that there may also be a connection between stress and diabetes onset.

One study by Fukunishi, Akimoto, Horikawa, Shirasaka, & Yamazaki (1998), with a sample of 600 persons, suggested that poor utilization of social support was associated with the onset of glucose tolerance abnormalities. These authors suggested that lack of social support from family, relatives, and friends, as well as other stress-related factors, were negatively correlated with glucose tolerance test results in persons not known to have diabetes. Despite these findings, stress is not discussed as a risk factor for diabetes onset during health care visits. However, with immigrants who believe in the relationship between diabetes and stress, stress should be discussed by nurse practitioners during office visits.

CASE STUDIES

The case studies that follow illustrate the problems in caring for immigrants with diabetes. These case studies were recorded following telephone interviews with chosen participants. The names and some minor details were altered in order to protect the privacy of the participants.

Case Study 1

Boris S. is a 75-year-old male refugee who emigrated with his family from Sverdlovsk, a large city in Russia, 8 years ago. Before emigrating, Boris worked as an engineer in a factory where he sat most of the day. He had almost no physical activity after work. He was overweight, liked to eat candy, and had no family history of diabetes. Boris had been diagnosed with diabetes in Russia 10 years previously. First, he had noticed that he was thirsty all the time. He asked people around him what they thought the cause could be, and they recommended he consult an endocrinologist. He went to a local endocrinologist, who did a blood sugar exam and sent him home stating that there was no problem with his sugar. Boris continued to suffer from excessive thirst, and people around him started to notice that he was drinking water all the time. Boris went to the endocrinologist once more, and the endocrinologist sent him to another place for a glucose tolerance test. "They let me drink sugar and then tested my blood every hour," stated Boris.

After this test, the physician diagnosed him with type II diabetes. The endocrinologist told Boris that the first time he visited he had pre-diabetes, but now his diagnosis was diabetes. The endocrinologist said that his diabetes was caused by working in the stressful environment at the factory and didn't mention that Boris was overweight. The endocrinologist gave Boris some Polish diabetes medication for 1 month. Boris didn't receive any specific education regarding his diabetes, and he was sent home without a glucometer. Every month he visited the endocrinologist to check his blood sugar and to receive his medication. He knew, though, that he should avoid simple carbohydrates in his diet, but he sometimes found that very difficult. Even today, every once in a while Boris eats food not recommended in his diabetic diet.

After Boris came to the United States, he was diagnosed with hypertension and coronary artery disease that required heart bypass surgery. In addition he has spinal stenosis, making it difficult for him to exercise because of the back pain. "Physicians here recommend physical activity such as walking and bicycling, but I can't do anything because of shooting pain in my spine and legs, and in addition I walk like on pillows and cannot feel my legs well because of my diabetes neuropathy, so I continue to be overweight. When my son came to visit me I noticed that he is getting big and I suggested to him immediately start to lose weight," stated Boris.

Now Boris is visiting his primary care provider every 3 months. He checks his blood glucose at home. Boris does not believe in natural remedies. His main diet now consists of vegetables, some fruits, oatmeal, buckwheat, and all kind of meats. His primary care provider gives him instruction regarding a diabetic lifestyle, and he tries very hard to follow those instructions.

Case Study 2

Marina P., 67 years old, emigrated as a refugee from Kiev in the Ukraine. She was diagnosed with diabetes 14 years ago in the Ukraine. Before emigrating, she worked as an accountant in a sewing factory. At work she sat most of the time and didn't have time for physical activity. As a result, she became overweight, but she didn't think that it was a health problem. For 2 years before she was diagnosed with diabetes mellitus, she felt thirsty all the time and had urinary urgency. Despite her symptoms, she did not seek medical help and continued to live with this "discomfort." Marina's friend, who was a physician, noticed that Marina frequently went to the restroom and suggested she have her blood sugar checked.

When Marina went to the clinic and checked her blood and urine, she already had diabetes in progression. The physician suggested that there was something wrong with Marina's pancreas and didn't mention a thing to her about weight and lifestyle. Initially her physician suggested a low-carbohydrate diet and prescribed medications. Then, after she did not feel better, she started to take a Hungarian medication for diabetes. She didn't have a glucometer at home; instead she checked her blood sugar once in a month at a local clinic.

At the time of her immigration to the United States 9 years ago, Marina had very high blood glucose, kidney problems, arthritis, neuropathy, and poor vision. It was suggested that she take insulin, but she insisted on taking oral medications. As a first step, Marina was referred to a dietitian, and her daughter helped her with translation. She received prescriptions for three different types of diabetes medications, and now her blood sugar is stable and within normal limits.

Marina received diabetes education from a primary care provider and dietitian and decided not to go to a diabetes support group. For now, her diet consists mostly of vegetables, buckwheat, and meat. She likes potatoes and used to eat them in every dish, but the dietitian asked her to reduce the amount of potatoes in order to preserve a healthy diet. She still needs to reduce her weight but finds it difficult because of severe arthritis and diabetic neuropathy. "Diabetes is distorting everything," said Marina.

These two case studies are examples of urban, educated immigrants who were diagnosed with diabetes before immigration to the United States. Because of their diabetes, these people have multiple complications, and in the United States, they continue complex treatment including blood glucose control and prevention of further complications of diabetes. Despite the fact that these two people were from different countries of the former Soviet Union—Russia and the Ukraine—they both had similar stories. Boris and Marina went to see a health care provider after their symptoms of diabetes—polyuria, poludipsia, and polyphagia—had persisted for a long time. These case studies show the poor awareness of diabetes, along with the absence of preventive measurements after diagnosis of pre-diabetes and diabetes. In the United States, Boris and Marina became more aware of their condition and achieved better glycemic control, but it was too late for preventing many of their diabetic complications.

In a Russian article, Sharafertdinov et. al. (1997) discussed the typical diet for many diabetes immigrant patients. The immigrants in his study preferred dishes with cereals such as buckwheat and grains (e.g., ray wheat) or whole wheat bread as a main dish. Nurse practitioners need to be aware that immigrants may prefer this specific diet and help them find healthy alternatives that meet their ethnic preference. For example, they can encourage the consumption of more vegetables and other healthy products available in stores in addition to the healthy grains in their native diet. In addition, nurse practitioners may inform their clients that although American restaurants, including fast food restaurants, may have healthy meals, they often offer large portions, too large for people who are trying to reduce their weight. Referral to a dietitian who is knowledgeable about this ethnic group may be very helpful for immigrants.

IMPLICATIONS FOR PRACTICE

As the worldwide incidence of diabetes increases, multiple studies have been conducted. The prevention and treatment of diabetes should involve a cultural approach because diet and lifestyle, major risk factors in diabetes, have strong cultural components. Studies conducted in the United States and other countries receiving immigrants show an increased risk of type II diabetes in this population. However, with proper education, diabetic complications may be prevented. Prevention of diabetes and its complications is essential for new immigrants who are poor and have limited access to health care. Nurses need to emphasize the importance of prevention and educate patients about issues such as stress, diet, lifestyle, pre-diabetes, metabolic syndrome, and other risk factors for diabetes and about the complications related to late diagnosis.

From this literature review of Russian clients and diabetes, two specific variables for this culture were identified: the use of natural remedies and stress. A nurse practitioner might be surprised that a Russian patient would refuse to accept the standard treatment for diabetes and instead prefer to take natural remedies. However, with appropriate cultural understanding and knowledge about those natural remedies, the nurse practitioner is better able to explain how natural remedies may be more helpful when combined with other treatment plans.

Stress is also a factor that, in Russian culture, is considered to be a main risk factor for diabetes. Nurse practitioners may forget to discuss stress as a risk factor for diabetes because they are more concerned about obesity and sedentary lifestyle factors that seem more important in preventing or treating diabetes. Most Russian-speaking patients, however, would appreciate it if a nurse practitioner would discuss stress-related risk factors with them. It is reasonable to discuss stress because these immigrants, having moved to another country to begin a new life, often experience tremendous stress.

Smith (1996) mentioned in her article another important point for nurses. She explains that immigrants often ask to see only physicians and not nurses or nurse practitioners. They may even become angry if, instead of physician, they spend time with a nurse. This reaction is understandable because in the former Soviet Union, the role of the nurse is mainly to obey the commands of physicians, and the nurses in those countries are usually not allowed to make decisions regarding patient care. In addition, immigrants may not know the role of nurse practitioners because in their former countries this specialty does not exist. Nurse practitioners need first to discuss with patients the role of nurses and nurse practitioners in the United States.

The literature review and case studies discussed here aim to help nurse practitioners understand why patients from the former Soviet Union need unique approaches to care. It may be very useful for the prevention of diabetes or diabetic complications, if immigrants visiting the clinic for any health problem also receive education or screening for diabetes. In addition, nurse practitioners who educate about healthy lifestyle habits, including a healthy diet, are a key element of the care management team in health promotion and maintenance.

Reviewing the literature about immigrants from the former Soviet Union and diabetes showed that little is known about diabetes prevention among those ethnic groups who have a clear predisposition to diabetes. Case studies were used to illustrate some of the problems that these people with diabetes face, but more studies are needed about diabetes rates among immigrants, their diet patterns, and the effect of specific diets on the development of diabetes.

REFERENCES

Adams, C. R. (2003). Lessons learned from urban Latinas with type II diabetes mellitus. *Journal of Transcultural Nursing, 14,* 255–265.

Aroian, K. J. (2001). Health and social service utilization among elderly immigrants from the former Soviet Union. *Journal of Nursing Scholarship, 33,* 265–71.

Ben-Noun, L. (1994). Shchihutmahalot chroniot vemaafyanim sociodemografiim ecel olim hadashim mihever haamim beshana harishona. [Chronic diseases in immigrants from Russia (CIS) at a primary care clinic and their socio-demographic characteristics]. *Harefuah, 127,* 441–445.

Brodov, Y., Mandelzweig, L., Boyko, V., & Behar, S. (2002). Is immigration associated with an increase in risk factors and mortality among coronary artery disease patients? A cohort study of 13,742 patients. *Israel Medical Association Journal, 4,* 326–329.

Brown, D. (2003) More studies need to examine habits within ethic groups. *Journal of the American Dietetic Association, 103,* 706.

Centers for Disease Control [CDC]. (2003, January 17). *Diabetes public health resource.* Retrieved November 6, 2003, from *http://www.cdc.gov/diabetes/projects/community.htm.*

Duncan, L., & Simmons, M. (1996). Health practices among Russian and Ukrainian immigrants. *Journal of Community Health Nursing, 13,* 129–137.

Fields, C. (2003). Applied Food Sciences announces weight loss benefits to its green coffee antioxidant extract. Natural product industry center. Retrieved July 8, 2003, from *www.npicenter.com/index.asp? action=NBViewDoc&DocumentID=4388.*

Fukunishi, I., Akimoto, M., Horikawa, N., Shirasaka, K., & Yamazaki, T. (1998). Stress coping and social support in glucose tolerance abnormality. *Journal of Psychosomatic Research, 45,* 361–369.

Hosler, A. (2003). Diabetes among immigrants from former Soviet Union. International diets. Retrieved June 5, 2003, from *www.dietconsultants.com/russian-diet.html.*

Ivanov, L. L., & Buck, K. (2002). Health care utilization patterns of Russian-speaking immigrant women across age groups. *Journal of Immigrant Health, 4,* 17–27.

Jimenez del Rio, M. (2003). Blueberry leaves extract: Diabetes & more. Retrieved July 8, 2003, from *www.annieappleseedproject.org/blubleavexm.html.*

Levetan, C. (2001). Diabetes prevention. How about now? *Clinical Diabetes, 19,* 34–38.

Manvelov, L. C. (1999). Saharnyi diabet kak factor riska celebrovaskulyarnyh zabolevanii. [Diabetes as a risk actor for cerebro-vascular accidents]. *Lechashii Vrach, 9,* 1–9. Retrieved July 8, 2003, from *http://www.osp.ru/doctore/1999/09/09.htm.*

Mehler, P. S., Scott, J. Y., Pines, I., Gifford, N., Biggerstaff, S., & Hiatt, W. R. (2001). Russian immigrant cardiovascular risk assessment. *Journal of Health Care for the Poor and Underserved, 12,* 224–235.

Meyerovich, M. (2003). American Medical Association. *Somatic symptoms among recent Russian immigrants.* Retrieved July 7, 2003, from *www.ama-assn.org/ama/pub/article/8401-1959.html.*

Ministry of Health. Russian Federation. (2003). *Phederal'naya celevaya programa—saharnyi diabet.* Retrieved July 17, 2003, from *http://www.minzdrav-rf.ru/in.htm?rubr=130.*

Mull, D. S., Nguyen, N., & Dennis, J. M. (2001). Vietnamese diabetic patients and their physicians: What ethnography can teach us. *Western Journal of Medicine, 175,* 307–311.

National Diabetes Information Clearinghouse. (2003, May 3). *National diabetes statistics.* Retrieved November 4, 2003, from *http://diabetes.niddk.nih.gov/dm/pubs/statistics/index.htm.*

Nikitin, Y. P. (1989). Problemasaharnogo diabeta v regionah Sibiri. [The problem of diabetes mellitus in the Siberian regions]. *Vestnik Akademii Meditsinskikh Nauk, 5,* 35–9.

Oystragh, P. (1980). Diabetes mellitus in Russian Jewish immigrants. *Australian Family Physician, 9,* 269–270.

Peyrot, M., McMurry, J. F. Jr., & Kruger, D. F. (1999). A biopsychosocial model of glycemic control in diabetes: Stress, coping and regimen adherence. *Journal of Health and Social Behavior, 40,* 141–158.

Popkin, B. M. (1998). The nutrition transition and its health implications in lower-income countries. *Public Health Nutrition, 11,* 5–21.

Rankin, S. H., Galbraith., M. E., & Huang, P. (1997). Quality of life and social environment as reported by Chinese immigrants with non-insulin-dependent diabetes mellitus. *Diabetes Educator, 23,* 171–176.

Rennet, G., Luz, N., Tamir, A., & Peterburg, Y. (2002). Chronic disease prevalence in immigrants to Israel from the former USSR. *Journal of Immigrant Health, 10*(4), 29–33.

Sharafertdinov, K. H., Mesheryakoba, V. A., Plotnikova, O. A. (1997). Izmenenie poslepishevoi glikemii pod vliyaniem nekotoryh uglevodosoderzhashih produktov u bol'nyh saharnym diabetom. [Change of postprandial glycaemia under effect of some carbohydrate containing food in patients with type II diabetes]. *Lechebnoe Pitanie, 1,* 27–30.

Sidorov, P. I., Novikova, I. A., & Solov'ev, A. G. (2001). Rol' negativnyh social'nyh i psichologicheskih factorov na poyavlenie i kurs lechenia saharnogo diabeta. [The role of unfavorable social and psychological factors in the onset and course of diabetes mellitus]. *Terapevticheskii Arhiv, 73,* 68–70.

Smith, L. (1996). New Russian immigrants: Health problem, practices, and values. *Journal of Cultural Diversity, 3,* 68–73.

Wheat, M. E., Brownstein, H., & Kvitash, V. (1983). Aspects of medical care of Soviet Jewish emigres. *Western Journal of Medicine, 139,* 900–904.

Zabina, H., Schmid, T. L., Glasunov, I., Potemkina, R., Kamardina, T., Deev, A., et al. (2001). Monitoring behavioral risk factors for cardiovascular disease in Russia. *American Journal of Public Health, 91,* 1613–1614.

CHAPTER 26

Making a Difference: The "Gift of Sight"

Jo Anne Latimer Grunow

This chapter is a description of how nurses might identify opportunities for health promotion programs serving vulnerable populations from personal experiences. On one sunny fall day in October 2002, I traveled to the LensCrafters store at Bellevue Square on the east side of Seattle for my annual eye exam. On this day, I had no idea that my routine visit would be a catalyst that would set in motion a collaborative community-wide interdisciplinary effort that would result in 150 school-aged children, at-risk for vision impairment, receiving the "Gift of Sight" (LensCrafters Foundation, 2004), an annual charitable vision program sponsored by LensCrafters.

I chose LensCrafters for my own use primarily because of their advertising campaign of a 1-hour return on prescription lenses. I was astonished by the personal service I received from Patti Rutten, a sales associate at the Bellevue store. Patti was not only extremely knowledgeable about all aspects of eyewear and fittings, she spent time explaining options, selecting and measuring frames, and answering questions. She also, patiently and empathetically, listened to the story about my father's recent death and my desire to recycle his three pairs of glasses. One option, Patti explained, was to donate my father's glasses to LensCrafters International (LensCrafters Foundation, 2004), one of the many charitable outreach programs sponsored by LensCrafters whereby needy people in third-world countries receive recycled glasses.

At my request, Patti also shared information about other LensCrafters charitable programs in the United States. I listened eagerly and took notes. Upon hearing about the 2003 annual Gift of Sight program in Washington State, I obtained the name and phone number of the regional LensCrafters captain, Alice Rowley, at the Redmond Town Center store. Patti indicated that two cities in the state, one in east and one in west Washington, would be chosen as recipients of the 2003 Gift of Sight program and that it would be necessary to write a letter of request to Ms. Rowley, outlining a community in need, in order to be considered among the many applicants. I gathered data about my assigned garden community (a local neighborhood our College of Nursing uses as a community health clinical site), in order to build a case for why it should be the next recipient of the Gift of Sight program.

GARDEN COMMUNITY

As a faculty member at the Seattle University College of Nursing, a Jesuit institution with a long tradition and mission of outreach to vulnerable groups, social justice, and service, I was the community liaison to one of five garden communities. Garden communities, composed of primarily low-income, immigrant families in the Seattle metropolitan area, are used regularly as sites for the community nursing clinicals in our curriculum, which begin in the junior year for nursing majors. Because I had supervised community assessments for a number of student groups, I was keenly aware of the needs of the vulnerable families and children in this community.

In 1999, a total of 857 households, made up of 2,568 people, were located within the census track of the community. Of these, 995 persons lived below the poverty level, and 1573 people lived at or above the poverty level (Public Health, Seattle and King County, 2000). In the below-poverty group, 12% of individuals were younger than 5 years of age, 10.3% were between ages 5 and 11, 16.9% were between ages 12 and 17, and 55.8% were between 18 and 64 (Public Health, 2000). Of 373 Year 2000 census tracts in King County, my assigned garden community was the fifth poorest (A. Glusker, personal communication, January 8, 2004). A primarily younger age group is represented among residents in the garden community, and only 4.7% of the 65–74 age group are living below the poverty level (Census Data, 2000).

The majority of residents living in this vulnerable community are Asian immigrants from Cambodia and Vietnam; however, a sizeable number are from Somalia. A multiethnic community, other racial and ethnic groups include but are not limited to whites, African Americans, Native Americans, Alaskans, and Hispanics/Latinos (Public Health, 2000). I knew from my clinical experiences with nursing students that in-depth vision exams and new eyewear were needed but would not be a priority for many families because of financial constraints.

GIFT OF SIGHT PROGRAM REQUIREMENTS

LensCrafters provided a window of opportunity that opened when I received a call from Alice Rowley, captain of the Gift of Sight program, on January 23, 2003, stating that LensCrafters had tentatively chosen our garden community as a recipient for the program, provided that the local school district would be able to accommodate their requirements. She gave a short deadline for response by the community. My first call was to the director of NeighborHood House, a major social services gateway for the garden community, to determine which school had the largest number of children (an elementary school). I then faxed a letter to the principal to describe the purpose and requirements for implementation of the program.

Annually, LensCrafters administrators select one or two economically disadvantaged communities in each state for the purpose of providing free eye examinations, frames, and lenses, which are made on site (LensCrafters Foundation, 2004). The target population is children in grades K through 12. Ms. Rowley suggested that teachers, school nurses, and parents identify those at-risk for vision impairment (as opposed to screening all children in the school) and directed the school to design and disseminate parental permission slips for minors and have them signed by one parent for submission on the day of screening.

The school would need to provide space for a 40-foot LensCrafters Vision Van, one of two such vans in the United States, which is literally a store on wheels, fully equipped to provide in-depth eye exams and provide frames and custom-made lenses on site. The Vision Van would need to be placed near a covered area where children could wait in line to be screened, fitted for glasses, and where paperwork could be expedited. Donations from the LensCrafters Foundation Grant, area businesses, and McDonald's ensured that the children were provided with lunch, jump ropes, and clowns to make the day an enjoyable experience. Two volunteer doctors of optometry from LensCrafters and 10 volunteer LensCrafters associates would implement the program, examining and fitting about 150 children each day over the 2-day period. The associates conducted intake interviews, helped with eye exams and fitted children for glasses, grinding lenses on site in the specially equipped van. The school had to arrange for the transportation of children and teens from various elementary, intermediate, and high schools; allow the absences from class in order to participate in the program; and provide interpreters, if needed, for non-English-speaking students. The principal of the elementary school with the largest number of students from the garden community immediately responded by contacting the heads of all schools with eligible students. Administrators, school nurses, parents, teachers, and children were told about the program and were provided with necessary information.

SIGNIFICANCE OF VISION PROBLEMS IN SCHOOL-AGED CHILDREN

An estimated 20% of school-aged children have undetected vision problems that interfere with academic performance. These problems may also have a negative impact on self-esteem and, if undiagnosed and untreated, may lead to a worsening of visual health (Children's Vision Information Network, 2004). The National Parent–Teacher Association (PTA), concerned about the typically limited vision screening programs in many school systems (i.e., testing only for distance vision) adopted a resolution at its annual convention in 1999, calling for widespread education of PTA members, school administrators, teachers, and health officials concerning the need for more comprehensive visual screenings in schools, screenings to be administered by qualified personnel. Such a resolution was deemed necessary to maximize children's opportunities for success in the classroom (National PTA Convention, 1999).

PROGRAM IMPLEMENTATION

On May 5th and 6th, 2003, 300 children and teens received eye examinations (150 received glasses) from the LensCrafters Vision Van in the garden community's high school parking lot. The students to be screened were driven to and from the high school by school nurses, who played an integral role in the success of the program. More than $38,500 in donated goods and services was provided by LensCrafters, including eye exams, custom-made lenses, and frames for the children and teens who participated in the program. Ms. Rowley reported that the 2003 program was so well organized that they would contemplate a return in 2004 for a 3-day period. She then related one story that exemplifies the personal rewards of the Gift of Sight program for LensCrafters employees.

> I can't begin to tell you what it means to us [LensCrafters employees] to be able to provide the Gift of Sight to children in need. There are so many stories to tell, but I will tell you one about this program that I will not forget. On one occasion, a 5-year-old girl who had just put on her first pair of glasses looked at the technician in utter amazement. As she studied the technician's face, she pointed to a brown dot on his face and said, 'What's that?" pointing to a freckle. All of us were moved to tears. How absolutely amazing it is to observe a child who can see clearly for the first time. With such vision impairment, one can only imagine what type of difficulty the child might have in completing schoolwork and moving forward in life. We receive many letters of thanks from children and parents who are so grateful for this special gift. It makes our work so rewarding to know that we can give back to the people in need within our communities.

As I walked away from the Vision Van area, I noticed children running about with glee, laughing and enjoying their new glasses. As I glanced to my right, I noticed a young girl, about 10 years old, sitting alone on a bench dressed in tattered, soiled clothing and white socks with holes. She had stringy hair that separated and fell around her oval face, and I could not take my eyes off her as she sat, bespectacled with new Armani glasses. She was staring, with a look of bewilderment and tears in her eyes, at the fine lines on her left hand. As the young girl held up the palm of her hand, fingers spread apart and carefully supported at the wrist with her other hand, she examined each crease with the precision of a scientist studying the veins of a leaf with a magnifying glass. As I walked away, I swallowed hard to hold back a dam of tears. It was at this moment that I fully realized the impact of Alice Rowley's story, which I had heard only minutes before. I felt privileged to have played a small part in this program and a profound sense of gratitude for the honor of being a nurse.

If you have ever doubted the impact that you, as one person, can make in the complex health care environment, perhaps this story will change your viewpoint. Armed with knowledge of community assessment concepts, community resources, collaboration, signs and symptoms, secondary prevention, characteristics of vulnerable populations, and communication skills taught in all baccalaureate nursing programs, you possess the basic know-how that will enable you to effect a positive change in health status for vulnerable populations. There is one more important attribute—you will need to care enough to take the time necessary to initiate the process of successful partnering and interdisciplinary collaboration (Mattessich & Monsey, 1992), a necessary component for community intervention. Never doubt that you, one person, can make a difference.

About LensCrafters

The Gift of Sight is one of a number of charitable vision programs conducted in the United States, Canada, and developing countries by LensCrafters, the retail division of the Italy-based Luxottica group. The corporation is unique in that it provides opportunities for employees (LensCrafters associates) to travel to third-world countries to hand deliver recycled glasses to needy individuals. The Gift of Sight programs are made possible by LensCrafters, their customers, volunteer LensCrafters associates, doctors, business partners, the Lions Clubs International, and local charities in the United States who donate time and/or money to the LensCrafters Foundation. To date, 3 million people have been recipients of the Gift of Sight programs.

The philosophy of LensCrafters is based on their belief in the importance of vision, a valuing of vision care, efficient service, the use of state-of-the-art equipment, and extensive training and certification of lab associates. Their strategic plan considers diversity awareness a moral obligation; therefore, they provide diversity education training programs to all employees nationwide.

The following list of resources will assist professionals in learning more about LensCrafters' charitable programs as well as other useful vision resources.

LensCrafters: Gift of Sight Programs

- ☐ Gift of Sight. Web site: *http://www.givethegiftofsight.org/index.html.*
- ☐ Halloween "Sight Night" free collection kits. Used glasses are collected, repaired, refurbished, classified, and distributed to people in developing countries. Schools, community

groups, and scout troops have collected more than 500,000 pairs of eyeglasses. Web site: *http://www.sightnight.org;* phone: 1-877-605-4242.

☐ Hometown Day. An annual program conducted by LensCrafters in US stores on the first Wednesday of December. Free eye exams and new glasses are given to preselected recipients in need. Agencies and individuals can contact a local store for information.

☐ Gift of Sight on site. Approximately 60,000 people receive new glasses and special vouchers from LensCrafters on an annual basis. Local charities forge partnerships with stores and assist in identifying recipients in need.

☐ Vision Vans. Two 40-foot Vision Vans, named "Seemore" and "Iris," which are stores on wheels, have fully equipped labs and travel continuously to various inner-city locations in the United States. Volunteer doctors and LensCrafters associates provide free in-depth eye exams, custom lenses, and frames to disadvantaged children in grades K–12.

☐ Outreach. LensCrafters associates visit nursing homes and hospitals to clean and adjust eyewear and conduct vision screenings at schools and area health fairs year-round.

☐ Donations. Donations of used glasses or monetary donations are welcome and can be made online. Web site: *http://www.givethegiftofsight.org/gos_get_involved.html.*

☐ LensCrafters store locator. Call 1-800-522-LENS.

OTHER VISION RESOURCES

☐ Lions Clubs International collects and donates recycled eyeglasses and sunglasses to needy people in developing countries. Web site: *http://www.lionsclubs.org/EN/ content/vision_eyeglass_sight.html.*

☐ Parents Active for Vision Education (PAVE), a grassroots, nonprofit parents' organization, provides information to parents, teachers, professionals, and others about vision-related learning problems. PAVE is committed to raising public awareness about the relationship between vision and learning for all age groups. PAVE received an award for their video *The Hidden Disability: Undetected Vision Problems.* Web site: *http://www.pavevision.org;* e-mail: info@pavevision.org; phone: 1-800-PAVE-988.

☐ Catalyst! Vision and Learning Kits, three-part toolkits, assist parents and educators in the areas of education, screening, and activities for learning-related vision problems (also linked on the PAVE Web site). Web site: *http://www.catalystvision.com.*

☐ College of Optometrists in Vision Development: Find a doctor or a certified fellow in the United States or internationally who specializes in developmental optometry. Web site: *http://www.covd.org/mem.html;* phone: 1-800-268-3770.

☐ Pediatric ophthalmologists can be found in local areas through the phone book.

REFERENCES

Children's Vision Information Network. (2004). *Vision and learning.* Retrieved January 13, 2004, from *http://www.childrensvision.com/learning.htm.*

LensCrafters Foundation. (2004). *Gift of sight.* Retrieved January 9, 2004, from *http://www.givethegift ofsight.org/index.html.*

Mattessich, P. W., & Monsey, B. R. (1992). *Collaboration, what makes it work: A review of research literature on factors influencing successful collaboration.* St. Paul, MN: Amherst H. Wilder Foundation.

National PTA Convention. (1999, June). *Resolution adopted at the national PTA convention: Learning-related vision problems education and evaluation.* Retrieved January 7, 2004, from Children's Vision Information Network Web site: *http://www.childrensvision.com/pta.htm.*

Public Health, Seattle and King County. (2000). *Census data* (Epidemiology, Planning and Evaluation Unit, SF3 Files). King County, WA: Author.

CHAPTER 27

Evaluation of Child Sexual Abuse Prevention Programs

Lauren E. Osterbur

The purpose of this chapter is to provide some evaluation of the literature on child sexual abuse prevention programs. According to Plummer (1999), child "sexual abuse prevention efforts are only 20 years old" (p. 79). It was not until the 1970s that people in this country became aware of or accepted that there was a child sexual abuse problem. Research was undertaken, and studies showed the devastating impact on victims. There was an uproar throughout the nation and a general consensus that something had to be done. Child sexual abuse prevention programs (CSAPPs) sprang up across most of the United States and Europe. In the haste to develop these programs, most of them were implemented without ever being tested and evaluated. Berrick & Gilbert (1991) explained, "The programs were not built on rigorous systematic testing of curricula. They sprang almost full blown out of a pressing need to respond to the alarming reports of child sexual abuse" (cited in Hanson, 1996, p. 4).

Evaluation of CSAPPs remains incomplete today. Prevalence rates of child sexual abuse have risen, but it is unclear if this is due to an actual increase in abuse or an increase in awareness and, thus, the amount of reporting. In 1992, Geffner stated that "both the incidence and the prevalence of child sexual abuse had reached epidemic proportions" (cited in Esser-Stuart & Skibinski, 1998, p. 88). By 1994, Sandberg noted that "typical estimates state that 20% of children will be sexually assaulted before the age of 18" (cited in Davis & Gidycz, 2000, p. 257). And more recently, in 1998, large-scale surveys indicated that prevalence rates ranged from about 10 to 60% (Reppucci, Land, & Haugaard, 1998). Finkelhor & Strapko (1992) commented that studies and programs had increased substantially without anyone critically analyzing the results. Once research began to appear in the professional literature, studies were noted to suffer from numerous shortcomings (Plummer, 1999, p. 79).

DEVELOPMENTAL APPROPRIATENESS

It seems common sense to teach children at their own developmental level, but in a rush to start teaching about sexual abuse, many programs forgot this detail. Often, programs present the same material to preschoolers that is taught to 12-year-olds. Hanson (1996) explains that "Children are limited in their learning capabilities, especially at younger ages, and therefore, child sexual abuse prevention programs need to provide developmentally appropriate lessons that a child at a particular age can understand" (p. 43). Some concepts that are taught are relevant to sexual abuse but simply are not appropriate for young children. For example, empowering skills are ineffective unless the child understands the concept of responsibility (McLeod & Wright, 1996). To effectively meet the learning needs of the children, programs should take into account the vocabulary and cognitive ability of each age group.

CULTURAL APPROPRIATENESS

Cultural appropriateness includes the entire spectrum of what makes people unique. This includes, but is not limited to, ethnicity, religion, language, lifestyle, and gender. These differences must be taken into account when a CSAPP is introduced into a particular community (Berrick, & Gilbert, 1991; Crisci & Torres, 1986; Fay, 1986; Hanson, 1996; Wurtele, 1987). This is of particular importance in the United States, where the minority ratio is shifting. According to Cushner et al. (1992), students from so-called minority cultural groups already make up more than 50% of the school populations in California, Arizona, New Mexico, Texas, and Colorado, and by the year 2020, it is projected that 46% of all students enrolled in public schools will be people of color (cited in Hanson, 1996).

Even though statistics show that the number of minority children in the school system is increasing, authors do not take into account how many of these children and their families have been assimilated into the dominant culture. Race does not necessarily dictate culture. CSAPPs need to take into account how each culture treats sexuality in order to prevent confusion among children who may learn about sexuality at a very young age. Korbin (1990) stated, "In some societies, sexualized behavior, such as fondling or kissing genitals, are [sic] normative child-rearing practice. In other societies, sexual contact between adults and children occurs during religious or ceremonial events" (cited in Wurtele, 1998, p. 502). For example, Ahn & Gilbert (1992) noted that many Vietnamese, Korean, and Cambodian families find it "permissible for a grandfather to touch his 3-year-old grandson's genitals with pride" (p. 423) (cited in Hanson, 1996, p. 30). Programs may unknowingly lead children to believe that they have experienced abuse when, in fact, what occurred may be perfectly acceptable for their culture. Finkelhor (1984) (cited in Hanson, 1996, p. 31) noted that it is important for children in programs to view themselves as a victim or potential victim in order to internalize the concepts taught. Actors on the stage or in videos and drawings in books should include adults and children from a variety of backgrounds.

SKILLS TAUGHT

Effective programs teach a variety of skills that are applicable to many situations. For example, assertiveness is a skill that may help a child say "no" to a potential abuser but will also help the child with other life situations. Programs that not only give children a chance to practice but that prompt discussion with parents and include information on dealing with bullies are more likely to result in the use of program skills because children are much more likely to encounter bullying than the threat of sexual abuse (Cox, 1998).

There are several questions to ponder when evaluating CSAPPs:

☐ Does the program teach skills such as saying "no" and telling a trusted adult?
☐ Does the program provide children with the opportunity to rehearse skills?
☐ Does the program teach children to identify specific individuals in their lives that they can turn to for help?
☐ Does the program provide options for the child responding to sexual abuse?" (Hanson, 1996).

PARENT AND COMMUNITY INVOLVEMENT

"An important component of more comprehensive programs is parent and community involvement, not only to gain parental support but also to successfully implement programs" (Jordan, 1993, p. 79). Almost every article in the CSAPP literature emphasizes the importance of parental involvement in achieving strong outcomes. McLeod & Wright (1996) believe "It is imperative that parents or other relatives of young children be involved in these programs so that prevention concepts can be reinforced in the natural home environment" (p. 75). They most likely used the word "imperative" because "evidence suggests that the involvement of parents (Binder & Mc-Neil, 1987; Wurtele, Gillespie, Currier, & Franklin, 1992) can lead to more persistence of the effects of training" (Cox, 1998, p. 35). Some would even go as far as to say that it is the duty of parents to talk with their children about sexual abuse. "Butler (1986) has found that 'parents are the major socializers of their children, the primary transmitters of family and religious values and attitudes. They can provide the daily, consistent teaching children need if abuse prevention education is to be effective'" (Hanson, 1996, pp. 12, 37).

Because sexuality is already a very sensitive topic, there is limited material teachers are allowed to discuss in the classroom. Where information is omitted in the classroom, parents need to fill in the gaps at home. "Parents are in a position to further explain to children when 'no' is an appropriate response and when it is not. Regarding prevention concepts such as touching, parents are, again, in a position to reassure children regarding nurturing touch and that it is never appropriate for an adult to sexually use a child" (Adams & Fay, 1986, cited in Hanson, 1996, p. 37). On the other hand, parents who leave child sexual abuse education up to teachers alone "may not know how to respond to their child's questions, may contradict accurate information, may not know how to correct any misconceptions the child may have, and may not recognize the signs that may indicate their child has been abused" (Hanson, 1996, p. 37).

RETENTION OF INFORMATION

Of the programs that have been evaluated, many show that the children retained knowledge from the lessons immediately afterward but that, weeks later, had already forgotten much of the material. Some authors have suggested that review sessions are necessary to maintain what gains are made (Plummer, 1984; Reppuci et al., 1998; Tutty, 1994). Reviews, sometimes called booster sessions, are helpful for older children and necessary for the younger age groups in order to help them retain the information initially learned. It is also important for programs to be of reasonable duration for the children to gain in knowledge (Cox, 1998). This means that short lessons carried out over a longer period of time are more effective than long lessons that occur only once or twice a year.

COST

"The treatment of sexually abused children is more difficult and quite costly when compared to implementing a child sexual abuse prevention program in a school system where large numbers of children can be impacted" (Hanson, 1996, p. 2). For example, in the 1980s, CSAPPs were offered to 4.6 million children enrolled in state-funded schools in the state of California at an annual cost of $11.4 million, or less than $7 per student. In contrast, treatment of a sexually abused child can cost between $5,000 and $8,000 annually (Daro, 1994; Hanson, 1996). Although it is exciting to think of the money that can be saved, while at the same time preventing child sexual abuse, we must be cautious about jumping to conclusions. "According to Wurtele & Miller-Perrin (1992), 'given the lack of evidence about whether these programs actually prevent abuse, the costs must be minimal to nonexistent to justify their continuation, let alone their expansion'" (Hanson, 1996, pp. 43, 81). Until it is proven that CSAPPs actually decrease the occurrence of child sexual abuse, it is not reasonable to allocate all funds to their implementation; some must be used for evaluation.

DECREASE IN CHILD SEXUAL ABUSE

The most accurate, but most difficult, method for measuring program effectiveness is to evaluate if there has been a decrease in child sexual abuse after implementation. The options for this evaluation are limited. It would be unethical to "test" children by pretending to be a perpetrator in order to note their responses. Another method would be long-term tracking (to adulthood) of children who have been through CSAPPs, perhaps interviewing them often to find out if they have been threatened with or experienced child sexual abuse. This would be too costly and also, perhaps, unethical. A less accurate but realistic method is to monitor incident rates (Wurtele, 1998). If programs are effective, then child sexual abuse incidence rates should decrease. The problem, though, is identifying which programs in particular were effective and which were not.

SCHOOL-BASED PROGRAMS

Most CSAPPs today take place in the classroom setting. There are many benefits to carrying out programs in a school environment. The school setting is appropriate for educating children about sexual abuse, given that their primary function is to inform and educate. Teachers have appeal as instructors, given their expertise as educators and that they have an established rapport with their students. Because teachers have ongoing relationships with students and their families, they also play a key role in identifying and supporting abused children. School-based programs are also appealing because they are able to reach large numbers of children of every racial, ethnic, and socioeconomic group in a relatively cost-efficient fashion (Wurtele, 1998).

There is a risk in accepting schools as the best environment for CSAPPs without evaluation. Cox (1998) explained that "Although children exposed to school-based prevention programmes were more likely to feel that they had been successful in protecting themselves and were more likely to disclose to someone about threats or assaults, they were not better able to limit the seriousness of assaults and in fact experienced more injuries" (p. 34). Further research needs to be done to determine the most appropriate setting for CSAPPs.

The "Who Do You Tell?" Program

The "Who do you tell?" program was first introduced in 1983 by the Calgary Sexual Assault Center and was updated and reintroduced by the Calgary Communities Against Sexual Assault in Canada. This program is taught to small groups (15–20) of children from kindergarten through grade 6. The learning objectives include understanding what sexual abuse is, identifying private body parts, learning assertive responses to unwanted touching, and naming adults they trust to tell if abuse occurs. The program consists of two 60-minute sessions. A variety of teaching strategies, such as stories, songs, videos, and role-plays, present several key messages. Slightly different formats are presented to each group so that age-appropriate materials and videos are matched to the developmental level of the children. Following the presentations, children are given the opportunity to ask for individual time to talk to the presenters. Teachers attend a 1-hour in-service that outlines the program and shows them how to recognize sexual abuse in children and how to respond to disclosures. A parent-information evening prepares parents for their children's participation in the program and provides them with information about child sexual abuse and how to respond to disclosures. A parent handbook is available that describes the program and issues related to child sexual abuse. Parent permission is required for children to participate. The cost for the program package has not yet been determined (Calgary Communities Against Sexual Assault, 2003).

The length of the program is a bit long for the 5- to 8-year-olds, who typically have an attention span of 20 minutes. The fact that there are two sessions is good in that repetition is needed at this age to retain information. The opportunity for parent involvement is present, but attendance is typically small (Tutty, 2000). Tutty explains that this "speaks to the continuing difficulty of involving parents in sexual abuse prevention programs. Because repetition of the concepts is vital to the material, parents are a logical target to reinforce these ideas, yet school-based programs have continually noted problems attracting parent participation" (p. 877).

Overall, children who participated in the "Who do you tell?" program had significantly higher levels of knowledge of both inappropriate and appropriate touch than children in the control group (Tutty, 2000). However, "the meta-analysis conducted by Rispens et al. (1997) concluded that the amount of instruction time and explicit training in self-protection skills have an impact on effectiveness. The 'Who do you tell' program may be improved by increasing both of these components" (Tutty, 2000, p. 295).

Child Assault Prevention Program

The Child Assault Prevention Program was originally developed in 1986 in Maryland as the Children's Primary Prevention Training Program but has since been revised and renamed. The program's objective is to increase children's sexual abuse prevention knowledge and skills. The program is offered to children in kindergarten through grade 3. Five lessons center on five interrelated storybooks entitled *Let's Talk About Touching, Private Parts, Surprises, Tell Someone,* and *Remember.* Each story contains specific rules and behaviors that a child can use if confronted with a potential abuser. Behavior rehearsals during the story and questions for use in follow-up exercises provide opportunities to practice the skills and concepts learned. An internal teacher who receives a manual teaches the program, and there is also a parent manual. The cost for the five storybooks, the teacher's manual, parent manual, and a demonstration video is $25 (Calgary Communities Against Sexual Assault, 2003).

However, books may not be the best idea for this age group. Kindergartners are just learning to read, and even the third graders may have difficulty with some of the vocabulary. Because there is only one copy of each book per class, the teacher reads the story aloud. This resolves the problem of lack of reading ability but creates another one; it may be difficult for the entire class to see the book, and children in this age group rely heavily on pictures. The role-play and follow-up exercises are essential to making this program at least somewhat appropriate. Lack of parental involvement is exacerbated by the fact that each kit only comes with one parent manual. Although there are many qualms about the use of this program with younger children, "the evaluation of the Child Assault Prevention Program indicated that the knowledge of the concepts treated in the prevention program by 8 to 9 and 11 to 12-year-old children increased from 48% to 59% and from 55% to 68%, respectively" (Krivacska, 1992; cited in Taal & Edelaar, 1997, p. 399). The price is very reasonable in that the larger the group, the more inexpensive it becomes. The cost for a group of 25 students would be $1 per student.

Good Touch/Bad Touch Program

This program is taught to children in kindergarten through grade 6. The topics covered include understanding abuse, how to prevent or interrupt abuse, and the fact that it is never right to hurt another child. The primary focus is sexual abuse prevention; however, physical abuse and bullying prevention are included in grade 3, and sexual harassment and emotional abuse are included in grade 5. Children learn five body safety rules: body ownership, how to say "no" to abuse, who can help them if they are abused, it's all right to ask adults questions about other adults' behavior, and sexual abuse is never a child's fault.

Materials and techniques such as role-plays reinforce the concepts and offer opportunities to practice the skills. The program is taught by an internal teacher who is either trained on site or by audiotape training kits, which are available in grade-specific or complete curriculum packages. Parents are referred to a Web site (*http://www.goodtouchbadtouch.com/talking_to_children.html*) that introduces the program and teaches them how to talk with children about sexual abuse, respond to disclosures, and recognize signs of abuse. There are also messages for children about different types of touch and sexual abuse. On-site training costs about $195/person or $1,450 for an audio training kit. The cost for curriculum materials is unknown (Calgary Communities Against Sexual Assault, 2003).

The curriculum is very specific to each age group and is developmentally appropriate. The Web site is a great resource for parents and allows them to be very much involved in the learning process. The cost is reasonable inasmuch as the same teacher presents the program every year or the audiotape training is reused many times. One of the negative aspects of the program is that "limitations in young children's attributional skills—that is, their abilities to judge a person's character or motivation—are hypothesized by de Young (1988) as the reason children have difficulty with the good touch–bad touch distinction" (Jordan, 1993, p. 77). There is a gray area of good or bad, right or wrong that is difficult for children to understand. The gray area may be different depending on cultural practices, thus parents would need to educate their children about touches or actions that fall into this area.

Stay Safe Program

The Stay Safe program (MacIntyre & Lawlor, 1991) is conducted in almost all Irish primary schools and has a great deal of support within the country (MacIntyre & Carr, 1999). The program is a culturally appropriate, developmentally staged CSAPP, specifically designed for the Irish educational context. It uses a multimedia format and focuses on cognitive, affective, and behavioral dimensions of learning (MacIntyre & Carr, 1999). The program teaches feeling safe and unsafe, bullying, wanted and unwanted touches, telling adults about negative interactions with victimizers and bullies, and dealing with strangers (MacIntyre & Carr, 1999). Parents are invited to a parent education meeting prior to implementation of the program, where they are asked to give consent for their children to participate. The meeting lasts for 3 hours and is also attended by community health care workers, including family doctors and public health nurses. Parents are given a guide to take home with them. Teachers attend two 4-hour training workshops, taught by a teacher experienced with the program and a mental health professional with child protection expertise. They, in turn, become the educators who implement the program for their classes. The program is conducted over 12 sessions for juniors and 10 sessions for seniors. Sessions are 30–40 minutes long, and 2 sessions are conducted per week. After each session, children are given Stay Safe homework sheets to complete at home and have signed by their parents.

The Stay Safe program is by far the most comprehensive CSAPP seen to date. It involves parents, teachers, and the larger community. Stay Safe is developmentally and culturally appropriate and uses a wide variety of media to reach individual children. Understanding the age group's attention span, the sessions are short in duration but are repeated to help children better retain information. Studies show that the Stay Safe program has a predominately positive and relatively enduring effect on the children who participate in it (MacIntyre & Carr, 1999).

Feeling Yes, Feeling No Program

This program was developed in 1980 by the Green Thumb Theatre for Young People in Vancouver, BC, Canada. The program consists of three 15-minute interactive instructional videos taped by the National Film Board of Canada in 1985 and is offered to children in grades 1 through 6. It is available in French as *"Mon Corps, C'est Mon Corps."* The videos include children from various ethnic backgrounds. The main objectives of the program are to help children identify responses to being touched, how children can seek help if touch leaves them feeling "no," and to identify some reasons why it is hard to tell about "no" feelings. The series of videos provides children the tools to protect themselves from sexual assault by strangers, family members, and other trusted people. Using the three videos as the starting point for instruction, the entire program can take 15 to 18 hours of classroom teaching. A facilitator's guide outlines role-plays, mime, art, music, and other activities that reinforce the messages from the videos. An adult "Feeling Yes, Feeling No" video is available for parents and teachers. A short one-time booster session is offered to further enhance children's ability to identify safe and unsafe situations portrayed in videotaped scenarios. The cost is $39.95 for the 78-minute family program video or $125 for the professional package, which consists of four videos (Calgary Communities Against Sexual Assault, 2003).

The Feeling Yes, Feeling No program demonstrates cultural appropriateness by offering the videos in two different languages and by portraying a variety of ethnicities in the videos. However, there is no mention of a distinction between videos shown to children in grade 1 versus children in grade 6. Because the material is generalized for 6- to 12-year-olds, the concepts and vocabulary used may be developmentally inappropriate for some of the children. Parental involvement appears minimal, but the program is cost-effective.

Women Against Rape: Child Abuse Prevention Program

Women Against Rape, in Columbus, Ohio, developed the Child Abuse Prevention (CAP) program in 1978. Facilitators delivered the CAP program throughout the United States and many other countries. In 1985, a French adaptation was created. The objective of the program is to prevent physical, psychological, verbal, and sexual abuse of young children. The program offers school workshops, taught by trained CAP facilitators, for children in preschool through grade 6, their teachers, and their parents. Classroom presentations are approximately 1 hour and include information and strategies to assist children and youth in resisting abuse. Topics covered include sexual, verbal, emotional, and physical abuse by peers (bullying); known adults; and strangers. Guided group discussions, narratives, and role-plays help students learn prevention/protection strategies such as assertiveness, peer support, a self-defense yell, and telling a trusted adult if abuse occurs. There is a 2-hour school workshop for teachers and a 2-hour family in-service for parents (Calgary Communities Against Sexual Assault, 2003).

The program is culturally appropriate for French children. Finkelhor & Strapko (1988) feel that "programs that actively involve children and occur over a long period of time, such as the Child Abuse Prevention (CAP) format, seem to yield a greater increase in children's knowledge than do programs that rely on children's passive participation and are brief exposures" (cited in Jordan, 1993, p. 77). CAP shows promise, both because it involves parents, teachers, and other adult community members and because it includes active research for additional evidence of program effects (Finkelhor & Strapko, 1988; Jordan, 1993; Nibert, 1987).

CONCLUSION

It is interesting that society thinks it appropriate to begin teaching children about sexual abuse before even talking to them about sexuality. Many younger children may not even know that there are anatomical differences between males and females. Tharinger et al. (1998) noted that fear that the program will be rejected by parents explains the lack of sex education programs in schools and cautions against the danger of this omission (Jordan, 1993; Krivacska, 1989; Tharinger, 1998). Perhaps it would be more beneficial, and less traumatic, to teach children some general principles about sex and sexuality before warning them about the danger of sexual abuse.

Further evaluation of the effectiveness of CSAPPs is needed, but there are also other avenues of approach besides focusing on the children. The general public, professionals, and parents should play important roles in child sexual abuse prevention, but, unfortunately, these groups have not received as much attention as have children. It is time to extend preventive efforts and target others, especially parents, to play a more active part in preventing child sexual abuse. Children should not be held solely responsible for prevention of sexual abuse (Wurtele, 1998).

Until CSAPPs are proven effective, it is incorrect and unethical to call them "prevention" programs. "To date, there is no evidence suggesting that these programs are helping to decrease the incidence of child sexual abuse" (Wurtele, 1998, p. 506). The word "prevention" misleads the public into thinking that implementing these programs will stop child sexual abuse. Wurtele & Miller-Perrin (1992) suggest that these programs be referred to as "personal safety programs" (cited in Wurtele, 1998). The public needs to know that child sexual abuse programs may prevent child sexual abuse, but there is no guarantee.

REFERENCES

Calgary Communities Against Sexual Assault (n.d.). *School-based violence prevention programs: A resource manual.* Retrieved May 25, 2003, from *http://www.ucalgary.ca/resolve/violenceprevention/ English/reviewprog/childsxprogs.htm.*

Cox, A. D. (1998). Preventing child abuse: A review of community-based projects II: Issues arising from reviews and future directions. *Child Abuse Review, 7,* 30–43.

Davis, M. K., & Gidycz, C. A. (2000). Child sexual abuse prevention programs: A meta-analysis. *Journal of Clinical Child Psychology, 29*(2), 257–265.

Esser-Stuart, J. E., & Skibinski, G. J. (1998). Child sexual abuse intervention: An exploratory study of policy concerns and implications for program development. *Journal of Child Sexual Abuse, 7*(2), 87–103.

Hanson, A. S. (1996). *Application of an instrument for evaluating child sexual abuse prevention programs.* Unpublished doctoral dissertation, University of Illinois, Urbana-Champaign.

Jordan, N. H. (1993). Sexual abuse prevention programs in early childhood education: A caveat. *Young Children, 48*(6), 76–79.

MacIntyre, D., & Carr, A. (1999). Evaluation of the effectiveness of the Stay Safe primary prevention programme for child sexual abuse. *Child Abuse and Neglect, 23*(12), 1307–1325.

McLeod, N. S., & Wright, C. (1996). Developmentally appropriate criteria for evaluating sexual abuse prevention programs. *Early Childhood Education Journal, 24*(2), 71–75.

Plummer, C. A. (1999). The history of child sexual abuse prevention: A practitioner's perspective. *Journal of Child Sexual Abuse, 7*(4), 77–95.

Reppucci, N. D., Land, D., & Haugaard, J. J. (1998). Child sexual abuse prevention programs that target young children. In P. K. Trickett & C. J. Schellenbach (Eds.). *Violence against children in the family and the community* (pp. 317–337). Washington DC: American Psychological Association.

Taal, M., & Edelaar, M. (1997). Positive and negative effects of a child sexual abuse prevention program. *Child Abuse and Neglect, 21*(4), 399–410.

Tutty, L. M. (1997). Child sexual abuse prevention programs: Evaluating Who Do You Tell. *Child Abuse and Neglect, 21*(9), 869–881.

Tutty, L. M. (2000). What children learn from sexual abuse prevention programs: Difficult concepts and developmental issues. *Research on Social Work Practice, 10*(3), 275–300.

Wurtele, S. K. (1998). School-based child sexual abuse prevention programs: Question, answers, and more questions. In J. R. Lutzker (Ed.). *Handbook of child abuse research and treatment* (pp. 501–516). New York, NY: Plenum.

CHAPTER 28

Healing Ministries in Health Care

*Medrice Coluccio, Retha R. Porter, and Kathryn A. Robbins**

Throughout time and across cultures, those practicing the healing arts have provided more than physical healing to the sick and ailing. Whether it is a shaman blocking a curse from an enemy tribe, a high priest of ancient Israel issuing a quarantine for lepers, a Knights Hospitaler caring for a plague victim, or a hospice nurse counseling a family, healers have always fulfilled many spiritual and social needs in their communities.

Although the needs of society have changed, the need for compassionate, dedicated health providers has never been greater or the calling higher. Immense challenges and opportunities face our modern-day healers, but for those dedicated individuals the rewards can be great. Individuals that are beneficiaries of a healer's skills obtain reciprocal value.

Nursing is a special calling of one's inner passion to provide care, teach, research, and promote opportunities for enhancing health to all populations. Nurses and their health care colleagues have an excellent opportunity to lead and make a difference in the ongoing health of a community. Facilitating a shared vision of improving health status is a lifelong gift to a community.

Providing exclusive care to only a certain population should not be an option. One of the more challenging and vulnerable populations to serve is that of the underserved and uninsured. In caring for these individuals, the care should be viewed from a holistic perspective. This includes attention to an individual's physical, emotional, and spiritual health. The holistic approach to caring for the whole person is a guiding light in caring for each person.

The health of our community is the pulse of our community. Strong economics, solid educational systems, cultural diversity, access to care, and healthy lifestyles are indicators of a healthy community. Nurturing and growing healthy populations enrich all of our lives.

HISTORY OF PEACEHEALTH

In 1884 in Nottingham, England, Margaret Anna Cusack, known as Mother Clare, founded a religious congregation of women, the Sisters of St. Joseph of Peace. The order originally worked with poor Irish women, but at the end of the 19th century, they came to the United States and have been providing health care in the Pacific Northwest since 1890. Their inspiration is to promote social justice as a path to peace (Ward & O'Connor, 2000).

---

*The authors are members of the congregation of the Sisters of St. Joseph of Peace.

One of the ways in which we actualize Mother Clare's dreams of peace and social justice is to provide health care services to underserved public communities. Mother Clare's vision continues over 100 years later as a vibrant and compassionate model of delivering health care (Vidulich, 1990). In 1976, the sisters consolidated their various health care ministries into a single not-for profit system called PeaceHealth. Today, PeaceHealth operates six hospitals, various medical groups, and other health services throughout Oregon, Washington State, and Alaska.

MISSION AND VALUES

The overarching PeaceHealth mission is the foundation of its health care ministry: to carry on the healing mission of Jesus Christ by promoting personal and community health, relieving pain and suffering, and treating each person in a loving and caring way (PeaceHealth, 2002). The related core values of respecting individual dignity and worth, stewardship, collaboration, and social justice are the impetus and focus of how PeaceHealth provides patient care through its many vital community ministries.

As members of the Sisters of St. Joseph of Peace, the values of PeaceHealth guide our actions in service to the community. We demonstrate respect for individual human dignity and the worth of each person with compassion, caring, and acceptance of individual differences. The exercise of ethical and responsible stewardship in the allocation and utilization of human, financial, and environmental resources is our responsibility. We value collaboration by welcoming the involvement, cooperation, and creativity of all who work together to promote the health of the community. Along with others, we build and evaluate the structures of our organization and those of society to promote the just distribution of health care resources.

SETTING

One of the regions that will be highlighted in this chapter is PeaceHealth's lower Columbia region. This region comprises St. John Medical Center, PeaceHealth Medical Group, and other related health services. The medical center serves a widespread geographical area of eight counties in southwest Washington State and northwest Oregon. The population served is approximately 200,000 people.

Providing for the poor and underserved is an integral part of the mission that physicians and other staff in PeaceHealth have embraced. Through their efforts, the ministry of the Sisters of St. Joseph of Peace, which began in the Pacific Northwest's logging camps and continued in the lower Columbia region for over 60 years, continues to be a vital force in the community.

Today, the Sisters' mission serves a population with significant challenges. The communities served in the lower Columbia region rank near the top, both in the state of Washington and nationally, with regard to unemployment, low income, and numbers of people uninsured. Domestic abuse, drug and alcohol addiction, and crime rates are increasing, as are the unhealthy life styles and conditions that arise out of these situations.

THE CALLING

Because of these external forces in the community, many citizens in the lower Columbia region have difficulty accessing appropriate care, and PeaceHealth has not closed its door to those in need. During the past 5 years alone, PeaceHealth has provided over 40 million dollars in charity and uncompensated care to this community. This amount is expected to double over the next 3 years.

PeaceHealth is not the only hospital affected by the growing needs of the community. In 1989, Washington State enacted legislation that prohibits any Washington hospital from denying access to emergency care because of patients' inability to pay. It also prevents hospitals from adopting admission policies that significantly reduce charity care. The same legislation directs each hospital to develop a charity care policy. The impact of uncompensated health care on hospital charges and continued access to health care in a community places new burdens and challenges on health care providers. In addition, the public's demand for state-of-the-art care, the latest technologies, and improved facilities puts even more strain on health care resources.

Despite these challenges, PeaceHealth is committed to continuing its mission by providing exceptional medical and compassionate care to all who enter its doors. These challenges are why we are committed to extending our mission beyond our doors and partnering with other organizations to foster the health of our community.

PARTNERING

Recognizing the need to creatively reach outside the walls to address these growing community needs, the St. John Medical Center has partnered with others in the community to proactively address these concerns. There are many examples of programs created together with others that have positively affected the community.

Parish Nurse Ministries

PeaceHealth's Interdenominational Parish Nurse Ministries began as a compassionate response to the changing health care needs in the community. The goal for this ministry is to respond to the health, wellness, and wholeness concerns of church congregations through the melding of hospital and parish nurse partnerships. Parish nurse coordinators are nurses with special training who work with local church congregations and are available to offer consultation to pastors, parish nurses, and health ministries interested in the start-up and continuation of parish health programs.

The history of parish nursing began in the early 1980s as the vision of a forward-thinking Lutheran pastor/chaplain in Parkridge, Illinois, at what was then the Lutheran General Hospital. Rev. Granger E. Westberg saw the integration of faith and health as the fundamental basis of a parish nurse ministry, creating partnerships with health care systems and the faith communities (Westberg, 1990). Since the inception of parish nursing, 7500 registered nurses have been trained in the United States. Their role focuses on the whole person, not only the physical but also the spiritual and psychological aspects of care. Programs are offered throughout the country that provide continuing education and spiritual growth to clergy, parish nurses, and allied health care professionals. Currently the American Nurses Association considers the ministry of parish nursing as a specialty for registered nurses (American Nurses Association, 2000).

Through individual and team approaches, parish nurses assess individual and/or congregational health concerns and serve in a variety of capacities: health counselor, educator, advocate, liaison, trainer, and healer. In these roles, parish nurses discuss individual health needs such as treatment availability, prevention, and wellness and provide reassurance during times of crisis. This provides invaluable support in patient decision making regarding health care issues. They offer information in the areas of domestic violence, alcohol and drug abuse, depression, cancer, diabetes, obesity, arthritis, childcare, senior daycare, and Medicaid.

The parish nurse can also provide clinicians with valuable information needed to provide the best medical care to individuals. Through various programs and literature offerings, parish nurses promote the relationship between faith, health, attitude, and lifestyle choices. They implement this approach to the healing of body, mind, and spirit in a variety of ways, including prayer, visitation (home, long-term care facility, or hospital), and providing a listening presence.

Parish nursing is a visible symbol of extending a healing ministry into the congregation and thus the larger community. This is seen in the advocacy parish nurses provide by identifying the medically underinsured, the vulnerable, and isolated members of the congregation. In response to specific needs, they also put parishioners in touch with appropriate community services, agencies, primary care providers, and fellow members of the congregation who might be able to help. The nurses recruit and supervise volunteers and provide information and education to assist them in their health ministry. Parish nursing is a successful example of a collaboration of dedicated individuals responding to the greater needs of the community.

Youth Mentorship Program

The Youth Mentorship Program evolved from the vision and passion of Sister Rose Marie Nigro, Director of Community Ministries at PeaceHealth, lower Columbia region. In response to the region's high number of school dropouts, Sister Rose began working with area high schools and community leaders to establish a program to encourage and assist high school students in their pursuit of higher education. The program helps at-risk high school juniors and seniors by providing opportunities to attend college, a goal that otherwise would be out of reach. The students in the program need financial help, as well as coaching, to attend college. Sister Nigro explains, "We try to target, not the kids with the best grades, but the ones who could not otherwise get scholarships. Those are the ones we want to give a chance."

To be accepted into the program, students must complete an essay about their goals and the barriers that could hinder them in achieving these goals. One student wrote, "My immediate goal is to obtain a master's degree in a computer-related field at the University of Washington. There are several barriers to reaching my goal, however. We have a single parent/single income home, with no child support. Although we have a great deal of love and faith, there isn't always enough money to meet our basic needs, much less college."

Once in the program, students are teamed with a mentor who assists them in understanding processes and opportunities for education after high school. However, the mentors do much more than that. Students have commented that their mentors have taught them about professionalism and life experiences.

The Youth Mentorship Program provides part-time employment, 10 hours per week. The students agree to set aside one third of their salary to save for their education after high school. PeaceHealth then matches these savings through scholarships to the school of the student's choice. Some of these students may also serve as teen volunteers at the medical center. This additional experience provides increased insight into their professional aspirations.

Both the Interdenominational Parish Nurse Program and Youth Mentorship Program came out of PeaceHealth's mission and ministry to the community. They provide unique opportunities for nurses and other health care professionals to make a far greater impact beyond that of their traditional roles.

Community Provider Opportunities

Increasing access to health care for the uninsured through development of a community free clinic that offers urgent care to vulnerable populations in cases where a primary care physician is unavailable, or as an alternative setting to the hospital emergency department, is the goal of a community team of providers. PeaceHealth's community providers are seeking greater access to primary care for populations that are uninsured.

Another initiative is to find a "medical home" to serve as a primary care resource for the recurrent underinsured users of the emergency department. To date, a community provider clinic that is federally reimbursed to care for these patients has been identified. This would align with the care continuum of the emergency department.

It is through this collaborative spirit that much can be accomplished. The beneficiaries of all these efforts are the vulnerable populations in this community. Chances of improving their health status are vastly improved by these outreach programs and services.

SUMMARY

Today, the need for accessible health care and related community programs continues to increase among the populations we serve. Along with our growing populations come growing social challenges. Increasingly, hospitals and health care organizations are called on to fill a vital niche in the social needs of their communities. Without this help, the most vulnerable may be overlooked. It is imperative that those in health care accept the challenge of creating programs and services that help educate and serve those who are most in need.

ACKNOWLEDGMENTS

This chapter is dedicated to Sister Rose Marie Nigro, Director of Community Ministries, PeaceHealth, lower Columbia region. Sister Rose's dedication and leadership in caring for vulnerable populations is an inspiration.

REFERENCES

American Nurses Association. (2000). *Scope and standards of parish nurse practice.* Washington, DC: American Nurses Association.

Vidulich, D. (1990). *Peace pays a price.* Washington, DC: Sisters of St. Joseph of Peace.

Westberg, G. E. (1990). *The parish nurse.* Minneapolis, MN: Augsburg.

Ward, J., & O'Connor, C. (2000). *A great love of peace.* Bellevue, WA: Our Lady Province.

Youth Mentorship Program. (2002). Conversation with Sr. Rose Marie Nigro—1994.

PeaceHealth Brochure, Bellevue, WA: PeaceHealth.

CHAPTER 29

Rural Appalachian Women: A Vulnerable Population

Carol M. Patton

The concept of vulnerability implies a higher than average risk of harm or neglect as well as social and health problems (Lancaster, 1999; Sebastian, 1999). Vulnerable populations frequently face actual and perceived barriers to health care, predisposing them to acute and chronic illnesses that ultimately lessen quality of life (Ludwig-Beymer, 1999, 2003; Spector, 2000). Vulnerable populations are at increased risk for developing many acute and chronic diseases, and they are also vulnerable because of barriers to health care services that leave gaps that result in health care disparities. In order to decrease vulnerability in patient populations, lessen health disparities, and provide culturally congruent, patient-focused care, it is imperative for advanced-practice nurses to become sensitive to and aware of the specific needs of identified vulnerable populations.

The purpose of this chapter is to provide a description of the Appalachian region and how the demographics (or characteristics of the people) of this mountainous area predispose its indigenous populations to vulnerability. Specifically, the chapter will describe the cultural context of rural Appalachia and the vulnerability of poor rural Appalachian women; then it will address how advanced-practice nurses can help improve the health status of these women.

APPALACHIAN REGION

Appalachia is a 200,000-square mile geographic region located in the eastern United States. This predominantly mountainous and rugged terrain is often referred to as the "Appalachian region." The Appalachian region comprises 13 states: Alabama, Georgia, Kentucky, Maryland, West Virginia, Ohio, Pennsylvania, New York, North Carolina, South Carolina, Mississippi, Tennessee, and Virginia (Appalachian Regional Commission, 2000). Portions of 12 states lie within this region, but only West Virginia lies completely within its borders (Purnell, 2003).

Topographically the Appalachian region consists of mountainous and rugged terrain, with a belt of mountains 2,000 miles long and nearly 360 miles wide (Appalachian Regional Commission, 2000). The population of this region is approximately 22 million, with approximately 42% of the total population living in rural areas. The nature and structure of the Appalachian region presents its inhabitants with barriers to health care that predispose them to vulnerability and health care disparities.

Potential demographic and cultural barriers have been identified in the Appalachian region, along with barriers preventing access to the health system. In Appalachia, the poverty rate is higher and the average socioeconomic status is lower than in the rest of the United States. The 1999 US census data report that 27% of the Appalachian region's 406 total counties are economically distressed compared with a national rate of 13% (Appalachian Regional Commission, 2000). For many reasons, there is little opportunity for Appalachian women to overcome conditions of poverty and harsh socioeconomic realities, but the primary reason is reported to be a lack of transportation. Rugged mountainous terrain can sometimes only be traveled by all-terrain vehicles, and roads are often impassable in the harsh winter months (Appalachian Regional Commission, 2000). Lack of knowledge regarding primary and preventive care, in addition to those barriers already mentioned, predisposes poor rural Appalachian women to health care disparities and vulnerability (Elnicki, Morris, & Shockor, 1995).

Cultural Origins and Historical Roots of Rural Appalachians

The culture of rural Appalachia is heavily rooted in long-standing traditions stemming from early ancestry. Early settlers in the Appalachian region were immigrants from northern Ireland, Scotland, Germany, and England. They came to the East Coast, primarily to New Jersey and Philadelphia. As these areas became more and more populous, living space decreased, and in the early 1700s immigrants from these groups began traveling west, making their way into the mountains of what is now known as the Appalachian region. Other culturally diverse groups that resulted in unique subcultures within the Appalachian region were Native Americans, African Americans, and a group known specifically to the Appalachian region as Melungeons. Melungeons are persons of mixed race, including African American, Native American, Mediterranean, Middle Eastern, and white ethnic backgrounds (Costello, 2000).

These early groups from the various culturally diverse backgrounds favored the mountains of the Appalachian region as their new home because, it is said, this new land reminded them very much of their former homelands (Appalachian Regional Commission, 2000). These early immigrants to what is now known as Appalachia found the region rich in abundant natural resources, and they began building their lives, working and farming the land (Roark & Wallace, 2000).

The early ancestral composition of Appalachia resulted in subsequent generations of proud, self-sufficient people with rich family and community traditions, tremendous pride in their heritage, a common phraseology distinct to Appalachian people, and what could be characterized as the most rugged of lifestyles. Within the Appalachian region there are also subcultures, and advanced-practice nurses should have an increased awareness of and sensitivity to key characteristics of Appalachian culture when providing health care to this unique and culturally diverse population (see Table 29.1).

APPALACHIAN WOMEN AS A VULNERABLE POPULATION

The topography and geography of the rugged Appalachian terrain is a barrier to health care for rural Appalachian women. Appalachian women are also at increased risk for health care disparities because their culture and heritage make it unacceptable for a woman to put her health care needs ahead of the daily needs of her family (Purnell, 2003) and because preventive health care is not a priority for them. It is reported that the people of Appalachia are less concerned about

TABLE 29.1 Characteristics of Appalachia

☐ Mountainous topography—many unimproved roads

☐ Tax bases may be and quite often are low, depending on industry. Predominant industry (and employer) is underground bituminous coal mines

☐ Public schools reflect low tax base, poor economics, lack of industrialization

☐ Extensive geographic and sociocultural isolation because of hilly mountainous regions and lack of public transportation—often results in economic disparities

☐ Many small settlements and communities with <2,500 habitants located throughout the region

☐ Limited formal education because of isolation from mainstream society and lack of financial resources and social support

☐ Traditional household is very patriarchal

their health and less engaged in health promotion initiatives than non-Appalachian people (Elnicki, Morris, & Shockor, 1995; Ramsey & Glenn, 1998; Tripp-Reimer, 1982; Tripp-Reimer & Freidl, 1977).

There is a strong correlation between socioeconomic status and health indicators for at-risk populations (Naidoo & Wills, 1998, 2000; Powell, 2000; Woolf, 1996). Poverty results in reduced access to health care, thereby increasing the vulnerability of the poor and the economically disadvantaged (Spector, 2000). Specifically, it has been described that lower socioeconomic status combined with lower educational status is an indicator for poorer health status and poorer patient outcomes (Green & Kreuter, 1999; US Department of Health and Human Services [DHHS], 2000; US Preventive Services Task Force, 1996). Rural Appalachian women fall into this category, with a likelihood of increased mortality and morbidity from major preventable illnesses. The predominant major illnesses of concern in this high-risk vulnerable population include, but are not limited to, heart disease, diabetes, obesity, cancer, and mental illness. This population is also vulnerable to injury and violence, limited access to health care, substance abuse disorders, and tobacco and smokeless tobacco addictions.

There is a paucity of research specifically aimed at effects of primary health care in Appalachian women. Variables that make Appalachian women a high-risk, vulnerable population are a lack of knowledge about primary care services and concern about high-risk behaviors. Specifically and particularly relevant is a lack of information among rural Appalachian women regarding the benefits of engaging in primary prevention and health promotion initiatives. Many Appalachian women do not seek preventive care and tend to seek acute care interventions only when they have suffered a disease or illness condition that affects their functional status to the point that they can no longer perform activities of daily living and act as caretakers of their families (Elnicki et al., 1995; Purnell, 2003; Tripp-Reimer, 1982; Tripp-Reimer & Freidl, 1977; Williams, Lethbridge, & Chambers, 1999).

In addition to the unique demographic characteristics of the people of the Appalachian region, poor rural Appalachian women also have other characteristics unique to women that must be considered by advanced-practice nurses in providing culturally sensitive, culturally congruent health care. Table 29.2 depicts key characteristics of rural Appalachian women that should be

TABLE 29.2   Key Characteristics: Women in WV and Southwestern PA

☐ Women are expected to take care of the house and assume responsibility for childrearing
☐ Women are seen as providers of emotional strength
☐ Older women are responsible for preserving Appalachian culture
☐ Women are viewed as "experts" in health care
☐ Women usually provide herbal remedies and folk medicines to their neighbors and relatives ("kin" or "kinfolk")
☐ Fewer Appalachian women who live in urban areas work outside the home
☐ Appalachian women marry young, usually by age 20
☐ Woman's primary obligation is to her family
☐ Incidence of emotional and mental health disorders 150 to 400% higher in rural Appalachian women than in the general population
☐ Many women ignore health care problems until their functional status is decreased or they experience complete physical incapacity

considered by advanced-practice nurses in providing health promotion and acute care to this high-risk, vulnerable population.

PRIMARY CARE NEEDS OF APPALACHIAN WOMEN

From a primary care perspective, there are 10 leading health indicators identified by the US DHHS in *Healthy People 2010* (US DHHS, 2000) that should be used as a foundation of care for poor rural Appalachian women. Table 29.3 identifies the leading indicators for health in the United States.

Although it is a challenge to provide primary care that focuses on primary and secondary levels of health promotion because of previous actual and perceived barriers to care, implementation of a practice model incorporating these identified leading health indicators can create opportunities for poor rural Appalachian women to engage in health-promoting behaviors. Engaging these high-risk, vulnerable women in primary care initiatives can facilitate health promotion and disease prevention behaviors, ultimately lessening the gap in health care disparities for poor rural Appalachian women. In addition, it is particularly relevant for the advanced-practice nurse working with poor, vulnerable, rural Appalachian women to develop culturally congruent strategies that maximize health outcomes, with the ultimate goal of facilitating the motivation and desire to sustain healthy lifestyles. The ultimate goal of advanced-practice nursing interventions in primary care is to empower these women to ultimately improve their health status by engaging them as well as their families and significant others in their own health care initiatives by addressing one or more of the leading indicators of health.

SUMMARY

The chapter has described the Appalachian region and how the Appalachian heritage of women living in this area continues to influence their primary care needs. It is relevant for advanced-

TABLE 29.3   Leading Indicators of Health in the United States

☐ physical activity
☐ overweight/obesity
☐ tobacco use
☐ substance abuse
☐ responsible sexual behavior
☐ mental health
☐ injury and violence
☐ environmental quality
☐ immunizations
☐ access to health care

Adapted from US Department of Health and Human Services, 2000.

practice nurses to embrace the cultural diversity of this high-risk population of women in order to more accurately assess, identify, and implement health promotion concepts so these women may live longer, healthier, productive lives without the burden of chronic disease states. The geography and topography of the Appalachian region subject its inhabitants to barriers to primary health care, health promotion, and disease prevention in many instances. It is incumbent on advanced-practice nurses to have an increased awareness of and sensitivity to poor rural Appalachian women in order to provide culturally congruent care, ultimately empowering them to have enhanced quality of life and fewer chronic disease states over their lifetimes.

REFERENCES

Appalachian Regional Commission. (2000). *Counties in Appalachia.* Retrieved December 14, 2003, from *http://www.arc.gov/index.do?nodeld=27.*

Appalachian Regional Commission. (2000). *Executive summary: Building on past experiences: Creating a new future for distressed counties.* Retrieved December 14, 2003, from *http://www.arc.gov/index.do?nodeld=1375.*

Costello, C. (2000, May 30). Beneath myth: Melungeons find roots of oppression: Appalachian descendants embrace heritage. *The Washington Post,* p. 44.

Elnicki, D. M., Morris, D. K., & Shockor, W. T. (1995). Patient-perceived barriers to preventive health care among indigent, rural Appalachian patients. *Archives of Internal Medicine, 155,* 421–424.

Green, L. W., & Kreuter, M. W. (1999). *Health promotion planning: An educational and ecological approach* (3rd ed.). Mountain View, CA: Mayfield Publishing.

Lancaster, J. (1999). Foreword. In J. G. Sebastian & A. Bushy (Eds.). *Special populations in the community: Advances in reducing health disparities* (pp. xiii–xv). Gaithersburg, MD: Aspen.

Ludwig-Beymer, P. (1999). Trends in health care delivery and contributions of transcultural nursing. In M. H. Andrews & J. S. Boyle (Eds.). *Transcultural concepts in nursing care* (3rd ed., pp. 262–282). Philadelphia, PA: Lippincott.

Ludwig-Beymer, P. (2003). Creating culturally competent organizations. In M. M. Andrews & J. S. Boyle (Eds.). *Transcultural concepts in nursing care* (4th ed., pp. 249–271). Philadelphia, PA: Lippincott.

Naidoo, J., & Wills, J. (1998). *Practicing health promotion: Dilemmas and challenges.* London: Bailliere Tindall.

Naidoo, J., & Wills, J. (2000). *Health promotion: Foundations for practice* (2nd ed.). Edinburgh: Bailliere Tindall.

Powell, S. K. (2000). *Advanced case management: Outcomes and beyond.* Philadelphia, PA: Lippincott.

Purnell, L. D. (2003). People of Appalachian heritage. In L. D. Purnell & B. J. Paulanka (Eds.). *Transcultural health care: A culturally competent approach* (2nd ed., pp. 73–89). Philadelphia, PA: F. A. Davis.

Ramsey, P., & Glenn, L. (1998). Risk factors for heart disease in rural Appalachia. *Family and Community Health, 20*(4), 71–82.

Roark, A., & Wallace, G. (2000). *Appalachian culture: A thumbnail sketch.* Retrieved December 14, 2003, from *http://pegasus.cc.ucf.edu/~abrice/roark.html.*

Sebastian, J. G. (1999). Definitions and theory underlying vulnerability. In J. G. Sebastian & A. Bushy (Eds.). *Special populations in the community: Advances in reducing health disparities* (pp. 3–9). Gaithersburg, MD: Aspen.

Spector, R. E. (2000). *Cultural diversity in health and illness* (5th ed.). Upper Saddle River, NJ: Prentice Hall.

Tripp-Reimer, T. (1982). Barriers to health care: Variations in interpretation of Appalachian client behavior by Appalachian and non-Appalachian professionals. *Western Journal of Nursing Research, 4*(2), 179–191.

Tripp-Reimer, T., & Freidl, M. C. (1977). Appalachians: A neglected minority. *Nursing Clinics of North America, 12*(1), 41–54.

US DHHS. (2000). *Healthy people 2010.* Retrieved October 4, 2002, from *http://www.health.gov/ healthypeople/about/hpfact.html.*

US Preventive Services Task Force. (1996). *Guide to clinical preventive services* (2nd ed.). Philadelphia, PA: Williams & Wilkins.

Williams, R. D., Lethbridge, D. L., & Chambers, W. V. (1999). Development of a health promotion inventory for poor rural women. In J. G. Sebastian & A. Bushy (Eds.). *Special populations in the community: Advances in reducing health disparities* (pp. 274–284). Gaithersburg, MD: Aspen.

Woolf, S. H. (1996). Principles of risk assessment. In S. H. Woolf, S. Jonas, & R. S. Lawrence (Eds.). *Health promotion and disease prevention in clinical practice* (pp. 3–19). Philadelphia, PA: Lippincott.

CHAPTER 30

Pregnant Women Who Use Drugs: A Disenfranchised Group

Bonnie H. Bowie

In health care, "vulnerable populations" normally refers to groups of people with increased risk for health-related problems such as higher morbidity and mortality rates, reduced access to care, and a diminished quality of life. Because of a specific characteristic (e.g., race, gender, disability, disease), the vulnerable group experiences discrimination, stigmatization, and a lack of power in personal, social, and political relationships (UCLA Center for Vulnerable Populations, 2003). In their article on risk and vulnerability, Rose & Killien (1983) proposed that the term "vulnerability" characterizes personal factors that interact with the environment to influence health.

Pregnant women who use drugs are vulnerable in several ways. When a woman becomes pregnant, her actions affect not only herself but also her unborn fetus. Pregnancy is viewed by many as a public domain. It is a source of joy to the community, but it also elicits a protective response toward both the woman and her helpless unborn fetus. As a result of this protectiveness, the pregnant woman's right to complete autonomy is often overlooked. If she uses drugs, it moves her into a population that frequently experiences discrimination and stigma. This chapter will explore three key areas that represent this population's vulnerability: personhood or autonomy, discrimination, and socioeconomic status.

PERSONHOOD

Rather than being a biological category, "personhood" refers to the moral and legal status granted by moral codes established by society. A "person" is a bearer of rights and responsibilities, is worthy of respect, and has moral responsibilities and legal standing (Newton, 1975). The debate as to whether a fetus has the full rights and standing as a person is beyond the scope of this chapter. For the purposes of this discussion, the focus will be on the pregnant women who use drugs as a class of people who have diminished personhood as a result of pregnancy.

Women who are pregnant may be surprised to hear open criticism regarding their unhealthy behaviors by friends, and even strangers, once their pregnancy is apparent. Behaviors such as eating unhealthy foods and smoking may be openly commented upon when a pregnant woman engages in them as people verbalize their concern for the unborn fetus. The right of an individual to make personal life choices is suddenly in question during pregnancy. In other areas of health and medicine, we acknowledge the right of the patient to consent to or refuse treatment and to ignore medical advice. However, when a fetus is present, the pregnant woman suddenly becomes a nonperson, and her personhood—her inherent rights as a human being—is stripped from her as the rights of the fetus are given priority.

Although there are certainly several behaviors and substances that can adversely affect the well-being of the growing fetus, none has been more openly condemned than the use of illicit drugs by pregnant women. In 30 states, charges have been brought against pregnant women caught using illicit drugs based on statutes ranging from child abuse to manslaughter (Tillett & Osborne, 2001). The most notorious of these cases occurred in South Carolina where it was hospital policy at the Medical University of South Carolina to screen high-risk pregnant women in labor for cocaine use without the woman's knowledge or consent (Gostin, 2001). For women who tested positive, police were notified and prosecution threatened, in order to provide "the necessary leverage" to force them into treatment (Gostin, 2001). The South Carolina Supreme Court held that the ingestion of cocaine during the third trimester of pregnancy constitutes criminal child neglect. However, the state's efforts to protect the fetus at the expense of the rights of pregnant women actually resulted in decreased admissions of pregnant women to drug treatment programs in South Carolina that give priority to pregnant women. In addition, not only did South Carolina's 1997 infant mortality figures increase, but so did the number of abandoned babies (Paltrow, Cohen, & Carey, 2000). The South Carolina judicial system's effort to protect the rights of the fetus seems to have had the reverse effect. Certainly the rights and personhood of the pregnant women were not taken into consideration under this system of targeted prosecution of pregnant women.

Although many professional organizations in the field of health care professional organizations now have position statements opposing drug screening of pregnant women for the intent of criminal prosecution (Foley, 2002), drug screening during the mother's birth experience, without the mother's consent, continues to be standard practice in many US hospitals. "Intrapartum" or newborn testing is assumed within the general consent for care, and most hospitals do not seek parental consent for newborn testing, citing its use as a medical diagnostic tool" (Washington State Regional Perinatal Outreach Program, 2003). In other words, when health care providers feel that an infant may be at risk for drug withdrawal and/or other adverse effects from exposure to drugs, they feel justified in ignoring the mother's right to informed consent and perform a drug screen without her knowledge. It is not uncommon, then, for a mother who has a history of drug abuse not to be informed about her infant's positive drug screen, the hospital's intent to notify Child Protective Services, and/or the intention to hold the infant for observation and/or treatment until this plan is a *fait accompli.* In other patient populations, health care providers would not consider taking action that would affect a woman's life so profoundly without informing her prior to initiating the plan. In addition, by taking action without the mother's knowledge or consent, the relationship of trust between patient and provider may be irreparably damaged, and the provider may lose his or her chance of facilitating the mother's entry into drug treatment. Establishing trust in the provider–client relationship is essential if a therapeutic relationship with meaningful communication is to evolve. When a client trusts a care provider, the client willingly places herself into a position of vulnerability and will be more apt to act on provider recommendations (Arnold & Boggs, 2003).

DISCRIMINATION

In this chapter, for the purpose of discussion, discrimination refers to the practice of treating a group of people with a specific characteristic(s) differently from another similar group of people. During the 1980s when Nancy Reagan launched her campaign entitled "Just Say No" (to drugs), "crack babies" were a prominent feature of American media stories, and criminal prosecutions of pregnant women with drug addictions occurred in record numbers (Reinarman & Levine, 1997). Interestingly, the number of crack babies, reported to be as high as 375,000 per year, was grossly exaggerated in the media. This only served to further stigmatize pregnant women who use drugs. As a result of this media attention, various charges were brought against pregnant women suspected of abusing drugs, including criminal mistreatment of a child, child abuse, child neglect, delivery of drugs to a minor, and even attempted murder (DeVille & Kopelman, 1998).

However, as Tillett & Osborne pointed out in their article on legal and ethical concerns, risks to the fetus are often competing (2001). For example, a pregnant woman may knowingly expose herself to an environmental hazard in her workplace because she cannot afford to lose her income and health care coverage. Currently our society does not prosecute a pregnant woman for knowingly exposing herself to an environmental teratogen or even to alcohol or cigarettes. According to the National Institute on Drug Abuse (NIDA), American women are almost 20 times more likely to drink alcohol or smoke cigarettes than to use cocaine during pregnancy (NIDA, 1995). The harmful effects from alcohol abuse, potentially resulting in irreversible brain damage to the fetus as well as other deformities, are well documented, and yet the lack of persecution of these women when compared with pregnant women who use illicit drugs is dramatic (Figdor & Kaeser, 1998).

In many populations, drug addiction is treated as a disease, and people are given the option of treatment. Conversely, a pregnant woman is often held to a higher standard of accountability for her actions because of the potential adverse effect to the fetus and is given jail time rather than treatment. In a 1989 Florida criminal prosecution case of a young pregnant woman named Jennifer Johnson, the judge presiding over the case stated that "pregnant addicts have a responsibility to seek treatment" and sentenced Ms. Johnson to 1 year of house arrest (Reinarman & Levine, 1997). This statement assumes what ethicists refer to as "duty of care" on the part of the pregnant woman or a moral and legal responsibility to ensure a healthy baby (Tillett & Osborne, 2001). The statement also implies that all pregnant women have access to contraception, prenatal care, and drug treatment. Unfortunately, for many women in the United States, access to basic health care services, as well as drug treatment, is sadly lacking. The availability of substance abuse treatment services for pregnant women has improved over the past decade, but demand continues to exceed supply, and it is not unusual for women to remain on waiting lists for weeks or months before being admitted to treatment (Fidgor & Kaeser, 1998). In some states, such as Idaho, there are no treatment programs available for pregnant women (Substance Abuse Issues Group, 2002).

Within the larger disenfranchised group of drug-abusing pregnant women is a group of women for whom additional causes of discrimination can be found: women of color. In their research on pregnant women who use illegal drugs in Florida, Whiteford & Vitucci (1997) found that incarceration is not a consequence for all pregnant addicts but, instead, reflects racial and/or ethnic and socioeconomic categories of prejudice. The authors found that pregnant women of color are 10 times more likely than white women to be prosecuted for illicit drugs. Whiteford & Vitucci found this statistic to be startling because drug use by pregnant minority women is comparable to such rates among white women.

In 1987, in an effort to protect the unborn, the Florida Department of Health and Rehabilitative Services issued a policy requiring mandatory reporting to the statewide Abuse Registry of all infants showing a positive urine screen. Yet only women who delivered at publicly funded hospitals were routinely screened for drug use, whereas private-paying patients seen outside county hospitals were not routinely screened for drugs (Whiteford & Vitucci, 1997). Whiteford & Vittuci stated that "our research suggests that laws jailing pregnant women for their addictions are concerned less with protecting the unborn than with punishing women for being poor, pregnant and addicted." (p. 1372).

SOCIOECONOMIC FACTORS

Violence in families and lack of social support affect a woman's sense of self and her coping mechanisms, leading to substance abuse as a method of coping (Kearney, 1999). Curry (1998) found that abused women used more alcohol and other drugs and had higher stress, lower self-esteem, and less partner support than did nonabused women. The lack of resources or skills to escape these environmental factors is of particular importance to women of color and/or women who live in poverty or are among the working poor (Kearney, 1999). Women, particularly women of color, are more likely than men to lack economic resources or employee benefits with which to purchase drug treatment, and they often are reluctant to leave their children in the care of others or risk losing custody (Kearney, 1999).

Sanders-Phillips (1998) emphasizes that policy makers and health care professionals need to examine the use of illicit drugs by women within the larger context of factors that affect health behaviors. Psychosocial and social variables such as social support, emotional support, and information sharing, as well as the provision of tangible goods and services, are associated with healthier lifestyle behaviors and choices (Sanders-Phillips, 1998). Conversely, lack of social support and higher levels of stress due to life events such as violence and poverty are associated with risky lifestyle behaviors such as alcohol, tobacco, and illicit drug use among women (Sanders-Phillips, 1998). Despite this information, a recent federal statute added to the Temporary Assistance for Needy Families Program (TANF) added a provision that denies individuals with drug felony convictions eligibility for food stamps and assistance from TANF unless the individual states enact legislation to opt out of or modify the ban (Paltrow et al., 2000). In addition, the statute states that if individuals violate any condition of their parole, they will be ineligible for TANF, food stamps, or supplemental security income (SSI) (Paltrow et al, 2000). On the surface, the statute seems reasonable; however, if a pregnant woman has been prosecuted, then, according to this statute, a relapse, which is a normal part of the addiction recovery process, will constitute a parole violation, and the pregnant or parenting woman will no longer be eligible for basic social supports. Our federal and state policies are adding to the stressful life events of this vulnerable population and possibly increasing their risky behavior choices, rather than facilitating positive social variables.

To compound this situation, Vazquez (2003) states that there is increasing evidence that prenatal (as well as postnatal) stressors, such as poverty, violence, and exposure to drugs, may lead to a permanent alteration of the normal physiology of neurotransmitter systems that mediate drug abuse and thus predispose the adult offspring of the stressed woman to self-administer psychochostimulants. In other words, the socioeconomic stresses that a pregnant women experiences are also experienced by her unborn child and may predispose that child to drug abuse later in life. During pregnancy, then, it is more important than ever for women who use drugs to receive assistance in locating treatment, safe housing, and health care for themselves, their unborn infants, and their other children.

SUMMARY

The title of this chapter refers to pregnant women who use drugs as a disenfranchised group; i.e., a group of people who have been deprived of basic rights and privileges. Loss of autonomy, discrimination, and socioeconomic variables unique to pregnancy serve to disenfranchise this vulnerable population. Much of the premise for this claim is based on the author's belief that not only is drug addiction a disease, rather than a lifestyle choice, but also that treatment, which includes care for the mother–baby dyad, should be readily available to all pregnant women who use drugs. The negative implications of drug abuse as well as other environmental factors for the mother and her infant are well documented, yet our current social, health, and political policies serve to further exacerbate these factors rather than diminish them. As health care providers, we are able to positively affect the health and well-being of the mother and her infant through the interventions we provide and by working to change social and political policy.

Implications for Practice

- ☐ Counsel pregnant women with regard to the adverse effects of alcohol, cigarettes, and illicit drugs.
- ☐ Establish hospital and clinic policies and procedures regarding screening and treatment referral that support the rights of the addicted pregnant woman while protecting the fetus and newborn.
- ☐ Use a reliable and valid questionnaire to screen *all* pregnant women for drug and alcohol use, regardless of race and socioeconomic status.
- ☐ Continue to offer and encourage prenatal care whether or not a substance-abusing pregnant woman has entered treatment.
- ☐ Always consider a woman to be at-risk for physical abuse when substance abuse is present and vice versa.

ACKNOWLEDGMENTS

The author wishes to acknowledge the support of the Women's Health Nursing Research Training Grant through the Center for Women's Health Research, University of Washington School of Nursing, in writing this chapter. In addition, special thanks to Marcia Killien, RN, PhD, FAAN, who is a true mentor as well as champion of nursing research in the area of women's health.

REFERENCES

Arnold, E., & Boggs, K. U. (2003). *Interpersonal relationships: Professional communication skills for nurses* (4th ed.). Philadelphia, PA: W. B. Saunders.

Curry, M. (1998). The interrelationships between abuse, substance use, and psychosocial stress during pregnancy. *Journal of Obstetric, Gynecologic, and Neonatal Nursing, 27*(6), 692–699.

DeVille, K. A., & Kopelman, L. M. (1998). Moral and social issues regarding pregnant women who use and abuse drugs. *Obstetrics and Gynecology Clinics of North America, 25*(1), 237–254.

Figdor, E., & Kaeser, L. (1998, October). Concerns mount over punitive approaches to substance abuse among pregnant women. *Guttmacher Report on Public Policy, 1*(5), 3–5.

Foley, E. M. (2002). Drug screening and criminal prosecution of pregnant women. *Journal of Obstetric, Gynecologic and Neonatal Nursing, 31,* 133–137.

Gabbe, S., Niebyl, J., & Simpson, J. (1996). *Obstetrics: Normal and problem pregnancies* (3rd ed.). St. Louis, MO: Hartcourt Health Sciences.

Gosten, L. (2001). The rights of pregnant women: The Supreme Court and drug testing. *Hastings Center Report, 31*(5), 8–9.

Kearney, M. (1999). *Perinatal impact of alcohol, tobacco, and other drugs.* Wilkes-Barre, PA: March of Dimes.

National Institute on Drug Abuse [NIDA]. (1995). Drug use during pregnancy. *NIDA Notes, 10*(1).

Newton, L. (1975). Humans and persons: A reply to Tristram Engelhardt. *Ethics, 85*(4), 332–336.

Paltrow, L., Cohen, D., & Carey, C. (2000). Governmental responses to pregnant women who use alcohol or other drugs: Year 2000 overview, part 1. *Women's Law Project and National Advocates for Pregnant Women,* October, 2000. Retrieved December 1, 2003, from *http://www.lindesmith.org/library/governmental_response_p1.cfm.*

Substance Abuse Issues Group. (2002). *Report to the governor's coordinating council for children and families, Idaho.* Retrieved December 5, 2003, from *http://www2.state.id.us/gcc/SubstanceAbuseRpt.*

Tillett, J., & Osborne, K. (2001). Substance abuse by pregnant women: Legal and ethical concerns. *Journal of Perinatal and Neonatal Nursing, 14*(4), 1–11.

UCLA Center for Vulnerable Populations. (2003). *Who are vulnerable populations?* Retrieved November 15, 2003, from *http://www.nursing.ucla.edu/cvpr/who-are-vulnerable.html.*

Vazquez, D. (2003). Maternal deprivation, brain stress circuits, and drug abuse. From *NIDA: The intersection of stress, drug abuse, and development.* Retrieved December 6, 2003, from *http://www.drugabuse.gov/MeetSum/stressabstracts.html.*

Washington State Regional Perinatal Outreach Program. (2003). *Maternal substance abuse screening initiative for providers.* Retrieved November 15, 2003, from *http://www.didyouask.org/clinical.*

Whiteford, L., & Vitucci, J. (1997). Pregnancy and addition: Translating research into practice. *Social Science Medicine, 44*(9), 1371–1380.

CHAPTER 31

Hepatitis B and Homeless Adolescents: Creating Educational Opportunities

Deborah Brown, Mary de Chesnay, and Debby A. Phillips

The number of homeless adolescents is increasing, and their health concerns are multiplying. Essential to the health of this community are awareness of common health problems and strategies to prevent illness. The incidence of hepatitis B among homeless adolescents, for example, is rising and has become a priority concern in this community. The hepatitis B virus (HBV), transmittable through any exchange of body fluids, causes a liver disease that can lead to jaundice, cirrhosis, liver failure, and liver cancer. Symptoms include jaundice, fatigue, fever, loss of appetite, nausea, vomiting, abdominal pain, and joint pain. Nurse practitioners working with this underserved population are in a position to help decrease health risks such as hepatitis B.

In this chapter, we describe a project designed to educate homeless adolescents about hepatitis B with a handout and educational video. The project and its description in this chapter fulfill the scholarly project requirement for the Seattle University master's degree in nursing, family nurse practitioner track. The project examines a health problem of relevance to advanced-practice nurses who work with vulnerable populations. Although such a project can take many forms, the choice here was to develop a video and handout that could be used both in future practice with homeless adolescents and by various agencies in the community already serving this population.

LITERATURE REVIEW

It is extremely difficult to achieve an accurate count of homeless people because of the nature of this transient and changing population. Although the number of homeless youths varies from night to night, estimates in King County, Washington, state that up to 2000 youths aged 12 to 24 are homeless, with 500 to 1000 teens homeless in Seattle each night. Furthermore, as extrapolated from national statistics, as many as 5000 youth aged 12 to 17 are homeless at some point during a year in King County. This number more than doubles if the 18- to 24-year-old age group is included, making as many as 10,000 adolescents homeless during a year in King County (Levine, 2001).

Homelessness is significantly associated with HBV infection (Alderman, Shapiro, Spigland, Coupey, Bashir, & Fox, 1998). Feldmann & Middleman (2003) found that "the prevalence and incidence of hepatitis B (HBV) and hepatitis C (HCV) are 10 to 12 times higher in homeless adolescents than among the general adolescent population" (p. 7). Moreover, Beech, Myers, & Beech (2002) found that 22% of homeless youth have positive serum markers of either hepatitis B or C, an alarmingly high figure.

In 2001, there were an estimated 79,000 new incidences of HBV infection in the United States (Center for Disease Control, 2002). The highest rate of infection was in the 20- to 29-year-old age group; however, in the homeless population, there are several other factors that increase the risk of acquiring HBV. Alderman et al. (1998) notes that common among homeless people, and homeless adolescents in particular, are a history of anal sex, anal receptive sex, prostitution, and sexual abuse, all of which are significantly associated with HBV infection. In addition, the most prominent risks for HBV infection among homeless adolescents are being homosexual or bisexual, having one or more episodes of crack use, being older (such as early 20s), and being male (Beech et al., 2002). Homeless youth are also at risk because they often do not attend school and may therefore miss opportunities to learn about HBV infection and prevention.

Homeless youths have an interest in learning techniques to reduce their risk of sexually transmitted infections (STIs) (Lifson & Halcon, 2001; Rew, Chambers, & Kulkarni, 2002). Rew et al. found that homeless teens in focus groups were eager to offer their suggestions for how to structure an STI educational program. They identified three main themes: need for knowledge, overcoming barriers, and respectful interventions. Most participants had some knowledge about STIs, but misinformation was also prevalent. Rew et al. found that educational needs included use of proper terminology, routes of transmission, signs and symptoms, and treatment options. Participants identified barriers that increase their STI risk such as present-moment attitudes (living in the present), feelings of invincibility, and the cost of condoms. Another barrier is drug and alcohol use, which reduces inhibitions and potentially increases unsafe behaviors. Moreover, the youths emphasized that respectful interventions are essential because they often feel that they are treated in a demeaning manner.

Although homeless youth have identified pamphlets and flyers as a "highly desirable" source of information (Rew et al., 2002, p. 172), the authors of such materials should keep in mind that a majority of homeless adolescents have less than a high school education (Lifson & Halcon, 2001) when writing the pamphlets so that the resulting document is geared to an appropriate level of understanding. In addition, pamphlet location is also important. In the study by Rew et al., focus group members asked that the pamphlets be placed in an inconspicuous place so they could avoid embarrassment when accessing them. However, flyers located in the room where the focus groups met were not noticed by participants, indicating that if the location is too discreet, the information may go unnoticed.

Despite the importance of hepatitis B education to public health, only 21% of the federally funded STI programs surveyed had developed and distributed written policies about preventing hepatitis B with vaccination, and only 27% had developed policies to encourage hepatitis B education activities (Fraser, Buffington, Lipson, & Meit, 2002). Although this lack of attention demonstrates the low priority status of hepatitis B infection, it also suggests significantly inadequate attention specifically addressing the needs of homeless adolescents. To begin to address this dearth of education and services, funds must be allocated to target homeless youth and providers, such as Healthcare for the Homeless. Professionals working with homeless youth need to be educated about health care concerns among homeless adolescents, safety and risky behaviors, and available community resources. In addition, homeless youth advocates are needed to seek wide improvements in health care, housing, and social services for this very vulnerable group (Feldmann & Middleman, 2003). Nurse practitioners have a responsibility to advocate for homeless youth by demanding and providing accessible and effective health care programs as well as hepatitis B education for adolescents and community health care providers.

Information about safer sex practices and safer intravenous (IV) drug use behaviors is much needed by the homeless adolescent community in order to prevent transmission of hepatitis B. Printed materials are an important component of educating this population about hepatitis B. These materials should be written at an appropriate reading level and should be made available in discreet locations that are accessible to young homeless people. Brief educational sessions may also prove helpful in teaching homeless adolescents about the risks and transmission of HBV and in subsequently reducing the incidence of risky behaviors and the rate of new infections. In addition, providing information about cessation of drug use as a risk reduction technique is essential. Furthermore, these youth often lack a regular health care provider. Health care access and available services should be part of this education to promote STI testing and general health care.

PROJECT PLAN

In order to address the lack of education about hepatitis B in the homeless adolescent community, Deborah Brown, the first author of this chapter, decided to create a handout and educational video about hepatitis B for distribution in local drop-in centers, shelters, and clinics serving homeless adolescents. In order to do this, she first conducted a literature search on the Internet and in medical journals. She then organized all of the pertinent information related to the description and sequelae of hepatitis B: modes of transmission, risk factors, and prevention into a Frequently Asked Question (FAQ) format. The handout she produced was was determined to be written at less than an 8th grade level by the Flesch-Kincaid Grade Level Analysis. FAQs included a variety of questions written in lay language appropriate to age. Two sample questions, with their answers, follow.

Why should I care about hepatitis B?

The liver is like the powerhouse of the body. It cleans out the waste in the body, keeping you healthy. When the liver is not working properly, the wastes and toxins are not being cleared out, and you will not feel well. Hepatitis B is the most common serious liver disease in the world. About 1 million people die every year from problems related to hepatitis B. It is 100 times more contagious than HIV (the virus that causes AIDS), which means that it is much easier to catch. Most new cases of hep B are in young people, like teenagers.

How can I protect myself?

There is a vaccination that works very well at protecting you from getting hepatitis B if you are exposed to it. A health care provider can give you a series of three shots that can prevent infection in almost everyone. Other ways to protect yourself are to use condoms for vaginal, anal, and oral sex every time. If you inject drugs, stop and get into a treatment program. If you can't stop, always use clean needles and works, and do not share them with anyone else. Do not share razors or toothbrushes, even if you know the person really well. When getting a tattoo or piercing, consider the risks and make sure that the tattoo artist or piercer cleans the equipment properly.

The 15-minute video script was based on this handout, paying special attention to presenting accurate information in a respectful manner, as requested by the homeless youth in the Rew et al. (2002) study. After the script was written, several non-nurses read through it and made suggestions about the content, language, and the appropriateness for homeless adolescents. The script was then edited based on these suggestions, and roles were assigned to each actor or actress in the video.

A friend of the author with a background in filmmaking worked as the videographer and editor for the project. Six friends who looked young participated as actors, and a date was set for filming. In the video, Deborah Brown portrayed an educator in a drop-in center for homeless adolescents. The actors (friends of the first author) portrayed homeless adolescents. The filming took place in an apartment made to look as much like a homeless drop-in center as possible. Artwork was removed from the walls, and a sign was displayed with "group rules." Each actor chose a seat in the room: on the couch, the chair, the beanbag, or the floor. Each participant signed a form granting permission to be videotaped and photographed for possible future distribution. The videographer signed a form granting permission to use the materials. First, the entire script was filmed once for rehearsal. Then each actor and actress filmed his or her portion of the video separately. These were later edited into a whole, along with some short clips and group shots that were added in as needed. The actors were compensated with pizza and beverages.

EVALUATION

At the end of the filming, the participants were asked their opinion of the project. The response was overwhelmingly positive. "It's much better than I thought it would be," said one actor. Another stated, "I'm really learning a lot." The group engaged in a lengthy conversation about hepatitis B, with the participants asking several in-depth questions that were beyond the scope of the video. For example, one participant asked about the transmission rate of hepatitis B with women who have sex with women. The participants all stated that this further increased their knowledge about hepatitis B and were grateful for the conversation.

Later, the film was edited with Final Cut Pro, a computer program. After each clip was viewed, the best takes were chosen for each piece. Smooth transitions were inserted between each clip, and a montage of the outtakes was created and set to music at the beginning of the film. After completing the editing, the group reconvened, and the final product was screened by the actors. After viewing the film, they gave verbal feedback about the video. "Very informative," "I didn't know much about it before," and "I learned a lot of new information about hep B by doing it" were some comments made by the participants. We then had further discussion about hepatitis B and other STIs and about the availability of current educational programs in the community.

After giving their verbal feedback, each actor and actress completed a written project evaluation, rating the effectiveness of several factors relating to the video. Each factor was rated on a Likert-type scale from 1 to 5. The following is an example of the type of questions and format used for the evaluation.

1. Was the material presented in a way that was easy to understand?

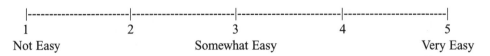

1	2	3	4	5
Not Easy		Somewhat Easy		Very Easy

On the written evaluations, everyone agreed that the material was presented in a way that was very easy to understand and that the nurse was very effective in portraying an instructor in the video. Most people said that the setting was somewhat representative of a drop-in center and that the video portrayed a respectful educational experience with homeless adolescents. All but one person stated that the video answered most, but not all, of their questions about hepatitis B. Overall, the response to the video was very positive; everyone said that the video would be a helpful tool for instructing homeless adolescents about hepatitis B. All participants agreed that written information, along with pictures, should be inserted throughout the film to highlight important information and enhance learning. Based on this suggestion, these were later inserted by the editor after the date of the screening.

Some aspects of this project went very smoothly. It was fortunate that there was a videographer/editor who was experienced in filmmaking and who was eager to work on this project. He had all of the necessary equipment, including cameras, lighting, computers, and the editing program. This made the production part of the project relatively easy. The actors and actresses were relaxed and comfortable talking about this potentially sensitive subject in front of a camera.

There are some things that could be done differently if the opportunity arises. For example, it would have been helpful to use real adolescents to read over the script and edit for content and language to be more certain that the script was written appropriately. The evaluation could not be completed the same day due to the need for editing. This meant that the group had to reconvene on a second day. It was not possible to tell the actors before the day of filming that it would require 2 days of their time, and one participant was unable to return for the viewing of the film. This also meant that the editing had to be done very quickly. With more time, a different final product might have resulted. Also, although the setting was not completely inappropriate, it would have been good to have created a space that was more representative of a homeless drop-in center than a living room. Ideally this could have been filmed at a shelter. Despite the changes that could have been made, the completed video was of good quality, and those involved are hopeful that it will prove to be a useful health education tool.

ACTION

The video will be distributed with the FAQ handout free of charge to those agencies that express interest and that serve homeless adolescents. It is hoped that these resources will educate homeless adolescents about hepatitis B, thereby decreasing the incidence of hepatitis B and related health problems in this community. Nurse practitioners are in a position to develop, distribute, and use these types of materials. Indeed, this can be an important aspect of commitment to the health of the community, especially to vulnerable populations.

REFERENCES

Alderman, E. M., Shapiro, A., Spigland, I., Coupey, S. M., Bashir, M., & Fox, A. S. (1998). Are there risk factors for hepatitis B infection in inner-city adolescents that justify prevaccination screening? *Journal of Adolescent Health: Official Publication of the Society for Adolescent Medicine, 22*(5) 389–393.

Beech, B. M., Myers, L., & Beech, D. J. (2002). Hepatitis B and C infections among homeless adolescents. *Family and Community Health, 25*(2), 28–36.

Feldmann, J., & Middleman, A. B. (2003). Homeless adolescents: Common clinical concerns. *Seminars in Pediatric Infectious Diseases, 14*(1), 6–11.

Fraser, M. R., Buffington, J., Lipson, L., & Meit, M. (2002). Hepatitis C prevention programs: Assessment of local health department capacity. *Journal of Public Health Management and Practice, 8,* 46–49.

Levine, S. (2001). *Data on homeless youth in King County.* Retrieved October 21, 2002, from *http://www.cityofseattle.net/humanservices/fys/homelessyouth/homelessykingcodata.htm.*

Lifson, A. R., & Halcon, L. L. (2001). Substance abuse and high-risk needle-related behaviors among homeless youth in Minneapolis: Implications for prevention. *Journal of Urban Health, 78,* 690–698.

Morbidity and Mortality Weekly Report-Centers for Disease Control. (2002). Achievements in public health: Hepatitis B vaccination—United States, 1982–2002. Retrieved November 22, 2003, from *http://www.cdc.gov/mmwr/preview/mmwrhtml/mm5125a3.htm.*

Rew, L., Chambers, K. B., & Kulkarni, S. (2002). Planning a sexual health promotion intervention with homeless adolescents. *Nursing Research, 51,* 168–174.

CHAPTER 32

Aboriginal Adolescents in Eastern Taiwan

Yun-Fang Tsai and Thomas K. S. Wong

The indigenous people who originally inhabited Taiwan are known as aborigines (natives). After people from mainland China immigrated to this island, some aborigines gradually moved from richer agricultural lands to less fertile areas. There are approximately 400,000 aborigines in Taiwan now. They include 10 different aboriginal tribes (see *http://visitnative.nat.gov.tw/group/ group.asp*), each with its own cultural practices. In general, their average household income is far below the average Taiwan farmer's income; their per capita income is less than 40% of that of the general population (Hsu, 1991). Moreover, their health status is worse than that of the rest of the Taiwanese population (Ko, Liu, & Hsieh, 1994).

About 162,000 Aborigines live in the eastern part of Taiwan, where they represent 25% of the population (Executive Yuan, 2000). In this area, the population consists of seven different tribes: Amis, Atayal, Bunun, Puyuma, Rukai, Paiwan, and Yami. Because of their cultural practices and characteristics, aboriginal people represent an important group in the health care system. Health promotion in aboriginal adolescents especially becomes a main focus for health care providers and researchers.

COMMON HEALTH PROBLEMS

Some studies have been done to explore the health problems among aboriginal adolescents in eastern Taiwan. Results indicated that this group is susceptible to chewing betel quid, smoking tobacco, drinking alcohol, and being adolescent mothers. All these factors can have a negative impact on health. We will emphasize betel quid chewing and pregnancy among adolescents in this chapter.

Areca Quid Chewing

Areca quid chewing is a popular habit in many countries (Kwan, 1976), especially in India, Southeast Asia, the Pacific Islands, and China. Areca quid chewing also has a history that goes back 1000 years in Taiwan, and it is a habit mainly of blue-collar workers or men with less education (Ko, Chang, Chang, & Hsieh, 1992). Excluding the fact that it provides feelings of well-being and helps overcome sensations of hunger and exhaustion (Wiesner, 1987), areca quid chewing is also a symbol of strength and machismo (Ko et al., 1992). Areca is an important

295

aboriginal sacrificial rite and is a part of their culture and customs. Some Taiwanese aborigines grow areca at home for their own consumption.

Because of the rapidly increasing population of chewers and the potential adverse effects chewing has on health, such as oral submucous fibrosis (Ko et al., 1992; Seedat & VanWyk, 1988a) and oral cancer (Seedat & VanWyk, 1988b)], areca quid chewing has become an important agenda for health authorities in Taiwan. Because the eastern part of Taiwan is in fourth place in Taiwan in betel sales, the issue of how to help these aboriginal adolescents keep away from chewing betel quid is very important there.

A previous study (Tsai, Wong, & Chen, 2002) surveyed 1461 junior high students in eastern Taiwan. Group 1 consisted of 896 nonaboriginal students and group 2 of 565 aboriginal students. These students were asked to fill out a questionnaire anonymously. The lifetime prevalence rate (49.8%) of areca quid chewing among the aboriginal students was derived from the percentages of those who were current chewers (9.7%), who had tried it but not become regular users (32.7%), and who had used it regularly and quit (7.4%). The difference between the lifetime prevalence rate of areca quid chewing between nonaboriginal students (20.8%) and aboriginal students (49.8%) was stark. Moreover, the prevalence of areca chewing was significantly different between boys and girls among the nonaboriginal group but not the aboriginal.

In the aboriginal student group, a student who used tobacco and alcohol was a likely candidate for acquiring the chewing habit. Analysis of the family traits indicated that an areca quid chewer is likely to grow areca at home and have family members and relatives as areca quid chewers. Analysis of the school environmental factors indicated that an areca quid chewer is likely to have close friends who are chewers and not to have close friends who disagree with the chewing habit. A logistic regression model confirmed that aboriginal student chewers are likely to grow areca at home, are tobacco smokers and alcohol drinkers, and have family members and close friends as chewers.

Tobacco smoking was found to be the most important risk factor for areca quid chewing in this study (Tsai et al., 2002). The carcinogenic effects of smoking have been shown to be synergistically enhanced by areca quid chewing (Warnakulasuriya, 1992). Alcohol consumption is another cofactor in the etiology of oral cancer (Binnie, Rankin, & Mackenzie, 1983). Together with areca quid chewing, it is deleterious to oral health (Binnie et al., 1983). In this study (Tsai et al., 2002), more than 50% of students had experienced alcohol consumption, and 40% of aboriginal students had experienced tobacco smoking. In addition, 26.3% of aboriginal students were shown to have had concurrent experiences of alcohol consumption, tobacco smoking, and areca quid chewing. The potential for developing oral cancer and further substance abuse by these students cannot be ignored. Recently, researchers (Yang, Chung, Yang, Hus, & Ko, 2001) also found that the risk of adverse birth outcomes such as low birth weight at full-term, preterm labor, and fetal malformation was five times higher among betel quid-chewing women than in nonusers after adjusting for maternal age. The impact of betel quid chewing on health is quite severe and long-term.

As stated by the authors (Tsai et al., 2002), there currently are some regulations for using illicit drugs (e.g., opium, morphine, heroin, amphetamines) in Taiwan. A monetary penalty or imprisonment is imposed when people are arrested. School education plays an important role in emphasizing the drawbacks of smoking, drinking, chewing areca quid, or illicit drug use. Those who drop out cannot benefit from such education. Moreover, a systematic intervention strategy has not yet been implemented.

Based on the results of this study, the authors (Tsai et al., 2002) suggested that a prevention program is desperately needed for the well-being of future generations. It should focus on 1) increasing adolescents' knowledge of substance abuse, 2) enhancing the ability to resist the pressure from peers, 3) improving adolescents' self-confidence, and 4) reducing the rate of alcohol, cigarette, and areca quid consumption.

ADOLESCENT PREGNANCY

Early pregnancy can have harmful effects on a girl in physical, social, and economic terms. It increases the fertility rate substantially and increases infant mortality, poverty, and downward social mobility for women (Remez, 1989). Adolescents are also a group at risk for acquiring HIV infection and sexually transmitted diseases (Hinhson, Strunin, & Berlin, 1990; MacDonald et al., 1990) because they have multiple sexual partners, frequent sexual activity, and unprotected sexual behavior. Finding ways to help young people form appropriate sexual attitudes and become adept in performing safer sex practices has become an urgent task for health care providers.

In 1985, a newspaper (Fang, 1985) revealed that one aboriginal village, Show-Lin, in Hualien County in eastern Taiwan, had a secret. Aboriginal parents in that village had been selling their adolescent daughters. Many of them became prostitutes. In the village where this was most prevalent, nearly 6 of every 10 households had sold their daughters into prostitution (Fang, 1985). Following this report, many journalists and research scientists went to this village to explore the phenomenon. They found that severe poverty was the main reason for this practice (Fang, 1985; Hsu, 1988).

Even 15 years later, adolescent sexual behavior remains a significant problem in eastern Taiwan. In 1999, adolescent women between the ages of 15 and 19 years accounted for 9 to 9.5% of the total births in Taiwan's eastern counties (Executive Yuan, 2000). Based on a preliminary study in the eastern area (Tseng, 1998), more than 50% of adolescent mothers with unplanned pregnancies were aborigines. Promoting safer sexual practices in aboriginal adolescents has become an urgent task in eastern Taiwan.

Using aboriginal nurses to provide information on sexual behavior may have potential as a means of promoting healthy sexual practices among aborigines. We have conducted a qualitative research design to explore aboriginal nurses' perceptions of reasons for the high prevalence of aboriginal teenage pregnancy (Tsai & Wong, in press) and potential strategies for resolving this problem (Tsai & Wong, 2003). A total of 14 aboriginal nurses participated in the intensive individual interviews, and 12 aboriginal nurses participated in the focus group interviews. Content analysis was used to analyze the data, and results were highlighted as follows.

Reasons for High Prevalence of Teenage Pregnancy

Six themes were identified in this study (Tsai & Wong, in press). These were restructuring of the family, communication difficulties, changes in social norms, discontinuity in school teaching, misuse of information, and vicious cycle.

Restructuring of the Family

Many participants mentioned that because of economic difficulties and trouble finding a job in eastern Taiwan, many aboriginal parents have left their villages and sought employment in the large cities, such as Taipei. Their children remain in the villages where they live with grandparents. In general, the children see their parents infrequently, because their parents work long hours in order to both support themselves in the cities as well as send money back to their family in their home community. For many aboriginal children, their immediate family members are their grandparents and siblings.

Communication Difficulties

Communication difficulties can be divided into two parts, language and ideas. Beginning in 1950, all schools in Taiwan were required to use Mandarin to teach their students. All media had to deliver their information only in Mandarin. This situation has not changed. Because of this policy, aboriginal adolescents may not have had the opportunity to learn their traditional language (or dialect), and as a result many are unable to speak it. On the other hand, their grandparents can only speak the traditional language. On the other hand, their grandparents can only speak the traditional language, having never learned Mandarin. This has created a situation where the generations experience great difficulty in communicating with each other. Although some of these families understand each other's language, their ideas are quite different across the generations. Grandparents hold more conservative ideas, while aboriginal adolescents are more open to new ideas.

Changes in Social Norms

Aboriginal tribes used to have their own specific social norms. For some tribes, their gods or ancestors held unlimited power; tribesmen respected their gods and ancestors and followed the regulations of the tribe. The chief was the most powerful person in the tribe. In recent times, for most of these tribes the traditional norms have been weakened or even disregarded. For example, in the past, premarital sex was banned because this behavior violated the morals of their gods or ancestors and was regarded with disgust by tribesmen. Such tribal norms do not exist in some tribes now.

In addition, organized religion also used to play an important role in aborigine society in Taiwan. In the past, the Christian church provided food and relief to community members because of poverty. The church gradually became a part of their lives. Aboriginal children were taught modern social norms through fellowship and by their ministers or priests. In recent times, the quest for money seems to have replaced the church in importance as a new social norm. Many aborigines express great concern about earning money. Money has at least two meanings—one is related to power and respect, and the other is related to compensation. For compensation, it is related to parents' intention. They think that they cannot go to school to become educated, but they can provide the money that allows their children to have a good education. Unfortunately, adolescents don't understand the meaning of their parents' behavior.

Peer pressure also influences adolescent sexual behaviors. Without the concept of self-protection and the prevention of pregnancy through the use of contraceptives, abortion seems to be an inevitable phenomenon.

Discontinuity in School Teaching

The quality of teachers and teaching seems to be causing difficulty for some aboriginal tribes. The high frequency of turnover in teachers has disrupted the continuity of students' education. As a result, children feel that they are being abandoned and that no one cares about them. In addition, schoolteachers are not well prepared to teach human sexuality.

Misuse of Information

In today's highly technical environment, it is very easy for adolescents to access information from the Internet, as well as through books, magazines, videotapes, and television programs. Most communities in Taiwan have access to electricity; most aboriginal families watch television frequently (Hsu, 1991). Videocassette recorders and personal computers are available in schools, libraries, and private households. It also is a very popular pastime for adolescents to frequent Internet cafes after school. All of these media can have an impact on their attitudes toward sexuality and sexual behaviors.

Vicious Cycle

The experiences related in this study show that most aboriginal adolescent girls get married after they find out they are pregnant. The majority of their husbands also are adolescents. It is difficult for young couples to support themselves financially without the help of their families. They may need to quit school and leave their hometown to earn money. The same thing may also happen to their children. This then becomes a vicious cycle. Women who were teenage mothers often find their daughters also become pregnant during adolescence. Establishing a family may not be a bad thing for adolescents who are seeking a caring relationship in their lives. Their husband or wife may provide some love that they previously felt they had not received and are eager to obtain. The search for this emotional support is one reason to form a family; however, a major problem for these young families is how to support themselves.

Resolving the Problem of Aboriginal Adolescent Pregnancy

Nine possible methods of dealing with the issue of teen pregnancy were identified (Tsai & Wong, 2003). They can be divided into three aspects: family, school, and society.

Family Aspect

Enhancing the sexual education of parents. Most participants believed that the family plays an important role with adolescent pregnancy among aboriginals. If parents can talk and discuss sex with their children, sex may not be a puzzle for adolescents. It can reduce their curiosity about sex and prevent trial and error experimentation. Therefore, parents' sex education is necessary and must be addressed.

Enhancing the understanding of older people about sex education in villages. As stated before, for many aboriginal children, their immediate family members are their grandparents and siblings. Based on participants' information, older people in villages seem to hold conservative ideas about sex. They believe that sex is unclean and disgusting. Therefore, they will not discuss this issue with their grandchildren. Without an open channel for discussion on sex, their children may not have a role model for learning about appropriate sexual attitudes and behavior. How to change the ideas of older people in villages is considered a key point for reducing the high pregnancy rate of aboriginal adolescents.

School Aspect

Improving sex education in school. Most participants believed that school is also an important place for aboriginal adolescents. Unfortunately, sex education has not been emphasized in the curriculum. Although textbooks have a chapter about the reproductive system, some teachers ask students to read this by themselves. In addition to the reproductive system, participants suggested adding content about condom use, the way to use contraception, and how to calculate the safe period.

Offering interrelationship courses for adolescents. As mentioned before, communication difficulty is a severe problem in the aboriginal family. Feelings of loneliness are strong for many adolescents, and some constantly seek the feeling of being cared for. It is easy then for them to have an intimate sexual relationship, and the probability of getting pregnant is increased. Moreover, peer pressure also influences adolescents' sexual behavior. Participants suggested that this problem could be resolved by offering a course on interpersonal relationships for adolescents. Helping adolescents reconsider the meaning of a close relationship, learning new ways to develop interpersonal relationships, and resisting peer pressure should be objectives of the curriculum.

Offering courses on gender issues for adolescents. Some participants mentioned that adolescents are at a stage of feeling curious about the opposite sex. How to interact with each other appropriately is a concern. Participants suggested that adolescents should be taught about respecting their own bodies and that their curiosity about the opposite sex should be explored. In addition, how to interact with the opposite sex is also important. The content should be included in the course on gender issues for these adolescents.

Improving sex education training of teachers. Many participants indicated that their schoolteachers did not teach any sex education, even though the textbook used did include a chapter on the reproductive system. The effectiveness of preparation of teachers on sex education is therefore questionable, and how to enhance their abilities to teach sex education is an essential topic.

Social Aspect

Advocating the sense of family in church. Participants suggested that the church would play an important role in discussing the meaning of a family. Adolescents then might understand the responsibility of being parents. Before they make a decision to form a family or have a baby, they could assess their abilities to fulfill the responsibility. This might reduce the pregnancy rate among adolescents.

Advocating social norms in church. Participants still believed that the church could play an important role in advocating the customary social norms. They expected people to understand that money is not everything, that children's education is important and takes time, and that parents must pay attention to it.

Discussing appropriate sexual behavior in adolescent church fellowships. Participants pointed out that peer support could be used in a positive way to prevent adolescent pregnancy. Appropriate sexual behavior could be advocated through church fellowships. Adolescents could discuss and share their concerns with others, and the support from others could help them reject inappropriate sexual behavior and avoid pregnancy.

CONCLUSION

Aborigines form the vulnerable portion of the population in Taiwan. The changes that have occurred in the aboriginal communities have resulted in health issues and concerns that must be addressed in the context of their own culture as well as the development of the Taiwanese majority society. Nurses, being the first point of contact with this vulnerable group, should acquaint themselves with different strategies for addressing these issues or concerns. With their effort, our society will gradually move toward health for all, no matter whether we are a minority or majority.

REFERENCES

Binnie, W. H., Rankin, V., & Mackenzie, I. C. (1983). Etiology of oral squamous cell carcinoma. *Journal of Oral Pathology, 12,* 11–29.

Executive Yuan. (2000) *1999 Taiwan-Fukien demographic fact book.* Taipei: Republic of China.

Fang, B. (1985, December 9). From different perspectives to talk about the consultation of aborigines. *Chinese Newspaper.*

Hinhson, R.W., Strunin, L., & Berlin, B. M. (1990). Acquired immunodeficiency syndrome transmission: Changes in knowledge and behaviors among teenagers, Massachusetts stateside survey, 1986 to 1988. *Pediatrics, 85,* 24–29.

Hsu, M. (1988). *A study of aboriginal parents' values: Using Show-Lin village of Haulein county as an example.* Unpublished master's thesis, Don-Hai University, Tai Chung, Taiwan.

Hsu, M. (1991). *Culture, self, and adaptation: The psychological anthropology of two Malayo-Polynesian groups in Taiwan* (p. 24). Taipei, Taiwan: Academia Sinica.

Ko, Y. C., Chang, T. A., Chang, S. J., & Hsieh, S. F. (1992). Prevalence of betel quid chewing habit in Taiwan and related sociodemographic factors. *Journal of Oral Pathological Medicine, 21,* 261–264.

Ko, Y. C., Liu, B. H., Hsieh, S. F. (1994). Issues on aboriginal health in Taiwan. *Kaohsiung Journal of Medical Sciences, 10,* 337–351.

Kwan, H. W. (1976). A statistical study on oral carcinomas in Taiwan with emphasis on the relationship with betel nut chewing: A preliminary report. *Journal of Formosan Medical Association, 75,* 497–505.

MacDonald, N. E., Wells, G. A., Fisher, W. A., Warren, W. K., King, M. A., Doherty, J. A., et al. (1990). High-risk STD/HIV behavior among college students. *Journal of the American Medical Association, 263,* 3155–3159.

Remez, L. (1989). Adolescent fertility in Latin America and the Caribbean: Examining the problem and the solution. *Internal Family Planning Perspectives, 15,* 144–148.

Seedat, H. A., & VanWyk, C. W. (1988a). Betel-nut chewing and submucous fibrosis in Durban. *South Africa Medical Journal, 74,* 568–571.

Seedat, H. A., & VanWyk, C. W. (1988b) Betel chewing and dietary habits of chewers without and with submucous fibrosis and with concomitant oral cancer. *South Africa Medical Journal, 74,* 572–575.

Tsai, Y. F., & Wong, T. K. S. (2003). Strategies for resolving aboriginal adolescent pregnancy in eastern Taiwan. *Journal of Advanced Nursing, 41,* 351–357.

Tsai, Y. F., & Wong, T. K. S. (In press). Aboriginal adolescents' pregnancy in eastern Taiwan. *Western Journal of Nursing Research.*

Tsai, Y. F., Wong, T. K. S. & Chen, S. C. (2002). Prevalence and related risk factors of areca quid chewing among junior high students in eastern Taiwan. *Public Health, 116,* 190–194.

Tseng, L. (1998). The adjustment of maternal role, stress and social support among adolescents' mothers in Hualien. Unpublished master's thesis, Tzu Chi Medical College, Hualien, Taiwan.

Warnakulasuriya, K. A. A. S. (1992). Smoking and chewing habits in Sri Lanka: Implications for oral cancer and precancer. In P. C. Gupta, J. E. Hamner, III, & P. R. Murti (Eds.). *International symposium on control of tobacco-related cancers and other diseases* (pp. 113–118). Bombay: Oxford University Press.

Wiesner, D. M. (1987). Betel-nut withdrawal. *Medical Journal of Australia, 146,* 453.

Yang, M. S., Chung, T. C., Yang, M. J., Hsu, T. Y., & Ko, Y. C. (2001). Betel quid chewing and risk of adverse birth outcomes among aborigines in eastern Taiwan. *Journal of Toxicology and Environmental Health, 64,* 465–472.

CHAPTER 33

Vulnerability Among Hospitalized Older Adults

Anna Zisberg and Heather M. Young

The population of our world is aging, and persons aged 85 years or older are the fastest growing segment (Health United States, 2002). Since 1990, the number of older Americans has increased by 12%. In the year 2000, persons aged 65 years or over accounted for 12.4% of the general US population (Health United States, 2002). These numbers will nearly double by the year 2030 when 20% of the population will be 65 years or older. Both the total number and the proportion of older adults is increasing. With greater longevity, the potential period of living with a chronic illness or disability has also increased. As a growing population and as the most significant health care consumers, persons over age 65 are becoming a more important focus of nursing and other health professions.

THE ISSUE OF FRAILTY

Frail hospitalized older adults are the focus of this chapter. In particular, definitions and risks for frailty will be described, and the relationship between hospitalization and frailty will be explored. Finally, nursing interventions for hospitalized elders will be presented.

Various authors in various fields have applied different definitions of frailty to diverse populations, yet currently there is no agreed-upon precise definition. However, Markle-Reid & Browne (2003), in a comprehensive analysis of the concept, identified seven indicators of frailty that recurred throughout the literature:

1. Functional impairment and dependency on others for activities of daily living
2. Poor physical health (chronic or acute illnesses)
3. Disability
4. Lack of strength and resilience
5. Poor mental health/functioning (cognitive impairment or depression)
6. Need for long-term care (to meet basic needs)
7. Old age (usually 85 years or older)

Fried et al. (2001) offer a slightly different set of criteria for frailty. These authors define frailty as the presence of three or more of the following criteria: unplanned weight loss (10 pounds or more in a year), weakness, poor endurance and energy, and slowness and low activity levels. The lack of a consistent definition yields a wide range of estimates of the prevalence and incidence of frailty. Fried et al. claim the prevalence of frailty is around 7% in older adults aged 65 years or more, yet Stolee & Rockwood (1981) report a frailty rate of 27% with a similar reference population.

A Working Definition of Frailty

For the purpose of this chapter, frailty will be discussed in terms of the potential for functional decline for various reasons. In order to be considered frail, a person must either suffer from a number of functional threats to independence (although no actual limitation needs to occur) or demonstrate reduced reserve capacity based on physical evaluation tests (e.g., declined upper extremity strength).

Risk Factors Related to Frailty

In their review, Markle-Reid & Brown (2003) identified six major conceptual models explaining the nature and occurrence of frailty. Three of them claim that the source of frailty is predominantly biological/physiological. Frailty may result from loss of skeletal muscle mass (Walston & Fried, 1994), reduction in aerobic capacity and metabolic changes (Campbell & Buchner, 1997), and problems with "structural (tissue) integrity," which refers to dysfunction resulting from disuse (Bortz, 1993). Two additional models bring in psychological and personal factors that pertain to attitudes (toward health), cognition, and spirituality (Raphael et al., 1995; Rockwood, Fox, Stolee, Robertson, & Beattie, 1994). The last model reviewed by Markle-Reid & Brown (2003) asserts that frailty is a social by-product of the interaction between older persons and their caregivers as determined by social norms, roles, and beliefs (Kaufman, 1994).

Stuck, Walthert, Nikolaus, Bula, Hohmann, & Becket (1999) conducted a comprehensive meta-analysis of 1283 articles, including empirical studies, in the field of frailty and functional status deterioration, looking for patterns identifying leading indicators and risk factors. Among the leading risk factors identified by the authors were depression (even when controlling for other intervening factors), alcohol consumption (in high dosage), cognitive impairment (especially orientation and memory loss), low physical activity, poor self-rated health status, smoking (both current and former), low frequency of social contact, both high and low body mass index (both extreme gain and loss of weight), and poor self-reported vision. Two additional risk factors that were slightly less predictive yet significant enough to mention were the number of medicines consumed and the incidence of falls in the past.

A group of additional background factors seem to play a significant role in the phenomenon of frailty. The ones that were found especially relevant are age, ethnicity, poverty, and lower educational attainment. Each was found independently to contribute to the risk of frailty (Johnson & Smith, 2002).

Frailty and Vulnerability

Data (provided by Medicare) reviewing the causes of mortality during a 7-year period identified frailty as an antecedent of death (47%). The typical trajectory of frailty is described as a steady progression of disability, with eventual complications such as pneumonia for about half of the population. In other words, frailty is one of the most substantial indicators of functional deterioration and often results in a progressive process ending in death (Lunney, Lynn, & Hogan, 2002; Young, 2003).

Frailty is also associated with an increase in instances and duration of hospitalization, nursing home placement, and greater use of formal and informal home services. This, in turn, places additional burdens on older persons, their caregivers, and health care resources (Gill et al, 2003; Kao & Stuifbergen, 1999). An analysis of health care expenditures shows that 27.4% of each year's Medicare expenditure is incurred by 5% of Medicare enrollees who died that year, suggesting a preexisting condition of frailty and high utilization by this at-risk group (Lunney et al., 2002).

Frailty is a dynamic condition, constantly evolving and developing. In this respect frailty constitutes the potential for deterioration in health and functional status. By considering frailty a risk factor for these changes, one assumes it does not necessarily and directly lead to the aforementioned adverse health outcomes. Hence, frailty may be amenable to intervention to reduce the negative sequelae of this condition. There are frail older adults who lead productive functional lives, but by virtue of their frailty, they are more vulnerable to a range of moderating factors that may "push" them beyond functionality and trigger a process of deterioration.

HOSPITALIZATION AS A FACTOR IN FRAILTY

Effects of Disease and Medical Interventions

Frail older adults are disproportionately represented as the largest group of consumers both within the health care system as a whole and as recipients of nursing care in particular. They have a higher frequency of primary care visits, consume 50% of all hospital care, use over 80% of home care services, and occupy 90% of all nursing home beds in the United States (Mezey & Fulmer, 1998). Chronic and acute health conditions commonly lead to hospitalization and are also factors that may trigger a downward spiral of function. Increased frailty and functional decline may result directly from certain health conditions (e.g., stroke, fractured femur) or they may be iatrogenic, resulting from health-related interventions (e.g., medication side effects, surgical intervention that may limit mobility and require a long period of recovery/rehabilitation) (Kane, Ouslander, & Abrass, 2004).

Effects of Hospitalization Itself

A less frequently acknowledged factor is the effect of hospitalization itself, beyond the effects of disease process and interventions. Some patients are admitted to hospitals with diagnoses that typically do not directly lead to general deterioration (e.g., pneumonia, urinary tract infection), yet they demonstrate general functional decline after a hospital stay. In other words, in some cases, as the health condition is cured, a new kind of deterioration is created, resulting from the hospital stay itself. This is a significant problem for hospitalized older adults. Of hospitalized elderly patients, 30–50% decline in their functional status during acute hospitalization (Sager & Rudberg, 1998).

Research on the adverse effects of hospitalization on the elderly population emerged in the early 1980s. McVey, Becker, & Saltz (1985) reported that approximately 30% of elderly patients in acute hospitals developed additional disabilities in activities of daily living (ADLs) while still hospitalized. A high prevalence of "new" disabilities in hospitalized older patients was demonstrated in a 1982 survey of 279 patients admitted to a community hospital. More than half of the patients aged 75 years and over required assistance with ADLs (Warshaw et al., 1982). Ten years later a prospective study on acutely ill medical patients conducted within the Hospital Outcomes Project for the Elderly (HOPE) in five hospitals nationwide yielded more scientifically robust results. Of 1279 hospitalized medical patients 70 years of age and older with nondisabling diagnoses, 32% experienced a functional decline in ADLs and 41% experienced a decline in instrumental ADLs at hospital discharge compared with their functional status 2 weeks before admission. Only half of the patients that showed decreases in functional status recovered fully as far as 3 months after discharge (Margitic, Inouye, & Thomas, 1993).

Currently, despite numerous past articles, technological advances in medicine and nursing, policies that limit hospital stays, and a substantial increase in professional attention to this subject, recent studies show approximately the same ratio of functional decline in hospitalized elders that there has always been. Counsell et al. (2000) reported functional decline in 35% of elderly patients in general medical units. Inouye, Bogardus, Baker, Leo-Summers, & Cooney (2000) showed a 26% mental functional decline and a 33% physical functional decline in the very same population. The risk factors leading to functional deterioration during a hospital stay (e.g., low cognitive status, prior functional decline, depression) also reflect the definitions and risks for frailty.

A variety of factors have been suggested to explain the role of hospitalization in the deterioration of frail older adults (Palmer, Counsell, & Landfeld, 1998; St. Pierre, 1998). These include the quality of care provided, organizational structures and culture, and the hospital environment itself. Suboptimal care can create and foster dependency. Age biases potentially "allow" for functional deterioration (e.g., incontinence, disorientation) by permitting functional loss among the elderly to be viewed as "normal" and "expected." Hospital cultures may put safety issues before the well-being and comfort of patients. Hospital routines can disrupt personal habits and routines, for example, waking patients up in the night to draw blood and having bathing and toileting schedules that do not reflect patient preferences. Finally, the depersonalization of patients, exaggerated bed rest, and a dramatic change in the environment are linked with functional decline.

Reducing Functional Decline in the Hospitalized Frail

Three major types of interventions targeting the prevention of functional decline of frail elders during acute hospitalization have emerged during the last 20 years: geriatric consultation, acute care units for the elderly, and various nurse-driven interventions.

Geriatric Consultation

Geriatric consultation is carried out by physician specialists or multidisciplinary teams, usually for target populations at high risk for functional decline. It is aimed at improving patient outcomes in medical and/or surgical units. The consultation process is focused on the restoration of patient function and on comprehensive discharge planning as well as on the management of certain geriatric conditions that are considered risk factors for frailty (e.g., decubitus ulcers, confusion). In some cases, standardized criteria have been developed to target frail hospitalized patients for geriatric consultation. Winograd et al. (1991) developed a set of screening criteria including confusion, dependence in the performance of an ADL, polypharmacy (more than six medications), disabling chronic illness, and a stressed care-giving system. Unfortunately, studies that examined this model of intervention and screening failed to show a positive impact on functional improvement when ADLs were used as the outcome criterion (Fretwell et al., 1990). Indeed, the overall effectiveness of this intervention remains unclear. Although many studies showed some effect on patients' functional status (Thomas, Brahan, & Haywood, 1993), others, based on large-scale samples, failed to show any change in functional decline (Reuben et al., 1995).

Acute Care Units for the Elderly

Acute care units for the elderly (ACEs) are an intervention strategy based on a multidisciplinary collaborative approach and patient-centered care. The ACE intervention generally involves specially designed units that provide a modified environment aimed at facilitating patient orientation and independence. The modifications of the physical environment may include carpets on the floors, calendars and clocks in sight to help with orientation, and directional signs to assist with navigation. Beds with floor lighting promote safety for transfers at night, and unnecessary clutter is removed from rooms and hallways. A large common activity room often serves as the hub of the unit, encouraging dining outside of rooms, socializing, and exercising. The units are intended for at-risk populations, identified in advance or upon admission.

These units focus care on relevant risk factors, paying special attention to nursing assessment and care plus specialized medical review protocols that stress nonpharmacological interventions. Primary care nurses have an expanded role in such units, being in charge of multidimensional assessment at the patient's admission, managing care throughout the hospital stay, serving as guides to other health professionals, and tailoring care to individual needs. Assessment is conducted daily by means of an interdisciplinary round. The focus is on improving or at least maintaining self-care abilities, continence, nutrition, mobility, sleep, and skin integrity. These units also offer careful, improved discharge plans and policies that anticipate gradually improving levels of functioning after discharge and match recommendations and interventions accordingly. Home planning begins with the patient and an informal network at the beginning of admission and is ongoing throughout the process of hospitalization to optimize the transition of care (Palmer et al., 1998).

An overall assessment of ACEs derived from numerous studies supported the validity and effectiveness of the ACE intervention, despite a few findings showing little or insignificant overall change (Counsell, Landefeld, & Palmer, 1996; Counsell et al., 2000; Landefeld, Palmer, Kresevic, Fortinsky, & Kowal, 1995). The most outstanding and unique achievements of this approach to care are in succeeding not only to diminish readmission and increase nursing home discharges but also to improve functional status upon and up to a month after discharge, compared with a control group (Covinsky, Fortinsky, Palmer, Kresevic, & Landefeld, 1997; Landefeld et al., 1995). The next steps in the ACE program implementation and evaluation will be to adapt the program to the steadily growing older population and to demonstrate cost-effectiveness on this larger scale.

Nurse-Driven Interventions

Nursing is taking a more central role in alleviating functional decline in older adults by introducing novel interventions. Most are in early stages of development and implementation and have yet to be thoroughly tested. In this chapter, the most promising two will be discussed, and others will briefly be mentioned.

The Geriatric Resources Nurse (GRN) model incorporates geriatric education, regularly scheduled geriatric clinical rounds with the geriatric care team, and routine monitoring for common geriatric syndromes, using a new role, the unit-based geriatric resources nurse. GRNs are staff nurses who acquire knowledge in gerontological nursing and serve as resources on gerontological care to the unit nursing staff. Besides providing direct care and supporting other nurses' work in the units, the GRN coordinates communication among primary nurses and the interdisciplinary team that includes advanced-practice nurses in geriatrics, physicians, and other health professionals (Francis, Fletcher, & Simon, 1998; Inouye, Acampora et al., 1993; Turner, Lee, Fletcher, Hudson, & Barton, 2001). The model introduces therapeutic protocols to manage the most common syndromes in older adult patients such as fall risk, urinary incontinence, sleep disturbance, impaired mobilization, and lowered functional status. The role of the GRNs has been adopted by many sites nationwide (Francis et al., 1998; Inouye, Acampora et al.,1993; Lopez, Delmore, Ake, Kim, Golden, & Bier, 2002; Phaneuf, 1996; Turner et al., 2001). The model is actually based on the belief that nurses are the health professionals who are the closest to the patients and hence are the most appropriate ones to take charge of managing patient outcomes in these settings. Two experimental studies evaluated the outcomes of this type of intervention, and both showed improvement in functional status upon discharge as a result of the interventions described. (Inouye, Wagner et al., 1993; Turner et al., 2001).

The second model is the Transitional Care model (Naylor, 2000; Naylor, Brooten, Jones, Lavizzo-Mourey, Mezey, & Pauly, 1994). The definition of transitional care is "safe and timely transfer of patient from one level of care to another, and from one type of setting to another" (Naylor, 2000, p. 1). The model was developed as an attempt to cope with shortening hospital stays in which care continuity and quality can be compromised. The model puts clinical experts at the center of patient care, placing them in charge of managing the continuity of interventions across settings (usually in the transition from hospital environment to home or nursing home). Services are provided by the nurse practitioners responsible for discharge planning both while the patient is in the hospital and when the patient goes home. This home care is accomplished through nurse visits in the period following discharge. It is important to note that the same nurse who planned the discharge provides the follow-up services. Protocols are evidence based and aimed especially at meeting the needs of frail adults and their caregivers.

An expansive long-term series of studies of this approach demonstrated a significant reduction in readmission rates and cost of care, but no differences were found in patient- and family-related outcomes such as satisfaction, depression, and functional status (Naylor et al., 1994; Naylor et al., 1999). This promising approach has yet to be widely adopted and discussed in the literature.

Two additional approaches to intervention are compelling. One creates special geriatric units and/or subunits under the full supervision of nurses. This approach aims at early rehabilitation, e.g., starting rehabilitation concurrently with treatment for the admitting condition. Early rehabilitation requires more nursing staff, and additional skilled human resources are a tenet of this approach. Nurses are more independent in decision making about patient rehabilitation needs and activities than they are in the previously mentioned interventions. Two studies used this approach (Boyer, Chang, & Gipner, 1986; Hamilton & Lyon, 1995). Both found significant improvements in functional status in patients admitted to those units compared with patients admitted to regular units.

The last intervention type is a Multidisciplinary Resource Utilization model for case management. The innovation of this intervention includes adding a new position of case manager and maintaining daily meetings of the multidisciplinary team to discuss each patient's unique needs, hospitalization, and discharge plan. While the other interventions targeted specific patients only, this intervention was an inclusive one and targeted all the patients admitted to the ward. A pilot study on a small sample did not yield any results to support the model (Trella, 1993).

CONCLUSION

Hospitalization is a significant issue for older adults, who are among the highest users of this service and who, once admitted, stay the longest. The mean length of hospital stay for persons 65 years or older is 6 days, compared with 4 days for the general population (Health United States, 2002). Frail adults who are hospitalized for acute health conditions may be discharged with improvements in their admitting condition, but they are at higher risk for functional decline and related chronic conditions that may result in repeated multiple hospitalizations, further deterioration, and, eventually, death.

In this chapter, factors and influences involved in the process were reviewed, from physiological to psychosocial and environmental factors. Accordingly, interventions were suggested to target risk factors. Comprehensive outcome evaluation of these interventions is not yet completed. The trends observed in this brief review of the interventions show that external counseling is less beneficial than intervention designed and performed by professionals who are in constant contact with the patients and their social environment. Continuity of care is also identified as a major influence here, across settings and periods of time. All models stress the importance of screening and early detection. The value of preventive intervention, used simultaneously with restorative strategies, is also demonstrated repeatedly. Multidisciplinary approaches are endorsed in many models and again show the value of coordination and cooperation among health professionals.

Additional research and practice are focusing on "successful aging" and the prevention of frailty or on improvement of functioning to avoid hospitalization altogether. These approaches focus on interventions such as immunizations, exercise, and other activities promoting health and function in older adults. Although beyond the scope of this chapter, the primary prevention of frailty is no less important or relevant.

REFERENCES

Bortz, W. M. (1993). The physics of frailty. *Journal of American Geriatric Society, 41*(9), 1004–1008.

Campbell, A. J., & Buchner, D. M. (1997). Unstable disability and the fluctuations of frailty. *Age and Ageing, 26*(4), 315–318.

Counsell, S. R., Holder, C. M., Liebenauer, L. L., Palmer, R. M., Fortinsky, R. H., Kresevic, D. M., et al. (2000). Effect of multicomponent intervention on functional outcomes and process of care in hospitalized older patients: A randomized control trial of ACE in a community hospital. *Journal of the American Geriatric Society, 48,* 1572–1581.

Covinsky, K. E., Fortinsky, R. H., Palmer, R. M., Kresevic, D. M., & Landefeld, C. S. (1997). Relation between symptoms of depression and health status outcomes in acutely ill hospitalized older patients. *Annals of Internal Medicine, 126,* 417–425.

Francis, D., Fletcher, K., & Simon, L. J. (1998). The geriatric resource nurse model of care: A vision for the future. *Nursing Clinics of North America, 33,* 481–496.

Fretwell, M. D., Raymond, P. M., McGarvey, S. T., Owens, N., Traines, M., Silliman, R. A., et al. (1990). The senior care study. A controlled trial of a consultative/unit-based geriatric assessment program in acute care. *Journal of American Geriatric Society, 38,* 1073–1081.

Fried, L. P., Tangen, C. M., Walston, J., Newman, A. B., Hirsch, C., Gottdiener, J., et al. (2001). Frailty in older adults: Evidence for a phenotype. *Journal of Gerontology: Biological Sciences and Medical Sciences, 56A*(3), M145–M156.

Gill, T. M., Baker, D. I., Gottschalk, M., Gahbauer, E. A., Charpentier, P. A., de Regt, P. T., et al. (2003). A prehabilitation program for physically frail community-living older persons. *Archives of Physical Medicine and Rehabilitation, 84,* 394–404.

Healthy United States (2002). *Healthy, health care, and disability—A profile of older Americans: 2001.* Retrieved February 23, 2003, from *http://www.aoa.gov/prof/Statistics/profile/profiles.asp.*

Inouye, S. K., Bogardus, S. T., Jr., Baker, D. I., Leo-Summers, L., & Cooney, L. M., Jr. (2000). The Hospital Elder Life Program: A model of care to prevent cognitive and functional decline in older hospitalized patients. *Journal of American Geriatric Society, 48,* 1697–1706.

Inouye, S. K., Wagner, D. R., Acampora, D., Horwitz, R. I., Cooney, L. M., Jr., Hurst, L. D. & Tinetti, M. E. (1993). A predictive index for functional decline in hospitalized elderly medical patients. *Journal of General Internal Medicine, 8,* 645–652.

Inouye, S. K., Wagner, D. R., Acampora, D., Horwitz, R. I., Cooney, L. M., Jr., & Tinetii, M. E. (1993). A controlled trial of a nursing-centered intervention in hospitalized elderly medical patients: The Yale Geriatric Care Program. *Journal of the American Geriatric Society, 41,* 1354–1360.

Johnson, J. C., & Smith, N. H. (2002). Health and social issues associated with racial, ethnic, and cultural disparities. *Generations, 26*(3), 25–32.

Kane, R. L., Ouslander, J. G., & Abrass, I. B. (2004). *Essentials of clinical geriatrics* (5th ed.). New York, NY: McGraw-Hill.

Kao, H. F., & Stuifbergen, A. K. (1999). Family experiences related to the decision to institutionalize an elderly member in Taiwan: An exploratory study. *Social Science and Medicine, 49,* 1115–1123.

Kaufman, S. R. (1994). The social construction of frailty: An anthropological perspective. *Journal of Aging Study, 8,* 45–58.

Landefeld, C. S., Palmer, R. M., Kresevic, D. M., Fortinsky, R. H., & Kowal, J. (1995). A randomized trial of care in a hospital medical unit especially designed to improve the functional outcomes of acutely ill older patients. *New England Journal of Medicine, 332*(20), 1338–1344.

Lopez, M., Delmore, B., Ake, J. M., Kim, Y. R., Golden, P., Bier, J., et al. (2002). Implementing a geriatric resource nurse model, *Journal of Nursing Administration, 32*(11), 577–585.

Lunney, J. R., Lynn, J., & Hogan, C. (2002). Profiles of older Medicare decedents. *Journal of American Geriatric Society, 50,* 1108–1112.

Margitic, S., Inouye, S., & Thomas, J. (1993). Hospital Outcomes Project for the Elderly (HOPE): Rational and design for a prospective pooled analysis. *Journal of the American Geriatric Society, 41,* 258–267.

Markle-Reid, M., & Browne, G. (2003). Conceptualizations of frailty in relation to older adults. *Journal of Advanced Nursing, 44*(1), 58–68.

McVey, L., Becker, P., & Saltz, C. (1989). Effect of geriatric consultation team on functional status of elderly hospitalized patients: A randomized controlled clinical trial. *Annals of Internal Medicine, 110,* 79–84.

Mezey, M., & Fulmer, T. (1998). Quality care for the frail elderly. *Nursing Outlook, 46*(6), 291–292.

Naylor, M. D. (2000). A decade of transitional care research with vulnerable elders. *Journal of Cardiovascular Nursing, 14*(3), 1–14.

Naylor, M., Brooten, D., Jones, R., Lavizzo-Mourey, R., Mezey, M., & Pauly, M. (1994). Comprehensive discharge planning for the hospitalized elderly: A randomized clinical trial. *Annals of Internal Medicine, 120,* 999–1006.

Naylor, M. D., Brooten, D., Campbell, R., Jacobsen, B. S., Mezey, M. D., Pauly, M. V., et al. (1999). Comprehensive discharge planning and home follow-up of hospitalized elders: A randomized clinical trial. *Journal of the American Medical Association, 281,* 613–620.

Palmer, R. M., Counsell, S., & Landefeld, C. S. (1998). Clinical intervention trials: The ACE unit. *Clinics in Geriatric Medicine, 14,* 831–849.

Phaneuf, C. (1996). Screening elders for nutritional deficits. *American Journal of Nursing, 96*(3), 58–60.

Raphael, D., Cava, M., Brown, I., Renwick, R., Heathcote, K., Weir, N., et al. (1995). Frailty: A public health perspective. *Canadian Journal of Public Health, 86*(4), 224–227.

Reuben, D. B., Borok, G. M., Wolde-Tsadik, G., Ershoff, D. H., Fishman, L. K., Ambrosini, V., et al. (1995). A randomized trial of comprehensive geriatric assessment in the care of hospitalized patients. *New England Journal of Medicine, 332,* 1345–1350.

Rockwood, K., Fox, R. A., Stolee, P., Robertson, D., & Beattie, B. L. (1994). Frailty in elderly people: An evolving concept. *Canadian Medical Association Journal, 150*(4), 4894–4895.

Sager, M., & Rudberg, M. (1998). Functional decline associated with hospitalization for acute illness. *Clinics in Geriatric Medicine, 14*(4), 669–679.

St. Pierre, J. (1998). Functional decline in hospitalized elders: Preventive nursing measures. *AACN Clinical Issues, 9*(1), 109–118.

Stolee, P., & Rockwood, K. (1981). *Report of the Saskatchewan Health Status Survey of the Elderly.* Saskatoon, Canada: University of Saskatchewan.

Stuck, A. E, Walthert, J. M., Nikolaus, T., Bula, C. J., Hohmann, C., & Beck, J. C. (1999). Risk factors for functional status decline in community-living elderly people: A systematic literature review. *Social Science & Medicine, 48,* 445–469.

Thomas, D. R., Brahan, R., & Haywood, B. P. (1993). Inpatient community-based geriatric assessment reduces subsequent mortality. *Journal of the American Geriatric Society, 41,* 101–118.

Trella, R. S. (1993). A multidisciplinary approach to case management of frail, hospitalized older adults. *Journal of Nursing Administration, 23*(2), 20–26.

Turner, J. T., Lee, V., Fletcher, K., Hudson, K., & Barton, D. (2001). Measuring quality of care with an inpatient elderly population: The geriatric resource nursing model. *Journal of Gerontological Nursing, 3,* 8–18.

Young, H. M. (2003). Challenges and solutions for care of frail older adults. *Online Journal Issues in Nursing, 8*(2), 5.

Walston, J., & Fried, L. P. (1994). Frailty and the older man. *Medical Clinics of North America, 83*(5), 1173–1194.

Warshaw, G. A., Moore, J. T., Friedman, S. W., Currie, C. T., Kennie, D. C., Kane, W. J., et al. (1982). Functional disability in the hospitalized elderly. *Journal of the American Medical Association, 248,* 847–850.

Winograd, C. H., Gerety, M. B., Chung, M., Goldstein, M. K., Dominguez, F., Jr., & Vallone, R. (1991). Screening for frailty: Criteria and predictors of outcomes. *Journal of the American Geriatric Society, 39*(8), 778–784.

CHAPTER 34

Vulnerability of Rural Nicaraguan Men: A Model of Endurance

Carl A. Ross

Although the environment affects human health in general, environmental health threats do not weigh evenly on all segments of the population. Unfortunately, there are many populations that are more vulnerable to environmental health challenges than others. Men are among these vulnerable populations, especially rural men. Most men who live in rural areas tend to be self-sufficient through farming or working in the fields as an employee of another individual. These are the mechanisms that enable him to provide financial support for himself and his family.

Nurses have always been in the forefront of providing health promotion and primary care in rural clinics. Many times these rural health care clinics are staffed by nurses who are inexperienced recent graduates, especially in Nicaragua. This chapter will address rural men as a vulnerable population, using rural Nicaraguan men as a model, and will help nurses and other health care practitioners who work in rural health care clinics become more adept at identifying and meeting their needs. To assist health care professionals, recommendations for developing specific strategies to promote the health and well-being of rural men will be made.

The mission of the Ministerio de Salud (Ministry of Health) of Nicaragua is to ensure that the population has access to health services that respond to their real and perceived needs and to see that the health system emphasizes health promotion and prevention with an integrated and humane approach (Ministerio de Salud [MINSA], 2003). Work is underway in Nicaragua to develop a new health care model that will approach health problems with a preventive, integrated, interprogrammatic, and participatory strategy that addresses risk factors. For now, the country's priority continues to be women and children, and in the new model, greater attention will be given to adolescents and the elderly. Men continue to be identified as a nonpriority group. Nicaraguan men are a vulnerable subculture that suffers from limited health care resources and limited access to those resources. Overall, men in Nicaragua have a life expectancy that is 5 years shorter than that of women and higher death rates from all the leading causes of death identified by the Pan American Health Organization (Pan American Health Organization [PAHO], 1998). In rural areas, the difference in life expectancy is 10 years, with women living longer. To assist Nicaraguan men with health and well-being it is imperative that health care professionals establish a public health program that focuses on primary prevention rather than the traditional diagnosis and treatment model.

The PAHO (PAHO, 1998) has identified Nicaragua as one of the poorest countries in Latin America. Significant problems exist with obtaining the everyday necessities of life, such as adequate water and sanitation. Health care in Nicaragua might be called a luxury. There is little access for the majority of the population who cannot afford to pay for usage, services, and supplies. As a result of the small percentage of monies made available for health care from the gross domestic product, Nicaragua's health care system continues to function with limited resources. In keeping with the mission of MINSA, initiatives for health care reform are moving from a "diagnose and treat" system to a system that responds to the real and perceived needs of Nicaraguan people. This health care initiative will emphasize a "promote and prevent" approach to health care.

Nurses need to understand what health and well-being mean to rural men in order to better provide comprehensive health care and empower them to be better consumers of health care. Through this understanding, nurses and other health care providers will be better prepared to assist these vulnerable individuals in meeting their spiritual, social, physical, political, and emotional health care needs.

INTRODUCTION TO NICARAGUA

Nicaragua is located in the middle of the Central American isthmus between the countries of Honduras and Costa Rica. The current population is approximately 4.3 million, with an active yearly increase of 3.1%. The country is divided topographically into three regions: Pacific, Atlantic, and central. The population is unevenly distributed, with the majority concentrated in the Pacific region. The Pacific region occupies 15.3% of the national territory but is home to 61.5% of the total population.

Nicaragua, as stated before, is cited by the PAHO as one of the poorest Third-World countries. The people of Nicaragua are ethnically mixed. Mestizos (a mix of Indian and Spanish ancestry) make up 69% of the population. Of the rest, 9% are black, 17% white, and 5% pure Indians. The life expectancy for males is 66 and for females 71 years. In the rural areas, life expectancy is almost 10 years lower, although females have a higher life expectancy than males. The overall mortality rate estimated for Nicaragua during the period from 1990 to 1995 was 10%, which is higher than the Latin American average of 7%.

The MINSA is the governing body that controls the national health care system of Nicaragua. The mission of this governmental agency is to ensure that 1) the population has access to health services that respond to their real and perceived needs and 2) the emphasis is on health promotion and illness prevention. Due to pressing health problems, the current system does not adequately address health promotion; it is still disease oriented. Men in Nicaragua only seek out health care at times of illness, not for health promotion. According to Nicaragua's health care plan, women and children should still be health care priorities, and greater attention should be given to adolescents and the elderly. Currently, men's health is not addressed as part of the national health plan. Work is underway to develop a new model that will approach health problems of men through a preventive and participatory strategy.

La Reforma, Jinotega, Nicaragua: A Rural Community

Much of the environment and geography of La Reforma is very similar to that of rural communities in the United States. La Reforma, Jinotega, is located about 125 miles north of Managua. La Reforma is a district equivalent to a county in the United States. There is no real central town or village. The area is populated with approximately 2500 people. The average family size is about eight members. Thus it can be projected that there are about 300 family units in the district. Local statistics show that about half of the population is below age 18 (MINSA, 1996).

Access to the district is confined to 4-wheel drive vehicles via dirt roads that are drivable during the 4 months of the dry season; however, during the remainder of the year—the rainy season—access is more difficult. The nearest city is Jinotega, and in the dry season, it is situated 90 minutes away from La Reforma.

La Reforma is typical of the western half of Nicaragua, with a predominantly mestizo population. La Reforma is entirely agricultural, producing mainly coffee, bananas, and vegetables as cash crops. The land is owned by individual families who farm plots varying from a few to 50 acres. A plot is insufficient to support a family unless it is about 5–10 acres. The terrain, being mountainous, is difficult to farm.

The residents of La Reforma are poor, with an average income of $1 to $2 a day in US dollars, which equals $300 to $600 dollars annually (Banco Central de Nicaragua, 1999). Larger coffee plantations, those above 10 acres, produce a better income. Most families live below the poverty level, and a few live in extreme poverty (Banco Central de Nicaragua, 2001).

Housing is crude and consists of basic planks on frame structures. Roofs are mainly wood and sheets of tin. Dirt floors are the norm, and furniture is basic and minimal. Cooking is done in iron pots on primitive clay wood-burning hearths; a simple clay dome located beside the main hearth serves as a bread oven. There are no chimneys, and smoke is vented directly into the rooms. The kitchen is usually located in the corner of the main family room. This room serves in most cases as the sleeping area, particularly for the children. Hammocks are pulled to the ceiling during the day and lowered at night as the family's beds. Animals are encouraged to stay outside; however, animals ranging from dogs and cats to pigs and chickens run freely through the house, leading to many disease processes. Despite these conditions the people are very proud, and the dwellings are kept as clean as possible.

The water sources are invariably contaminated because animals are allowed free access by necessity. This problem is further compounded by the generally poor disposal of human waste. Some families have constructed pit latrines, but many have not. Human feces are also used for fertilizer. If the water source is a stream, it is often contaminated along its entire length by animals, stock, and families living upstream. The problems of water supply and poor sanitation are the most important factors in causing disease.

The food found in La Reforma is similar to that found in other parts of the country. The staple diet is rice and beans. The range of foods available to this community is varied, but the author's initial cursory opinion is that nutrition here is suboptimal in general. Some families have a pig or a cow, but most have chickens.

The most important health problems in La Reforma are intestinal disease, respiratory disease, and subtle malnutrition. These account for 60% of health problems. If problems of childbirth and sexually transmitted diseases are included, then 80% of the health issues faced in the region can be accounted for. Other problems include bacterial infections of the skin due to poor cleanliness, accidental injuries, and burns. Men's health issues in the rural community are hypertension, diabetes, arthritis, gastritis, prostatitis, and depression. Dental and eye health are poor and need to be addressed (PAHO, 1998).

ROBERTO CLEMENTE CLINIC OF LA REFORMA

Built by the Pittsburgh Rotary Club in collaboration with the Rotary Clubs of Managua and Jinotega, the Roberto Clemente clinic is situated in a compound shared with the local two-room school. The clinic is well constructed, with concrete walls and a tin sheet roof on steel rafters. It is the first solar building in the country. It consists of four main areas. The first three are a central receiving room, a consultation room that frequently serves as an examination room, and a larger examination room that is suitable for emergencies, minor surgery, and childbirth. This room also contains a small area that is used for laboratory specimen analysis, medication storage, and a rudimentary filing system. The fourth room serves as the living quarters for the two resident health care workers.

The Roberto Clemente Clinic provides health care for seven communities, a total population of 2797 people. MINSA either staffs the clinic with two auxiliary nurses or a nurse and physician who have one year of training. They work at the clinic to fulfill their service requirement following the completion of their education. The staff consists of hardworking, intelligent, and dedicated health care professionals. They rapidly identify community health problems and conduct health education programs addressing these health problems. Visiting doctors from the city of Jinotega are often sent to the clinic to deal with more complex patients.

OVERCOMING VULNERABILITY: A MODEL OF ENDURANCE

Rural Nicaraguan men live in a world of endurance (Ross, 2000, 2002) that results from the social structure. The main themes of this endurance model, the themes that nurses and health care providers must keep in mind when caring for rural Nicaraguan men, address health in several ways.

1. Health is being able to function and meet the responsibilities to self, family, and community.
2. Health is believing that you will be cared for by God.
3. Health is composed of five dimensions: spiritual, physical, mental, family, and community.
4. Health is withstanding the hardships of poverty, limited access to health care, and inadequate health care supplies.
5. Economic, environmental, work, and worldview factors guide rural Nicaraguan men's health care practices.

The model that was developed to illustrate the model of endurance is depicted in Figure 34.1. The model represents the manner in which the main concepts and themes are interrelated and dynamic. The five themes are complex and interrelated. These themes affect the way man defines health and well-being and the manner in which he maintains and restores health and well-being. In the center of the model shown in Figure 34.1 is a circle identifying the main emic definition of health: health as function. The five dimensions of health as described by rural Nicaraguan men in the author's dissertation (Ross, 2000) are shown as a circular border with no definitive beginning or end. The significance of this circle is that no one dimension of health can be altered without affecting the other dimensions. Each dimension is equally important in maintaining the homeostasis that ultimately leads to health and well-being.

In the model, the rural Nicaraguan man and the dimensions of health are surrounded by a thin halo that represents the health care provider. The majority of rural Nicaraguan men believe that health care providers are extensions of God. Health care providers have the ability to affect all dimensions of health in their attempt to assist these men in attaining, regaining, and main-

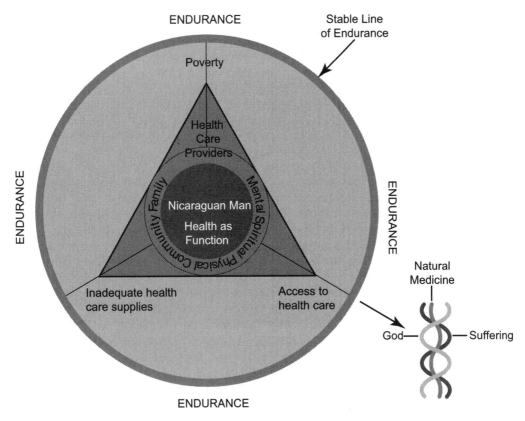

FIGURE 34.1   Model of Endurance

taining their health and well-being. The rural Nicaraguan man and these dimensions of health are suspended in a triangle representing the limitations of the social situation. The three social structure limitations located at each corner of the triangle are poverty, access to health care, and inadequate health care supplies. Each of the dimensions of health is touching the triangle, showing that each dimension of health is affected by the social structure. The triangle is also suspended in the middle of a circle, illustrating the world of endurance in which the Nicaraguan man lives. The circle's border is a thick line representing the stable line of endurance. If this line were dissected, three interwoven strands (see inset), representing the dynamic and interrelated properties of these elements by which the rural Nicaraguan man endures, would be revealed. The three elements inherent in endurance are God, natural medicines, and suffering. The interwoven strand representing God is larger than the strands representing natural medicines and suffering. God is viewed as the main resource for enduring and as the provider of natural medicines and strength during suffering, the other two elements associated with endurance. All lines starting from the center of the model outward are connected, showing the interconnectedness of the concepts and comprehensiveness and dynamic relationship of the model. No one concept stands alone in the model. One can follow any line that is connected to the Nicaraguan man and trace it out to the stable line of endurance. Another important component of the model is the representation of shapes selected for each of the major concepts. The Nicaraguan man is represented by a circle suspended in a triangle, which is then suspended in another circle of endurance. The circles represent the connection between earth and heaven, and the triangle represents the passion the Nicaraguan man experiences, based on the social situation of La Reforma and Nicaragua.

According to Ross (2002), the following is a cultural example illustrating the use of the endurance model. Rural Nicaraguan men frequently reported that they would go to the clinic when they experienced pain and burning on urination and pain located in the flank area lasting approximately 2 weeks. Men would not travel to the clinic immediately because to do so would take them away from their work. When they arrived at the clinic they encountered one of two situations: either the clinic was closed, or the antibiotics were not available to treat what was most likely a urinary tract infection. If the physician was at the clinic, the doctor would write them a prescription for the antibiotic. Due to the inadequate supply of medications, the man would have to go to Jinotega (approximately 90 minutes away via bus) to purchase the antibiotic. Because of their poverty, these men did not have the money to take the bus or purchase the antibiotics. As a result, they would return home from the clinic to suffer further from the symptoms of a urinary tract infection, pray to God for healing and for strength to endure, and use natural medications such as *Llanten* and *Bejuco de Sangre*. *Llanten* alleviates acidic urine and *Bejuco de Sangre* alleviates kidney pain. One can also see how the factors of poverty and culture can affect the health and well-being of these men. The rural Nicaraguan man has a strong spiritual dimension of health that gives him faith that God will provide him with strength to endure the discomfort in order to continue to work. These men thank God for the natural medicines He has provided them. A strong cultural value of family is seen when one is ill; the nuclear as well as the extended family and community assist and provide for each other during a time of need. Mental health is maintained knowing that the family and community will assist him until he can return to work.

This substantive model has been generated and grounded from the data obtained through interviews, fieldwork, and field notes. The Model of Endurance explains the process of endurance that rural Nicaraguan men undergo in order to maintain or regain an optimal level of health and well-being and to overcome issues of vulnerability. The process of endurance is not simple and is not achieved without much work and sacrifice. The goal of these men, despite the inherent social and cultural limitations, is to maintain an optimal level of health and well-being. Being healthy means being able to function to meet their responsibilities. Meeting responsibilities for God, self, family, and community leads to an optimal state of well-being.

CONCLUSION

Nurses and other health care providers need to be active in developing creative and comprehensive care for vulnerable populations. They need to know the definition and meaning of health and well-being as viewed by various populations. An understanding of this definition helps nurses to plan and provide culturally competent care to rural Nicaraguan men. Rural men as a vulnerable population have cultural needs that must be recognized by practitioners to assist them in restoring or maintaining their health and well-being. In order to assist rural men with their health, nurses working in the rural clinic environment need to incorporate programs that promote function and facilitate spiritual, family, and community health. In order to encourage these rural men to use the clinic, health care practitioners need to provide health care delivery that prevents extended time away from work. Health care practitioners caring for rural men need to provide programs that facilitate health for the family and the community. The clinic nurses can play a key role in the education of other health care practitioners who are members of the health care team involved with caring for these rural men.

REFERENCES

Banco Central de Nicaragua. (2001). *Informe annual.* Managua, Nicaragua: Banco Central de Nicaragua.

Ministerio de Salud [MINSA] (2000). Prioridades del programa de subsidios de investigacion de la Organizacion Panamericana de la Salud. *Buletin Epidemiologico, 1*(1), 10–14.

Pan American Health Organization [PAHO]. (1998). *Health in the Americas.* Washington, DC: PAHO.

Ross, C. (2000). Caminando mas cerca con Dios [A closer walk with thee]: An ethnography of health and well-being of rural Nicaraguan men. Unpublished doctoral dissertation, Duquesne University, Pittsburgh.

Ross, C. (2002). The theory of endurance of Nicaraguan men. *Home Health Care Management Practice, 14*(6), 448–451.

Transgender Health: Improving Access to Better Care

Kerry L. Clark

Please keep in mind that although many of us do suffer greatly from the same things that plague other marginalized communities—discrimination, violence, low self-esteem, substance addiction, unemployment and poverty, depression, and high suicide rates—being transgendered is not, in and of itself, a problem (Transcend, 2003).

There is most certainly a privilege to having a gender. Just ask someone who doesn't have a gender, or who can't pass, or who doesn't pass. When you have a gender, or when you are perceived as having a gender, you don't get laughed at in the street. You don't get beat up. You know which public bathroom to use, and when to use it. People don't stare at you or worse. You know which form to fill out. You know what clothes to wear. You have heroes and role models. You have a past (Kate Bornstein, 1994).

There is a growing awareness of the issues facing transgender men and women in the health care community. In the past several years it has come to the attention of providers, researchers, educators, government agencies, and policy makers that there is not only a need to better understand their health care needs but to examine the barriers that prevent transgender persons from obtaining appropriate, comprehensive care. What may prove to be a significant barrier is the social stigmatization of gender identities that fall outside the norm. We as health care providers unwittingly contribute to the stigma in that we ourselves are limited in our knowledge and lack the ability to provide inclusive, sensitive care. A significant body of research has emerged with regard to access limitations, but often, transgender issues are buried within the data collected regarding the lesbian, gay, and bisexual (LGB) population. The unique needs of the transgender population warrant more thorough investigation to identify barriers to care and offer guidelines to assist health care providers, policy makers, and, most importantly, the transgender community itself.

The purpose of this chapter is to raise pertinent questions about our responsibilities as health care providers to this marginalized group of men and women and to explore the social implications of access. The nursing values of health care for all, cultural competence, and commitment to education are critical when providing care to the transgender community.

TRANSGENDER IDENTITY AND ISSUES IN HEALTH CARE

What It Means to be Transgendered

"Transgender" is a relatively new term that broadly describes any individual exploring gender identity or who has transitioned from his or her birth gender. Transgender identity was previously referred to as transsexual because it describes altering one's biological sex. Today the term "transgender" may also include those individuals who self-identify as transsexual, intersexed, or transvestite. Frequently in the literature these terms are used interchangeably, but not all transgender persons fit the traditional concepts of what is defined as transgender (Bockting, & Cesaretti, 2001; Lombardi, 2001). Transition occurs from male to female (MtF) and female to male (FtM). Individuals may be preoperative or postoperative in their transition. However, not all transgender men and women choose surgical interventions (i.e., genital reassignment) to complete their transition and may instead opt for other less invasive measures such as hormone administration. Transgender men and women can identify themselves as heterosexual, homosexual, or bisexual (Bockting, Robinson, & Rosser, 1998; Transcend, 2003). Transgender identity has evolved in such a way that it includes many "isms" related to sexuality. Roen (2002) describes this evolution as a societal mechanism in which "violating gender codes" (p. 507) becomes a necessity in order for an individual to be included as part of a larger, supportive community. Subsequently, the transgender community is often labeled as part of the larger LGB populace. This is where many transgender men and women have found acceptance and support, but this type of labeling also poses a problem for many in the context of gathering accurate health data. For the purposes of research, studies have traditionally grouped LBG and transgender (LGBT) persons together. In 1999, the American Public Health Association (APHA) began promoting policies that would increase awareness of the need for transgender-specific research. In doing so, the association brought significant attention to the unique health care needs of the transgender population, as well as stressing that transgender men and women must not be blindly categorized into LGB issues (Craft & Mulvey, 2001; Fox, 2002; Gay and Lesbian Medical Association, 2001).

Health Care Issues

Transgender individuals face an array of issues related to health. Most notable is that they are much more frequently subject to discrimination and violence than are their LGB counterparts. Lombardi, Wilchins, Priesing, & Malouf (2001) conducted a transgender violence study in San Francisco over a 12-month period and found that over 50% of respondents ($n = 402$) reported being victims of harassment and violent crime, including verbal abuse, stalking, rape, and physical assault. Economic discrimination is one of the strongest predictors of transgender violence. In work situations, when transgender adults disclosed their identities, they were fired, harassed, and intimidated by supervisors and coworkers. Additional studies conducted in New York and San Francisco have shown there is a high incidence of homelessness, lack of education, sexually transmitted diseases, drug and alcohol abuse, suicide attempts, and depression among transgender populations. Combined, these issues have far-reaching implications with regard to how health care is accessed and how it is delivered in a system unprepared to deal with the issues in a sensitive manner. (Feldman & Bockting, 2003; Lombardi et al., 2001; Nemoto, Luke, Mamo, Ching, & Patria, 1999).

BARRIERS TO ACCESS

Social Stigmatization

It should come as no surprise that transgender men and women are subjected to considerable social prejudice. Much like the LGB communities, they suffer from overt job discrimination, sexual harassment, violence, and social isolation. Heterosexist and homophobic attitudes prevail in our society, with an even more antagonistic view of those challenging traditional gender roles and identity. Hereck (2000) reported that surveys conducted in the United States showed considerable negative attitudes and disgust toward those considered homosexual, whether they were in fact a member of the LGBT community or simply perceived as such. What makes these attitudes especially troubling is the fact that attitudes of sexual prejudice strongly correlate with hate crimes and other forms of violence against persons who make up these communities (Lombardi et al., 2001; Transcend, 2003).

Economic Marginalization

The Gay and Lesbian Medical Association (GLMA) reports in their *Healthy People 2010 Companion Document for LGBT Health* (2001) that poverty is a frequent reality that accompanies the transgender experience. This is due in part to job discrimination, lack of education, and rejection from family members. Many transgender persons are unable to afford basic medical services and are denied health insurance. They therefore must rely on emergency departments for care because they lack primary providers. Those facing economic hardship may resort to trading sex for money or housing. The few individuals who are granted health care coverage, either through a public agency such as Medicaid or through private employer insurance, are not guaranteed coverage for treatment of transgender-related issues. In fact, many institutions will exclude coverage on the grounds that treatments are cosmetic or experimental (Fox, 2002; GLMA, 2001; Spade, 2003).

Provider Discrimination

One of the most critical and often ignored barriers to accessing health care is the relationship between transgender persons and providers. Insensitivity on the part of health care professionals is consistently cited as a reason that transgender persons do not access services. Doctors, nurses, and other medical staff often fail to acknowledge or respect the identities of transgender men and women. One example would be refusing to use "she" as the pronoun when addressing MtF clients. Furthermore, health care professionals receive little or no education with regard to the specific health needs of transgender individuals. Providers are therefore universally ill prepared to offer comprehensive, sensitive care and may impart negative biases and inappropriate stereotypes when confronted with transgender identity and sexuality (Beatty, Gruskin, Hsi, Jillson, Neisen, & Ross, 2003; Fogarty, 2003; GLMA, 2001; Lombardi, 2001).

There is a widely held view in the medical community among providers and researchers that transgenderism is a pathological medical condition with underlying mental illness. The American Psychiatric Association includes gender identity disorder (GID) as a diagnosis in the DSM-IV. However, in order to be approved for sexual reassignment or body alteration, GID must be documented. To obtain such a diagnosis requires an integrated approach to patient management, but this may not be appropriate for all simply based on gender identity (Spade, 2003).

Policy, Law, and Research

According to Boehmer (2002), a review of research related to the LGBT population spanning 20 years found that transgender individuals were the least-studied group. It was found that less than 10% of over 3700 articles published were transgender specific. LGBT research lacks data unrelated to sexually transmitted diseases in that most, if not all, studies focused on the issue of homosexual transmission of HIV. Boehmer (2002) states that these findings "point to the dominance of a biomedical paradigm that narrowly understands LGBT health in relation to sexual behavior" and recommends that "sexuality needs to be expanded to include the recognition of sexual orientation and transgender identity as cultural and social categories that shape all health experiences" (p. 1129). Boehmer's view is supported by the APHA policy, which now supports public health outreach and research to address transgender health by asking for federal support for funding and by imploring public agencies and providers to show sensitivity and respect. Research aimed at understanding the needs of transgendered persons is needed to provide evidence-based practice measures (Beatty et al., 2003; GLMA, 2001).

Transgender individuals are universally denied legal protection and are excluded from consideration under most civil rights laws, even in the event they are granted a GID diagnosis by a qualified provider. This leaves them especially vulnerable, unable to take legal steps when denied treatment or Medicaid coverage for genital reassignment surgery. Transgender individuals are also excluded from receiving protection under the Americans with Disabilities Act. Although Medicaid is approved to fund surgical interventions, policies are inconsistent, and judgments are ruled on a case by case basis. Most transgender people do not have the financial means to cover prohibitive legal fees, nor do they receive adequate representation when filing cases in US courts (Fox, 2002; GLMA, 2001).

IMPLICATIONS OF DENYING ACCESS

Public Health Policy

Barriers that transgender men and women face indicate the necessity for confronting current policy shortcomings. Yet, from a policy standpoint, are we ever going to reverse discrimination when there are varying opinions on whether such actions are plausible or justified? Let us look at the stated goal to eliminate health disparities in *Healthy People 2010*. In public health this is said to be the defining policy publication that makes recommendations to monitor and improve the health of those populations identified as at risk. The Department of Health and Human Services (DHHS) now specifically names sexual orientation as an indicator for disparities in health or health care services. According to Fox (2002), sexual orientation, named as a population in the document for the first time in its history, includes LGB individuals but fails to acknowledge transgender individuals within their definition. Therefore, it can either be argued that the lack of epidemiological data has kept the transgender population out of public health policy or that federal agencies fail to see that transgender is not simply a sexual identifier but encompasses a broader cultural definition beyond gender conformity and pathological components.

Unfortunately, by excluding transgender people as a population worthy of monitoring, *Healthy People 2010* misrepresents the need for further study and further perpetuates barriers to access. In 2001, the GLMA responded to the challenge of the *Healthy People 2010* omission by publishing the *Healthy People 2010* Companion Document of LGBT Health. Although not approved by the DHHS, it provides a thorough review of the literature and was compiled through the efforts of LGBT consumers, health care providers, educators, and researchers, serving as a reminder that transgender health must be included in our public health care agenda. Future public health care policies that are inclusive of transgender issues must be cultivated if we are to see change and improvement in the barriers that LGBT people confront in accessing care (Craft & Mulvey, 2001; Fox, 2002; GLMA, 2001).

It has been argued that LGBT health issues are no different than non-LGBT health issues, with the exception of sexual orientation. The argument is that focusing on LGBT issues pushes the envelope of civil liberties, diverts health care funding inappropriately, and bolsters the political platform of gay rights. These arguments may also serve to prevent large-scale studies from receiving funding, perpetuating the idea that such a small portion of our society does not necessitate population-based surveys and research that drain public funds (Boehmer, 2002; GLMA, 2001).

Gender Identity

Although homosexuality has long been removed from the American Psychiatric Association diagnostic manual as a mental disorder, GID remains an active diagnostic tool. For many transgender people, this inclusion in the DSM-IV offers a viable option for receiving insurance reimbursement for treatment. Critics remain steadfast in their opposition to the diagnosis as a means to punish those in society that challenge gender norms or wish to deviate from their assigned biological sex. The GLMA (2001) provides an overview that recognizes a cultural definition of gender as well as a biological one and distinguishes gender nonconformity from pathology. Health care providers should not confuse sexual orientation with sexual perversion. Instead, providers must be reminded that gender is defined by individuals, and it is their definition that makes it authentic for them (Fogarty, 2003; GLMA, 2001; Spade, 2003).

RELEVANCY AND RECOMMENDATIONS FOR NURSING

Honoring Nursing Values

In nursing, we assume the value system of the profession. To be a nurse is to practice in concert with a code of ethics that promotes caring in a variety of settings, serving a diverse range of cultures and individual needs. Care should reflect our professional dedication to human dignity, social justice, altruism, advocacy, and patient autonomy. Because heterosexism and homophobia are a part of our culture, we can expect these biases to filter into nursing practice, disrupting the nursing process and undermining professional values. Unless we are acutely aware of our own biases, we will not be able to attend to the needs of our transgender clients. Further, we sabotage the building of trust if our clients do not feel safe in disclosing their gender identity.

Open empathic communication promotes dignity and respect. If the client has experienced discriminatory treatment when accessing health care in the past, it may take more time to establish trust. Be patient when asking questions, and allow the client to set the tone. The following scenario involving a transgender client provides some examples of how nurses can approach communication, promote client advocacy, and serve as role models for others when caring for clients.

Imagine that you are the RN at a busy community clinic. You notice a male sitting in the waiting area wearing female attire. You double check the client sign-in sheet to make certain who you will be seeing next. When you call out the name Karen Jones, the male client stands up and proceeds towards you. "Hello, are you Karen Jones?" The client nods and says, "Yes." This is an opportunity for you to introduce yourself and guide the client to the exam room. Once inside the room, you politely ask how the client wishes to be addressed. Often we forget the importance of acknowledging how the client's name is pronounced, if they prefer to be addressed in a more formal manner such as Ms. Jones, or what pronoun they prefer. The client replies that using Karen is fine, and that she is female identified. Once name and appropriate pronoun have been established, you can begin your assessment by inquiring why the client is visiting the clinic today. While charting notes during intake, you notice that the client's chart bears the name "Thomas." Before leaving the client, you take a moment to confirm that Karen would like the chart changed to reflect the new name. Before the doctor is to see the client you make certain that he or she is aware of Karen's preferences and of the change of name on the chart.

When you return to the front area you hear two staff members making inappropriate remarks about the client. One of them states that she refuses to address the client as a female. The comments are being made in a public area where other clients can hear what is being said. The best way to approach this type of situation is to gently remind your coworkers that client privacy is at stake, and it would be better if they discontinued their discussion. Perhaps at a later time that day you can sit down with each of them and explore the issue further by emphasizing that client care is the priority, and it must be done with equal respect to each individual regardless of their gender identity. As a follow-up, you may ask that a meeting or in-service be provided to all staff to provide education, communication strategies, and increase awareness of transgender issues (Fogarty, 2003; Gray, Kramer, Minick, McGehee, Thomas, & Greiner, 1996).

Cultural Competency

The development of the skills necessary to achieve cultural competency in practice are offered throughout nursing education and are reinforced professionally through continuing education. Although we have been repeatedly oriented to respect diversity of ethnicity, religion, and disabilities, issues surrounding sexual orientation and gender identity are overlooked when considering cultural awareness. LGBT persons cross all socioeconomic, ethnic, and religious groups, yet somehow they are rarely acknowledged during cultural competency training. Fogarty (2003) refers to this population as "the invisible minority" (p. 11). Nurse educators claim that knowledge regarding sexual orientation and gender identity is nonexistent in nursing curriculua as well as in the workplace. Gray et al. (1996) reported that heterosexist theories and textbooks are used throughout nursing education. They simply omit mention of gender identity beyond what is traditionally held acceptable in a male and female context. Society in general has historically discriminated against LGBT people, and this has manifested as antagonism and insensitivity in the health care community. Therefore, in order to develop a true sense of cultural competence in professional practice, nurses and other health care providers must continually examine their own personal values and stereotypes. Not until nurses become comfortable with their own attitudes regarding sexuality and gender identity can they possibly provide competent, quality care to clients with identities different from their own values and beliefs (Misener, Sowell, Phillips, & Harris, 1997).

Conclusion

Health care needs change. Although embedded within the LGB data, the barriers that transgender individuals currently face are not insurmountable. Social stigmatization, economic marginalization, provider discrimination, and lack of appropriate policy can be eradicated if health care providers, researchers, and policy makers employ strategies set forth by the GLMA and the APHA. Opponents to policy change must be challenged to more closely examine the authenticity of gender identity in our diverse communities. Transgender men and women should enjoy the same rights and privileges as anyone else using the health care system. We cannot allow providers to deny them quality care or to bar access through discriminatory practices such as stereotyping and heterosexist and homophobic attitudes. The exclusion of LGBT civil rights protection must be confronted as a threat to public health. Transgender persons are socially and medically marginalized, unable to enjoy the same legal recourse as other vulnerable populations. Nurses are in a unique position to touch the lives of transgender people. In clinics, communities, hospitals, and schools, nurses must reach out to these patients and acknowledge transgender identity. We must examine our own attitudes. Discriminatory practices must not be tolerated. We must advocate for the vulnerable to obtain health care. Finally, we must be leaders who set a tone of acceptance that is inclusive of the transgender experience in all the contexts of health care.

References

Beatty, R. L., Gruskin, E., Hsi, A., Jillson, I. A., Neisen, J., & Ross, M. (2003). Bridging science and practice in LGBT health. *Clinical Research and Regulatory Affairs, 20*(2), 229–246.

Bockting, W. O., & Cesaretti, C. (2001). Spirituality, transgender identity, and coming out. *Journal of Sex Education and Therapy, 26*(4), 291–300.

Bockting, W. O., Robinson, B. E., & Rosser, B. R. (1998). Transgender HIV prevention: A qualitative needs assessment. *AIDS Care, 10*(4), 505–526.

Boehmer, U. (2002). Twenty years of public health research: Inclusion of lesbian, gay, bisexual, and transgender populations. *American Journal of Public Health, 92*(7), 1125–1130.

Craft, E. M, & Mulvey, K. P. (2001). Addressing lesbian, gay, bisexual, and transgender issues form the inside: One federal agency's approach. *American Journal of Public Health, 91*(6), 889–891.

Feldman, J., & Bockting, W. (2003). Transgender health. *Minnesota Medicine, 86*(7), 25–32.

Fogarty, S. (2003). Culturally competent care for the invisible minority. *Michigan Nurse, 76*(6), 11–13.

Fox, C. E. (2002). Difficult challenges for Healthy People 2010: Putting policy into practice: A commentary. *Clinical Research and Regulatory Affairs, 19*(2), 119–123.

Gay and Lesbian Medical Association [GLMA]. (2003). *Healthy People 2010 companion document for LGBT health: Access to quality health services.* Retrieved October 18, 2003, from *http://www.glma .org/policy/hp2010/PDF/Access.pdf.*

Gray, D. P., Kramer, M., Minick, P., McGehee, L., Thomas, D., & Greiner, D. (1996). Heterosexism in nursing education. *Journal of Nursing Education, 35*(5), 204–210.

Hereck, G. M. (2000). The psychology of sexual prejudice. *Current Directions in Psychological Sciences, 9*(1), 19–22.

Lombardi, E. (2001). Enhancing transgender health care. *American Journal of Public Health, 91*(6), 869–872.

Lombardi, E. L., Wilchins, R. A., Priesing, D., & Malouf, D. (2001). Gender violence: Transgender experiences with violence and discrimination. *Journal of Homosexuality, 42*(1), 89–101.

Misener, T. R., Sowell, R. L., Phillips, K. D., & Harris, C. (1997). Sexual orientation: A cultural diversity issue for nursing. *Nursing Outlook, 45*(4), 178–181.

Nemoto, T., Luke, D., Mamo, L., Ching, A., & Patria, J. (1999). HIV risk among male-to-female transgenders in comparison with homosexuals or bisexual males and heterosexual females. *AIDS Care, 11*(3), 297–312.

Roen, K. (2002). "Either/or" and "both/neither": Discursive tensions in transgender politics. *Journal of Women in Culture & Society, 27*(2), 501–523.

Spade, D. (2003). Resisting medicine, re/modeling gender. *Berkeley Women's Law Journal, 18,* 15–37.

Transcend. (2003). Transforming community: Resources for trans people and their families. Retrieved October 13, 2003, from *http://www.transgender.org/transcend/guide.sec118.htm.*

CHAPTER 36

Open the Door: Primary Care for Youth with Autism Spectrum Disorder

Kathryn S. Deane

This chapter aims to provide practitioners with a way to approach clients with autism spectrum disorder (ASD) in order to facilitate positive experiences and outcomes. Research has shown an increase in the number of children with ASD. It affects an estimated 2 to 6 individuals per 1000 (Centers for Disease Control, 2003; United States Department of Education, 2002). Given this statistic, it is almost certain that family practitioners will treat clients with this disorder for routine health care management and will therefore need to know how to communicate effectively with and increase comfort levels for these clients. This is crucial for the child with ASD because a change in daily routine (e.g., a health care visit) can be perceived as a threatening situation and create anxiety, agitation, noncompliance, and physical aggression (Fairfax County Public Schools, 2004). Practitioners should do everything possible to make health care visits routine in order to instill trust and facilitate lifelong involvement in primary care. This is especially significant for individuals who will be independent as adults. To do this, the practitioner must understand the clinical presentation of ASD and the factors that influence the effectiveness of care, such as the health care environment and the approach to examination.

CLINICAL PRESENTATION

ASD is designated a spectrum disorder, meaning that there is a variance in the degree of symptoms; each child is unique within the diagnostic criteria. Although research does not indicate a racial, ethnic, or psychosocial link, it is four times more prevalent in boys (Blackwell & Niederhauser, 2003). Impairments are evident in social interaction, communication, and language, and a restrictive range of behaviors, interests, and activities is displayed (American Psychiatric Association [APA], 2000). Cognitive levels can range from above average intelligence to profound mental retardation, with up to 80% having mental retardation (Fombonne, 1999). The degree to which an adult with autism can lead an independent life is related to intelligence and the ability to communicate. It is estimated that approximately 15 to 20% of individuals with ASD will be able to acquire at least some degree of partial independence (Friedlander, Yagiela, Paterno, & Mahler, 2003).

Despite highly publicized claims, scientific evidence does not support a link between the measles/mumps/rubella (MMR) vaccine or any combination of vaccines as a cause of autism (CDC, 2003). Genetic factors and brain abnormalities at birth are among the most recognized

causes of autism and current research suggests autism primarily results from a genetic susceptibility that involves multiple genes (CDC, 2003; Courchesne, Townsend, & Saitoh, 1994; Courchesne, Yeung-Courchene, Press, Hesselink, & Jernigan, 1988).

Factors Affecting Children with ASD

The child with ASD experiences the world in a vastly different way than does a typical developing child. The practitioner must understand key factors that profoundly affect these children in order to maximize the efficacy and comfort level of the examination. These include
abnormal social skills, communication difficulties, sensory integration disorders, and the effect
of changes in puberty.

Abnormal Social Skills

A universal trait of ASD is abnormal social skill development. The younger child demonstrates this with abnormal eye contact, aloofness, failure to orient to name, failure to use gestures
to point or show, a lack of interactive play, and a lack of interest in peers, among other behaviors
(Committee on Children with Disabilities, 2001). These children are often observed playing in a
side by side manner rather than in a reciprocal manner with peers.

As these children age, they fail to develop relationships to an appropriate developmental
level. They show a lack of social or emotional reciprocity and do not seek out others for enjoy-
ment or to share interests or achievements. This is demonstrated by a lack of showing, bringing,
or pointing out objects of interest to other people (APA, 2000).

Communication Difficulties

The communication abilities of children with autism fall within a broad range, and skills can
range from no verbal communication to high verbal capacity (Kuhn, 1991; Turnbull, Turnbull,
Shank, & Leal, 1995). Communication deficits can include the inability to comprehend verbal
communication, to communicate verbally, and/or discern or decipher nonverbal communication.
Problematic behavior is often used to express needs a child is unable to verbalize, and therefore
it should be viewed as a communication method (Kuhn, 1991).

Among verbal children, there is often an inability to initiate or sustain conversation with others and to integrate words and gestures. Language tends to be rote, repetitive, and lacking in
meaning. Answering questions, especially if they are open ended, is challenging. There is often
inappropriate use of personal pronouns such as using "you" for "I," lack of directional verbs
(e.g., "give" and "take"), and a lack of understanding that words can have multiple meanings.
Echolalia and abnormal patterns of speech volume, pitch, and rate are also often heard (Ho,
Keller, Berg, Cargan, & Haddad, 1999). Children with high verbal capacities are often subject to
unreasonably high expectations. They present as high functioning but can have serious deficits
in many areas. This can lead to frustration and negative behaviors.

Individuals with ASD often interpret words and phrases quite literally and are described as
"concrete." Colloquialisms, clichés, innuendo, and sarcasm are often misunderstood or misin-
terpreted by ASD children. This is important for the practitioner to note because a common tac-
tic used to gain cooperation with children is to make a game of the examination, for example,
making bird sounds as they examine the ear. With children with ASD, this can have the opposite
effect and cause distress because they may believe they actually have a bird in their ear.

Generalization

Generalization is also a problem for children with autism (Grandin, 2002). Transferring similar experiences and social skills from one context to another is challenging. For example, the average developing child who is told not to be disruptive in the dentist's waiting room will most likely transfer their understanding of appropriate behavior to other waiting rooms. In contrast, for children with ASD, it is likely that they perceive different waiting rooms as completely different environments. Behaviors expected at the dentist have no application in a new environment, and guidelines must be reintroduced. Because of this inability to generalize, children with ASD crave routine. New experiences or environments are unpredictable, and fear of the unknown can create significant anxiety.

Sensory Integration Disorders

Sensory integration disorders are very common in ASD. Sensory input structures are usually intact, but difficulty occurs as the child tries to process sensory intake and respond to task and environmental demands (Dunn et al., 2002). As a result, many children with ASD either over- or underreact (Grandin, 2000). For example, in the medical environment, many children cannot tolerate bandages, dressings, arm-boards, and blood pressure cuffs, and certain noises and smells can trigger inappropriate behaviors. Some autistic people are bothered by visual distractions and fluorescent lights; they can see the flicker of the 60-cycle electricity (Grandin, 2000). Some examples of sensory difficulties are illustrated in the following accounts.

> My hearing is like having a hearing aid with the volume control stuck on "super loud." I have two choices: turn the mike on and get deluged with sound or shut it off. Mother sometimes acted like I was deaf. Hearing tests indicated that my hearing was normal. I can't modulate incoming auditory stimulation." (Grandin, 2000, p. 9)
>
> Dr. Marek's kitchen was a nightmare. The kitchen had fluorescent lights and yellow walls, the worst combinations ever. Even from the doorway, I could see light bouncing off everything. In my tense state everything climbed to hyper, vision included. There were no whole objects in that room, just shiny edges and things that jumped off the yellow walls like sunshine on water. Dr. Marek wanted me to go in there and be blind. Forget it! (Gillingham, 2003, p. 15)

Puberty

Some adolescents and teens with ASD make major gains during puberty, but psychiatric illnesses such as anxiety disorders, mood disorders, attention-deficit hyperactivity disorder, and obsessive-compulsive disorder can become more prevalent (Friedlander et al., 2003). Seizures may appear, and the sudden growth, changes in physical appearance, and growing sexual drive can create anxiety for the autistic young person (Friedlander et al., 2003; Haracopos & Pederson, 1992). Addressing issues present in adolescence and promoting a healthy self-image can help to alleviate potential feelings of depression and loneliness for the person with ASD (Koller, 2000).

Sexuality

Emerging sexuality and confusion regarding sexual issues are exacerbated by communication issues and lack of social skills. Socialization is often desired but elusive because of developmental and communication deficits. The lack of understanding of social norms and inability to empathize can lead to a young autistic person trying to touch, kiss, or hug strangers or undress and masturbate in public. Defeats in connection with attempts to establish friendships or love affairs and/or rejection of sexually motivated physical contact can lead to frustration and result in aggressive or self-mutilating behavior. Affected teens may also withdraw into themselves or even give up sexuality entirely (Haracopos & Pederson, 1992). Thus appropriate education about sexuality and development is critical to the creation of the adolescent's positive self-esteem (Koller, 2000).

In order to optimize effectiveness, it is important for the dialogue between parents and professionals concerning sexuality to begin early, before it becomes a major issue or problem, preferably by the age of 10 years. Because many parents do not know what to expect, they are very surprised when sexual behaviors appear. If they are prepared for these in advance, they will be less traumatized when they occur and more likely to discuss concerns with professionals as they arise (Society for the Autistically Handicapped, 2003).

OFFICE VISITS

Because autism is a spectrum disorder, individuals vary greatly in the severity and type of issues they struggle with, and the practitioner must address issues pertinent to that particular individual. To achieve this, the practitioner can engage in preplanning, modification of the environment, and creating an accommodating appointment routine. It is important to preplan for the client with ASD because deviations from normal daily schedules can be distressing and cause adverse behavior (Souders, Freeman, DePaul, & Levy, 2002). Techniques used include assessment, priming, visual supports, and social stories. Cooperation with the caregiver is integral to the success of the implementation of such routines.

A preliminary assessment of the ASD child and his or her family should be completed prior to the initial health care visit or interaction. A short conversation, either in person or by phone, with a caretaker prior to the clinical visit can make a significant difference in the efficiency and quality of the visit. This assessment includes the child's communication, social, sensory, and behavioral skills, and successful strategies for compliance (Souders et al., 2002).

Assessment also serves to identify triggers that precipitate problem behaviors typically exhibited by children with ASD, including biting, spitting, head butting, scratching, pinching, punching, slapping, kicking, screaming, flopping to the floor, stripping, and property destruction. The practitioner should discuss protocols that can be used to alleviate such behaviors in the event they occur (Souders et al., 2002). Knowing what works for each particular child is invaluable and can alleviate stress for both the child and the practitioner.

Priming is a technique used to familiarize the child with elements he or she is likely to find troublesome. A preview activity is presented prior to the appointment to introduce potentially distressing materials or task processes. The action is presented in a nondemanding manner, preferably in an environment the child views as safe. By doing this, anxiety is decreased through familiarization and exploration (Wilde, Koegel, & Koegel, 1992). For example, a child who finds a blood pressure cuff distressing would be given a cuff to use at home prior to the health care appointment.

Visual supports are used so individuals can anticipate and predict upcoming activities, experience easier transitions, and understand expectations (Dunn, Saiter, & Rinner, 2002). Helpful visual supports for the health care visit include visual schedules and social stories. Visual schedules tell the client with ASD what activities will occur and in what sequence. A common format is a list of daily activities with a corresponding photograph or drawing. This is significant in that many individuals with ASD think in pictures rather than words (Grandin, 2002). It is recommended that the parent present the child with a full day's schedule that includes a detailed description of the office visit. If this is not possible, a detailed schedule of the exam should be written by the practitioner and reviewed by the child when he or she enters the office.

Social stories were created by Carol Gray for individuals who have difficulty understanding appropriate social interaction. In social stories, appropriate social behaviors are presented in the form of a story that provides a model for desirable actions and teaches routines and correct social responses in a nonthreatening manner. They are presented prior to the addressed social situation. The formula for writing a social story is a specified balance of certain sentences. Descriptive sentences (2–5) describe where the situation occurs and why, and they usually contain words such as "usually" and "sometimes" to encourage generalization. Perspective sentences (2–5) are statements that describe a person's internal state, such as knowledge, thoughts, feelings, beliefs, opinions, motivation, and physical condition/health. They are most often used to help the individual with ASD to understand the feelings, reactions, and responses of others in the situation being addressed. Directive sentence (1) describes desired responses to social situations (Gray, 2003; Kuoch & Mirenda, 2003). An example of a social story for the child who has a history of difficulties in the waiting room would read like this:

> My name is John. Sometimes I go to the doctor. People sit in the chairs while they wait to see the doctor. Sometimes I don't feel calm when I have to wait. It is important for me to keep my body in the chair while I wait. This helps to keep myself and other people safe. My mom can help me to stay calm. She can give me a hand held video game to play. I can sit still and play the video game and wait. Mom likes it when I keep my body calm at the doctor's office. I will try to wait calmly until it is time for me to go to the examination room.

Modification of Environment and Examination Technique

The competent practitioner, being aware of communication difficulties and sensory integration issues in children with ASD, can implement strategies to decrease stress and increase comfort. These include modifying exam rooms, providing adequate equipment and staffing, and modifying exam techniques (Dalrymple, Porco, & Chung, 1993; Souders et al., 2002).

Examination rooms can be distressing for the ASD child. They often contain toys, bright colors, magazines, and other stimuli that can create distress and lead to negative reactions and outbursts. By modifying the setup of the room, problem behaviors can often be reduced or eliminated (Dalrymple et al., 1993). To achieve this, the examining room should be uncluttered, with supplies and equipment set up ahead of time and screened from view prior to the patient entering the exam room (Souders et al., 2002). If possible, try to have an alternative light source or use the newest bulbs possible to reduce the flickering of fluorescent lights. Incandescent lights used in conjunction with fluorescent lights can also reduce stimulation (Grandin, 2002).

The practitioner can encourage generalization by conducting health care visits in different locations. One way to do this is to use different examining rooms for subsequent visits. However, be sure to prepare the child for such an occurrence and provide reassurance: "We are going into a different room than last time. It will have the same things in it—a stethoscope, an examining table. You were safe in the last room, and you will be safe here too."

Additional equipment and staffing requirements should be considered. For example, if the child spits, then gowns, gloves, and goggles should be used. If the child is large, aggressive, or requires restraint for a procedure such as phlebotomy, IV insertion, or immunization, an appropriate number of trained helpers should be identified and available (Souders et al., 2002). Furthermore, it is important to keep a familiar person, such as the caretaker, in the room because this can help alleviate stress in a time of crisis (Dalrymple et al., 1993).

If immunizations, phlebotomy, or IV insertion is anticipated, apply a lidocaine hydrochloride cream disk (lidocaine 2.5%/prilocaine 2.5%).The disk, applied 1 hour before the anticipated procedure, has been shown to decrease discomfort for invasive procedures (Fradet, 1990; May, Britt, & Newman, 1999; Walco, Cassidy, & Schechter, 1994).

Small changes in the examination technique can go a long way toward facilitating a good exam. These include modifications to communication, allowing tactile exploration, and scheduling. It is important to remember that children with ASD have varying degrees of communication disorders. Some nonverbal children and adults cannot process visual and auditory input at the same time. For these children it is important not to give an auditory and visual task at the same time. Avoid long strings of verbal instructions because sequencing can be very difficult for this population no matter what their verbal abilities (Grandin, 2002). Give one direction at a time. Also, remember that this population is very literal, so keep language concrete.

For example, a problematic statement would be, "Your mom can have a seat. Hop up on the table, take off your shoes and shirt, and let's take a look at you." First, it is a string of directions that can be difficult to follow. Second, if a child thinks a practitioner is only going to "look" at him and then proceeds to perform a hands-on examination, mistrust of the practitioner can result. The practitioner may be viewed as a liar in that he or she said one thing and did another. A preferred way to communicate would be to offer direction as each task is completed: "Get up on the examining table," then "Take your shirt off," then "Take your shoes off," and then "Now I am going to examine you."

Explain each procedure before it occurs: "Now I am going to look in your ear" or "Now I am going to weigh you." Give reasons for each action. For example, when weighing the child tell him or her about the importance of monitoring weight. Without a reason, expected actions may be viewed as meaningless and arbitrary, and the child may resist. It can help to write down the instructions on a piece of paper or use picture lists depending on the verbal level of the child. Furthermore, if a child is stressed or agitated, he or she may not listen or process words until he or she is calm (Vicker, 2003).

If the child is verbal, then the practitioner should strive to establish rapport. Children with ASD often get fixated on certain topics, and expressing interest can serve to establish trust. Furthermore, having the child talk about what he or she is interested in can not only relax the child, but it can also serve as a diversion during the more distressing parts of the exam (Vicker, 2003). In older nonverbal children and adults, touch is their most reliable sense (Grandin, 2002). Allow them to touch instruments, if possible, before using them. This can provide reassurance.

Waiting for long periods can be difficult for a child with ASD. Try to schedule appointments at the beginning of the day or at the very end when wait times will not be as long. Also, allow for extra time in the event the child needs time to calm down.

Record Keeping

In addition to the standard information included in the medical record, it is a good idea to keep unique information about the child with ASD in his or her chart. This could include, but not necessarily be limited to: autistic severity; special features; developmental level; likes and/or fetishes; dislikes and/or phobias for food, drink, activities, or objects; any special needs; and social circumstances (Van Der Walt & Moran, 2001). This information can serve as a quick reference for the primary care practitioner and other health care providers involved with the child's care.

A positive experience for the child with ASD can have long-lasting effects, as can a negative one. Understanding ASD and modifying the environment and examination techniques can be invaluable in providing a positive experience for these children. The competent practitioner has the ability to turn a perceived threatening and frightening experience, such as a health care visit, into one that is positive and comforting.

It is the duty of a practitioner to reach out to these clients to help them achieve the best health possible. Children with ASD are like clients with cultural differences; their world is vastly different from that of the typical developing child. Respecting these children is paramount. This is done by acknowledging and accepting their differences. By instilling routine, comfort, and trust, the practitioner can facilitate lifelong involvement in health care for the ASD client.

REFERENCES

American Psychiatric Association (APA). (2000). *Diagnostic and statistical manual of mental disorders* (4th ed.). Washington, DC: APA.

Blackwell, J., & Niederhauser, C. (2003). Diagnose and manage autistic children. *Nurse Practitioner, 28*(6), 36–43.

Centers for Disease Control. (2003). *Autism spectrum disorders.* Retrieved December 22, 2003, from *http://www.cdc.gov/programs/defects6.htm.*

Committee on Children with Disabilities. (2001). The pediatrician's role in the diagnosis and management of autistic spectrum disorder in children. *Pediatrics, 107*(5), 1221–1227.

Courchesne, E., Townsend, J., & Saitoh, O. (1994). The brain in infantile autism: *Posterior fossa* structures are abnormal. *Neurology, 44,* 214–223.

Courchesne, E., Yeung-Courchene, R., Press, G. A., Hesselink, J. R., & Jernigan, T. A. (1988). Hypoplasia of cerebellar vermal lobules VI and VII in autism. *New England Journal of Medicine, 318,* 1349–1354.

Dalrymple, N., Porco, B., & Chung, J. (1993). *Instructional modules on autism.* Bloomington, NJ: Institute for the Study of Developmental Disabilities.

Dunn, W., Saiter, J., & Rinner, L. (2002). Asperger syndrome and sensory processing: A conceptual model and guidance for intervention planning. *Focus on Autism and Other Developmental Disabilities, 17*(3), 172–186.

Fairfax County Public Schools, Department of Student Services and Special Education. (1995). *Program for students with autism.* Fairfax, VA: FCPS.

Fombonne, E. (1999). The epidemiology of autism: A review. *Psychological Medicine, 29*(4), 769–786.

Fradet, C. (1990). A prospective survey of reactions to blood tests by children and adolescents. *Pain, 40,* 53–60.

Friedlander, A. H., Yagiela, J. A., Paterno, V. L., & Mahler, M. E. (2003). The pathophysiology, medical management, and dental implications of autism. *Journal of the California Dental Association, 31*(9), 681–691.

Gillingham, G. (2003). *Understanding sensory sensitivities and developing supports and accommodations based on the book autism: Handle with care.* Retrieved December 12, 2003, from *http://www.autism-mi.org/aboutautism/general7.html.*

Grandin, T. (2000). *An inside view of autism.* Retrieved November 20, 2003, from *http://www.autism.org/temple/inside.html.*

Grandin, T. (2002). *Teaching tips for children and adults with autism.* Retrieved November 6, 2003, from *http://www.autism.org/temple/tips.html.*

Gray, C. (2003). *Social stories guidelines.* Retrieved May 17, 2004 from *http://www.thegraycenter.org/Social_Stories.htm#The%20Social%20Story%20Guidelines.*

Haracopos, D., & Pedersen, L. (1992). Sexuality and autism: Danish report. Retrieved December 10, 2003, from *http://www.autismuk.com/index9sub.htm.*

Ho, P. T., Keller J. L., Berg, A. L., Cargan, A. L., & Haddad, J., Jr. (1999). Pervasive developmental delay in children presenting as possible hearing loss. *Laryngoscope, 109,* 129–135.

Koller, R. (2000). Sexuality and adolescents with autism. *Sexuality and Disability, 18*(2), 125–136.

Kuoch, H., & Mirenda, P. (2003). Social story interventions for young children with autism spectrum disorders. *Focus on Autism and Other Developmental Disabilities, 18*(4), 219–228.

Kuhn, P. M. (1991). Response to "Effective Communication With Autistic Children." *Rehab Nursing, 16*(2), 19–22.

May, K., Britt, R., & Newman, M. M. (1999). Pediatric registered nurse usage and perception of EMLA. *Journal Society of Pediatric Nursing, 4*(3), 105–112.

Souders, M. C., Freeman, K. G., DePaul, D., & Levy, S. E. (2002). Caring for children and adolescents with autism who require challenging procedures. *Pediatric Nursing, 28*(6), 555–562.

Society for the Autistically Handicapped. (2003). *Sex education for people with autism: Matching programmes to levels of functioning.* Retrieved December 23, 2003, from *http://www.autismuk.com/index9sub1.htm.*

Turnbull, A. P., Turnbull, H. R., Shank, M., & Leal, D. (1995). *Autism in exceptional lives: Special education in today's schools* (pp. 327–361). Englewood Cliffs, NJ: Merrill-Prentice Hall.

United States Department of Education. (2002). *Twenty-fourth annual report to congress on the implementation of the individuals with disabilities education act.* Washington, DC: DOE.

Van Der Walt, J. H., & Moran, C. (2001). An audit of perioperative management of autistic children. *Paediatric Anaesthesia, 11,* 401–408.

Vicker, B. (2003). *Aiding comprehension of individuals with autism spectrum disorders during one-on-one interactions.* Retrieved December 22, 2003, from *http://www.iidc.indiana.edu/irca/communication/aidingComprehension.html.*

Walco, G. A., Cassidy, R. C., & Schecter, N. L. (1994). Pain, hurt, and harm: The ethics of pain control in infants and children. *New England Journal of Medicine, 331,* 541–543.

Wilde, L. D., Koegel, L. K., & Koegel, R. L. (1992). *Increasing success in school through priming: A training manual.* Santa Barbara, CA: University of California.

C H A P T E R   3 7

Vulnerability in Woman with Infertility

Cheryle G. Levitt

The prevalence of infertility in the United States has been consistent at approximately 10 to 15% (Martin, 1994) of the reproductive population, about six million women and their partners (Hart, 2002). Infertility, often unexpected and complex, is usually an undesirable diagnosis or identity (Olshansky, 1987b) and has multiple effects reaching well beyond the physical ramifications of the condition (Woods, Olshansky, & Draye, 1991). Recurrent emotional responses include grief, depression, anger, guilt, shock, denial, and anxiety (Dunkel-Schetter & Lobel, 1991). A transitional life experience bounded by a physiological beginning and end, infertility is uniquely defined in terms of time and meaning for each individual. The physiological culmination of infertility, meaning the final physical inability to conceive or the decision to end attempts to achieve pregnancy, may not signify the actual or true ending of the diagnosis for women. The transitional, experiential aspect of infertility, therefore, may be open-ended. Life transitions involving health may be enhancing or have potential for risk (Meleis, Sawyer, Im, Messias, & Schumacher, 2000), and a measure of increased vulnerability is directly associated with a transitional experience.

Vulnerability has been described as an experience within the process of transition, a "quality of daily lives uncovered through an understanding of clients' experiences and responses during times of transition" (Meleis et al., 2000, p.12). Within a human population, vulnerability has also been defined within a particular group as increased relative risk or susceptibility to adverse health outcomes (Flaskerud, 1998). The connotation of vulnerability suggests a potential or true situation of need, risk, or suboptimal condition for individuals or a population. A conceptual model for vulnerable populations that uses a community health perspective (Flaskerud & Winslow, 1998) is applicable to women with infertility and further defines their relative risk for adverse health outcomes.

This chapter discusses infertility as a vulnerable transitional period in a woman's lifetime. Data analysis from a qualitative study of women who were infertile and subsequently pursued international adoption revealed a period of intense vulnerability and identified women who experience infertility as an at-risk population requiring attention and awareness on the part of health professionals (Levitt, 2002). Certain aspects of the experience identify closely with the Vulnerable Populations Conceptual Model (VPCM) (Flaskerud & Winslow, 1998), validating further both the conclusion of the vulnerability in infertility and conceptualization of the model.

REVIEW OF THE LITERATURE

Vulnerability

The conceptualization of vulnerability in terms of health relates to it as a situation in human life, occurring at different times, that results in potential or actual risk of developing adverse outcomes (Flaskerud, 1998). Groups with increased potential for vulnerability are generally identified based on their access to resources (e.g., financial, environmental, and social), both in the family and in the community at-large. Typical groups with higher inherent susceptibility to vulnerability include women, children, the poor, the handicapped, immigrants, the homeless, people of color, the elderly, gay men and lesbians, and those with a diagnosis of a mental illness (Flaskerud, 1998; Gelberg, Anderson, & Leake, 2000; Katerdahl & Parchman, 2002). In addition to predisposition within a particular group, a change in health status resulting in a sudden acute or serious chronic condition or a potentially terminal disease is also a stimulus for the development of a vulnerable state. Illness-related vulnerability is influenced by and susceptible to (or at relative and varying amount of risk from) factors stemming directly from the problem itself or from preexisting environmental, social, or personal issues directly or indirectly affecting the situation. Those groups with a predisposition to vulnerability, such as the elderly, immigrant populations, and the homeless, are further affected by health conditions, which increase their need for assistance.

Research into vulnerable populations is relatively recent, and it is mainly within the past decade that models have been developed and refined that enable the close analysis of populations with predisposing, enabling, and need components (Gelberg et al., 2000) and have provided a framework for examination within a community health services perspective (Flaskerud & Winslow, 1998). It is advantageous to examine population groups rather than individuals in terms of their vulnerability in order to coordinate responses that best fit the needs of a particular group and that allocate resources most effectively. A model that includes social structure and physical characteristics, aspects of relative risk, and resource availability and then relates these to health status enables the development of more specific clinical practice interventions to assist a particular group.

The Behavioral Model for Vulnerable Populations divides characteristics of populations into predisposing, enabling, and perceived and evaluated need components, and this is further subdivided into traditional and vulnerable domains. Gelger, Anderson, & Leake (2000) studied the homeless population's use of health services and the outcomes of this use by measuring health outcomes with this model. This community is known to be highly vulnerable to both immediate and long-term chronic adverse health conditions. Results showed support for the model and demonstrated 1) improved outcomes for those with longer periods of homelessness and improved coping mechanisms, 2) a reluctance of the homeless to seek services, and that 3) the use of care did not have a major impact on health outcomes given both the harshness of their environments and the quality of health services available.

Katerndahl & Parchman (2002) applied the behavioral model to study people with panic attacks in a study that used 96 panic sufferers and 96 control subjects. The findings found significance in the identification of vulnerability in those with panic attacks as opposed to the control group (who had no history of panic), supporting the hypothesis that the experimental group was a vulnerable population.

The VPCM identifies resource availability in terms of socioeconomic and environmental resources and relative risk by exposure to risk factors (Flaskerud & Winslow, 1998). Resource availability is subdivided into the concepts of human capital (income, jobs, education, and housing), social connectedness (integration, social support, equality, and marginalization), social status (power to have impact on political decisions and distribution of resources), and environmental resources (access to health care and quality of that health care) (Flaskerud & Winslow, 1998).

This chapter describes the application of parts of the VPCM as one basis for understanding some of the increased vulnerability of women with infertility. Particularly pertinent to infertility are the aspects of social connectedness and environmental resources. Social connectedness or integration, as proposed by Flaskerud & Winslow (1998), refers to individuals who are marginalized, stigmatized, and discriminated against by society. Their social integration is incomplete, social inequality is prevalent, and their vulnerability stems from a lack of, or limited connection to, the resources available to fully accepted members of society. I have applied and extended this theoretical explanation to include a population of women who, by virtue of infertility, exhibit vulnerability in that they feel marginalized and disconnected and have imposed upon themselves a stigma because they have not achieved pregnancy, which they see as their right and role as a woman.

Infertility

The diagnosis and history of infertility has been described as a psychogenic illness (when all organic etiologies have been ruled out) (Mazor, 1984; Seibel & Taymor, 1982), a stressful experience (Stanton & Dunkel-Schetter, 1991), and a life crisis (Berger, 1980; Bernstein, 1990; Bresnick, 1981; Cook, 1987; Menning, 1980). Potential effects of infertility relate to physical symptoms, self-esteem, career identities, self-concept, body image, marital communication, sexual relationships, expectant life goals, family relationships, social support systems, religious beliefs, and spiritual practices (Bernstein, 1990; Clark, Henry, & Taylor, 1991; Woods et al., 1991). Although women experience infertility in terms of being unable to physically conceive a pregnancy, the cause of the problem may lie with either partner, and the diagnosis affects both members of the couple (if an active partner is involved).

Infertility is not a single event but a complex process that has been characterized by varying levels and intensities of stress. A review of empirical and descriptive studies by Dunkel-Schetter & Lobel (1991) shows inconsistency in both the psychological manifestations reported as well any sort of sequencing. Emotional and psychological effects are variable; what is consistent is the aspect of the negativity of the infertility experience. Descriptive studies have identified loss of control and effects on self-esteem, identity, beliefs, and social functioning. Loss of control stems from the effects of treatment on health, life routines, scheduling of future life events, and an uncertain future. Less emphasized, but still present in some reports, is loss of autonomy over decisions pertinent to major areas of life and effects on women's career identities (Olshansky, 1987a). The discrepancy between the present and the ideal self, the effect on sexual functioning, and the view of oneself as impotent were prevalent. Further research is needed on the duration of the multiple effects of infertility, especially given the transitional nature of the condition.

Couples with a history of infertility who perceive it as stressful report experiences of loss, possible bereavement, and the "work" (Sandelowski, 1995) and "identity" (Clark et al., 1991; Olshansky, 1987a) of living through infertility. These life experiences have the potential to alter subsequent parenting transitions and the meaning that parents attach to normative events throughout their parenting experiences (Schechter, 1970). This again indicates the open-ended nature of infertility, because the effects last beyond the physiological condition.

Olshansky (1987a) used grounded theory to explore the meaning of infertility, finding that taking on an "identity of self" as infertile was the basic social process. Symbolic rehearsals of becoming pregnant or becoming a parent, and informal followed by formal viewing of the self as infertile, progressed to an expansion of the identity. Managing this identity, which did not necessarily mean relinquishing it, was via one of three modes: overcoming, circumventing, or reconciling. Remaining "in limbo" was a fourth option but not one viewed as managing the identity as infertile. The result, that the identity is pushed to the periphery during the management phase, is significant in the acknowledgment that the identity of "being infertile" does not necessarily disappear once pregnancy or adoption occurs; therefore it may influence subsequent parenting.

The characterization of infertility as a negative life transition associated with possible longer-term effects such as depression, lowered self-esteem, and issues of identity resolution makes the examination of the vulnerability of women with this condition important for health professionals.

Transitions

Viewed as a transitional phenomenon because it is a time-limited and defined period, infertility as the loss of an assumed natural ability to procreate is described as a detour on the journey toward parenthood (Sandelewski, 1995). Transitions can be viewed as a disruption in a person's individual reality (Schaper, 2001) or a period of uncertainty (Selder, 1989), and they may create opportunities for positive change and enhanced well-being. They may also carry the potential for increased risk of negative processes or outcomes. Transitions result from and in changes in health status, life situations, assumptions, opportunities, relationships, and environment (Meleis et al., 2000). Within a transition there are different times and varying levels of perceived or actual vulnerability.

Schumacher & Meleis (1994) identify the centrality of transitions within nursing experiences. The quality and consequences of transitions are influenced by meanings, expectations, level of knowledge and skill, environment, level of planning, and emotional and physical well-being.

Meleis et al., 2000, identified qualitative studies that used transitions as a framework for examining life experiences, and through the analysis of the results, the components of transitions emerged. The studies included becoming an African American mother (Sawyer, 1999); the menopausal transition (Im, 1997); parents and diagnostic transitions (Messias, Gilliss, Sparacino, Tong, & Foote, 1995); and family caregiving (Schumacher & Meleis, 1994). This research enabled an expansion of the theoretical framework of transitions to identify types and patterns of transitions, properties of experiences, transition conditions, and process indicators. Especially meaningful to the study of infertility are the inhibitors to transition: meanings, cultural beliefs and attitudes, socioeconomic status, preparation and knowledge, and community and societal conditions. Transitions require adjustments, some of them major, so that the skills needed for coping and adapting can be developed. Infertility is an example of one such transition.

RESEARCH: WOMEN WITH INFERTILITY
WHO LATER PURSUED ADOPTION

A qualitative study was conducted using grounded theory of women who were diagnosed with infertility and later pursued and became mothers through international adoption (Levitt, 2002). The first phase of the study centered on the women's experience of infertility. It is a secondary analysis of that data that is presented here. Thirteen women were interviewed and asked to describe their experiences during infertility as a diagnosis and during treatment until they decided, or it was decided for them, to cease treatment as the solution to becoming a mother.

Emotions of Infertility

Participants in the study were very emotional when discussing their past experiences of infertility, crying openly despite the passage of 1 or 2 years. Infertility was perceived as a temporary, unnatural condition but an open-ended one because the schedule was flexible by necessity. One participant stated that infertility had its own calendar and all else in her life revolved around it. The irony of the infertility period was that despite the intense physical activity and emotional involvement required for success, there was a very passive, submissive form of involvement and participation for the women and/or couples involved. There were limited options for treatment. There was a progression in intensity and severity for those choices, and the ending was uncertain. The participants were instructed what to do by their physicians, and there was little room or opportunity for negotiation. The cycle of trying, hoping, coping during the wait, "failing" the test, grieving, then regrouping and trying again was repeated month after month, time after time. The constant was the women's perseverance. To be placed in such a passive role was not easy for women who had achieved success professionally and in their private lives. They persisted however, some for years, trying to achieve their goal of a pregnancy, despite the potential threats to health from the treatments. Their vulnerability to future adverse health outcomes is realized and expressed by women during treatment. This suggests a higher relative risk for future, unknown health conditions. One woman stated:

> It only took me two or three years before I stopped the standard fertility treatments because they turned me inside out. I'm firmly convinced that all this stuff is cancer-causing and we're going to see in probably another 10 to 20 years a lot of women dropping at a rate that you wouldn't believe. I'm firmly convinced that you cannot do those kinds of things to your body and survive it. So every step of the way was very difficult for me.

Women were resentful of both the physical changes wrought on their bodies during this time and of their increased personal vulnerability to the possibility of unknown risks, both current and future, in order to achieve their goal of pregnancy.

Marital Distance

Significant marital distance demonstrated the threats to relationships during infertility. All but two participants spoke of increased marital distance, loneliness, and the actual expectation of unhappiness because infertility is an unhappy, unnatural state.

"The issue of infertility was a huge insult to my husband and it was very difficult for him. Blaming is a non-issue on these cases, but he felt very offended. I think he was somewhat pleased when the issue stopped being the quality of his sperm and the quality of my age."

There have been reports (Fleming & Burry, 1988; Menning, 1980) of marital satisfaction and of growing closer during this stage, but this was not found in this study. Instead there was much spoken about the isolation and need to "keep things inside." On the surface, life appeared the same, but underneath was sorrow and discontent. When asked if they concentrated on their relationship with their spouse during this time, women recalled such attempts but also reported not focusing specifically on it because they had other goals. This is consistent with Olshansky's (1987b) findings that infertility is a "full-time job," making other life roles and responsibilities secondary. This shifting of life priorities affected careers, friendships, marriages, and family roles and responsibilities.

Feelings and Emotions

The feelings and emotions remembered during this time were uniformly negative, but there were degrees, ranging from "difficult and frustrating" to "devastating." Participants used many words to describe this time: unexpected, devastating, hopeless, depressing, disappointing, and frustrating. They reported feeling inferior and sensitive and wanting to be alone and to suffer by themselves. "Few highs and many lows were the norm," stated one participant. There was grief work that was unresolved, as evidenced by the crying and regret expressed openly and repeatedly. Despite all participants having achieved eventual motherhood through adoption, several expressed real regret, persisting to the present, over never becoming pregnant and never achieving motherhood through pregnancy. This was described as being a separate issue from being a mother to their current child(ren). The least negative description was that infertility was "a sensitive time for me that was too painful to share with others while I was going through it. . . . It's certainly not a pleasant experience. The most frustrating part was basically because we never found the problem. We were always looking, searching. . . . I didn't want to feel good about it, you know? The point wasn't to feel good about it and be resolved. You just wanted it to succeed. You didn't want to be reconciled to being infertile."

The resolution to transitions includes the development of coping and adaptation skills. Women who have faced infertility speak of not wanting to adjust, to accept or to assimilate the challenges into their lives. They did not want to be or stay infertile and felt that assimilation of the identity would have signified defeat or, at least, a comfort they were unable to justify or accept. The only sustaining and remotely positive emotion expressed was hope, but it was sporadic and muted, as this participant recalled. "The period between when you get the treatment and you wait for the (pregnancy) test, I wouldn't even allow myself to think it was happening. I wanted to hope but was afraid to hope because it was too risky. Later while waiting (for the adoption) I felt real hope and that felt good."

Social Isolation and the Need for Privacy

The majority of participants carefully preserved their privacy, preferring to cope alone or with a few chosen and supportive family members or friends. Participants reported recalling an intense need for this privacy. Repeatedly, they declared their desire to travel this journey alone or with one select family member or friend. Some went to a support group initially but said it did not help; instead, it reinforced their loneliness. Two participants said that support groups at the end of their infertility treatment assisted them with closure. One participant, who was single at the time of her infertility and adoption but married at the time of the study, stated that although she was single and alone in her decision to have a child, she never went through a treatment alone. She always had her mother or a friend at the hospital with her, and this made it bearable. As this participant said:

> I really grieved the experience of not being pregnant. I felt the loss of control over the inability to have a child to be overwhelming. At the time I didn't have much information about infertility diagnoses and treatment processes, and didn't have many people to talk to about our experience. The infertility part was private; something we shared only with immediate family and very few close friends. It was very isolating and difficult but I couldn't have handled the talking about it.

In terms of community support, participants discussed the difficulty of living in a young, pro-life, vibrant, and fertile community that was focused on family and children. Most participants recalled that it was difficult to be around children, and some discussed the negative impact of living in such an environment during their struggle with infertility. Self-protective measures such as avoidance—not attending community affairs such as baby parties—were a common step that was taken. Participants recalled how difficult it was to visit the homes of friends with children, so women often refused or invented excuses and chose solitude or isolation over misery and disappointment. Self-protection also took the form of distraction, which they achieved by immersing themselves more deeply into their work, investing time in their homes, and trying new hobbies and classes. They consistently stated that these activities were secondary to the fertility schedule. They also stated that they knew intellectually that infertility was, by definition, a temporary state of being and that knowing this provided help and solace.

The lack of social connectedness is described within the VPCM (Flaskerud & Winslow, 1998) as social marginalization, inequality, incomplete integration, and decreased or no family support. Women with infertility did not want social connections or integration into a group, yet they felt alone, isolated, and vulnerable to the unknown risks and future without a pregnancy or children. Women reported "missed opportunities" and frequently avoided social situations as a form of self-protection. This became a cycle however, because creating solitude did not help them feel better, yet their fears of sadness in public were perceived to be more pervasive, more threatening or difficult than being alone. Participants reported changes in their perception of and roles within some social relationships and knew this was a result of their inability to interact and respond in the same way they did before their infertility.

Cessation of Treatment: Closing the Door

Cessation of fertility treatments constituted the physical closure of the infertility period for all participants but not necessarily the emotional closure. Despite the difficulties and anguish unanimously expressed when describing their fertility treatment, most participants also recalled ambivalence when deciding to end it. One participant said: "Finally the doctor said to us, 'Close the door.' I mean, the wailing that went on within me. I never really dealt with that mourning completely even within myself and we never really did any kind of closure for that period. But I have trouble to this day dealing with it."

Cessation of treatment meant failure to conceive, closure of the option to have a biological child, and surrender of the role of biological mother. It was a decision made with trepidation and fear of the future. One participant stated that "It was very easy for me to begin fertility treatments but very hard to stop them. I felt like I was giving up. It was very hard for me to admit failure. Part of me has a regret that I was never able to get pregnant."

Conversely, treatment cessation also constituted an end to the acute physical and emotional suffering caused by the treatments and ended somewhat the identity of infertile as defined by the rigors of the treatments. It also paved the way for the consideration of other options for parenting, which included adoption. "Once I stopped the fertility treatments, it was a lot easier to prepare emotionally for parenthood."

The cessation of treatment signaled an end to the active pursuit of pregnancy but did not close the door of complex and conflicting emotions, unfulfilled wishes, and hopes for resolution of the infertile state. The vulnerability of the women during the time of ending treatment shifted to the need to accept the possibility that pregnancy might never occur and that their goal of parenting was at least deferred until other options could be explored.

CONCLUSION

Infertility represents an open-ended transitional time in a woman's life, a time where intense physical and emotional needs create a vulnerability to increased relative physical and psychological risk and issues with social connectedness and integration. The experience of infertility has a profound effect on a woman's self-image, identity, and outlook on the present and future, which is consistent with the finding of Meleis (1975) that significant transitions have effects on one's sense of self. Cessation of treatment does not end the infertility period for women, and, indeed, studies exploring women who became new mothers after a period of infertility (Olshansky, 2003) indicate that they have increased vulnerability to depression. Given mothers' reports that they still carried the "identity of infertility" after they became mothers, further research is recommended on the progression and resolution of other aspects of the infertility experience, including the social integration issues.

Health professionals should recognize the vulnerability to physical and emotional health risks and the social integration issues in women with infertility. Nurses have an opportunity to interact regularly with women while they receive their treatments, and counseling is advised as an option for women and their partners before beginning, during, and possibly after infertility treatment. In addition, knowledge of the signs of emotional stress and depression are important so that women with potential risk for further emotional issues can be identified.

REFERENCES

Berger, D. M. (1980). Couple's reactions to male infertility and donor insemination. *American Journal of Psychiatry, 137,* 1047–1049.

Bernstein, J. (1990). Parenting after infertility. *Journal of Perinatal & Neonatal Nursing, 4*(2), 11–23.

Bresnick, E. R. (1981). A holistic approach to the treatment of the crisis of infertility. *Journal of Marital and Family Therapy, 7,* 181–188.

Clark, L. F., Henry, S. M., & Taylor, D. M. (1991). Cognitive examination of motivation for childbearing as a factor in adjustment to infertility. In A. L. Stanton & C. Dunkel-Schetter (Eds.). *Infertility: Perspectives from stress and coping research* (pp. 157–180). New York, NY: Plenum.

Cook, E. P. (1987). Characteristics of the biopsychosocial crisis of infertility. *Journal of Counseling and Development, 65,* 465–470.

Dunkel-Schetter, C., & Lobel, M. (1991). Psychological reactions to infertility. In A. Stanton & C. Dunkel-Schetter (Eds.). *Perspectives from stress and coping research* (pp. 29–57). New York, NY: Plenum.

Flaskerud, J. H. (1998). Vulnerable populations. In J.J. Fitzpatrick (Ed.). *Encyclopedia of nursing research.* New York, NY: Springer.

Flaskerud, J. H., & Winslow, B. J. (1998). Conceptualizing vulnerable population's health-related research. *Nursing Research, 47*(2), 69–78.

Fleming, J., & Burry, K. (1988). Coping with infertility. In D. Valentine (Ed.). *Infertility and adoption: A guide for social work practice* (pp. 37–41). New York, NY: Haworth.

Gelberg, L. A., Anderson, R. M., & Leake, B. D. (2000). The behavioral model for vulnerable populations: Application to medical care use and outcomes for homeless people. *Health Services Research, 34,* 1273–1302.

Hart, V. A. (2002). Infertility and the role of psychotherapy. *Issues in Mental Health Nursing, 23*(1), 31–41.

Katerdahl, D. A., & Parchman, M. L. (2002). Understanding ambulatory care use by people with panic attacks: Testing the behavioral model for vulnerable populations. *Journal of Nervous and Mental Disease, 190*(8), 554–557.

Levitt, C. (2002). *Maternal role attainment through intercountry adoption.* Unpublished doctoral dissertation, Duquesne University, Pittsburgh, PA.

Martin, M. (1994). Infertility. In A. H. DeCherney & M. L. Pernoll (Eds.). *Current obstetric and gynecologic diagnosis and treatment* (8th ed.). Norwalk, CT: Appleton & Lange.

Mazor, M. D. (1984). Emotional reactions to infertility. In M. D. Mazor & H. F. Simons (Eds.). *Infertility: Medical emotional and social considerations* (pp. 23–35). New York, NY: Human Sciences.

Meleis, A. I. (1975). Role insufficiency & role implementation. *Nursing Research, 24,* 264–270.

Meleis, A. I., Sawyer, L. M., Im, E. O., Messias, D. K. H., & Schumacher, K. (2000). Experiencing transitions: An emerging middle-range theory. *Advances in Nursing Science, 23*(1), 12–28.

Menning, B. E. (1980). The emotional needs of infertile couples. *Fertility & Sterility, 34,* 313–319.

Messias, D. K., Gilliss, C. L., Sparacino, P. S., Tong, E. M., & Foote, D. (1995). Stories of transition: Parents recall the diagnosis of congenital heart defects. *Family Systems Medicine, 3*(3/4), 367–377.

Olshansky, E. (1987a). Identity of self as infertile: An example of theory-generating research. *Advances in Nursing Science, 9*(2), 54–63.

Olshansky, E. (1987b). Infertility and its influence on women's career identities. *Health Care for Women International, 8*(2,3), 185–196.

Olshansky, E. (2003). A theoretical explanation for previously infertile mothers' vulnerability to depression. *Journal of Nursing Scholarship, 35*(3), 263–268.

Sandelowski, M. (1995). A theory of the transition of parenthood of infertile couples. *Research in Nursing and Health, 18,* 123–132.

Sawyer, L. M. (1999). Engaged mothering: The transition to motherhood for a group of African-American women. *Journal of Transcultural Nursing, 1,* 14–21.

Schaper, A. M. (2001). *A life transition theory: Women's postpartum negative experiences.* Unpublished doctoral dissertation, University of Wisconsin, Milwaukee.

Schechter, M. D. (1970). About adoptive parents. In E. J. Anthony & T. Benedek, (Eds.). *Parenthood: Its psychology & psychopathology* (pp. 355–371). Boston, MA: Little Brown.

Schumacher, K. L., & Meleis, A. I. (1994). Transitions: A central concept in nursing. *Image, 26*(2), 119–127.

Selder, F. (1989). Life transition theory: The resolution of uncertainty. *Nursing & Health Care, 10*(8), 432–451.

Seibel, M. M., & Taymor, M. L. (1982). Emotional aspects of infertility. *Fertility & Sterility, 37,* 137–145.

Stanton, A., & Dunkel-Schetter, C. (Eds.). (1991). *Infertility: Perspectives from stress and coping research.* New York, NY: Plenum.

Woods, N. F., Olshansky, E., & Draye, M. A. (1991). Infertility: Women's experiences. *Health Care for Women International, 12,* 179–190.

UNIT V

TEACHING-LEARNING

All of the health disciplines must become transcultural. We are living in a multicultural world. If we don't educate ourselves as to how we can provide culturally sensitive care to all people, people will not want to use the system or [will] find it inappropriate.

Madeleine Leininger

Source: Interview with Dr. Leininger—University of Nebraska Web site, retrieved 2/27/04.

CHAPTER 38

Teaching Nurses About Vulnerable Populations

Mary de Chesnay

There are many ways to teach nursing students how to work with vulnerable people, and there are numerous activities students can engage in to gain practice in providing culturally competent care. The purpose of this unit is to present some ideas for faculty with regard to the use of these strategies or to inspire them to devise similar learning activities for their own students. For students who read this unit, it is hoped that they find some of the experiences presented inspirational with regard to their own fieldwork.

For any activity designed to prepare nurses to provide culturally competent care, it is critical to emphasize two things: to know oneself and to show respect for others. First, the best thing nurses can do to prepare for working with vulnerable people is to *know themselves*. The more a person knows and acknowledges his or her own biases, the more easily the nurse can put these aside and concentrate on the patient as a person instead of a stereotype. Ethnocentric bias is a term derived from anthropology and refers to the notion that one's own cultural beliefs, practices, folkways, values, and norms are the right ones. Ethnocentric biases develop from our experience of living within our own cultures: growing up in families, attending educational institutions with certain emphases, and interacting with people we like or do not like. Ethnocentrism is neither good nor bad, it just is. To acknowledge that we all have biases simply indicates that we are human. Human beings tend to get in trouble when they act toward others as if their own way is the only right way or when they confuse bias with truth.

How do we learn to deal with ethnocentric bias? It is essential to recognize a particular feeling or attitude as bias and then critically examine all of our own values and beliefs, particularly in terms of how we see others who are different from ourselves. This principle of self-examination relates to everyone, not just to members of majority groups. It might be helpful to apply the general system theory concept of multifinality, which holds that there are many ways to the same end. Appreciating that other ways of achieving the goal might be equally effective and valid is a key component of self-awareness.

The second thing nurses can do to prepare for working with vulnerable people is to learn to *show respect*. Novices tend to expend large amounts of time and energy trying to learn cultural material quickly so that they can interact "appropriately" in terms of superficial gestures, such as making eye contact or not, shaking hands or not, or touching arms. Yet, despite the best of intentions, these actions can sometimes be interpreted as mocking the group. Being yourself, yet doing your best in terms of showing the most respect according to your own cultural standards, is more likely to be understood by the patient as respectful than is trying gestures or expressions that are obviously not your own.

Another key point in providing culturally competent care is to reframe compliance or adherence in light of the patient's or group's cultural norms, values, and folkways. For example, students might not understand food taboos and offer pork to a Muslim or Jewish patient, then wrongly interpret the patient's rejection of pork as loss of appetite. Many Arabs and Jews do not observe the dietary laws but many do, and it is important to ask. The patient and family are the best teachers of their culture. The point is to ask and not to assume.

WHY TEACH NURSING STUDENTS ABOUT VULNERABLE POPULATIONS?

Global demographics are changing as populations evolve into ever more complex societies. Demographics of individual countries change rapidly as people move within their countries or from one country to another to find food, jobs, or simply better lives for their families. The nursing profession cannot afford for its practitioners to be isolationist in the way they treat patients and families. Neither can we afford to ignore communities. Community-based care and focus on populations are aspects of nursing that students need to learn in order to provide cost-effective, culturally competent care.

The kinds of experiences students have in their basic educational programs can improve their confidence. In this chapter, two models from different universities are presented. Although both universities happen to be private, the strategies and activities are universal and can be adapted by anyone interested in helping students develop or improve cross-cultural interpersonal relations. In Chapter 39, "Preparing Nursing Professionals for Advocacy: Service Learning," a third service learning model is presented from a different point of view. Many schools have implemented similar programs on behalf of the vulnerable populations of their own or international communities. Web sites for the schools are a good source of information.

WHAT SHOULD STUDENTS LEARN?

Nurses need experiences that teach them to be comfortable with people different from themselves, and this requires interaction with many kinds of people. It is not sufficient to review the literature and write papers on vulnerable populations. Writing papers is useful but can be an empty intellectual exercise if not combined with developing competence at talking with people. Fieldwork is an excellent way to develop interaction skills.

Students need to develop an understanding of culture and become aware of their own ethnocentric biases. They need to do so within a safe context in which they will not be criticized by their faculty for attitudes they hold but rather coached to develop new ideas or views about the vulnerable. For example, it is not useful to berate students who believe that all homeless people should take menial jobs in order to get off the street. Instead, they should be guided to understand the complexities of homelessness and why even menial jobs are not an option for many people.

Even though the statistical information on vulnerable populations often becomes obsolete before it is printed because the health disparities in this country increase with population increases, students still need to know who the vulnerable are and recognize the health disparities of the vulnerable populations in their communities. Students should be encouraged to review the literature critically for applicability to vulnerable populations and to formulate practices that better serve the vulnerable.

Finally, students should learn how to reverse vulnerability. Nursing means not only curing and preventing illness but also strengthening the patient's resources so that the patient becomes less vulnerable. Once trendy, the term "empowerment" has fallen out of favor because it has a patriarchal connotation, but the notion that people can be helped to attain autonomy is still useful in teaching students to care for the vulnerable. Perhaps a more appropriate intervention is helping the patient develop or increase resilience. Everyone has strengths, and focusing on strength rather than weakness is a good therapeutic technique.

MODELS OF SERVICE LEARNING

Duquesne Model

Duquesne University is a small liberal arts institution founded in 1878 and operated by the Spiritans, an order of priests with strong service ties to developing countries in Africa and South America. Through its school of nursing, Duquesne confers undergraduate and graduate degrees, including the Ph.D., and a variety of certificate and continuing education programs. During the author's tenure as dean of the school from 1994 to 2002, the faculty created a variety of programs and experiences for students and faculty in order to operationalize the service mission of the university. Two major outreach programs (local and international) are particularly relevant to the education of nursing students in caring for people from vulnerable populations, and these programs involved students at all levels: baccalaureate, master's, and doctoral.

Nurse-Managed Wellness Centers

The first outreach program was initially funded by the school of nursing and later by a grant from the US Department of Housing and Urban Development (HUD.) The faculty member who coordinated the gerontological clinical nurse specialist track in the master of science in nursing (MSN) program created a model for outreach into the community by starting a wellness clinic in a high-rise apartment building designated for senior citizens (Taylor, Resick, D'Antonio, & Carroll, 1997). Students and faculty conducted many health-screening and health-promotion activities. The model was evaluated as successful by residents, staff, faculty, and students, with the result that the clinic was replicated later in a federally funded project to expand services to African Americans in the poor neighborhoods near the university.

With the success of the prototype center, two additional centers were opened in the African American communities called the Hill District and East Liberty (Resick, Taylor, & Leonardo, 1999). Later, the Visiting Nurse Association in Butler County, Pennsylvania, adopted the model for a rural community north of the city. To prepare for the expansion of the clinic, the faculty used ethnographic methods to gain access to the community, to establish rapport with civic leaders and community residents, and to identify areas of need that the school of nursing could fulfill (Resick, Taylor, Carroll, D'Antonio, & de Chesnay, 1997). The community members initially had reservations about the proposed clinic because they perceived previous experiences, when outsiders had come into the community for various research projects, as disrespectful to them. However, by using the principles of ethnographic research and the methods of participant observation and interviewing, the faculty found ways to involve the community in planning so that when the second clinic opened, the community members reported that they felt a sense of ownership.

As of this writing, the original clinic and the Hill District clinic are thriving and provide a continuous educational experience for students and a practice setting for the nurse-practitioner faculty. Faculty and students conduct health assessments, medication evaluations, teaching presentations, exercise classes in the form of dance therapy, and other health promotion activities. One of the projects at the clinics involved creating a chart audit system for measuring outcomes. This experience provided graduate students with the opportunity to apply theory to the practice of nursing in a functioning practice setting and allowed them to test the validity and reliability of the audit tool in a real setting in a way that would be used by the staff (Resick, 1999).

When necessary, staff refer residents to their primary care providers and, in some cases, directly to the emergency room. Students who rotate through the clinics obtain a sophisticated understanding of the health care issues of the elderly in the two independent-living high-rises, one predominantly white and the other predominantly African American. Through the clinics, students learn firsthand the issues of the elderly as a vulnerable population.

Other activities in the local communities were initiated at the request of the community leaders, who had identified problems. One highly successful program was one that taught cardiopulmonary resuscitation (CPR) to residents of all ages. A research project was conducted by faculty to examine community knowledge about CPR, and the results were helpful in developing the CPR programs (Winter, 2001). Classes were conducted by certified faculty in the community centers, and people of all ages completed the course.

Center for International Nursing

The Center for International Nursing was created in 1992 (Carty & White, 1993; White & Smith, 1997) to provide an administrative structure within which students and faculty could conduct educational programs, service projects, and research abroad. Initially, the Center's focus was Nicaragua, but later the Center expanded to South America, Africa, and Europe in order to complete specific initiatives. During the time period from 1994 to 2002, over 130 students at all levels completed international projects, and every year, 6 to 10 undergraduate students completed part of their community health nursing clinical requirement in a barrio in Managua in conjunction with Duquesne faculty and faculty in the sister school, *Universidad Politecnica de Nicaragua* (UPOLI) (L. Cunningham & S. Colvin, personal communication, August 2000). The students conducted community assessments, performed health assessments, intervened in referrals to the community health clinics, and conducted health fairs to teach the community residents a variety of health promotion techniques. On another project, one of the critical care faculty taught part of the trauma content to students in a hospital in Managua (C. Ross, personal communication, September, 1999).

Due largely to the publicity about the activities of the Center, the nursing school was approached by the Pittsburgh Rotary Club, who wanted to begin an international health project. They built a clinic in partnership with the Rotary Clubs of Managua and Jinotega in a northern community of Nicaragua near the city of Jinotega. When the community residents were asked what they wanted to name their clinic, they indicated that they wanted it named for the late member of the Pittsburgh Pirates baseball team, thus, *La Clinica de Roberto Clemente.* Clemente died in a plane crash while trying to deliver medical supplies after the Managua earthquake of 1972 and is still revered in Nicaragua. This clinic is used by nurse practitioner faculty as a clinical site for graduate students, and the community was the site of an ethnographic study on men's health conducted as dissertation research by a doctoral student, as described in Chapter 34 in this book (Ross, 2000).

A second international study was conducted as action research by a doctoral student who worked in Peru on the clean water project run by the Sisters of Mercy (Zolkoski, 2000). Other doctoral students have conducted independent studies in Nicaragua and served as teaching faculty for some of the programs offered to the local nurses and physicians.

Faculty made a commitment to the sister school (UPOLI), and many other projects were conducted with the poor of Nicaragua. The emphasis on the "train the trainer" approach meant that the faculty tried to work with the local nurses as much as possible; many projects were accomplished with the support of the sister school faculty. The study described in Chapter 17 of this book, "Child Health in a Barrio of Managua," was an outcome of the work conducted under the auspices of the *hermanamiento* (sister school relationship). Many other projects and programs have been conducted and are too numerous to mention here.

Online Doctoral Program

Concurrent with the increasing international visibility of the Duquesne University School of Nursing, the faculty became aware of the desire of nurses in developing countries to improve nursing education for their people. Dr. John Murray, the university president, challenged the deans to experiment with distance learning strategies, and the faculty chose to meet his challenge by creating opportunities for nurses in developing countries to earn Duquesne's Ph.D. in nursing through synchronous Web-based courses, coupled with residency on campus during the summers. The first course was taught by Dr. Jeri Milstead in summer of 1997 (Milstead, 1998). Although some international nurses applied to the program, we as faculty were surprised at the popularity of the program among nurses who lived within driving distance of the university. Many lived in medically underserved areas where they needed to continue working because there was no one to replace them or because they still had children at home, but they were highly motivated, and the program became extremely competitive.

Seattle University Model

MSN Program

The Seattle University College of Nursing has demonstrated a long tradition of consistent fit with the mission of the university to promote social justice by serving the poor. In response to changes in health care during the 1980s, faculty revised the master's degree program to teach advanced-practice nurses to work with vulnerable populations (Vezeau, Peterson, Nakao, & Ersek, 1998). Originally developed as a clinical specialist program, the faculty recognized the need for nurse practitioners and added a family nurse practitioner track and, more recently, an innovative second-degree immersion track for people with college degrees in other disciplines who wish to be nurses.

In the current MSN program, N502 is dedicated to working with vulnerable populations. Students examine the issues related to a population of their choice. Ch. 10, "Applying Leininger's Culture Care Theory: The Oromo of Seattle") and Ch. 43, "Graduate Fieldwork with Vulnerable Populations") are examples. Chapter 10 is an elaboration of the work the author completed in the course. Chapter 43 describes the teaching and learning strategies for the course with examples from students' fieldwork.

Many experiences in other courses (for example, the clinical courses and the thesis/scholarly project) enable the students to develop comfort and skill at working with diverse patients, families, and communities. For the thesis or scholarly project, the students are expected to develop projects significant to their own future roles as advanced-practice nurses and to vulnerable populations.

BSN Program

Chapter 40, "Neighborhoods and Nurses: An Integrated Undergraduate Curriculum," includes a description of the activities students complete in the garden communities of Seattle. Garden communities are the poor neighborhoods scattered around the city in which students spend a good bit of clinical time. In addition, faculty are assigned to each community and provide clinical supervision and support. The undergraduate course on vulnerable populations is a two-credit required course, originally developed by Dr. Jenny Tsai, in which the students conduct fieldwork by interviewing persons different from themselves in order to develop comfort with and competence at interacting with culturally diverse people and groups.

Faculty have many creative techniques for helping students work with vulnerable people. For their community health course, Dr. Helen Miske has taken senior students to Belize, where they live with local families and give direct care in a variety of health care settings. Special experiences in developing empathy for the homeless are directed by Dr. Suzanne Gillette, who guides students in exercises to help them see what it feels like to have limited transportation options (S. Gillette, personal communication, January 2004). Dr. Kathy Carr, an internationally known nurse-midwife, is helping draft a training manual for cervical cancer screening in areas with low resources (Camacho Carr & Sellors, 2004).

Key Components of Educational Experience

A plan for teaching nursing students how to care for vulnerable populations might include the following:

☐ Identify the vulnerable populations within the community. If international nursing is an interest of the school, then faculty might capitalize on their own international research or service experiences. Sister school relationships such as the Duquesne *hermanamiento* could provide wonderful opportunities for faculty and student exchanges, service learning projects, or collaborative research with nursing faculty in other countries.

☐ Develop a set of guidelines for students to follow for their fieldwork with the expected outcomes clearly stated. (The Instructor Guide for this book has sample syllabi and detailed guidelines.) Outcomes should include an expectation for improved self-awareness.

☐ Designate key faculty to coordinate or guide the process. Not every faculty member will want to be involved, but it is essential to have at least one faculty champion for each project.

☐ Establish the need for specific projects in concert with stakeholders who are key members of the population.

☐ Decide whether service learning projects will be part of the curriculum and conducted within specific courses or whether they will be freestanding as people express interest. One way to focus on vulnerable populations without major curriculum changes is to allow students to use independent study courses for fieldwork.

☐ Design and implement a small-scale project that can be funded through existing resources. Later, after individual faculty have established a track record, more sophisticated projects can be funded through grants and contracts.

☐ Evaluate the projects not only in terms of student satisfaction and learning but also in terms of benefits to the population.

☐ Consider evaluation data carefully before designing subsequent projects.

SUMMARY

The models presented here have several characteristics in common that contributed to their effectiveness in meeting the objectives of the courses and programs. Characteristics of successful experiences for students include opportunities for developing self-awareness, fieldwork that enables them to develop communication skills and exercises in interacting with people different from themselves, and review of available literature on the population of interest. Although these experiences are challenging, the students generally rate them as positive. In many cases in which students have traveled to be immersed in another culture, they indicate that their experiences were life-changing. The success of these service learning programs demonstrates that providing such opportunities at undergraduate and graduate levels is a crucial aspect of nursing education with regard to vulnerable populations.

REFERENCES

Camacho Carr, K., & Sellors, J. (In press). Cervical cancer screening in low resource settings using visual inspection with acetic acid (VIA). *Journal of Midwifery and Women's Health.*

Carty, R. & White J. (1993). *Nicaraguan-American nursing collaborating project.* Washington, DC: American Association of Colleges of Nursing, 37–38.

Milstead, J. (1998). Preparation for an online asynchronous university doctoral course: Lessons learned. *Computers in Nursing, 16*(5), 247–258.

Resick, L. (1999). Challenges in measuring outcomes in two community-based nurse-managed wellness clinics: The development of a chart auditing tool. *Home Health Care Management and Practice, 11*(4), 52–59.

Resick, L., Taylor, C., & Leonardo, M. (1999). The Nurse-Managed Wellness Clinic Model developed by Duquesne University School of Nursing. *Home Health Care Management and Practice, 11*(6), 26–35.

Resick, L., Taylor, C., Carroll, T., D'Antonio, J., & de Chesnay, M. (1997). Establishing a nurse-managed wellness clinic in a predominantly older African American inner-city high rise: An advanced practice nursing project. *Nursing Administration Quarterly, 21*(4), 47–54.

Ross, C. (2000). *Caminando mas cerca con Dios* [A closer walk with Thee]: *An ethnography of health and well-being of rural Nicaraguan men.* Unpublished doctoral dissertation, Duquesne University, Pittsburgh, PA.

Taylor, C., Resick, L., D'Antonio, J., & Carroll, T. (1997). *Advanced Practice Nursing Quarterly, 3*(2), 36–45.

Vezeau, T., Peterson, J., Nakao, C., & Ersek, M. (1998). Education of advanced practice nurses serving vulnerable populations. *Nursing and Health Care Perspectives, 19*(1), 124–131.

White, J., & Smith, C. (1997). Developing an international nursing partnership with Nicaragua. *International Nursing Review, 44*(1), 13–18.

Winter, K. (2001). Bystander CPR in two Pittsburgh communities. *Cultura de los Cuidados, 5*(9), 82–89.

Zolkoski, R. (2000). *Clean water for Chimbote, Peru: Transcultural nursing in participatory action research.* Unpublished doctoral dissertation, Duquesne University, Pittsburgh, PA.

Preparing Nursing Professionals for Advocacy: Service Learning

Lynda P. Nauright

Paralleling the women's movement, nursing in the 1960s and 1970s was evolving from the ethic of loyalty to the physician and hospital to a new ethic of patient advocacy. Modern nursing, which began on the battlefield of the Crimea (1854–56), had always been ingrained with a military metaphor. Nurses wore uniforms, caps, and cloaks. Different schools had unique insignia, and stripes were added as the student progressed up the ranks (Winslow, 1984).

Consistent with the military theme, loyalty to the commanding officer and strict obedience to his orders were a major part of the nursing ethic. The Nightingale pledge, written in 1893, states, "with loyalty, I will endeavor to aid the physician in his work" (Davis & Aroskar, 1978, pp. 12–13). Charlotte Aikens' classic text on nursing ethics, published in 1916, states:

> Loyalty to the physician is one of the duties demanded of every nurse, not solely because the physician is her superior officer, but chiefly because the confidence of the patient in his physician is one of the important elements in the management of his illness, and nothing should be said or done that would weaken this faith or create doubts as to the character or ability or methods of the physician (p. 44).

The moral power of this reasoning was compelling. Nurses were concerned about the well-being of their patients and were taught repeatedly that the "faith" that people have in a physician is as much a healing element as is any medicinal treatment. Thus even if the physician blundered, the patient's confidence was to be maintained at all costs. Parsons' (1916) text states: "If a mistake has been made in treating a patient, the patient is not the person who should know it if it can be kept from him, because the anxiety and lack of confidence that he would naturally feel might be injurious to him and retard his recovery" (p. 32).

From the beginning of the 20th century, some thoughtful nurses questioned and debated among themselves where such loyalty should end (Where does loyalty, 1910), and as early as 1932, Annie Goodrich spoke of modifying, if not abolishing, militarism in nursing (Goodrich, 1932). But the Code for Nurses accepted by the American Nurses Association (ANA) called for nurses to verify and sustain physicians' orders, sustain confidence in the physician, and report incompetence or unethical conduct "only to the proper authority" (A Code for Nurses, 1950, p. 196). The International Congress of Nursing (ICN) passed a similar code in 1953 (ICN, 1953).

However, in the turbulent 1960s and 1970s, a diminishing confidence in the medical profession, or perhaps just a more realistic view of it, coupled with rising consumerism and feminism, brought about changes in perspective for both nurses and patients. Leaders of the patients' rights movement turned to nurses for assistance in securing fundamental rights of patients: informed consent, the right to refuse treatment, and the right to have full information about diagnosis and prognosis.

George Annas, an attorney and author of *The Rights of Hospital Patients* (Annas, 1975), explicitly attacked the military metaphor and called for nurses to accept the new role of patient advocacy. He was not disappointed. Nurses enthusiastically embraced the role of patient advocate. The nursing literature of the 1970s and 1980s is replete with discussions of advocacy as an essential role of the nurse and with the concept of advocacy as an appropriate philosophical base for nursing.

Nursing codes of ethics were revised as well. In 1973, the ICN dropped all mention of loyal obedience to the physician's orders and stated, "The nurse's primary responsibility is to those people who require nursing care" (Davis & Aroskar, 1978, pp. 13–14). The 1976 revision of the ANA Code for Nurses specifically required nurses to protect the "client" from the "incompetent, unethical or illegal practice of any person" (ANA, 1976, p. 8). Gone from the revised code were rules obliging the nurse to maintain confidence in physicians or obey their orders. In fact, the word physician does not even appear in the Code.

Given that patient advocacy is a nursing value, how then do we prepare students to be patient advocates, to care about advocacy, and to exercise social responsibility? One method is through learning strategies such as service learning. Service learning is defined as educational experiences in which students participate in a service activity that meets community needs within the framework of a specific credit-bearing work. Service learning evolves from a philosophy of education that emphasizes active learning and is directed toward encouraging social responsibility (Mueller & Norton, 1998). Service learning connects thought and feeling in a deliberate way, creating a context in which students can explore how they feel about what they are thinking and what they think about how they feel. (Ehrlich, 1995). Service learning opportunities in which students are able to use their skills and knowledge to help the community while furthering their learning are powerful tools for teaching students to be advocates. After participating in a course using service learning, one student wrote, "Before taking this class, I did not have any idea of the importance of personal involvement. Having graduated 20 years ago, I was 'trained' to do tasks, not think too much, and be a good girl. Thank God times have changed. I have been helping myself as well as others by volunteering. The time that I have spent at [a homeless shelter] has given me a broader understanding of the word 'care.'"

BENEFITS OF SERVICE LEARNING

One obvious benefit of service learning is that it meets actual community needs, but there are many others. Service learning fosters caring for others, allows students to experience firsthand how vulnerable populations are affected by public policy, and helps them develop empathy with diverse individuals. Reflection on the experience is a critical component of service learning and fosters moral development and enhances moral decision making.

This direct participation with vulnerable populations often causes students to develop a better understanding of self and their own strengths and weaknesses. They develop skills in problem solving, critical thinking, leadership, and ethical decision making. An increased sense of civic responsibility, increased political and global awareness, and development of cultural competence may also be outcomes (Mueller & Norton, 1998).

Benefits also accrue to the institutions who engage in service learning. The foundation of an effective service learning program is a balanced long-term partnership between communities and institutions of higher education. This "hands-on" community involvement enhances institutional visibility, may appeal to potential donors, and helps minimize the traditional separation between "town and gown" (Pellietier, 1995).

In Their Own Words: Impact of Service Learning on Students

For several years the author taught an undergraduate policy course that had a service learning component. Students were allowed to choose a vulnerable population, interact with the people in it, identify a political or policy issue that affected it, and advocate with state or federal legislators on its behalf. Just the simple act of interacting with vulnerable populations and becoming personally involved in actions on their behalf is a life-altering event for students. Students were encouraged to reflect on their experiences and to record their reflections in a journal. Their journal reflections of the impact of service learning make the case far better than any narrative written by faculty.

Students interacted with vulnerable populations in a variety of ways: volunteering with the American Red Cross, the Georgia State Council on Maternal and Infant Health, the Georgia State Nurses' Association School Health Task Force, children's shelters, food banks, Planned Parenthood, the Salvation Army, refugee programs, the State Council on Aging, AIDS outreach programs, and various agencies serving the homeless with shelters, health clinics, treatment centers for addiction, and educational programs.

Volunteer activities were challenging and rewarding. One student reported on her day building a house with Habitat for Humanity volunteers: "We had to dance around large families of baby mice. We made walls until all the prepared materials were gone. This was inside an unheated warehouse but we kept on swinging those hammers. . . . We got pretty good! My family all want to come another time and try it."

After coaching a blind young woman about interviewing for jobs over the phone, a student reports, "By the 4th call, she was amazing! She had poise and confidence that surprised both of us. Needless to say, she made several appointments for job interviews. It made me feel incredibly good to have made such a difference in this young lady's job search."

Some students spent time lobbying at the state capitol. "I feel like I've already accomplished so much as far as learning about the legislative process, and a usually politically inert person (me), while not quite yet an activist, is becoming a real source of information to my peers. You can be sure I'll be at the capitol following bills next year." Another student attending a legislative hearing where misinformation was being given about access to clinics wrote, "I wanted to scream! I had to speak up. After I spoke, I felt so empowered. The representatives actually were listening to me. I'm so glad we had this experience. Who knows what kind of fires have been lit!"

One student who worked in a mobile clinic that visits shelters and places where homeless people congregate to provide health care services, observed, "I've begun to recruit my friends into volunteering with the Task Force [for the Homeless]. I laugh to myself at the crusader I've become."

Some activities led students to move past their comfort level. A female student volunteering at the Union Mission wrote, "When I walk into that building I feel so AFRAID. I can't imagine what the people feel like who have to live out there on those streets."

Reading about vulnerable populations was another assignment. After reading Randy Shilts' 1987 book, *And the Band Played On,* a student wrote, "My personal reaction to this book is one of shock, anger, frustration, and fear. I am afraid because the political system does not work when the groups who are being injured are not represented in the political parties. . . . I have a fuller understanding of the intricacies of the political system and the effect it can have on health care delivery (or non-delivery!). Another important lesson learned from reading this book was the importance of being politically aware, both as a citizen and a nurse."

Students often acknowledged their own behaviors and attitudes as part of the problem. In a particularly poignant and candid journal, this student acknowledged his contribution to the spread of HIV: "As a gay male who has been active within the gay community during the entire timeframe of this book [*And the Band Played On*], I was devastated at times by my own complicity in the affair. I knew there was a fatal illness going around. This knowledge did not stop me from engaging in unsafe sexual practices. It was actions such as mine that helped spread AIDS to every corner of the globe."

Another student, who read *Rachel and Her Children* (Kozol, 1988), commented:

> This book has heightened my awareness of homelessness. In the past, I felt no pity for the homeless. I would pass them on the street and turn my head in the opposite direction to avoid looking them in the eyes. I believed all homeless people were lazy male bums who wanted to stay intoxicated all day. I thought their homelessness was their own fault, and therefore asked, why should I help them? I never realized that the majority of the homeless are families with small children. As a result of the insight I have gained, I have decided to volunteer at Our House [a child care center for the homeless].

On the same subject, another student wrote:

> Because of Kozol's book, there has been a major adjustment in my attitude toward the homeless population. This change in attitude will not only affect my personal life but will have an enormous impact on my nursing practice. My apathy has been replaced by empathy, which will come across when I am caring for homeless people. . . . Armed with the information given to me in this book, I as a nurse, can be a respected voice in the community advocating the plight of the homeless.

From a third student came this insight: "The stories in *Rachel and Her Children* saddened, angered, and most of all, frustrated me. Kozol effectively exposed the deplorable plight of the homeless in our society and I was not at all prepared for what I read. When I finished the book, I was not at all proud to be a member of a society which treats people so inhumanely on such a routine basis." Similarly, a fourth student reported "Reading this book was excruciatingly difficult for me. I had to stop frequently because I felt so much sadness and so much pain. These people are real and have had to endure so much—the squalor, the red tape nightmare, hunger, sickness, fear and despair. I feel so ashamed—of our government, of our cities, of our citizens and of myself."

After the experience of interacting with vulnerable populations, interceding on their behalf, and even reading about them, students reported new insights that were life-changing. Their journals were touching and insightful.

After Senior Day at the state capitol: "The image I had of the frail old person was shattered by the group I saw at the capitol" and "When I first started this course, I did not think it would be very useful. I have changed my thinking. This is only one small area where we can make a big impact."

One of the biggest eye openers, as mentioned before, was the plight of the homeless, as stated by two students: "Last year I began working in the homeless clinic to meet a class requirement. This was my first introduction to the homeless. I began to realize that these men and women were individuals much like myself" and "How can this situation we call homelessness but [that] includes joblessness, hopelessness, nutritionessless [sic] and respectlessness [sic] be happening in what is supposed to be the greatest country in the world? It is mind-boggling and heart-wrenching and irrational."

Students welcome the opportunity to be advocates. Using service learning, especially with vulnerable populations, is an effective way to teach advocacy and to expose students to experiences that will affect the way they look at vulnerable clients and the way they practice nursing. An additional benefit is the recognition by students that political awareness and activism are a critical part of the nurse advocacy role.

REFERENCES

Aikens, C. A. (1916). *Studies in ethics for nurses*. Philadelphia, PA: Saunders.

American Nurses' Association (1950). A code for nurses. *American Journal of Nursing, 50*(4), 196.

American Nurses Association [ANA]. (1986). *Code for nurses with interpretive statements*. Kansas City, MO: American Nurses Association.

Annas, G. (1974). The patient rights advocate: Can nurses effectively fill the role? *Supervisor Nurse, 5*(7), 21–25.

Annas, G. (1975). *The rights of hospital patients: The basic ACLU guide to a hospital patient's rights*. New York, NY: Discus.

Davis, A. J., & Aroskar, M. A. (1978). *Ethical dilemmas and nursing practice*. New York, NY: Appleton-Century-Crofts.

Goodrich, A. W. (1932). *The social significance of nursing*. New York, NY: Macmillan.

International Congress of Nursing [ICN]. (1953). International code of nursing ethics. *American Journal of Nursing, 53*, 1070.

Kozol, J. (1988). *Rachel and Her Children: Homeless families in America*. New York, NY: Fawcett Book Group.

Mueller, C., & Norton, B. (1998). Service learning: Developing values and social responsibility. In D. M. Billings & J. Halstead (Eds.). *Teaching in nursing education*. Philadelphia, PA: Saunders.

Parsons, S. E. (1916). *Nursing problems and obligations*. Boston, MA: Whitcomb & Barrows.

Pellietier, S. (1995). The quiet power of service learning: Report from the National Institute on Learning and Service. *The Independent, 95*(2), 6.

Shilts, R. (1987). *And the Band Played On: Politics, people and the AIDS epidemic*. New York, NY: St. Martin's.

Where does loyalty to the physician end? [Letter to the editor]. (1910). *American Journal of Nursing, 10*(1), 274, 276.

Winslow, G. R. (1984). From loyalty to advocacy: A new metaphor for nursing. *The Hastings Center Report* (pp. 32–40). Hastings on Hudson, NY: Hastings Center.

CHAPTER 40

Neighborhoods and Nurses: An Integrated Undergraduate Curriculum

Sharon Jensen

The American Association of Colleges of Nursing (AACN) defines the essential knowledge, values, and professional behaviors expected of the baccalaureate nursing program graduate (AACN, 1998). Professional education includes the liberal arts, professional values, core competencies, core knowledge, and role development. Within professional values, altruism, autonomy, human dignity, integrity, and social justice are mentioned. Educational efforts must be designed to support student learning and provide experiences that facilitate development of these values. Ethics, human diversity, global health care, and health care systems and policy are core knowledge. Professional development includes advocacy, accountability, and participation in activities that advance the profession. The combination of these three areas of professional development defines professional nursing practice. They all play a role in educating nurses to advocate for vulnerable populations.

The best practice for teaching these essential characteristics is to provide academic experiences in the real world. Active learning strategies, service-learning opportunities, and community-based experiences provide a rich environment for learning. Attention to three areas: academic rigor, service to the community, and purposeful civic learning provides multidimensional learning (Howard, 2001). Programs that incorporate challenging placements, include frequent opportunities for reflection, and maximize diversity are the most effective (Eyler & Giles, 1999), especially when working with vulnerable groups.

Curriculum design is dynamic. Its constant changes are based on feedback, growth over time, the assimilation of new elements, and the discarding of old ones. Regardless of how the curriculum is organized and the courses are structured, attention to and congruence with the overall aims, purposes, and objectives are most important. As nursing curricula are built, the conceptual framework should consider student and faculty characteristics, the knowledge desired, and the demography in which the school resides (Bevis, 1989).

CURRICULUM FRAMEWORK

Student and Faculty Characteristics

Seattle University is the largest and most diverse independent university in the Pacific Northwest, with a student population of 6300 and a faculty of 400. There are 283 students enrolled in the undergraduate nursing program; 9% are male. The average age is 23 years; 39% of students identify themselves as Asian/Pacific Islander, Africa American, Hispanic, multicultural, and unknown. Although not as diverse as the student population, of the 25 full-time, tenured/tenure track faculty, 12% are from ethnic groups, and 8% are male (Seattle University School of Nursing, 2001).

Community Demographics

Seattle University sits on a 46-acre metropolitan campus located on the edge of downtown. It is situated near many large hospitals and health care facilities. The school is geographically accessible to four low-income housing areas. Funding for these housing programs comes from the US Department of Housing and Urban Development. In 2002, 91% of the households earned less than 30% of the median income for the Seattle metropolitan area (less than ~$15,000 for a single-person household). Each of the four communities has from 481 to 715 units, housing a total of 5448 people in low-rise apartment-style units. Thirteen percent of these residents are disabled, and 83% of heads of household identify themselves as African American, Asian/Pacific Islander, Native American, or "other." Many are immigrants and refugees, and 15% of heads of household speak languages other than English as their primary language (Seattle Housing Authority, 2002). Minors account for 44% of the population, and 12% are elderly (age >61 years) adults. Many of the heads of household are women. A fifth housing unit farther from campus is visited by students and is managed by King County.

Some characteristics of the population in these neighborhoods that make them vulnerable are being poor and/or low income, being of a minority race and/or ethnicity, having a female head of household, being either very young or elderly, being disabled, and having immigrant or refugee status. Vulnerability implies that these populations are more sensitive to risk factors that can negatively affect their health (Lundy & Janes, 2001). The goals of the nursing students at the university are to build resilience and provide resources to these clients (Swanson & Nies, 1997).

CURRICULUM DESIGN

Health, client (individuals, families, and communities), environment, and values are the key concepts in the nursing program at Seattle University. In terms of a framework for studying vulnerable populations, individual, family, and community perspectives are integrated from the beginning (Aday, 2001). There are seven encompassing program objectives. The objectives that relate to vulnerable populations include to

- □ provide direct care in a variety of health settings
- □ develop teams and partnerships with clients, community members, and other health care providers to facilitate health communities
- □ apply leadership principles and management strategies
- □ commit to service, diversity, and social justice

The nursing program is seven quarters in length, beginning the spring quarter of sophomore year. The courses are integrated across specialties (obstetrics, pediatrics, mental health, medical–surgical), client focus (individuals, families, communities), and settings (communities, schools, long-term care, hospitals). Students work in a neighborhood of their choosing over the span of five quarters. Students are introduced to the concept of health, not disease, as the primary concern of nurses. Methods of health promotion and risk reduction are introduced in the early courses and continue through the curriculum.

The Northeastern University Model (Matteson, 1995) was used to organize the community theme for the courses. The model focuses on delivery of care in the community to provide opportunities for students to

☐ participate in the lived experience of health and illness,
☐ encounter diversity in a natural setting,
☐ make clinical judgments informed by social, cultural, legal, political, ecological, and epidemiological factors, and
☐ collaborate with clients, providers, and community residents.

Courses that include the community experiences are, in order of sequence:

☐ Foundations of Professional Nursing (values clarification)
☐ Health Assessment and Intervention I (beginning community assessment)
☐ Health Assessment and Intervention II (teaching project in public schools or Head Start programs)
☐ Promoting Wellness in Altered States of Health I (attend a community meeting)
☐ Promoting Wellness in Altered States of Health II (visit a community agency)
☐ Health Care in Communities (theory)
☐ Health Care in Communities (clinical: 10 hours/week)
☐ Contemporary Issues with Vulnerable Populations (fieldwork)

COURSE EXPERIENCES

Foundations of Professional Nursing theory forms the basis for thinking about nursing from a broad perspective. Concepts include community-based care, cultural congruence and competence, values-based practice, and caring. Systems theory is introduced in addition to the curriculum concepts of nursing, health, client, and environment. Western values are compared with global values. Public health goals are introduced through *Healthy People 2010,* with focus on environmental quality, immunization, and access to health care. Students explore concepts of health promotion and disease prevention.

The Spirit Catches You and You Fall Down (Fadiman, 1997) is used as a springboard for discussion questions, e.g., Is there a culture of medicine in the United States? Why? What is the promotion of social justice? Additionally, basic interpersonal communication and group process skills are practiced in small groups for 2 hours per week. Communication skills for community-based practice (listening, establishing trust, forming partnerships, collaboration, and negotiation) are learned.

Health Assessment and Intervention I introduces students to their community. Students use the Anderson & McFarlane (2000) model of community assessment to become acquainted with the community core and community subsystems and to analyze perceptions. They assess age, gender, ethnicity, culture, income, and family size of residents in the communities in which they've chosen to work. Students all perform a "windshield survey" (a term used in community health nursing to describe informal observations of the neighborhood done by driving through). The students then break into pairs to investigate a subsystem more deeply. They meet with a key informant and ask questions such as "What do you like about living in your community?" The pairs present their findings to the group; additionally a notebook with resources is collated as a reference for future quarters of study. Group discussion helps students identify similarities and differences between communities. They discuss the question "How has your experience in the community affected your understanding of the root causes of social/health problems?" and respond to the statement "There is important knowledge only found in the community." They examine risk factors within the community that might make residents vulnerable.

Health Assessment and Intervention II places students in public schools and Head Start programs that are either in the community or nearby. This project is based on the Michigan Model (Howard, 2001) of combining academic learning with community service and purposeful civic learning. Some objectives are to

- assess culturally diverse students in a public school or Head Start program
- perform risk assessment in a public school or Head Start program
- identify *Healthy People 2010* goals for appropriate age group
- increase respect for others
- increase awareness of personal beliefs and biases
- increase awareness of self and community
- value differences with communities, families, individuals
- avoid assumptions about others

Pairs of students develop, implement, and evaluate a teaching project, spending a total of 21 hours on it. Their activities are reported and revised through Web-based assignments. The Anderson & McFarlane model (2000) is used to provide a visual representation and to reinforce their previous learning about assessment. Assignments guide students through the teaching and learning process and ask questions such as "How are you developing cross-cultural communication skills?" and "What incongruities exist between healthy lifestyles in the community and environment and cultural practices?" Attention is paid to age, gender, ethnicity, culture, income, and the family size of the children and adolescents in each student's project population. They examine risk factors and lines of defense for their clients.

In the next two quarters, the clinical experiences are hospital based, so the community assignments take up fewer hours. Promoting Wellness in Altered States of Health I asks students to return to the community to participate in a community activity three times over the quarter, for 90 minutes each time. Repeated community assignments create an immersion experience in the neighborhood. The questions raised are "Was the activity in which you participated culturally sensitive? Why or why not?" and "How does this activity address the needs of vulnerable people in your community?"

Promoting Wellness in Altered States of Health II assigns students to compare what postdischarge services are available to a hospitalized client with similar services available in the low-income neighborhoods. Students compare their client's profile with the county, state, national, or international incidence/prevalence of the disease (age, race, gender). They identify *Healthy People 2010* goals that relate to their client. Students visit an agency in the neighborhood and discuss barriers to services and associated costs after investigating types of insurance, eligibility, funded services, and reimbursement. The focus is on resources between hospital and home. Also, students collate and synthesize the community resources and assessment data through this point in time and share it during a presentation made to the students who are preparing to go into their neighborhood for the first time. This provides an opportunity to review their knowledge of the community and share it with beginning students.

Following this course, students are immersed in community experiences with the Health Care in Communities theory and linked clinical (10 hours per week) course. The course objectives include

- ☐ Demonstration of critical thinking in planning, implementing, and evaluating community health nursing interventions (such as advocacy, collaboration, health education, and community organization) with vulnerable families and populations
- ☐ Examination of human values in relation to vulnerable families and populations
- ☐ Examination of the professional role of advocacy for vulnerable families and populations
- ☐ Examination of legislative and health policy issues related to the health and health care of families and populations
- ☐ Analysis of select community health issues from a health policy perspective; participation in the professional role of advocacy for vulnerable families and population
- ☐ Advocacy for quality health care for vulnerable families and populations

By this point, the students are familiar with the neighborhood, feel more comfortable entering into the community, and have some ideas about the strengths and needs of the community. The theory part of the course addresses global health care in addition to neighborhood issues. A systems and policy perspective is incorporated at a higher level. Families and populations are the focus of the course, and a family's cultural patterns and values are assessed. The Anderson & Mc-Farlane (2000) model is used by students to design, implement, and evaluate a project in the community for a given population. Health fairs, community clinics, health promotion activities, and health screening are all examples of the types of activities in which students are involved.

A two-credit Contemporary Issues with Vulnerable Populations course is taken concurrently. Themes that have been integrated through the curriculum are given more focused attention. Students interview a person who is culturally different from themselves and who considers him- or herself a member of a vulnerable population. These interviews are shared with others in the class to increase awareness of the multiple dimensions of vulnerability in the US context. Self-reflection, advocacy, empowerment, collaboration, and community organization with vulnerable populations are techniques that students implement and evaluate. Students develop sensitivity to social justice by working with vulnerable populations. Increased awareness of the roles of social justice and political action is promoted.

BARRIERS TO COMMUNITY LEARNING

Students

With all of the advantages, however, some barriers are present. Students may be reluctant to move to the community setting because there is a mismatch between the community and the traditional role of nurses as reflected in the media. Students may be disappointed at the low-tech, slower-paced delivery of care. The communities often take students out of their comfort zone into neighborhoods that are much different from those in their personal lives. Establishment of a partnership with a community requires a time commitment. Not only does it take longer to get to and from neighborhoods, but it also takes time to develop the trust and relationship of the community (Matteson, 1995).

At the end of their community immersion, one group of students ($n = 30$) was asked to share their experiences and thoughts on community collaboration and communication. Students noted that they felt the community thread was lost during the two acute-care quarters when the focus was on hospitalized clients. They wanted better coordination of assignments, better flow from quarter to quarter, and more hands-on care in the community with other providers, such as visiting nurses or hospice. They also wanted more collaboration among themselves and they asked for assignments that built on the work of previous students, along with more involvement and collaboration with the actual community members. It is difficult, however, to balance these needs for more community experiences with the demand to produce the nursing generalist.

With regard to the Health Assessment and Intervention II course, students overwhelmingly agreed that they liked working with the same small group (of about 12) of children in the community over time and commented on the availability and helpfulness of the faculty. They mentioned Head Start and public schools as a good learning environment. The experiences that were more structured and organized were generally better received by students.

To evaluate student learning, knowledge, skills, and attitudes, a variety of tools are used. The course following their community immersion is Senior Synthesis, which is a course emphasizing synthesis of material learned earlier. Reflections on vulnerability from these senior-synthesis course journals ($n = 19$) are included as examples of outcomes of student learning through the curriculum.

"I have become accustomed to applying the essential values such as equality, justice and human dignity and others to my practice."

"My hope is that I can channel my strong personal beliefs into creating health care policy changes in society."

"Promoting diversity will empower and awaken the mind to envision new roles for nursing in the future."

"People are vulnerable when they are receiving health care. I feel I have it in me to advocate for my patients' rights."

Faculty

Faculty members may also find themselves out of their comfort zone, as Matteson (1995) puts it, "out of the towers and into the streets." Change is required to move from the traditional block of community experiences to the longitudinal experiences that disrupt the traditional curriculum. Faculty are required to retool their skills. Countless hours are spent as the curriculum is revolutionized; creative energy and commitment are required. Coordination and collaboration among all faculty are required as communication across courses and levels occurs.

Faculty ($n = 10$) who have been involved in teaching the integrated courses were surveyed for their responses to questions on community collaboration and communication. As with student interviews, the faculty included coordination of assignments and gaps and redundancies in assignments as areas needing improvement. There was difficulty coordinating placements because multiple levels of students were using the same facilities in one time period. A funded faculty liaison role was created for each community to coordinate student activities and serve both as a coordinator and point person for communication with the community. It became apparent that it was essential for faculty to be knowledgeable about the entire curriculum, holding students accountable for previous knowledge and building on that foundation.

The course syllabi were developed to make explicit expectations for each course, linking entering and exiting behaviors from course to course. There was debate on how to promote student to student collaboration and whether to use continuing versus new assessments and projects from quarter to quarter. For example, some faculty encouraged the use of previous students' assessments to minimize the burden on service providers; others thought that students should create their own knowledge and learn from discovering their own assessment. The lack of nurses to serve as role models in community settings created issues about how to best supervise students and in which settings to place them. One community notebook was lost, making the assessment resource unavailable for the community student group for assignments.

Positive thoughts were also expressed. Faculty liked being able to work with the same group of students on projects over quarters. When possible, the faculty were given placements in the same communities; this served to promote trust with the community and students. The faculty liked the assessment focus from the beginning of the nursing program. They also thought that the Head Start and public school experiences nearer the beginning of the curriculum were positive. Faculty noted that students entered their community immersion experiences as seniors with knowledge of culture and vulnerable populations. The students and community members knew each other, and students were more confident. Students saw the importance of the family, the individual, and the community in all settings and delivered more holistic care.

Communities

Barriers can also occur at the community level. Many of these communities are used to having "do-gooders" enter into projects funded by grant money and then leave as quickly as they came once the project is completed. Communities may resent those who enter the community if they have had previous experiences with providers who are culturally insensitive. Social injustices may be projected on students and faculty. Building trust takes time. In many cases, it must be earned (Matteson, 1995).

Potential neighborhoods, religious institutions, and community programs were initially evaluated as a focus for the community-based curriculum. Neighborhoods were chosen because of previous contacts and identification of providers who could be of assistance. In new neighborhoods, the faculty needed to learn about the key people with knowledge of the neighborhood and access the "gatekeeper." Sometimes this person was obvious, sometimes less so. The suitability of the neighborhoods as learning experiences was assessed. Many neighborhoods had services with which the nursing school could link; other relationships needed to be expanded and developed. It was essential to identify service providers in the neighborhoods who supported the student activities. In return, the providers asked for a continuing commitment from the school.

As students began work in the neighborhoods, it became clear that the goals for the school had to be shared with the community; the best case was when a calendar was established along with the objectives and activities for each course. The focus of students was health; data on the health of the community was unavailable, so data needed to be gathered and limitations recognized. The consistent presence of faculty in the communities was important, but scheduling and workload issues often meant the faculty members had to change. This created some confusion about who was responsible for maintaining communication with the neighborhood because the service providers frequently related to an individual faculty member with whom they had formed a relationship rather than the person who might be teaching the course during a given quarter. There was also the issue of consistency of students in community over summers and breaks. Community service providers wanted students available for activities during these times. Service providers appreciated opportunities for sharing information with us and each other and liked being invited to activities such as when we presented the results of the community assessment. A mechanism for expressing ongoing concerns was negotiated; some gaps in communication occurred as people and processes changed.

Positives in the community include the quality of the service. Knowledge of the community has grown through more complete assessments. Projects were implemented with appreciation for the complexity and social structure in which they were framed. Students considered issues of communication limited knowledge of English and the need for accurate translations as they encountered diversity in the community setting. Residents and families with whom the students worked received services to which they would not have otherwise had access. Service providers developed links to resources at the College of Nursing and Seattle University. Clients, providers, and community residents learned to collaborate with students. Data related to the health improvement impact of these projects are somewhat difficult to measure, however. As work in these neighborhoods proceeds, outcomes measurement should be included in the conversation.

Neighborhoods and Nurses

Integrating community issues, promoting social justice, encouraging cultural competency, and reducing vulnerability are part of a continuing process. The advantages of creating links across specialties, clients, and care settings are balanced with the challenges of coordination and communication within and between courses. Assessment, nursing process, health promotion, teaching and learning, and public health goals are threaded through the curriculum to create opportunities to reinforce important learning. Faculty learn to connect individual, family, and community issues that cross traditional boundaries. Communities interact with students to promote the education of culturally sensitive nurses and to receive higher quality care. Partnerships can be created to promote student learning about vulnerable individuals, families, and communities over time and across settings.

REFERENCES

Aday, L. A. (2001). *At risk in America: The health and health care needs of vulnerable populations in the United States.* New York, NY: Jossey-Bass.

American Association of Colleges of Nursing. (1998). *The essentials of baccalaureate education for professional nursing practice.* Washington, DC: AACN.

Bevis, E. O. (1989). *Curriculum building in nursing: A process* (3rd ed.). New York, NY: National League for Nursing.

Eyler, J., & Giles, D. E. (1999). *Where's the learning in service learning.* San Francisco, CA: Jossey-Bass.

Fadiman, A. (1997). *The spirit catches you and you fall down.* New York, NY: Farrar, Straus and Giroux.

Howard, J. (2001). *Service-learning course design workbook. Michigan Journal of Community Service Learning.* Ann Arbor, MI: University of Michigan.

Lundy, K. S., & Janes, S. (2001). *Vulnerability: An overview. Community health nursing: Caring for the public's health.* Boston, MA: Jones and Bartlett.

Seattle Housing Authority. (2002). *Annual population report: 2002.* Seattle, WA: Seattle Housing Authority.

Seattle University School of Nursing. (2002). *Seattle University School of Nursing self study report.* Seattle, WA: Seattle University.

Swanson, J. M., & Nies, M. A. (1997). *Cultural influences in the community: Other populations in community health nursing* (2nd ed.). Philadelphia, PA: W. B. Saunders.

CHAPTER 41

Fieldwork on Vulnerable Populations

Mary de Chesnay, Jenny Hsin-Chun Tsai, Jennifer Wagner,
Kelly Sehring, Clare Fontana, Katie Poinier, and Linda Frothinger

Seattle University is a Jesuit institution that is committed to fostering students' concern for social justice to promote a just and human world. To embrace the Jesuit tradition, the nursing faculty decided to include a theory course in the revised undergraduate curriculum to enhance students' ability to work with vulnerable populations and to advocate for justice in health care. Jenny Hsin-Chun Tsai (the second author of this chapter) was given a brief course description and the charge of designing the course. She developed the course and taught it twice. Basic content included the concept of vulnerability, associated risk factors, and intervention strategies such as ethics, advocacy, and empowerment.

The literature has suggested that the creation of vulnerability goes beyond the effects of individual characteristics (e.g., weight, age, gender). Many associated factors lie in the broader societal context and are embedded in the culture that its people use to make sense out of their life, decide their actions, and make judgments about the behaviors of others (Aday, 2001; Bezruchka, 2001; Butterfield, 1990; Langston, 1995; Sebastian, 2000). Everyone is immersed in his or her own culture and people participate in the construction of vulnerability in different ways and with different levels of consciousness. For example, some people unconsciously use particular words or phrases to joke about certain groups, and some engage in social and political actions for or with certain groups. Thus to enhance students' abilities to advocate for social justice for the vulnerable, not only do the students need to know about the theories and literature central to the construction of vulnerability, but more importantly, they need to increase self-awareness; that is, develop consciousness of their own participation in the construction processes.

To that end, articles and in-class activities were selected to guide the students in acquiring theoretical understanding about vulnerability and the health care of vulnerable populations. Fieldwork and critical reflection papers were included to help students apply their knowledge to real cases (with which they may or may not be familiar) and to critically examine the students' own values, beliefs, and assumptions and how they influence their attitudes and behaviors toward people from the group selected for the fieldwork. Since 2002, the course has been taught by another faculty member who continues the tradition of demanding extensive self-reflection and detailed reports on fieldwork experiences. Following are the guidelines. The remainder of the chapter includes excerpts from students' work in their own words.

GUIDELINES FOR FIELDWORK

The purpose of the fieldwork assignment is to help students gain an understanding of the nature of vulnerability from the point of view of a person who is culturally different from themselves and who considers himself or herself a member of a vulnerable population, whether or not the person feels vulnerable personally. It is critical to the experience to interview someone from a different racial or ethnic group or a group that is different based on state of health (e.g., frail elderly, person with history of substance abuse) from the interviewer. For the purposes of the exercise, students were asked to consider members of minority groups as vulnerable. Questions had to do with learning about the person's culture from their point of view and about their experiences with the American health care system. Fieldwork reports are detailed papers that describe the person, the context of the interview, and the student's analysis. Detailed guidelines can be found in the instructor's guide for this book.

David (interviewed by Jennifer Wagner)

David is a colleague of a friend of mine. David is a 21-year-old homosexual Caucasian male born in the United States who works at a clothing store and attends classes at a local community college. David is "not quite sure" what he plans for his future. He has lived in the same town his entire life. He lives with two male friends in a three-bedroom apartment and enjoys going to karaoke clubs on weekends and playing video games (when there's not too much homework to do). His family lives close by and they are all very close. He has one younger sister who is 18 and he sees his family quite often.

The interview with David was conducted at a small coffee shop that he chose as a meeting place. He did not feel comfortable being audio-taped but was open to my taking notes during the interview and I assured him that his real name would not be used. He seemed comfortable answering my questions and quite often led the conversation himself by going into stories or explanations. After some general conversation, I felt comfortable asking David when he knew that he was a homosexual and what it was like growing up. He knew he was a homosexual around 8 years old when he realized that he had an attraction to male classmates. He said it was very hard because he tried to make himself "see the attractiveness" in female classmates, but it "just wasn't there." He had several short relationships with females during high school but they were never sexual. He would kiss them when they wanted to but he did not become aroused. He said he knew for sure that he was homosexual in middle school but was too afraid to tell anyone until after he graduated from high school. David said that he did not know anyone who was homosexual and didn't know who to talk to because he was uncomfortable talking to his family about it: "we don't talk about that kind of stuff."

After graduation, David met another homosexual male when he was working in the mall. They began dating and it was the first time he became open about his homosexuality. He brought his boyfriend home and told his parents that he was "gay." He then laughed and said that his parents were quiet for a moment and then his father said, "Well, I thought you might be," and this was the end of the conversation. David feels very lucky to have such open parents and says that many of his friends "were not that fortunate." He has several friends whose parents do not speak to them anymore because they are homosexual.

He told me that he felt his successes in life are due to support from his family and hard work. David said that he doesn't quit anything and that he works hard at whatever he does. He also said that he had excellent grades in high school and is continuing to get good grades at the community college. He hopes that he will be able to get a scholarship to attend a university.

David said that the only things he has ever been held back from included things like attending a university or going on a senior class trip to Mexico because his parents do not have enough money and all of his money goes to rent and food. I asked him if there were any other factors and he said that being a homosexual has kept him from getting certain jobs. He said that he could never really be sure, but he did notice that his male interviewers would sometimes get uncomfortable around him: "It's pretty obvious when people meet me that I am gay, I just have that walk and talk."

David indicated that men sometimes call him "faggot" as he's walking by or give him nasty looks. He also said that he feels harassed by policemen whenever he gets pulled over or after leaving a club. He feels that they "look at [him] funny" because he is a homosexual. He then explained that other than this, he feels generally lucky because he has not been "beaten up" and that he has many friends, both "straight" and "gay," who don't care about his sexual orientation.

David said that he has only had one bad experience with the health care system and that it happened with his general practitioner. When he was 19 and at the doctor for a checkup, his doctor made the assumption that he was sexually active and began asking him questions about his sexual practices in order to assess if he was being safe (i.e., condom use, etc.). David said that he told his doctor that he knew about safe sexual practices and his doctor said "yes, but STDs are a serious concern with homosexuals, especially HIV and I want to make sure that you fully understand the potential consequences of your actions." David said that he is not sure if the doctor was reprimanding him for being a homosexual or was just very concerned for his health, but he said he felt very uncomfortable during the rest of the appointment. He says that he doesn't let discrimination "get [him] down," and that it is "their issue" if they have a problem with him.

David's advice to me as a nurse is "just continue to be open to everyone because really, we're not all that different . . . don't judge people "for who they are attracted to, what race they are, or what color their skin is, and treat them all with the same respect, then [I] will make a great nurse."

David has taught me much about homosexuals as well as other vulnerable populations. People of vulnerable populations only feel vulnerable when others discriminate against them. There are members of vulnerable populations who may never have felt discriminated against and then there are others who feel ashamed, angry, or alone as members of a particular vulnerable population. I also learned that we, as health care workers, should treat everyone (as David stated) with respect. Respect is the main value to focus on when working with vulnerable populations as a nurse, doctor, or any other health care provider. I learned I should not make assumptions about a person based on being a member of a particular population.

I learned much about the homosexual population from David. He really helped me to see that homosexuals are not that different from the rest of us. They fall in love, they date, they have friends, and their lives are basically the same as anyone except that they have a different sexual orientation. The sexual practices of homosexuals are no more dangerous than the sexual practices of heterosexuals. All those who are sexually active are at risk for STDs and HIV and everyone who is sexually active must practice safe sex practices to prevent contracting or spreading such diseases.

I do not feel as though I had many problems with the interview. It went very smoothly from start to finish and I think it really helped that we met at a place that David chose in order to help him be more comfortable. In addition, I believe that because we were talking over coffee, it made it feel more like a meeting between friends rather than an interview. He was very open to my questions and his nonverbal communication showed me that he was comfortable. He smiled quite a bit during the interview and did not lean away from me and he made eye contact when he was speaking. I really enjoyed this experience and I feel as though David may have benefited from the interview as well by being able to tell someone about his experiences and have them learn from it.

Kiya (interviewed by Kelly Sehring)

Kiya is a forty-eight-year-old African American female who is the mother of two children; a daughter who is thirty-one and a son who is twenty-five years old. Kiya was born and raised in a major Northwest city and she is the third generation of her family to reside in this region. Her uncle was the first African American mayor within the region. The interview was conducted at Kiya's place of employment. The location allowed me the opportunity to assess her environment in a professional context—giving me a picture of her daily life. For example, I noticed that her computer has an ergonomic keyboard and glare shield, which says to me that she pays attention to her own well-being. Several plants adorn the room, her desk faces outward below a large window, and the décor is rich with African artwork such as batik tapestries and other woven textiles that hang comfortably on the walls. Family pictures are visible on the multiple surfaces of a wide array of file cabinets and desk space.

Kiya reported being very close to her family, especially the women, including her grandmother, mother, sister, and aunts. She described the women of her family as "dedicated community activists" who are involved with activities such as participation in the civil rights movement, who serve as advocates for school-based programs in low-income areas, and who are active in a local community organization trying to have new traffic signals placed at high-risk intersections. The family also had an early involvement with the Black Panthers through participation in their breakfast programs. Community activism was a central theme within her family and influenced her career choice. Kiya works for a local housing agency that is renovating a low-income community. She identified her mother and aunts as "heroes" and early motivators for her continued involvement with vulnerable populations.

Kiya was a student in the first African American history class offered in her high school; however, she grew up with an appreciation of African American history from her family. She talked at length about the inadequate historical documentation of her culture. Kiya described her decision to change her major from psychology to humanities while at college, because although she wanted to provide counseling and support to high-risk populations, she felt that learning theories from Caucasian psychologists would not adequately address the cultural experience of minority populations.

Kiya describes herself as an extremely spiritual person and it is apparent that she has assumed a sense of wisdom about the world. She does not subscribe to a particular organized religion, however she regularly meditates and practices mindfulness in daily activities. She recently traveled to Egypt with her mother and sister, and she described Egypt as feeling like "home" during visitations to the pyramids and surrounding monuments. Kiya mentioned several times the importance of listening to elders, from whom she has received guidance and inspiration.

In response to a question about her experiences with the health care system, Kiya firmly expressed her preference for a female doctor who is from a minority population. Her current physician is a Japanese female, whom she feels can "understand where she is coming from" better than a Caucasian male or female, and to whom she feels more open to sharing her concerns. She expressed the view that older African Americans delay treatment due to mistrust of the health care system. This notion is based upon health care providers' arguable reluctance to discuss home remedies, which she stated were common in the African American culture, as well as a pervasive element of discomfort in placing one's life into the hands of the majority culture.

Themes of advocacy and spirituality were dominant in my interview and I had a personal revelation about the complexity of choosing a health care provider when one is from a minority culture if a basic foundation of respect and trust is still under construction. Kiya exemplifies leadership, dedication to service, and empowerment within the African American community. While it is important for nurses to address health disparities of African Americans, it is crucial also to include examples of success and triumph.

Duffy and Marie (interviewed by Clare Fontana)

I was fortunate enough to be able to interview an elderly couple, Duffy (80) and Marie (74) who live in a suburb of a bustling Pacific Northwest metropolis. They have been married for over 50 years and have many family and friends that live in the area. Recently, Duffy has undergone several medical procedures, and although has recovered quite well from them he has not maintained his independence and relies on his wife for help in activities of daily living. Marie has remained active by walking and swimming several times a week and she cooks meals for her husband and her grown son who lives with them. She also is consistent in keeping both of them on their medication regimen. We met in their home on a Friday afternoon to discuss their views on health and health care, and the use of both preventative measures and medical treatment in caring for their population, the aging. We also discussed how health and health care have changed, what they have received as treatments in the past and how it has affected them today and as they continue to age.

Marie and Duffy are native to the Pacific Northwest. Marie's parents were of Norwegian decent. Her father fished the west coast for a long time. Her mother is college-educated and raised three children while maintaining a home, and being involved with many services in the community. Duffy, one of nine children, was raised in the same manner. Both his parents worked hard taking advantage of the opportunities in America after emigrating from Ireland. The couple is comfortable in the city and have developed a strong and intricate support network of family and friends.

When talking about the health care system as they were growing up, they both commented "everything seemed to be taken care of back then. If you were sick, you went to the doctor, or he came to see you. Our doctor lived up the street and knew all the kids, when they were born and what was wrong with them at any given time. He would come over to check up on us . . . you just don't see that any more." "We are privileged to be able to be at the same doctor, the three of us (Duffy, Marie, and Duffy's older sister Meg) . . . it feels like they (the doctors) are very lenient and available to see us. If I have an appointment, but Meg is not feeling well and I bring her along, Dr. S doesn't mind. They are so good about asking about all of us. It makes me feel established, like they really do care about what my health is like. . . . It is wonderful to be in a professional situation and have the doctor say . . . 'If you were my mother . . .' and that's what I want for someone to take care of me like I was their mother. You know they have a real interest in you."

Financing health care was the next big topic to emerge. We discussed the fact that people are living longer these days, not because of better health per say but because of medications that increase the longevity of one's life. "We are so lucky to have a pension plan, and I (Marie) get a small check from social security. . . . I did not work enough in my life to qualify for a large amount, but it is enough. We do ok because we can sit down and plan ahead. One of our biggest expenses is buying medication. In that sense it would seem that maybe if we were able to prevent our diseases then our income would be a little more cushy, but I just don't know what people do who don't qualify for Medicaid or Medicare and who haven't really planned ahead. Even some people who worked all their lives and set money aside wouldn't have enough to pay for assisted living or a nursing home. Meg had set aside $10,000, but even that wouldn't allow her to make it through a year in a nursing care facility and then what would she do? I mean she has us to help her out, and we are getting by ok. . . . I just don't know if I could handle taking care of another person. . . . The other thing that has really worked for us is that J. our son has taken us up to Canada to buy our medicine and really we have probably saved $700.00 over the year! I don't know why they [the government] have not put a cap on the amount these companies can charge. It seems silly that they are allowed to charge so much. . . . I know that they spend a lot to discover these drugs but . . . it leaves us pretty helpless."

In talking with Duffy and Marie I began to understand their fears and concerns about health care and aging. They grew up in a time where the doctor was a neighbor and most of the care was given by someone familiar with the family's situation and resources were readily available. This is the kind of care this population is still seeking. Health to them involves the family as well as the individual. Marie and Duffy felt that a huge part of their health that is important to them is being able to support their children and grandchildren; to encourage good habits like reading, education, social participation, and especially familial involvement. They have helped to create a strong support network within the family thus empowering the individual members to help each other helping the whole in turn. Their advice to me as a health care worker was to address the individual in the context of the family. They found it very important to them that their primary care provider was aware of how the couple was doing physically and mentally together. They indicated that a third person who should be included in the health circle for Marie and Duffy is Meg because she is in the same population and in the family circle and is reliant on Marie and Duffy for social, family, and health-related interactions. The provider can also get a better sense of what stressors and resources a person has by understanding the context of their living situation and support system.

Belief system seemed another area that influences health and the way people of this generation approach the health care system. Approaching health care through the mentality of this generation brings about paternalistic model of health care. They want someone to tell them how to make the pain go away. They feel that they do not know enough about medicine or the system in general to be able to navigate through it. Marie is very inquisitive into parts of the care that they receive, but admits that at times it is overwhelming and "not worth the stress of trying to understand it all. . . ." Reviewing the different reasons why Marie and Duffy were receiving particular treatments and how the treatments could be incorporated into their daily routine was helpful in relieving some of that stress. For example we examined what diabetes is and how it affects the body on a day-to-day basis in a somewhat simplified explanation and this seemed to encourage the continuation of taking the medication that is helping to control this particular disease process. We also examined lifestyle changes that would help decrease the negative effects of this disease, such as exercise and diet. Duffy admitted that he has struggled with a weight problem for some time, but that in understanding how obesity complicates the process of diabetes he has decided to put more effort into eating good foods and doing modified exercise movements to keep up his mobility and strength.

What Marie and Duffy appreciated the most about our conversation was that someone took the time to go over their concerns about their health. Like they said "we manage ok . . ." but for them it was comforting to be able to talk to someone who is interested in what they had to say and to have their health practices reinforced. Marie commented at the end of the interview that "taking time with us is so important . . . everything is done so quickly these days, by phone or email, etc. I love to sit and talk with people because that is how I know they care. . . ." This was a reminder to me that the reason for my becoming a nurse was to be able to impact the lives of people around me through health care, and what better way to approach that than helping people become advocates for their own health.

Sarah and Mary (interviewed by Katie Poinier)

I interviewed a Caucasian lesbian couple who have been together for approximately five years. Each of them is in her early thirties, and both women are employed and insured through their respective employers. Neither of the women has any chronic health conditions. Sarah is currently pregnant and will deliver her child a few months after the interview. I participate on a sports team with Mary and when I told her about my class, she was eager to be interviewed. The interview was conducted prior to one of our weekly games. Sarah and I were sitting on a bench, and Mary was standing facing us. It was a very relaxed, casual atmosphere.

Both women were raised in California, but in very different environments and families. Mary has known that she was gay since she was about fourteen years old. Her parents are quite conservative, especially her father. In spite of her parents' beliefs, her experience of her sexuality was always that it was very normal. During her teen years she found herself in the unique situation of having many friends who were also gay. This provided her with a good network of friends she could turn to for support and an environment in which she did not have to lie to anyone about who she really was. She felt comfortable going out in public settings, and did not feel she had to hide her sexuality.

Sarah knew she was gay at age nineteen, and experienced several social and personal relationship difficulties before and after coming out. She did not enjoy the same special situation that Mary had. She did not have to endure any taunting during her high school years, but her brother is very religious and continues to have an extremely difficult time coping with the fact that Sarah is gay. Her parents attended support groups for parents of children who are homosexual.

Both women experienced at least some amount of confusion regarding their sexuality, and each turned to drugs at some point in her life to relieve the stress they experienced. They both explained the feeling of having to put some life plans on hold in order to deal with their sexuality. For example, Sarah's mother passed away when she was sixteen, so she didn't have the emotional capacity to handle coming out until later in her life. Mary was confused in terms of what was expected of her regarding her education. She regrets not being pushed to attend a university.

Despite the social tensions and issues surrounding each woman's sexuality, each of them had some strong role models. Mary had her close network of friends, and a few older lesbian women in school provided guidance and support. Sarah had her aunt as a role model. In college, the manager of the women's center provided her with a role model for a lesbian relationship. It was through her experiences and friendship with the manager that she realized that her sexuality did not have to be something that interfered with her life.

The social and psychological aspects of a patient's personality are acutely important in terms of his or her perception of care provided. One's lifestyle often has everything to do with one's health, and reflects his or her very definition of health. Choices regarding one's vocation, living arrangement, exercise, diet, community activities, and social group influence one's health status and are a result of one's definition of health.

Mary and Sarah having a child together is a socially unconventional arrangement since they are a homosexual couple. They have made regular visits for prenatal care throughout Sarah's pregnancy. On a number of occasions when visiting their provider, the women have arrived separately due to schedule constraints. During one visit, after waiting in the admission area, Sarah, who arrived first, was taken into the exam room. She alerted her provider and the unit secretary to the fact that Mary would be arriving any time, and that she wanted Mary to be in the exam area as soon as possible. The provider responded, "Sure, I'll bring him back as soon as he gets here." The idea that only a heterosexual couple would have a baby seems to be ingrained, though it is clearly not the only scenario. Having known Sarah and Mary for the few months that they had been coming in for prenatal care, the provider was aware that they were a gay couple. Sarah said she was taken aback at this statement, and interpreted it to be a harmless slip-up on the part of the provider; but she felt disappointed and overlooked when her provider was not mindful of her sexuality in that moment. She had chosen a provider she felt was quite open-minded and was clearly aware of her sexuality, yet was not thinking of her as an individual on that particular day.

Filling out admission forms is often a challenge, and it is sometimes difficult to place oneself into a category, inevitably leading to situations in which a patient cannot find a category box to check on the intake form. For example, when Sarah fills out forms for prenatal visits, she never checks the "single" or "married" box. She is neither one of these, as they are defined legally and socially. She is not single but is in a long-term, committed relationship that she and Mary intend to last throughout their lifetimes. But this is not enough to place a mark in the "married" box since committed, lifelong homosexual relationships are not recognized as legal marriages in the state in which they live.

By virtue of the admission form, Sarah has become invisible. There is no established category into which she falls, and as a result she is therefore something of a nonentity. She and Mary both say that the forms one must fill out are incredibly main stream—except for the "other" box; a nondescript grab bag term. Sarah and Mary feel disappointed that they are not represented, though they do not believe that they will receive poor care because of their sexuality.

Sexual health issues can be overlooked by health care professionals who know that their patients are homosexual. For example, Sarah's primary care provider told her that because she has sex with women, she does not need to get an annual pap smear. This provider's dismissal of the importance of annual health screening based on her sexuality fails to recognize Sarah as a woman who has potential risk for developing cervical cancer at some point in her lifetime solely because she is a woman who has had multiple sexual partners. Sarah's provider believes that the fact that she is homosexual somehow exonerates her from what is regularly a routine prevention measure for other women. Since cervical cancer is a disease that is treatable if detected early, the provider's dismissal of a regular examination that would detect this disease represents bias toward lesbian women.

Sarah and Mary are at risk for health problems because they are marginalized and have not received the treatment that many heterosexual women in the same situation receive. It is not just that they are overlooked because of their sexuality. It is a disappointing to me that health care providers are generally not aware of their own biases and that patients are mistreated because of these biases. This fieldwork experience inspires me to acknowledge the biases that exist and seek a more just system in which all people are recognized as being equally deserving of respectful, conscientious health care.

Carrie (interviewed by Linda Frothinger)

Carrie, a single mother, lives with her 2½-year-old son, her father, stepmother, brother, and stepsister in a comfortable middle-class home set on a quiet street, with a beautiful view. As I sit with Carrie on her couch, I absorb everything about this young woman, knowing that my 44 years in age could easily influence her choice of words. After all, her father is younger than I am, and my own daughter is just five years younger than Carrie. Since some of my life experience includes time spent with single moms, I find that this influence does not lean toward a negative bias, but rather indicates insight into this population of women. I keep in mind the potential for my own biases based on my age and the fact that I was married before having children. I watch and listen to Carrie as she sits comfortably, legs folded beneath her, ready to share her experiences. She has a truly beautiful disposition, unintentionally charismatic, quiet spoken, yet confident of her words. She smiles at certain recollections, tossing her shoulder length hair aside with an easy laugh, quickly replacing it with an earnest expression. Is she suddenly recollecting the seriousness of what she is saying to me? At times, I feel the maturity of an adult and at other times the carefree attitude of a teen. Carrie, I believe, is in transition between the two roles she assumes as a young mother.

Carrie was 18 years old when she became pregnant. She did not receive prenatal care until well into her fifth month of the pregnancy, after developing a clot in her leg. Soon after this, she developed shingles. "I had a lot of complications with this pregnancy," Carrie states. "I hemorrhaged after delivery, and then when "Tyler" was born a month 'premature,' and the couple who was going to adopt him was standing right there, and he could hardly eat, well, I wasn't going to give him up. See, I was going to give him up for adoption." Carrie pauses as she considers the course of events. "Well, first, I was going to have an abortion, then I decided to give him up for adoption, but when he was born 'premature,' I couldn't give him up." We spoke a little about the decision she made to keep Tyler, and how she handles the challenges of raising a child alone. This conversation eventually steers back to the pregnancy and her prenatal care: "I had a doctor I didn't like. He was awful. He didn't care what I said, what I told him, how I felt. I found him after someone told me about the clinic he worked at and that it was a good clinic. It was a good clinic, but he wasn't nice at all. He didn't care about me. But, he was the only one who could be there when 'Tyler' was going to be born." Carrie pauses and then continues, "And then he wasn't even there! But, that's okay, because I didn't like him anyway." Carrie smiles, her eyes telling me that she is okay with this outcome. She swings her head to the side, tossing her hair, catching the sun just right as she continues. I realize with her comments that this relationship with her physician could have easily been addressed through some simple understandings. Had the physician had an understanding that Carrie has her own challenges and is just in need of his professional care, the relationship might have taken a different course. Had the physician understood the fact that beneath the tough exterior of this young woman was a terrified teen, and he was the person she had turned to for guidance . . . had he understood that Carrie is a person with a need for an empathic ear . . . these thoughts consume me as we continue.

"It was a good thing Tyler was premature, that's all I can say. He had to stay in the hospital for a month. I can't imagine taking him home after just a couple of days." Carrie's eyes indicate the severity of her feelings with regard to this issue. This was my opportunity to ask about the nurses. "The nurses were great. They taught me so much. I never would have known how to do any of that stuff—how to hold the baby, how to put a diaper on him, how to dress him, how to feed him. They tried to teach me how to breast feed him, but he wouldn't do that. He wouldn't eat from a bottle either, so they put a tube down his nose to get food to his stomach." The wonderment of this statement appears like a revelation as Carrie continues.

"I didn't like the nurse practitioner. . . . She started telling me every reason why not to keep Tyler 'He'll have this. He'll have that.' She kept telling me about how sick he was. She told me he was going to have all this stuff wrong. But then the nurses came in and told me he was going to be fine; that he wasn't sick at all, just small, and they helped me learn how to take care of him." The nurses' regard and respect for Carrie are evident through her slight smile as she pauses.

I commented: "He sure looks like a healthy guy now. . . . Tyler moves around like any other 2½-year-old boy, playfully talking to the dog and his toys." "He is," Carrie smiles back. "He's big. His Dad's not big, but he sure is. His Dad is only 5′9″ and weighs 150 pounds." Carrie's later comments suggest a connection with Tyler's dad, but not a relationship. Then she continues, "Tyler's dad is being deployed next month. . . . I have health insurance for Tyler because his dad is in the military, but they don't make it easy. I have to go a long way just for immunizations—he has all his immunizations. And they want me to use the hospital near the base if Tyler needs emergency care! I can't do that . . . I don't have health insurance, but Tyler is covered. . . . Through DSHS, I'm trying to get some money from his dad for support. And, I'm getting money and food stamps. But, otherwise, I don't have any health insurance. . . . It's too hard. . . ." The burden of this issue is quickly replaced with a new idea. Carrie continues, "On Sunday, I'm moving out to my own apartment . . . plus, I just found out that [employer's name] is cutting back my hours. Working about twenty hours a week will just pay for my rent. Tyler and I will just have a one-bedroom apartment. It's small, but big enough for us. So, I won't have any money for [health] insurance."

Our interview continues to jump around from one issue to the next; issues Carrie faces on a daily basis, and with this understanding, I am humbled by the fact that Carrie knows so much about things I know so little. We talk about her life, her choices, her desires and dreams, and she brings up the idea of going back to school. Carrie wants to be a nurse.

As Carrie considers the notion of school *and* raising Tyler *and* working, she appears defeated, resigned, sensing the magnitude of this undertaking as a single mother. We consider the fact that her dad is unemployed, but wants to help Carrie, her brother who does help Carrie babysit, and her stepmother, who is currently the primary breadwinner of the family. Carrie says this is why she wants to move out. ". . . because Tyler doesn't know who to listen to. My dad tells him something, then I do, then my stepmother. My brother and stepsister tell him stuff too. He doesn't know who the boss is?!? We steer our conversation back to the idea of going to school. Carrie considers the idea of first getting an associate degree from the community college. Working in steps lessens the magnitude of what is required to become a nurse practitioner. Carrie says she will be a good nurse practitioner. I believe she will be a better nurse practitioner than the one she experienced at the time of Tyler's birth, and I know she has the stamina and strength, along with the will to do so. I hope she will.

During our time together, I sensed an internal strength in this young woman who has learned from a difficult childhood, who has grown as a result of an enormous transition from a small town to a major city at the age of fifteen and who has evolved with her sudden and simultaneous introduction to adulthood and parenthood.

Most of this interview was Carrie sharing her story, requiring from me only an occasional question, statement, or confirmation of my understanding. I learned from this experience more than I could have ever imagined before going into this interview. Yet, I believe we both learned from this experience. Carrie was eager to share, talking at length, this account only a brief illustration of a young mother's life and her experiences with the American health care system. However brief, the implication exists that young mothers do fall through the cracks with respect to health care, specifically the "Carries" who are in transition from teen to adulthood, and whose families can lend some financial support, but not provide total support. Resources to meet the needs of this population of women could be focusing on their development into caring and successful parents, especially when I consider Carrie's desire to earn a degree in school and to continue being a mom. This could be a feasible and measurable outcome with the right resources in place to help these young moms during and after delivering their babies. But mostly, this could be achieved through addressing this population with respect and empathic care. Knowledge with humanity is a powerful tool.

CONCLUSION

From the excerpted interviews, it is clear that these students learned the basic principles of providing culturally competent care and did so with an attitude of self-reflection and awareness of their own ethnocentric biases. The tone of respect and openness to new ideas and diversity of cultures is apparent in how they approached the people they interviewed. The original reports were more detailed and included more analysis, but these excerpts provide a framework for cultural competence that can be summarized as follows. Learning how to provide culturally competent care has less to do with what one does or does not do and everything to do with how one approaches the patient. Demonstrating respect, establishing good rapport, and knowing how to listen are critical. Suspending judgment about lifestyles that are different from one's own enables one to learn from the patient. Being aware of one's own biases makes it possible to recognize assumptions about people as biases and not truth.

REFERENCES

Aday, L. A. (2001). *At risk in America: The health and health care needs of vulnerable populations in the United States* (2nd ed.). San Francisco, CA: Jossey-Bass.

Bezruchka, S. (2001). Societal hierarchy and the health Olympics. *Canadian Medical Association Journal, 164*(12), 1701–1703.

Butterfield, P. G. (1990). Thinking upstream: Nurturing a conceptual understanding of the societal context of health behavior. *Advances in Nursing Science, 12*(2), 1–8.

Langston, D. (1995). Tired of playing monopoly? In M. L. Andersen & P. H. Collins (Eds.). *Race, class, and gender: An anthology* (2nd ed., pp. 100–110). Belmont, CA: Wadsworth.

Sebastian, J. G. (2000). Vulnerability and vulnerable populations: An overview. In M. Stanhops & J. Lancaster (Eds.). *Community and public health nursing* (pp. 638–665). St. Louis, MO: Mosby.

CHAPTER 42

Graduate Studies Approach to Vulnerability

Debby A. Phillips and Jane W. Peterson

The Seattle University College of Nursing developed a master of science in nursing (MSN) program in 1992 to help meet the increasing need for master's-prepared nurse clinicians and managers. Strongly influenced by Seattle University's Jesuit heritage, commitment to social justice, and congruent with other Seattle University educational program foci, the MSN faculty determined that the graduate program should broadly and specifically address the well-being of vulnerable populations, including people living in poverty, refugees, diverse ethnic groups, and other marginalized populations. The college of nursing developed a curriculum for the advanced-practice nurse leading to certification as a Community Health Clinical Nurse Specialist (CNS) Among Vulnerable Populations (Vezeau, Peterson, Nakao, & Ersek, 1998). Central to the curriculum was Nursing Care of Vulnerable Populations (N502), a first-quarter, three-credit theory course. N502 provided the foundation for development of subsequent courses that elaborated on the concept of vulnerability and vulnerable populations.

Since 1992, the college has added additional advanced-practice specialties including, Family Nurse Practitioner, Psychiatric Mental Health Nurse Practitioner, and Spirituality and Health. Evolving to meet the needs of the nurse practitioner programs and of a more explicit focus on culture and how it relates to vulnerability and to nursing, N502 was revised and is now titled, Culture, Vulnerability, and Nursing. It continues to be a foundational course in the MSN program. What follows is a description of N502 in its earliest and latest forms.

N502: NURSING CARE OF VULNERABLE POPULATIONS

A primary objective in the initial N502 course was to identify vulnerable populations and to analyze multiple factors that contribute to vulnerability. Field experience and seminar discussions focused on nursing strategies to promote wellness in families, communities, and populations.

Aday's (1993) *At Risk in America* provided a theoretical basis for the early N502 course. It used an epidemiological framework to predict populations at risk, to analyze the concept of vulnerability, and to study vulnerable populations. The main components of her framework are social status, social capital, and human capital.

Several other texts supplemented the Aday text. *Mama Might Be Better Off Dead: The Failure of Healthcare in America* (Abrahams, 1993) pulls together vulnerability, epidemiology, and health care by describing a poor African American family in Chicago faced with serious illnesses and countless barriers to even minimal accessible health care. *Epidemiology in Nursing Practice*

(Harkness, 1995) emphasizes population-based decision making and the need for nurses to incorporate epidemiological principles in their practice. Lastly, *Poverty: Opposing Viewpoints* (Koster [ed.], 1994) was used to discuss poverty from many different viewpoints, pressing students to critically think through the issue, reflect, and question strongly held perspectives.

Teaching Methods

Immersion in the concept of vulnerability required that students first explore their values and beliefs related to vulnerability. Students then compared their view to Aday's theory, gaining insight into meanings of vulnerability and of belonging to a vulnerable population. Epidemiology was used to help students focus on social context, on populations versus individuals, and on preventive health care. Debates and class discussions were and continue to be an integral part of the course.

Fieldwork and Logs

To better understand vulnerability and to explore the needs of vulnerable people, each student identified a group with whom he or she was unfamiliar. Praxis, or the bringing together of theory and practice, was enabled by fieldwork. Students were encouraged to participate in non-clinical activities in hopes of moving them away from their comfort zone and into a space where they were unfamiliar learners. Early N502 fieldwork activities included handing out food at a food bank, reading stories to abused children, playing basketball with inner-city children, and serving lunch to drop-ins at an outpatient psychiatric day center. Students kept a log of their 30 hours of fieldwork. Logs included activities, participant observations; description and analysis of thoughts and feelings related to unfamiliar beliefs and behaviors; and description of possible actions or changes based on exposure to a new perspective.

For example, a student in a shelter for abused children ages 0–5 years began her log with the self-assured entry, "I arrived for an orientation to the program . . . I met some of the children and practiced a fire drill with them. I am confident that this will be an exciting and interesting experience." By the middle of the quarter she reported, "Hard work!" The student noted that the shelter staff were interested in her insights regarding a child who was slow in developing. Describing her feelings as "overwhelming," she wondered if she could make any difference in the child's life, and she was concerned about his development into adulthood. The log entries documented the student's growing comfort with the new environment and with unfamiliar people and issues until she was faced with "two new boys in the class" and "aggression" at recess. She reflected on the new skills that she needed to address aggressive behavior in young children and on abuse in terms of risk and vulnerability. The student reached a turning point when she met the program director of 20 years who described her many "success" stories. Inspired by the director and by her own experiences, the student continued at the shelter and did her MSN scholarly project on this work.

Synthesis/Framework Paper

Students' work on vulnerability was synthesized in a paper proposing a framework for studying a vulnerable population. Each paper included a literature review, analysis of vulnerability, and a diagram and explanation of the student's conception of vulnerability. For example, Watters (1998) explored vulnerability in Native American groups and did her fieldwork with the Suquamish people of the Pacific Northwest. She used Aday's (1993) concept of "being wounded," and expanded it to included political, personal, environmental, religious, cultural, and biological sources of vulnerability.

> The Web Framework of vulnerability appears to work with the Native American population. Vision a spider web with the strongest part being in the middle of the web. Herein lie those who are at the lowest risk of vulnerability. Outside forces such as a challenge to tradition or ill health, threaten to break the strands holding the web together. Layers of strands may break away until the core or middle of the web is exposed to high a risk of vulnerability. Branching out and providing anchors of support for the entire web framework are environmental, emic and etic views of self and views of others, and adaptive ability. Positive factors in these areas will strengthen the anchors and negative factors will weaken them, making them prone to breaking. The Suquamish, with whom I did field work, appear to be adaptive to the pressing "white" culture around them, maintaining their own identity, yet able to successfully find and maintain jobs outside the reservation. Their view of self as a nation is strengthened by the legends of their Chiefs Kitsaps and Seattle. Others outside their culture are not viewed as threats. The environment or natural resources available to them such as their timber, land and fishing grounds provide a rich source of economic stability and cultural identity. The Sioux, on the other hand are to be more vulnerable using this framework. They lack natural resources, have difficulty staying in the work force and experience high rates of depression (Kilborn, 1992). The Sioux's anchor threads are thus weaker and their society more vulnerable to injury.

Spiraling out from the center in interconnected threads are human resources (schools, jobs, income, housing, health care availability), social resources (family structure, lifestyles, marital status, community, cultural and language heritage, religion), and non-negotiable factors (age, gender, genetics dictating heath). Like the web, each resource and the non-negotiable factors affect each other. They are interwoven and cannot be separated. For example, the Suquamish have good schools, tribal housing, and access to health care. These help strengthen weaker threads where lack of jobs or lower incomes may threaten to break the web. The Suquamish are about 600 members strong; living in a relatively small area that is accessed quickly by car. This has helped to promote strong community bonds, which in turn nourishes the younger generation in the absence of traditional family forms of mother and father nuclear family. Grandparents, uncles, and aunts help to watch and raise children.

Ethnicity is like the spider that repairs and watches over the web. This is one absolute binding element that Native Americans have. If ethnicity is squashed or ignored, broken threads cannot be repaired and the web will collapse into decay. Programs within the Native American communities, as well as outside, need to promote ethnic identity, sensitivity, pride, and ultimately survival of the web's integrity.

Chief Seattle of the Suquamish once said, "This we know: All things are connected like the blood that unites us. We did not weave the web of life; We are merely a strand in it. Whatever we do to the web, we do to ourselves" (Chief Seattle, 1854).

N502: Culture, Vulnerability, and Nursing

In 2001, N502 was revised in order to broaden the exploration of vulnerability to include the concept of "culture" and to explicate the interconnections between culture, vulnerability, and nursing. To allow space for this addition, N502 was increased to four credits and the majority of epidemiology content was moved to another graduate course.

Several core concepts provide frameworks or heuristics for analyzing and understanding cultural difference, marginalization, and vulnerability. Initially, students read Narayan's (1988) article, "Working Together Across Difference: Some Considerations on Emotions and Political Practice." Key concepts in this article that are particularly useful before beginning fieldwork are "epistemic privilege," "methodological humility," and "methodological caution." Narayan describes epi-stemic privilege as the theoretical belief that "members of oppressed groups have a more immediate, subtle and critical knowledge about the nature of their oppression than people who are non-members of the oppressed group" (p. 35).

Following from this belief, Narayan (1988) argues that outsiders to a group should act with methodological humility, that is

> the "outsider" must always sincerely conduct herself under the assumption that, as an outsider, she may be missing something, and that what appears to her to be a "mistake" on the part of the insider may make more sense if she had fuller understanding of the context. (p. 38)

Moreover, Narayan urges the outsider

> . . . to sincerely attempt to carry out her attempted criticism of the insider's perceptions in such a way that it does not amount to, or even seem to amount to, an attempt to denigrate or dismiss entirely the validity of the insider's point of view (methodological caution). (p. 38)

The concepts, "insider" and "outsider" (Narayan, 1988), "othering" (Canales, 2000), and "allostatic load" (Kendall & Hatton, 2002; Kneipp & Drevdahl, 2003), Apple's (1997) and Fine's (1997) work on whiteness, and Natadecha-Sponsel's (1993) work on ethnocentrism are used to help students understand how being (culturally) different from the "norms" of US society is connected to vulnerability. Other theoretical heuristics that are used to understand culture and vulnerability are gender, race, class, and heterosexism (Allman, 1992; McIntosh, 1992; Schroeder, 2003; Stevens, 1995).

To move these concepts from theory to outcomes, students are asked to read nursing research articles such as Tashiro's (2002) work on the effects of mixed race identity, Choi's (2002) examination of ethnocentrism in understanding adolescent depression, Kendall and Hatton's (2002) analysis of racism as a source of health disparities in children with ADHD, Meleis and Hatter-Pollara's (1995) examination of stereotypes and their consequences for Arab Middle Eastern women, and Tsai's (2003) work on the effects of immigration on Taiwanese immigrants to the United States.

Two books provide personal accounts of some of the societal causes and consequences of vulnerability in the United States related to health. Abrahams' (1993) book provides intimate details about the effects of race, poverty, and gender on health. *The Spirit Catches You and You Fall Down: A Hmong Child, Her American Doctors, and the Collision of Two Cultures* (Fadiman, 1997) demonstrates cultural insensitivity and ethnocentrism at it worst despite the good intentions of Western medicine and committed health care professionals.

Teaching Methods

A heavy emphasis is placed on careful, critical readings of the journal articles and texts, and on classroom discussion. Fieldwork related to a selected cultural group or vulnerable population and regular written work and analysis, including discussion questions, cultural identity paper, and a final paper are used to synthesize course readings, discussion, literature review, and fieldwork.

Fieldwork, Log, and Presentation

Fieldwork continues to be a central aspect of N502. Students are encouraged to work with people with whom they are unfamiliar and are reminded that these are not experiences where they will "do" nursing in the strictest clinical sense. They are participatory experiences where students learn subtle, and not so subtle, interpersonal and respectful ways to "do" nursing in a broad sense. SU CON's regular involvement in five, low-income communities in the Seattle area have facilitated the practical aspects of fieldwork for 30 students, such as accessibility. Recent student experiences included participation in English as second language (ESL) classes, citizenship classes, Boys' and Girls' Club leadership group, ESL computer labs, homeless women's day shelter, therapeutic riding (horses) center for developmentally delayed children, AA meetings for women in the county jail, alternative school program for boys with ADHA, WIC clinic, Latino health resources center, Teen Feed and Street Links van for homeless adolescents, and day shelter for Native Americans.

As mentioned earlier, students document their experiences, activities, interactions, and reflections in a fieldwork log. For example, a student assisting in a community center ESL class with mostly female students from Somalia, Eritrea, Mexico, Ukraine, India, and Iran, describes that "Academic classes are far more regimented than this class, which often erupts in a babble of conversation. . . . Sue [teacher] said she's decided against a firmer approach because the class represents social time for many. . . . Many students have formal education, but a significant majority do not and Sue's choice to compromise on classroom demeanor may better meet their needs. I see a clear analogy to everything we've studied about caring for patients in cultural context" (Crawford, 2001).

In a later log entry, Crawford (2001) describes working with Fadima, Nadija, Fazra, and Maryann and notices that

> . . . despite the veils and underclass social role, they aren't particularly shy in the all-female small group. We read the embarrassing pilgrim story, taking turns line by line. . . . They sound out better than getting meanings. I've noticed that their tongues handle English sounds more easily than do speakers of Southeast Asian languages. Somali, as translated in the alphabet is vowel heavy. The last exercise involved grammar, present, and past tenses in simple verbs. . . . I consulted Sue, but found that my backward gestures for past tense is what she uses. I thought of how heavily the medical interview depends on chronology and exact location and sequencing to separate indicator symptoms from red herrings. (p. 1)

Log entries like these assist the students with their fieldwork presentations and final papers. In the presentations, students are asked to describe their fieldwork, describe ways that the particular group is created as vulnerable or culturally "different" in US society, describe implications for themselves and for their professional practice, and prepare one or two discussion questions.

Cultural Identity Paper

Students are asked to synthesize readings and discussion from the first four weeks of the course and from their life experiences, to write a paper about their cultural identity. Criteria for the paper are: describe your cultural identity including gender, class, sexual orientation, age, ethnicity, religious/spiritual orientation, heritage, nationality, and other factors influencing your identity; describe one or more experiences that you have had with racism and/or whiteness, sexism and/or heterosexism, and classism; and discuss how their cultural identity, influencing factors, and the experiences support and/or constrain their nursing practice.

Fieldwork Analysis and Nursing Care Paper

This final paper allows students to organize, analyze, and critically evaluate their fieldwork. Criteria for paper are: to describe, in a detailed way, the group she/he worked with and her/his experience; describe theoretical positions on ways that this particular group is created as vulnerable or culturally "different" in US society; synthesize and describe findings from individual fieldwork interactions, observations, epidemiological data, the literature; and describe implications of her/his fieldwork and analysis for nursing practice and for the discipline of nursing.

In general, N502 students take significant steps in understanding that people in the US are born into a society that creates certain people as vulnerable and different due to dominant norms and institutional practices. For example, a student teaching citizenship classes at a health and resource center for Latino immigrants critiqued the norms of transportation availability. Clifton (2003) argued that

> [f]or Latinos seeking medical attention, transportation is another significant barrier [to accessibility]. Reasons for lack of personal transportation among Latino immigrants include low economic status (cannot afford costs related to vehicle ownership), lack of the English skills necessary to pass the State Licensing Exam, and lack of immigrant status necessary to obtain the paperwork for legal ownership of a vehicle. Many Latino immigrants depend on public transportation, which can be a confusing and inadequate alternative. Each of my students average 5–7 hours a week simply traveling to and from citizenship classes. One woman is brought to the center by her husband and young children who wait outside for her in the car during every two-hour lesson. They drive 44–60 minutes each way. (p. 4)

Students are also encouraged to synthesize theoretical positions from class readings, other literature, and fieldwork experiences. Hibbs (2003) for example, examined his dominant social position as a white, male, native English speaker in relation to the immigrants that he worked with in Talk Time, a class where non-native English speakers practice language skills. He describes,

> While considering ways to make the group more interactive, I realized that as a graduate student, an American, and a male, the group could possibly view me as being intimidating or unapproachable. Recognizing my "whiteness," my "maleness," and my "American-ness" was a difficult process. After reading "Othering: Towards an Understanding of Difference" (Canales, 2000) and "Working Together Across Difference" (Narayan, 1988), I became cognizant of my ascribed identity. This self-awareness led me to want to step outside of my own shoes and into others to see myself the way they do. Canales (2000) describes this process as "role taking," which is "imagining the world from the perspective of another" (p. 19).
>   Recognizing my dominant position in the group was the first step in changing group dynamics. The second step was to encourage the group members see me as equal. Canales (2000) describes this process as "inclusionary othering, . . . an attempt to create a transformative rela-

tionship in which the consequences are consciousness raising, sense of community, shared power, and inclusion" (p. 25). . . . I printed out a list of Vietnamese and Chinese phrases. I . . . greeted members with "Sin chow," and "Nee haow," which is simply hello. . . . I think they really appreciated that I was making an effort. Instead of viewing me as the critical American graduate student, I was now viewed more as a potential friend and imperfect linguist, who still has a lot to learn. (pp. 3, 4)

N502 students were also encouraged to examine the relationships between vulnerability and cultural differences. Hester (2003) critiqued the Women, Infant, and Children (WIC) program held at a low-income, multi-ethnic health center. She notes, "Aside from the measurable effects of poverty on individuals, it may be even more powerful to examine the qualitative effects that one's involvement in a government run program like WIC has on an individual" (p. 4). She asked important questions like,

What does it feel like to have to rely on a federal program for food? How does it feel when everyone at the grocery store knows you receive WIC checks? What is it like to have little or no choice in what foods you have access to? What is it like to eat food that you have never been exposed to during your life as a non-nature resident? (p. 4)

Critiquing the cultural sensitivity of the WIC program, Hester (2003) argues that,

. . . I quickly learned that WIC was far from a culturally sensitive program. Foods available to participants were extremely limited and included eggs, cereal, juice, cheese, milk, and peanut butter or beans. . . . From the perspective of many Asian-American immigrants, these food are not congruent with their traditional eating patterns. Specifically, milk and other dairy products are not customarily eaten by most Asians. . . . Rice, which is a staple for most people in the world, is not included in the WIC program. This is also the case for other traditional foods such as soy products. . . . (p. 5)

Implications of fieldwork findings and analysis for nursing practice and for the discipline is emphasized throughout the course and is a crucial gestalt for the last section of the final paper. Students address the individual level to the global level. For example, Aas (2003), who participated in Talk Time at an Asian counseling center, described

. . . it is important to know something about the individual history of each Asian immigrant we care for. The term "Asian" refers to 28 separate countries and includes over 50 islands (Dhooper, 2003). Despite commonalties in social structures and belief systems, there is enormous diversity across these cultures. In the Talk Time group, one participant works for a low-wage in a restaurant and lives with just one brother. Another man is a teacher who retired long before immigrating. He . . . has myriad affluent, professional family members in the area. . . . While both individuals can benefit from a chance to practice conversational English, their remaining needs may vary considerably. (p. 9)

Addressing implications for the nursing discipline, Hopkins (2003), who volunteered in a citizenship class, argues that,

As a discipline, nurses must become advocates for the vulnerable populations we serve. One of the first hurdles we face is to overcome our "ironic detachment," a term coined by Iris Young

(Schroeder, 2003, p.181). Although many nurses are relatively informed and critical thinkers, we are often apathetic when it comes to creating change in society. This fieldwork experience has made me realize how important it is to speak up for refugees who have no voice in our society. If we do not, someone else will, and what they decide may not be in the best interest of this population. Drevdahl (2002) supports this notion as she writes, "Finally, the complexity of the global culture demands that we be involved in political activism, including being knowledgeable about global trends in health care, understanding political processes and promoting policy changes that affect health" (p. 18). One of the many issues I will advocate for is increased opportunities for U.S. citizens to participate in "role taking" (Canales, 2000). . . . children could be exposed to new cultures and ways of thinking that will hopefully lessen creation of vulnerable populations in U.S. society in the future. (p. 8)

Summary

The concept of vulnerability is integral to the SU and CON mission and it is threaded throughout the MSN graduate curriculum beginning with N502: Culture, Vulnerability, and Nursing. Students are encouraged to build on understandings gained in N502 and to think about the final paper as a possible beginning for their MSN scholarly project or thesis. Evanson (1997), for example, used the framework she developed in one of the earlier N502 classes in her thesis, *Identification of Domestic Violence by Public Health Nurses Before and After an Education Program*. She used her framework to "examine the risk of vulnerability to the population of DV victims, utilizing existing knowledge gained from a review of literature" (p. 14). Evanson found that by not using such a framework to screen women, "health care workers not only fail to help battered women, but actually do further harm to them, and thereby increase their overall vulnerability" (p. 56).

Initially, student reception to N502 varies from "Why do we have to know this, it's not nursing," to "This is great. It should be taught everywhere." By the end of the class, the majority of students are thankful for the personal growth and self-reflection necessitated by N502 and for their newfound understandings. Moreover, most students seem to feel empowered to address vulnerability in their nursing practice and on a societal level.

References

Aas, E. E. (2003). Nursing care paper: Asian immigrants. Unpublished paper, Seattle University College of Nursing.

Abraham, L. K. (1993). *Mama might be better off dead. The failure of healthcare in America*. Chicago, IL: University of Chicago Press.

Aday, L. A. (1993) *At risk in America: The health and health care needs of vulnerable populations in the United States*. San Francisco, CA: Jossey-Bass.

Allman, K. M. (1992). Race, racism and health: Examining the "natural facts." In J. Thompson, D. Allen, & L. Rodrigues-Fisher (Eds.). *Critique, resistance, action: Working papers in the politics of nursing* (pp. 35–52). New York, NY: NLN.

Apple, M. W. (1997). Consuming the other: Whiteness, education, and cheap french fries. In M. Fine, L. Weis, L. C. Powell, & L. M. Wong (Eds.). *Off white: Reading on race, power, and society* (pp. 121–128). New York, NY: Routledge.

Canales, M. K. (2000). Othering: Toward an understanding of difference. *Advances in Nursing Science, 22*(4), 16–31.

Chief Seattle (1854). Speech given during treaty negotiations. In Jeffers, S (Ill.). *Brother Eagle, Sister Sky: a message from Chief Seattle.* New York, NY: Dial Books.

Choi, H. (2002). Understanding adolescent depression in ethnocultural context. *Advances in Nursing Science, 25*(2), 71–85.

Clifton, R. A. (2003). Fieldwork analysis: Latino immigrants. Unpublished paper, Seattle University College of Nursing.

Crawford, T. (2001). Fieldwork log. Unpublished paper, Seattle University College of Nursing.

Dhooper, S. S. (2003). Health care needs of foreign-born Asian Americans. *Health & Social Work, 28*(1), 63–73.

Drevdahl, D. J. (2001). Home and border: The contradictions of community. *Advances in Nursing Science, 24*(3), 8–20.

Evanson, T. (1997). Identification of Domestic Violence by Public Health Nurses Before and After an Education Program. Unpublished Masters thesis, Seattle University College of Nursing.

Fadiman, A. (1997). *The Spirit catches you and you fall down. A Hmong child, her American doctors, and the collision of two cultures.* New York, NY: Farrar, Straus, and Giroux.

Fine, M. (1997). Witnessing Whiteness. In M. Fine, L. Weis, L. C. Powell, & L. M. Wong (Eds.). *Off white: Reading on race, power, and society* (pp. 57–65). New York, NY: Routledge.

Hester, K. (2003). Fieldwork written analysis and nursing care paper. Unpublished paper, Seattle University College of Nursing.

Harkness, G. A. (1995). *Epidemiology in nursing practice.* St. Louis, MO: Mosby.

Hibbs, D. (2003). Asian immigrants as a vulnerable population. Unpublished paper, Seattle University College of Nursing.

Hopkins, M. (2003). Fieldwork written analysis and nursing care paper. Unpublished paper, Seattle University College of Nursing.

Kendall, J., & Hatton, D. (2002). Racism as a source of health disparity in families with children with attention deficit hyperactivity disorder. *Advances in Nursing Science, 25*(2), 22–39.

Kneipp, S. M., & Drevdahl, D. (2003). Problems with parsimony in research on socioeconomic determinants or health. *Advances in Nursing Science, 26*(3), 162–172.

Koster, K. (Ed.). (1994). *Poverty: Opposing viewpoints.* San Diego, CA: Greenhaven Press.

McIntosh, P. (1992) White privilege and male privilege: A person account of coming to see correspondences through work in women's studies. In M. L. Andersen & P. H. Collins (Eds.). *Race, class, and gender* (pp. 70–81). Belmont, CA: Wadsworth.

Master of Science in Nursing. Seattle University New Program and Changes in Existing Program Proposal. Fall 1992 (Submitted by Maureen Niland, Constance Nakao & Janet Claypool).

Meleis, A. I., & Hatter- Pollara, M. (1995). Arab Middle Eastern women: Stereotyped, invisible, but powerful. In D. L. Adams (Ed.). *Health issues for women of color: A cultural perspective* (pp. 133–163). Thousands Oaks, CA: Sage Publications.

Narayan, U. (1988). Working together across difference: Some considerations on emotions and political practice. *Hypatia, 3*(2), 31–47.

Natadecha-Sponsel, P. (1993) The young the rich and the famous: Individualism as an American cultural value. In P. R. Devita & J. D. Armstrong (Eds.). *Distant mirrors: America as a foreign culture* (pp. 46–53). Belmont, CA: Wadsworth.

Schroeder, C. (2003). The tyranny of profit: Concentration of wealth, corporate globalization, and the failed US health care system. *Advances in Nursing Science, 26*(3), 173–184.

Seattle University School of Nursing. Self Study Report to National League for Nursing Accrediting Commission, Fall 1997.

Stevens, P. E. (1995). Structural and interpersonal impact of heterosexual assumptions on lesbian health care clients. *Nursing Research, 44*(1), 25–30.

Tashiro, C. J. (2002). Considering the significance of ancestry through the prism of mixed-race identity. *Advances in Nursing Science, 25*(2), 1–21.

Tsai, J. H. C. (2003). Contexualizing immigrants' lived experience: Story of Taiwanese Immigrants in the United States. *Journal of Cultural Diversity, 10*(3), 76–83.

Vezeau, T. M., Peterson, J. W., Nakao, C. & Ersek, M. (1998). Education of advanced practice nurses: Serving vulnerable populations. *Nursing and Health Care Perspectives, 19*(3), 124–130.

Watters, E. K. (1998). Threads of a web: Vulnerability of the native Americans. Unpublished paper, Seattle University College of Nursing.

CHAPTER 43

Graduate Fieldwork with Vulnerable Populations

Debby A. Phillips, Robyn Bennetts, Tyler Free, Natalie Keilholz, and Deborah Parr

The excerpts in this chapter reflect papers written by master's degree nursing students to complete requirements for a required course, N502: Culture, Vulnerability, and Nursing, taught by the first author and described in the previous chapter. Students do extensive reading on the social context of vulnerability, including poverty, racism, white privilege, heterosexism, and other societal factors that mark particular people as not the "norm." In fieldwork with vulnerable people, the students move away from a solely individual focus and consider societal factors that significantly contribute to vulnerability in the United States. The four excerpts below illustrate this movement.

HOMELESS WOMEN (ROBYN BENNETTS)

I conducted fieldwork at a shelter for homeless women. Although the women with whom I worked shared the experience of being homeless, they faced their own unique challenges that led to homelessness: domestic violence, child abuse, mental illness, chronic physical illness, addiction, low-income employment, the experience of profound loss (death, employment, and social support), legal difficulties, and stress. The women varied in terms of whether they had experienced poverty throughout their lives or just recently. Regardless of the duration of their poverty, all of the women were at a place in their lives where they lacked power to change their circumstances. Some actively worked to improve their situations, whereas others seemed to have accepted homelessness and poverty as their fate.

The shelter provides ways the women can regain some power over their circumstances. They make their own breakfasts and receive points for doing chores. The points can be redeemed for clothing and hygiene items in the shelter. Each day provides opportunities for the women to regain power over their minds and bodies. There are Alcoholics Anonymous (AA), Narcotics Anonymous, and codependency meetings to open the door to addiction recovery for those who need or want to participate. Community meetings and tea time provide a means of gaining social support. Exercise classes and weekly health talks encourage the women to strengthen their bodies. Prayer groups and inspirational readings encourage the women to strengthen their souls.

There were several commonalities of violence, substance abuse, and mental illness among the women at the shelter, and these conditions are interconnected. Violence was a pervasive theme.

Violence perpetrated by partners left women in the precarious situation of being forced to choose between abuse and homelessness, only to find that shelter life is equally as dangerous at times. One woman told me that, although she did not want to return home to her abusive husband, at least when she was at home, she knew who the enemy was, and there was only one.

Physical and sexual childhood violence was also a common experience among the shelter women, and they spoke about it casually, as if it were just part of growing up. The consequences of childhood abuse are enormous (Felitti, 2002). Many of the women in the shelter reported being depressed or anxious. Others had slipped into a reality only evident to them. Goodman, Saxe, & Harvey (1991) hypothesize that there is a need to move beyond seeing mental illness as a risk factor for becoming homeless and recognize that homelessness itself is a risk factor for emotional disorders as these people experience the effects of isolation and segregation.

The problems of substance abuse were apparent among the women in this shelter. Clatts (1993) points out that the women he interviewed described their experience of crack and cocaine in terms of feeling powerful in relation to men. There are fewer women at the shelter at the beginning of the month when they get their "checks." Those living with addictions may spend all of their money on drugs and alcohol and then return to the shelter feeling sick and exhausted when the money is gone.

There are many structures built into our society that make coming out of homelessness extremely difficult. Abraham (1993) paints a compelling picture of the complexity of survival on the streets. There are numerous rules and regulations that at times do not even seem to make sense. Homeless women must navigate a complicated system. Sometimes it becomes so overwhelming that they give up and accept being homeless as their fate. The message sent is that these women have done something "wrong" in becoming homeless and that they do not deserve the same degree of autonomy granted to those in the dominant culture. There are a number of women in the shelter who have jobs yet cannot afford housing because they earn low salaries (Valle, 1994).

Professional Implications

I went into this fieldwork experience thinking that I was aware and sensitive to the homeless, but I have a long way to go. In an effort to prove that I did not consider myself better than anyone else, I tended to minimize differences and inadvertently did the opposite. By not recognizing the privilege in my life, I denied the fact that those who are vulnerable must overcome many more serious obstacles to survive. I also considered myself to be nonjudgmental but realized I am constantly making assumptions without even realizing I do this. I never thought that a woman in a homeless shelter went to work all day. I never thought that child abuse was an underlying issue in the lives of an extraordinary number of women. My previous job involved working with gay men, but for some reason I never thought that women attending a homeless shelter might possibly be anything but heterosexual. I never thought that a society as supposedly advanced as ours could have a system that is complicated to the point of absurdity. The most important thing I have learned from fieldwork is that we are a product of our environment.

What should nurses do to prepare to work with the homeless? Avoid making assumptions about the homeless. Look at the whole person. Ask the sensitive questions. Find out the nature of the environment in which people live their lives. Be persistent in asking these questions because one does not necessarily gain trust on the first visit, especially from patients who have learned not to trust. Implement care plans with realistic treatment goals. If transportation, medication management, or even rest is not an option, then those are the realities for the patient. Find a way for these women to regain power over their lives. This means working together with them on care plans and listening to their ideas and goals to instill hope of improving their situations. Become aware of the issues surrounding homelessness; good will is not enough. Advocate for the homeless. Although there were many issues facing the women with whom I worked, I cannot get past my feelings about the level of child abuse experienced by these women. It feels like child abuse is a "dirty little secret," and we have got to do something to change this. Advocate at every level by being more observant with our young patients, asking the important questions of our adult patients, and fighting for legislation to protect our children rather than the perpetrators of abuse.

ADHD AND VULNERABILITY (TYLER FREE)

I conducted my fieldwork in a school designed to serve adolescents with special needs. The school serves 32 students, ranging in age from 7 to 14 years. A certified special education teacher and two assistants staff each of the four classrooms. The goal is to reintegrate each student back into the "regular" school setting after their special needs have been identified and adequately addressed. Many of the students have been diagnosed with severe emotional and behavioral disorders, and several have attempted suicide. The one diagnosis that was consistent among many of the students was attention deficit hyperactivity disorder (ADHD). Of the 32 students, all of whom are boys, 20 had been diagnosed with ADHD.

I attended the school every Wednesday afternoon and assisted with the physical education class, participating in soccer, basketball, and football. One day I demonstrated how to accurately throw a spiral on the football. Another day I instructed the students on the proper defensive technique in soccer. Because discipline was not my responsibility, I feel that I developed a close connection with many of the students. The students understood that I would not punish or judge them, and they seemed to feel comfortable opening up with me. I had not previously spent a lot of time with special needs children, and having the opportunity to get to know these students was personally rewarding. The students have many teachers, classmates, and their parents, but many do not have a friend. As Eric (all names used are fictitious) told me last week, "Kids in my class are nice, but they're not really my friends." I would like to think that the students saw me as a friend.

ADHD is one of the most common reasons that children are referred to mental health practitioners. In the United States, it is recognized as the most prevalent childhood psychiatric disorder (Barkley, 1990). The prevalence of ADHD in children is estimated at 5% (Krueger & Kendall, 2001). ADHD is defined as "a persistent pattern of inattention and/or hyperactivity-impulsivity that is more frequent and severe than typically observed in individuals at a comparable level of development" (American Psychiatric Association, 1994). Distraction and disorganization create major problems in learning and, because children with ADHD take longer to finish an assignment, they feel different and are viewed as different by their peers (Kendall, Hatton, Beckett, & Leo, 2003). Chris told me about his school experiences before attending the school: "I was slow at everything, and everyone in my class knew it."

Experiencing problems with behaving and following rules was another major theme that emerged in the study (Kendall et al., 2003). These problems included breaking things, throwing things, cussing, and fighting. Because of their impulsivity, children with ADHD are often unable to control their behavior and express their emotions in an acceptable manner. I did not witness acts of violence at the school, but on two occasions, I arrived just after a student had attacked a teacher.

Krueger & Kendall (2001) interviewed 11 adolescents with ADHD to discover how adolescents experience it. The study participants developed an identity that centered around the stigmatizing beliefs and negative attributes of ADHD. Chris yelled out to a teacher, "Why do you want me to focus? You know I'm not like that." Kruger & Kendall also found that children with ADHD often feel a lack of empowerment. Ben expressed feelings of lack of empowerment after returning to class late from physical education. "I couldn't help it. I didn't know what was going on. How was I supposed to know?"

Hartman (1999) uses a metaphor to explain ADHD: there are farmers and there are hunters. Children with ADHD have a great ability to make instant decisions and to act upon them. Their impulsivity makes them perfect hunters. The rest of society is made up of farmers. Farmers are structured and live by routine. Unfortunately for the hunters, our society is built around order and structure. When a hunter is unable to learn farmer skills, he is unable to survive in the farmer's world. Children with ADHD are often in an educational environment in which they feel like failures.

Canales (2000) describes the process of "othering," in which members of a nondominant group are judged against a mythical norm. Children with ADHD are aware of their label as "other." For example, Chris told me that he likes the school "so much more" than his previous school. He told me how his classmates used to tease him because they knew he would "go off." Here, Chris was no longer surrounded by farmers, forced to live in the farmer's world.

ADHD has been characterized as a white middle-class disease (Kendall & Hatton, 2002). ADHD symptoms in many nonwhite children are often viewed as a product of poverty and violence. Instead of receiving a proper diagnosis of ADHD, many nonwhite children are misdiagnosed and consequently do not receive appropriate treatment. At the school, 30 of the 32 students were white.

Professional Implications

Recognize that ADHD in not a disorder limited to whites and males. This narrow-minded awareness of ADHD ignores minorities and females that may be in need of services. Understand the negative perception that our society has of people with ADHD. Shame and stigmatization are attached to ADHD and may act as a barrier. For example, parents may not wish to discuss their child's difficulties in fear of having the label "ADHD" placed on their child. Discuss ADHD in an open and nonjudgmental way. Disclaim the notion that ADHD is synonymous with being bad.

Recognize that symptoms may not be obvious. At the school, symptoms of ADHD ranged from violence to social isolation. Stereotypes may act as an obstacle in properly diagnosing children with ADHD. Be familiar with the classic symptoms, but remain open to the fact that ADHD presents in different forms.

Be familiar with the current knowledge of ADHD, including medicines and behavioral prevention programs. It is estimated that as many as 80% of children diagnosed with ADHD are on some form of medication (Frame, 2003). Understand, however, that medication may not always be appropriate.

Refer children with ADHD to behavioral specialists who can help them with their behavioral and emotional problems. Consider the emotional impact on the family when developing treatment plans. Studies have shown that ADHD in children predicts depression in mothers (Kendall et al., 2003).

See children with ADHD in a well-planned and warm environment. Be patient, and provide an appropriate level of stimulus. For example, offering a child with ADHD a video game with which to play during an office visit may make the visit much easier for the nurse, the parent, and the child.

My experience at the school exposed me to a group of individuals with whom I had no previous experience. I learned a lot about children with ADHD and look forward to helping this population in my future practice. My fieldwork enabled me to practice what Canales (2000) calls role-taking. Role-taking is where one attempts to see the world from the "other's" perspective. Although I will never understand exactly how children with ADHD experience the world, I feel that role-taking enabled me to better understand the difficulties that children with ADHD encounter on a daily basis.

CHILDREN WITH DISABILITIES AND HIPPOTHERAPY (NATALIE KEILHOLZ)

I was drawn to explore the meaning of disability in order to better understand my husband's sister, diagnosed with spina bifida. For this reason, I chose to spend my fieldwork at a riding center that is committed to nurturing children and adults with disabilities through the use of horse therapy, also called "hippotherapy." The Greeks recognized the therapeutic value of the horse from 460 BC, and the field of hippotherapy, derived from the Greek word "hippos," meaning "horse," was developed by the Germans in the 1960s (Schwartz, 2000). Hippotherapy is a therapeutic treatment that "provides a controlled environment and graded sensory input designed to elicit appropriate adaptive responses from the client," and it results in improvements in motor function (Heine, 1997).

I worked with two boys, Tyson and Alex (pseudonyms), ages 2 and 4 years. Although these children were diagnosed with autism and cortical blindness, the riding center cares for people with a variety of conditions, including cerebral palsy, stroke, muscular dystrophy, multiple sclerosis, spina bifida, and traumatic brain injury. Both of the riders I assisted were small for their age, lacked complete muscle control, and possessed limited vocabularies. Despite these "disabilities," they maintained enormous smiles, constant laughter, and exuded a radiance of delight throughout class.

For 2 hours each Wednesday morning, I worked with Tyson and Alex, on horses, in individual hippotherapy classes. During each class, I aided the physical therapist with a variety of tasks, such as leading the horse, playing games, singing songs, socializing with the rider, and maintaining rider safety by walking alongside the horse. Under direction of the therapist, I controlled the horse's course (making circles and figure eights) and walking pattern (increasing and decreasing speed) to challenge the child's postural abilities and strengthen trunk muscles. Depending on skill level, the children were asked to reach and pet the neck of the horse, to change positions on the horse from sitting forward to sitting backward, or to ride quadruped (on hands and knees), because these activities improved motor control, trunk stability, pelvic control, motor planning, and sensory input (Heine, 1997). Alex was encouraged to speak, using real words to communicate his needs, while Tyson was urged to strengthen his muscles and improve his flexibility. For Tyson and Alex, ability plays a role in their identity development. The center attempts to deconstruct this concept of disability through emphasizing the child's riding achievements. The therapist and I continually praised Alex and Tyson for their excellent riding. After all, it takes courage to sit on a 1000-pound animal.

Parents of disabled children are also members of a vulnerable population. One morning, when Alex's mother phoned in to cancel 10 minutes before hippotherapy class, everyone was frustrated. However, I later learned that she had four other children to care for and realized that her life must be extremely complex.

Professional Implications

Consider each child on an individual basis and use his or her name. Teach new parents to break down social stereotypes by providing informational resources and support groups. Educate people outside of the health care setting. For example, schoolchildren should be taught not only to overcome their fears and stereotypes but also to embrace differences in their peers, perhaps by learning about simple physiological development. Emphasize the strengths of the children and refer patients to programs, such as the center, that nurture all aspects of the child, encouraging social contact, strengthening self-esteem, and improving physiological functioning.

My experience at the center has led me to discard the concept of "normal." Every child has his or her own way of living life, of interacting and surviving in society. Because the children I worked with had minimal language development, I felt frustrated at being unable to communicate or connect with them because I have grown up in a society that relies heavily on language. I soon realized that the children relied not on words but on body language and facial expressions. Tyson would turn his head and smile when he liked a song I sang or make kissing noises to say goodbye. Alex would laugh and say "bah! bah!" to point out something exciting. When I began my fieldwork at the center, I viewed these children as small fragile creatures with whom I could not speak. Today, I see not their fragility but their strength, and I have learned from them the many facets of personhood.

FEMALE INMATES AND SUBSTANCE ABUSE (DEBORAH PARR)

I participated in 14 AA meetings for female inmates at a downtown jail in a major city in the Pacific Northwest. Meetings were held at the jail on Sunday and Thursday, for 90 minutes each day, and included two to five volunteers from the AA community with between 6 and 16 inmates attending. There was little continuity among attendees from meeting to meeting. AA members attend one meeting per month. Women from two of the three wings of the jail are selected to attend each meeting; the wings designated to attend vary meeting to meeting. During the period of my fieldwork, I was the only person consistently in attendance at every meeting.

Jails are very noisy places made of cinder block and concrete. The doors are remote controlled and make a jarring clang when opened or shut. Remote cameras tape the activity in the meeting room and rotate noisily throughout the meeting. Shouts can be heard from inmates in the recreation area. The meeting room has 4 tables and 20 plastic chairs. The volunteers set the chairs in a circle and determine the number of inmates who can attend the meeting. Some volunteers are comfortable with a large group; others limit the attendance to 12. Volunteers conduct a modified AA meeting, and the format varies with each group. A volunteer begins the discussion, sharing what alcoholism was like, what happened, and what it is like now in sobriety. Inmates are then encouraged to share their stories, keeping the focus on their problems with alcohol or drugs.

I was initially very uncomfortable with the environment: the noise, the camera, even the toilet without a seat. Nothing really prepared me for such an alien experience—being locked up with women who seemed very different. I wondered if I had anything of value that I could share that would be helpful to these women. I had never been to jail, was never arrested, never sold my body, and never used IV drugs; in so many ways I did not believe I had anything to offer. Over the course of my fieldwork, I found that sharing my time and my attention was valuable to the women. One night on my way to the jail, I backed into a car opposite my driveway. After exchanging insurance information, I continued on my way to the jail. I told the women at the meeting that I was a little rattled and described what happened. Several of the women were profoundly moved that I would still come to the jail to see them after getting into an accident. They hugged me.

Through repeated exposure, I became comfortable with both the physical and the emotional environment. Seeing a room of women dressed in red (which indicates having a felony charge) no longer caused me to feel apprehensive. Instead of seeing the clothes, I was able to see the women. They are among some of the most vulnerable women in our society and are often seen as "expendable, evil, women gone bad, incapable of change" (Singer, Bussey, Sone, & Lunghofer, 1995, p. 103). They are further marginalized within the corrections system because their needs have been overshadowed by the needs of the male inmate population. More than 94% of the corrections population is male (Phillips & Harm, 1998).

Women in the corrections system are predominantly poor, addicted, and survivors of abuse. They have limited education, coexisting mental health disorders, a history of homelessness, and frequently participate in trading sex for money or drugs. These women often have limited access to health care prior to being incarcerated (Fickenscher, Lapidus, Silk-Walker, & Becker, 2001). The victimization experienced by these women has left them wary of others, distrustful, and suspicious.

Jail policies contribute to the frequency with which women are reincarcerated. Upon completing their sentence, women can choose to be released at 12:01 AM on their release date. Many women choose this option and are released to the streets in the middle of the night. The bars are still open, and drug dealers wait in the park one block west of the jail. Buses are not running, and they have no way to get home. Women often report that they want to stay clean, but they don't have anyone picking them up at midnight and find themselves high before they even see their children. If the jail were to release inmates at 6:00 AM, the women would have different options.

The inmates do not have free access to telephones. Making collect calls labels the woman on the phone as being in jail and severely limits resources she can access. Many organizations do not accept collect calls from the jail. The inmates are caught in a bind. Frequently, they need to arrange treatment and housing as a condition of being paroled, but they do not have access to free telephone use to make the arrangements.

Several times during my fieldwork women expressed gratitude for being in jail. One woman with extensive gang tattoos was happy to be on her way to prison because that meant that she had a better chance of not being killed. She reported being targeted because of her tattoos and that no neighborhood was safe for her. On other occasions women reported being grateful because, while in jail, they were not using drugs. They believed that outside of jail they did not have any hope of staying clean and sober, that drugs were just too plentiful in their home environment for them not to use.

Women are further marginalized when they are convicted of a felony, and most drug offenses are felonies. Once convicted the women are ineligible for public housing, Title IV cash assistance, and food stamps (Phillips & Harm, 1998). They cannot get federal student loans for school. There are racial disparities. For example, driving under the influence is a misdemeanor, and those in jail due to DUI were exclusively white middle-class women, whereas those serving time for drug offenses were more often women of color. Although DUIs are life-threatening offenses, the penalties are less severe, and these inmates retain their eligibility for public support and public housing upon leaving jail.

Professional Implications

As a result of fieldwork, I have developed a better understanding of these women and the lengths to which they must go to survive. The behaviors that I witnessed at the beginning of my fieldwork, the confrontations between inmates and conflict between inmates and AA volunteers, are less threatening to me now. Rather than being afraid of the women as I was at the beginning, I now see them as, if not sisters, at least fellow suffering alcoholics and addicts. I have firsthand experience with substance abuse, and viewing the behavior in terms of 12-step programs makes it more understandable and gives me a framework in which to approach these women. I intend to work with substance abusers, and I gained understanding of the unique needs of incarcerated women.

REFERENCES

Abraham, L. K. (1993). *Mama might be better off dead: The failure of healthcare in America.* Chicago, IL: University of Chicago.

American Psychiatric Association. (1994). *Diagnostic and statistical manual of mental disorders* (4th ed.). Washington, DC: American Psychiatric Association.

Barkley, R. A. (1990). *Attention deficit hyperactivity disorder: A handbook for diagnosis and treatment.* New York, NY: Guilford.

Canales, M. K. (2000). Othering: Towards an understanding of difference. *Advances in Nursing Science, 3*(2), 31–47.

Clatts, M. C. (1993). Poverty, drug use and AIDS: Converging issues in the life stories of women in Harlem. In B. Bair & S. E. Cayleff (Eds.). *Wings of gauze: Women of color and the experience of health and illness* (pp. 328–339). Detroit, MI: Wayne State University.

Felitti, V. J. (2002). The relation between adverse childhood experiences and adult health: Turning gold into lead. *Permanente Journal, 6*(1), 44–51.

Fickenscher, A., Lapidus, J., Silk-Walker, R., & Becker, T. (2001). Women behind bars: Health needs of inmates in a county jail. *Public Health Reports, 116,* 191–196.

Frame, K. (2003). Empowering preadolescents with ADHD: Demons or delights. *Advances in Nursing Science, 26*(2), 131–139.

Goodman, L., Saxe, L., & Harvey, M. (1991). Homelessness as psychological trauma: Broadening perspectives. *American Psychologist, 46,* 1219–1225.

Hartman, T. (1999). Whose order is being disordered by ADHD? *Tikkun, 14*(4), 17–21.

Heine, B. (1997, July). *An introduction to hippotherapy.* Retrieved October 17, 2003, from *http://icanride.org/hippo.html.*

Kendall, J., & Hatton, D. (2002). Racism as a source of health disparity in families with attention deficit hyperactivity disorder. *Advances in Nursing Science, 25*(2), 22–39.

Kendall, J., Hatton, D., Beckett, A., & Leo, M. (2003). Children's accounts of attention-deficit/hyperactivity disorder. *Advances in Nursing Science, 26*(2), 114–130.

Krueger, M., & Kendall, J. (2001). Descriptions of self: An exploratory study of adolescents with ADHD. *Journal of Child and Adolescent Psychiatric Nursing, 14*(2), 61–72.

Phillips, S. D., & Harm, N. J. (1998). Women prisoners: A contextual framework. *Women & Therapy, 20*(4), 1–9.

Schwartz, M. (2000, August 8). *Hippotherapy explained.* Retrieved October 17, 2003, from *http://www.americanequestrian.com/Reference/ref.hippotherapy.htm.*

Singer, M. I., Bussey, J., Sone, L., & Lunghofer, L. (1995). The psychosocial issues of women serving time in jail. *Social Work, 40,* 103–112.

Valle, I. (1994). *Fields of toil.* Pullman, WA: Washington State University.

UNIT VI

POLICY IMPLICATIONS

If a free society cannot help the many who are poor, it cannot save the few who are rich.

John F. Kennedy

Source: Bartleby.com, retrieved 2/27/04.

CHAPTER 44

Literacy and Vulnerability

Toni M. Vezeau

Effective health care requires skills on the part of providers as well as clients. Providers must have a strong knowledge base and successful communication skills that match the needs of their clients. Clients must be able to take in information, make sense of it, apply it to their own situation, and retain the information for future use. These skills are the hallmarks of literacy. Without literacy as a basic client skill, there is little chance that health care interactions will meet intended goals. This chapter presents literacy as a primary driver of vulnerability in health care. The discussion explores the current status of literacy skills in the United States, links to Aday's (2001) Model of Vulnerability, client and provider aspects of the problem, and recommendations for current practice.

WHAT IS THE STATUS OF LITERACY IN THE UNITED STATES?

The National Adult Literacy Survey (NALS), conducted in 1992, defined literacy as the use of printed information to maneuver in society, meet one's goals, and to develop one's knowledge and abilities (Kirsch, Jungeblut, Jenkins, & Kolstad, 1993). Doak, Doak, & Root (2001) modified this definition to include comprehension and retention of verbal and gestural information. The NALS is the largest study on adult literacy in the United States ($n = 26,000$). This study went far beyond establishing the reading grade level of participants and tested their performance in three areas.

- ☐ Prose literacy: the printed word in connected sentences and passages; implies skill in finding information and integrating information from several sections of the text
- ☐ Document literacy: structured prose in arrays of columns and rows, lists, and maps; implies skill in locating information, repeating the search as often as needed, and integrating information
- ☐ Quantitative literacy: information displayed in graphs and in numerical form; in addition to locating information, this skill implies that one can infer and apply the needed arithmetic

Participants were tested on a variety of tasks encountered at work, such as signing a mock Social Security card and filling out personal information on a simple job application.

The NALS data suggest that one quarter to one third of American adults are functionally illiterate, and approximately an equal number have marginal literacy skills that disallow full

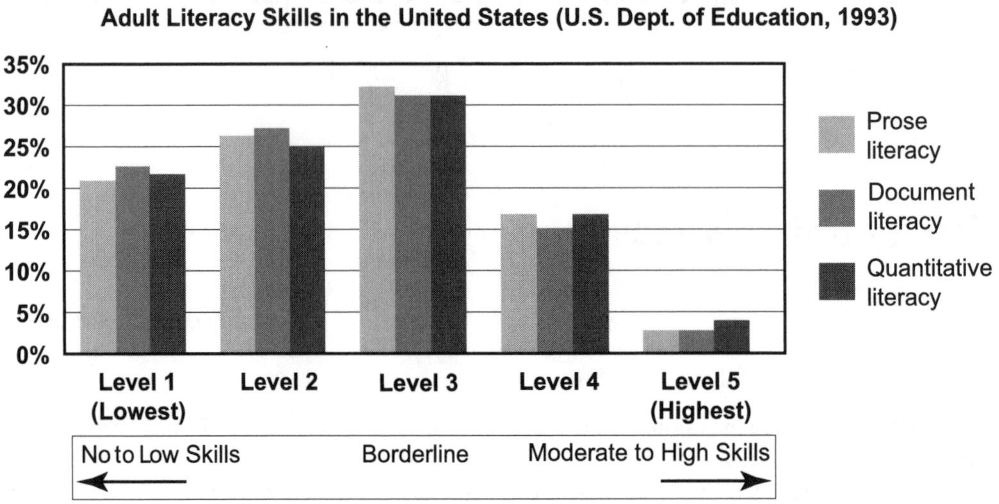

Adult Literacy Skills in the United States (U.S. Dept. of Education, 1993)

FIGURE 44.1   Adult Literacy Skills in the United States

Adapted from U.S. Department of Education, Office of Educational Research and Improvement, National Center for Educational Statistics, 1993.

functioning in society. Essentially, half of the adult population in the United States has poor to nonexistent skills in reading, listening, and computation (see Figure 44.1). The NALS survey also revealed that 5% are learning disabled and 15% speak English as a second language, if at all. However, the majority of study participants were white and born in America. Although education correlated with literacy, generally those adults who had a 10th grade education read at the 7th to 8th grade level. Participants receiving Medicaid had an average of a 5th grade reading level. One third of the NALS sample demonstrated basic functionality in understanding and using written information. Only 20% of the sample demonstrated proficiency in handling information to perform complex reading and computation tasks.

The NALS data suggest that certain groups fair much worse in their literacy skills (subfunctional) than the general population. Of those adults who tested at the lowest reading level, 41–44% were poor, 33% were over age 65 years, 25% were immigrants, 62% did not finish high school (disproportionately represented by minority groups), 12% had physical, mental, or health conditions that prevented working and schooling, and 75% of this group had a mental health problem. Participants at the lowest literacy level had difficulty performing the usual tasks of daily living that are based on printed information and in performing complex tasks requiring following directions and computation. Interestingly, the group considered to have no or minimal functional literacy did not acknowledge themselves as vulnerable, related to their illiteracy. This group noted that they could read "adequately to very well," and less than 25% of these participants stated that they received help with information from family and friends. Could it be true that persons with low literacy are not vulnerable in American society?

WHAT IS THE RELATIONSHIP BETWEEN LITERACY AND HEALTH VULNERABILITY?

Kirsh et al. (1993) discussed literacy as currency in the United States because those with less literacy are much less likely to meet the needs of daily living and pursue life goals. It is likely, then, that illiteracy can create health risks and exacerbate existing health conditions.

Literacy as a Predictor of Vulnerability

Aday's (2001) Model of Vulnerability and Health posits that, while all humans are vulnerable to illness, segments of the community are much more vulnerable to ill health in terms of initial susceptibility and in their response to health problems. Illiteracy is related to each of Aday's (2001) predictors of vulnerability. Persons with poor reading skills who are unable to perform basic literacy functions, such as reading a bus schedule or following directions in completing a task, generally have low social status outside of their immediate social ties. Social status has been correlated with poor health (Duncan, Daly, McDonough, & Williams, 2002) in that those persons with low status are more likely to use disproportionately more health care services for a wider range of ailments, receive substandard care and less information about their illness, and be presented with fewer options. Similarly, the NALS data are congruent with Aday's third driver of vulnerability, lack of social capital, in that persons who are illiterate are more likely to be single or divorced, live in single-parent homes, and be only loosely connected within their own communities.

Additionally, Aday addresses the relationship of vulnerability to health care access, cost of care, and quality of care. Accessing care most often requires complex language skills for tasks such as identifying and evaluating possible providers of care. Clients must negotiate appropriate entry points into the system, contact and communicate their needs to obtain an appointment, locate and travel to the provider, interpret written materials, and use clock and calendar skills. Access to care is seriously challenged when clients have poor literacy skills.

Consequences of Vulnerability

Quality of Care

Literature of the last decade has documented well how illiteracy has affected the cost of care and the quality of care (Baker et al., 2002; Institute of Medicine [IOM], 2003). Literacy (and illiteracy) is a significant component of client adherence to care regimens and of the number of hospitalizations in numerous health contexts: pregnancy, diabetes, AIDS, asthma, sexually transmitted diseases, women's health, mental health, advanced age, cardiac surgery, rheumatoid arthritis, and prostate cancer. Payer status and status as a rural resident or immigrant is also affected by literacy. Without exception, the populations just cited have a high prevalence of illiteracy in proportions that mirror NALS data. These studies noted that persons with literacy problems did not understand instructions and demonstrated less comprehension of their illness or condition.

Costs

Healthy People 2010 (US Department of Health and Human Services, 2000) notes that the consequences of illiteracy are poorer health outcomes and increased health care costs, as much as four times greater for those clients who read at or below the 2nd-grade level than for the general populace. Baker et al. (2002) reported that clients with documented low literacy had a 52% higher risk of hospital admission compared with those having functional literacy, even after controlling for age, social and economic factors, and self-reported health. Client illiteracy was the highest predictor of poor asthma knowledge and ineffective use of metered-dose inhalers (Williams, Baker, Honig, Lee, & Nowlan, 1998).

Acknowledging the pervasive influence of illiteracy on the quality of care in the United States, the IOM has identified literacy as one of the top three areas that cut across all other priorities for improvement in our nation's health. The IOM states that literacy is required for self-management and collaborative care, the other two priority crosscutting areas.

Redefining Literacy

Since the mid-1990s, the medical literature has used a new term, "health literacy," to address the literacy problem. The Ad Hoc Committee on Health Literacy for the Council on Scientific Affairs of the American Medical Association (AMA) defined an individual's functional health literacy as "the ability to read and comprehend prescription bottles, appointment slips, and other essential health-related materials required to successfully function as a patient" (AMA, 1999). The National Health Education Standards added to this the understanding of basic health information and the ability to effectively handle the health care system and understand consent forms (Williams, 2000). Health literacy has now become the preferred term for this intersection of health concerns and literacy skills. Williams is articulate in describing the complexity of this dilemma that requires listening, analytical, decision-making, computation, and application skills.

International health care work has addressed health literacy in the terms above for a much longer time, from the 1960s on. Interestingly, the issues discussed in international literature correspond well to current Western health literature. Watters (2003) summarizes well the health care implications of no or low literacy in international work: increased use of the health system and increased cost, late entry into care secondary to poor interpretation of symptoms, poor participation in preventive care, shame over literacy status (which affects self-identification of literacy needs to care providers), medication errors related to literacy errors, and inconsistent shows at appointments. Each of these health concerns related to literacy has been documented in the United States (AMA, 1999; Baker, 1999).

In summary, research has supported Aday's theoretical work on health vulnerability. It is clear that literacy strongly influences the health of individuals and populations. The problems with literacy, however, are jointly owned and created by clients and providers. It is important to understand the specific literacy problems of clients and how providers have contributed to these problems.

How Does Illiteracy Specifically Increase Health Risk of Clients?

Clients with no or low literacy cannot read or interpret pamphlets, directions on prescribed or over-the-counter medications, or diet instructions. A mismatch of vocabulary and skill is just one of the problems. Lack of comprehension of graphics and pictures poses additional and, for many clients, insurmountable challenges (Doak et al., 2001). Literacy has many components, such as decoding, comprehension, and retention of information, and it is not a free-standing skill. It requires integration of related life skills to navigate the health care system, effectively perform self-care, and make health care decisions.

Components of Literacy

Reading involves a synthesis of both language and thinking skills. These skills include decoding words, literal comprehension, and the use of logic, inference, and critical thinking.

Decoding

Text and oral language require decoding—the identification of the meaning of clustered letters or sounds. The skill is complex, requiring the word to be in the client's vocabulary and for the client to have had previous exposure to the word in meaningful situations. Simple variations in such things as type size or font can impair this decoding process. Poor readers generally decode one word at a time, and they often have great difficulty putting words together (Doak et al., 2001). This difficulty disallows extraction of meaning from a sentence or group of sentences. Effective decoding skills in good readers are often displayed by categorical thinking; poor readers have difficulty recognizing categories and understanding category labels. Listings of care providers by specialty in a telephone book or on a sign, even if the words themselves can be decoded individually, challenge the poor reader. Often the groupings are not meaningful. Poor readers skip over large or unfamiliar words. Instructional client literature is rife with commonly skipped words such as "avoid," a hard word for poor readers to decode, or uncommon words such as "grapefruit" or "pharmacy." The inability to decode language effectively creates risk for clients with literacy problems. They find it difficult to understand instructions or explanations, even if they are written or stated in simple language.

Clients at the most risk for problems with decoding, obviously, are those who speak English as a second language or who do not speak English at all. Census 2000 data found that almost 250,000 people living in the United States spoke no English at home, and one in five households preferentially spoke a second language in addition to English (US Census Bureau, 2000a). The national press release stated that "55% of the people who spoke a language other than English at home also reported they spoke English 'very well.' Combined with those who spoke only English at home, 92% of the population age 5 and over had no difficulty speaking English" (US Census Bureau, 2000b). The NALS data is consistent with the supposition that clients who demonstrate literacy skills that are less than functional do not perceive themselves to be at risk (Kirsch et al., 1999).

Comprehension

Once words are broken down and identified, comprehension is a separate and complex task. Comprehension requires that the message be logical to the receiver and that it be written in recognizable language; also, the receiver must have previous experience with the concepts communicated. For example, a pamphlet addressing the importance of the use of prophylactics when having intercourse with strangers may not be understood by those with no or low literacy. Many clients may be unfamiliar with the words or lack previous experience seeing, using, or hearing about others' use of condoms.

Poor readers may miss an implicit health message ("take before surgery" or "take when playing sports") and be unable to infer from factual data. Pamphlets and brochures often rely on the graphical representation of information that would generally be misunderstood by clients with no or minimal literacy (Doak et al., 2001). Often, information is taken literally. Directions to clients to "push fluids" on children, not eat a specific food, or to take medications by a certain route are often misunderstood. Providers have cared for clients who inserted oral tablets into ear canals or rectums, at times with calamitous consequences. Reading for clients with literacy problems is hard, unpleasant work. Such clients may fatigue quickly and miss subsequent necessary information regarding timing of dosages and the need for follow-up.

Recall

Recall, both short-term and long-term, is another component to literacy. Even if words are accurately decoded and generally understood, recall may be faulty in high-risk illiterate clients. Often providers give instructions in time-compressed and environmentally chaotic situations. Recall entails attention to the message to facilitate the necessary chemical changes that carry messages in the brain and lay down information for storage (Doak et al., 2001). Dry, solely verbal or written information is unlikely to be recalled by clients with literacy problems. Certainly clients already ill, in pain, or having certain mental issues such as depression or attention disorders will have difficulty with recall.

Auditory Mode

The erroneous assumption has been made that if clients cannot read, then they should certainly be able to follow audio- and videotapes, effectively bypassing the literacy issue. There are components to audiovisual education strategies that potentially could assist low-literacy clients: simple language, additional sensory modes of input, increased interest of message, and diversity of voices and examples. Limited research on the effectiveness of such methods with low-literacy clients is promising. However, audio- and videotaping generally ignore the decoding aspects of literacy by using large words and unfamiliar terms. It may be hard for clients to comprehend information that does not relate to their situation directly. Clients do not control the pace of the message, recall aspects due to informational overload (Doak et al., 2001; Hahn & Cella, 2003).

Influence of Illness or Health Conditions on Literacy

Health and health care add unique aspects to the concern for client literacy. Just as literacy skills affect health care, health care can affect literacy skills, temporarily or long-term. Some examples are anesthesia due to surgery, blood loss, and acute pain, any of which may temporarily impair one's decoding, comprehension, and recall skills. Long-term (sustained) medical conditions can often interfere with mentation, cognition, and attention. Delayed mental development, neurological conditions such as Alzheimer's disease, cerebrovascular accidents, and psychological disorders such as depression or anxiety may affect literacy skills and the ability of the client to interact effectively with providers. Understandably, clients who have sensory impairments will likely have literacy difficulty. Visual difficulties were noted in the 20% of the NALS sample who tested at the lowest level of literacy (Kirsch et al., 1993).

Medications may also negatively affect the ability of clients to effectively use their literacy skills, increasing their risk. Drug categories such as opiates, anticonvulsants, antidepressives, glucocorticosteroids, some antihypertensives, and thyroid and ovarian hormones are but a few that regularly affect information processing.

HOW DO HEALTH CARE PROVIDERS INFLUENCE THE LITERACY PROBLEM?

Clients come to providers with their own unique characteristics and abilities related to health literacy. Providers, in their listening, speaking, and written interactions with clients, generally have ignored the literacy variable in care and, in most cases, increased the literacy challenge for their clients (Doak et al., 2001; Hohn, 1998). The literature shows several threads addressing how providers have influenced health literacy: readability of client health education texts, measurement of clients' reading levels in specific health care settings, and client–provider communications.

Readability of Written Educational Materials

It has been documented in the literature since 1988 that the readability of written health care instructions, booklets, and informed consent forms have not matched the skills of clients in a general care population (Root & Stableford, 1999). Health education materials have been tested, but often only a few at a time. Doak et al. evaluated 1234 pieces of health education literature and found that over half were written at or above a 10th grade level. It is important to remember that the education levels of clients do not generally match their reading levels. On testing, reading skills average four to five grades lower than the level of educational attainment. This means that if a client population has a mean of 10th grade education, most education materials in current use would outstrip the clients' skill level (Doak et al., 2001) (see Figure 44.2). Studies have found that discharge instructions and client education materials are written well above a 9th grade level of difficulty (Gannon & Hildebrandt, 2002; Hayes, 2000).

Consent forms, contracts, and commonly used self-reporting diagnostic tools are consistently found to be written above a 9th grade reading level. For example, clients who read at a 6th grade level and below did not demonstrate comprehension of 54% of the items on the Beck Depression Inventory; good readers displayed difficulty with a third of the items (Sentell & Ratcliff-Baird, 2003). Similarly, in a study of 1014 adults who completed the Baltimore STD and Behavior Survey, 28% read at or below the 8th grade level; this group showed a high error rate in comprehending survey items. The error rate in item comprehension decreased significantly as the literacy level increased ($p < 0.0001$) (Al-Tayyib, Rogers, Gribble, Villarroel, & Turner, 2002).

Studies investigating the literacy challenge of informed consent forms have consistently rated such forms as being at or above a 12th or 13th grade reading level and have noted that institutional review boards typically do not take the reading difficulty of consent forms into account (Raich, Plomer, & Coyne, 2001). When institutional review boards do, the effect is generally to lower the reading level by one grade (Raich et al., 2001).

Provider–Client Interactions and Communication

Provider interactions with low-literacy clients are just beginning to be studied. Provider-client interactions are influenced by the perceptions of both client and provider. As stated previously in this chapter, the US Census Bureau literacy data and NALS data indicate that persons with low literacy tell others that they read well enough to meet their needs. However, it is important to understand that such clients generally do not self-identify or discuss their literacy status because of the stigma associated with illiteracy (Parikh, Parker, Nurss, Baker, & Williams,

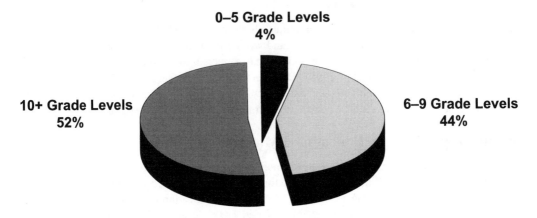

FIGURE 44.2   Readability of Health Education Materials

*Adapted from Doak, Doak, & Root, 2001. Readability levels of 1234 health care materials.

1996). Not only do low-literacy clients not admit to difficulties with literacy to their care providers, they may also hide their need for help from their spouses and families (Parikh et al., 1996).

Stigma and Shame

Stigma is both self-imposed in the form of shame and evident in how providers interact with clients. Baker et al. (1996) interviewed clients who tested as having no to low literacy. These researchers found that their participants held a deep sense of shame, which was reportedly worsened by health care providers who became distressed or irritated when clients had difficulty filling out forms or reading instructions. In many cases these clients avoided seeking care because of such stressful interactions with their care providers.

Myths and Misidentification

Providers generally are not knowledgeable about illiteracy and interact differently with clients who admit to literacy problems. There are a number of common myths held by providers (Doak et al., 2001, p. 6): "Illiterates are dumb and learn slowly if at all," "Most illiterates are poor, immigrants, or minorities," and "Years of schooling are a good measure of literacy level." Research refutes each of these myths (Doak et al, 2001). A person's measurement of intelligence does not correlate strongly with literacy skills; correlation with income level is higher. Years of schooling show the amount of education to which the person was exposed, not the skill level achieved.

Providers may also incorrectly believe that they can identify which clients need extra support related to their literacy needs. Bass, Wilson, Griffith, & Barne (2002) conducted a study to see if medical residents could correctly identify those with low literacy out of a pool of 182 clients. The residents identified 90% of the clients as having no literacy problem. Of this client group, 36% tested as functionally illiterate. On the other hand, 3 of 182 clients *were* thought to have literacy problems when they did not test as such. This study suggests that providers seriously underestimate the literacy problem in their client groups.

HOW CAN PROVIDERS DECREASE HEALTH RISKS OF ILLITERACY?

The literature reports a variety of approaches to decrease the vulnerability of clients related to illiteracy. Currently, many Web sites developed by private and public agencies exist as clearinghouses to guide clinicians on preferred approaches to working with low-literacy clients.

Identification

Many studies have emphasized a personal approach in discreetly asking about literacy status (Feifer, 2003), but considering the breadth of the literacy problem and the reading demand placed on clients in the United States, a systematic approach to address literacy in a client population is indicated. It is now recommended that literacy should be a measured at baseline as part of routine primary care; this is comparable to the many other baselines obtained in the course of quality health care. A number of tools exist to efficiently screen clients.

☐ The Rapid Estimate of Adult Literacy in Medicine (REALM) is a 2-minute test to measure recognition and the ability to pronounce common health care words (Davis, Long, & Jackson, 1993).

☐ The Test of Functional Health Literacy in Adults (TOFHLA) uses hospital-written materials to test both reading comprehension and basic computational skills. This test takes much longer to administer, from 20 to 25 minutes. A shortened version (S-TOFHLA) has recently been tested and has been found to take about 10–15 minutes to administer.

Davis et al. (1998) provide an excellent discussion on evaluating the pros and cons of multiple screening tools and overcoming obstacles in a primary care setting. Although it takes time and other resources to obtain literacy measures, proper identification of client literacy levels can give clear guidance in effective client education.

For those providers that do not routinely screen, it is important to note that asking blunt questions about reading abilities may not yield accurate responses. As discussed previously, clients with low literacy generally do not disclose their difficulties related to reading. Clients often conceal their literacy problems or may be unaware of their level of difficulty. Schultz (2002) identifies potential indicators of literacy problems: reading text upside down, difficulty orienting to a brochure, making excuses for not reading in front of others (e.g., forgot glasses), mispronouncing words (for English speakers), reluctance to ask questions, missed appointments, difficulty following verbal instructions, relying on family members to fill out forms, and tiring quickly when reading text. When providers identify such client behaviors, it is important for them to explore the issues.

Education Strategies

Low-literacy clients may learn better when information is offered in multiple formats such as audiovisual materials, pictographs, and small group classes (if they are thoughtfully constructed and pretested) (Houts, Wismer, Egeth, Loscalzo, & Zabora, 2001). However, it is important to understand that changing the mode of communication alone does not decrease the literacy demand of the message. The decoding, comprehension, and recall components remain the same. However, if there is careful use of language, appropriate use of pictographs and vignettes, client control over the pacing of the information, and provider follow-up to assess comprehension and to individualize the message, then these strategies can be successful (Houts et al., 2001).

Readability of Written Materials

The readability of written materials can be vastly improved. Both the IOM (2003) and *Healthy People 2010* (US DHHS, 2000) list evidence-based health communication as a high priority item for the improvement of health care. Multiple tools exist to assess the reading level of materials (Doak et al., 2001). SMOG, FOG, Flesch, and Fry and are among the most frequently used readability tools. However, evaluating the reading level demanded in text has encountered much criticism in recent years. The tools just noted evaluate aspects of reading demand such as word familiarity, length of sentences, punctuation, and number of prepositional words. However, recent reports in the literature show that new formulae are being developed that address the many other variables that affect readability. The Singh Readability Assessment Instrument also includes the legibility of the text, the interest level, and the style of writing (Singh, 2003).

The NALS data and the expense and importance of written materials in today's health care environment show the need for testing and evaluating written materials in a systematic fashion prior to their use (IOM, 2003; National Cancer Institute, 2003; US DHHS, 2000).

Improving Literacy Through Health Care

Potential strategies to address illiteracy in health care address how to identify and work with individual clients so that providers' styles of oral and written communication fit with their clients' skill levels. However, these approaches may essentially skirt the core issue of client vulnerability. As reviewed in this chapter, literacy problems themselves create health risks. By using methods that ignore or accommodate the literacy deficit, providers essentially perpetuate the illiteracy problem. This approach, in which providers address the consequences of such core problems as illiteracy, perpetuates the predominant tertiary care focus in our system of health care. Literacy affects the lives of our clients in foundational ways: the creation of social stigma and prejudicial attitudes; ability to navigate within complex systems throughout society, including and beyond health care; housing; and money management. Literacy is a core driver of vulnerability in America and needs to be addressed as a foundational aspect of health.

The literature review presented here found few clinical interventions or recommendations that spoke directly to the need to improve client literacy skills. Miles & Davis (1995) recommended that health care providers partner with neighborhood organizations and schools, in which the opportunity to become literate initially foundered.

International literature has already reported programs in which the development of literacy is in tandem with health care interventions. Watters (2003) presents a fascinating model, integrating linguistics, literacy, nursing, community partnership, and anthropology, that shows potential for use in the United States. Watters reviews the international programs, citing one in Nepal that noted the initially greater cost of a combined maternal nutrition and literacy program compared with the cost of simple administration of vitamin A. However, the combined approach of nutrition and literacy decreased infant and child mortality by one half. Such programs can help the community first gain the needed tools of literacy and subsequently provide long-term health benefits and decreased vulnerability in the community. As Baker (1999) states, in America, this would require a paradigm shift. Rather than compartmentalizing the skills needed to decrease health vulnerability, health care providers could actively work to address core issues that lead to clients' need to access care.

SUMMARY

Functional illiteracy directly creates health vulnerability in clients. Illiteracy is pervasive in client populations, and clinicians cannot rely on education level or self-disclosure to identify those clients with this need. Those clients with the greatest health needs are the same clients who do not have the tools to navigate the complex US health care system. Current provider communication styles and materials greatly mismatch client literacy skills. Solutions addressing this intersection of health care needs and illiteracy have been client focused and micro level. This chapter proposes that providers need to partner with communities to develop literacy skills in their members in order to decrease their health risk. International models may provide examples for trial in the United States.

REFERENCES

Aday, L. A. (2001). *At risk in America: The health and health care needs of vulnerable populations in the United States* (2nd ed.). San Francisco, CA: Jossey-Bass.

Al-Tayyib, A. A., Rogers, S. M., Gribble, J. N., Villarroel, M., & Turner, C. F. (2002). Effect of low medical literacy on health survey measurements. *American Journal of Public Health, 92*(9), 1478–1480.

American Medical Association (AMA). (1999). Health literacy report of the Council on Scientific Affairs. Ad Hoc Committee on Health Literacy for the Council on Scientific Affairs. *Journal of the American Medical Association, 10*(6), 552–557.

Baker, D. W., Parker, R. M., Williams, M. V., Pitkin, K., Parikh, N. S., Coates, W., et al. (1996). The health care experience of patients with low literacy. *Archives of Family Medicine, 5*(6), 329–334.

Baker, D. W., Gazmararian, J. A., Williams, M. V., Scott, T., Parker, R. M., Green, D., et al. (2002). Functional health literacy and the risk of hospital admission among Medicare managed care enrollees. *American Journal of Public Health, 92*(8), 1278–1283.

Baker, D. (1999). Reading between the lines: Deciphering the connections between literacy and health. *Journal of General Internal Medicine, 14,* 315–317.

Bass, P. F., III, Wilson, J. F., Griffith, C. H., & Barnett, D. R. (2002). Residents' ability to identify patients with low literacy skills. *Academic Medicine, 77*(10), 1039–1041.

Davis, T. C., Long, S. W., & Jackson, R. H. (1993). Rapid estimate of adult literacy in medicine: A shortened screening instrument. *Family Medicine, 25*(6), 391–395.

Doak, C. C., Doak, L. G., & Root, J. H. (2001). *Teaching patients with low literacy skills* (2nd ed.). Philadelphia, PA: Lippincott.

Duncan, G. J., Daly, M. C., McDonough, P., & Williams, D. (2002). Optimal indicators of socioeconomic status for health research. *American Journal of Public Health, 92*(7), 1151–1158.

Feifer, R. (2003). How a few simple words improve a patient's health. *Managed Care Quarterly, 11*(2), 29–31.

Gannon, W., & Hildebrandt, E. (2002). A winning combination: Women, literacy, and participation in health care. *Health Care of Women International, 23*(6–7), 754–760.

Hahn, E. A., & Cella, D. (2003). Health outcomes assessment in vulnerable populations: Measurement challenges and recommendations. *Archives of Physical Medicine and Rehabilitation, 84*(4Suppl2), S35–S42.

Hohn, M. National Institute for Literacy Fellowship. (1998). *Empowerment health education in adult literature: Guide for public health and literacy practitioners, policy makers, and funders.* Retrieved 12/5/03, from *http://www.nifl.gov/nifl/fellowship/reports/hohn/HOHN.htm.*

Houts, P. S., Wismer, J. T., Egeth, H. E., Loscalzo, M. J., & Zabora, J. R. (2001). Using pictographs to enhance recall of spoken medical instruction. *Patient Education and Counseling, 43*(3), 231–242.

Institute of Medicine [IOM]. National Academy of Sciences. (2003). *Priority areas for national action: Transforming health care quality.* Washington, DC: National Academy of Sciences.

Kirsch, I. S., Jungeblut, A., Jenkins, L., & Kolstad, A. (1993). *Executive summary of adult literacy in America: A first look at the results of the National Adult Literacy Survey.* Retrieved December 6, 2003, from *http://nces.ed.gov//naal/resources/execsumm.asp#litskills.*

Miles, S., & Davis, T. (1995). Patients who can't read. Implications for the health care system. *Journal of the American Medical Association, 274*(21), 1677–1682.

National Cancer Institute. (2003). *Clear and simple: Developing effective print materials for low-literate clients.* Retrieved 12/3/03, from *http://www.nci.nih.gov/cancerinformation/clearandsimple.*

Parikh, N., Parker, R., Nurss, J., Baker, D., & Williams, M. V. (1996). Shame and health literacy: The unspoken connection. *Patient Education and Counseling, 27*(1), 33–39.

Raich, P. C., Plomer, K. D., & Coyne, C. A. (2001). Literacy, comprehension, and informed consent in clinical research. *Cancer Investigation, 19*(4), 437–445.

Schultz, M. (2002). Low literacy skills needn't hinder care. *RN, 65*(4), 45–48.

Sentell, T., & Ratcliff-Baird, B. (2003). Literacy and comprehension of Beck Depression Inventory response alternatives. *Community Mental Health Journal, 39*(4), 323–331.

Singh, J. (2003). Research briefs reading grade level and readability of printed cancer education materials. *Oncology Nursing Forum, 30*(5), 867–870.

US Census Bureau (2000a). *Language use, English ability, and linguistic isolation for the population 5 years and over.* Retrieved 12/3/03, from *http://www.census.gov/population/cen2000/phc-t20/ tab01.xls.*

US Census Bureau (2000b). *Nearly 1-in-5 speak a foreign language at home; most also speak English 'very well.'* Retrieved 12/3/03, from *http://www.census.gov/PressRelease/www/releases/archives/census_2000/001406.html.*

US Department of Health and Human Services. (2000). *Healthy people 2010: Understanding and improving health.* Boston, MA: Jones and Bartlett.

Watters, E. K. (2003). Literacy for health: An interdisciplinary model. *Journal of Transcultural Nursing, 14*(1), 48–54.

Williams, M., Baker, D., Honig, E., Lee, T., & Nowlan, A. (1998). Inadequate literacy as a barrier to asthma knowledge and self-care. *Chest, 114,* 1008–1015.

Williams, M. V. (2000). Definition of health literacy. Message posted to National Institute for Literacy list server. Retrieved December 7, 2003, from *http://www.nifl.gov/nifl-health/2000/0439.html.*

CHAPTER 45

Medically Disenfranchised: Workers Without Health Insurance

Mari Van Court

According to the Cambridge Advanced Learner's Dictionary, disenfranchisement is "taking away power or opportunities from a person or group." Medically disenfranchised workers are those without health insurance coverage either as a result of working for an employer who does not offer health insurance benefits or as a result of the premium cost of offered insurance being more than they can afford. As a result they do not have the opportunity to access medical services that others with health insurance are granted. This study seeks to analyze this situation for such workers in terms of what they say about their experience.

I have long had a casual interest in this topic. Three recent events, however, served to catalyze casual interest into a call to action. As a registered nurse working at a local urgent care center, I took care of a 24-month-old with severe sinus and ear infections and bilateral ruptured tympanic membranes. The parents reported that the child had been sick with fevers for over a week and had green drainage from both ears for 5 days. They reported that the child alternated between crying and screaming and extended periods of sleep. Initially angered about their apparent lack of caring for this child, I inquired why they had waited so long before seeking treatment. They responded that they "did not have medical insurance, and the clinic required a cash deposit of $54.00 prior to being seen." The father had to wait until his next paycheck before they had the money to have the child seen.

The second event involved a young married couple who experienced a miscarriage that resulted in a hemorrhage and surgery. The medical bills for this event totaled more than $8,000. Both the husband and wife had full-time jobs; however, neither of their employers offered health insurance. Their combined monthly income just covered their bare sustenance needs. Because their combined wages were $85 higher than 200% of the federal poverty limit, they were ineligible for any state or charity assistance. Without health insurance or charity assistance, they were responsible for the total bill for services without the benefit of the write-offs and discounts available to those with health insurance. Subsequently, the majority of the hospital bill was turned over to a collections agency, resulting in a further deterioration of their financial situation.

I myself then experienced an unexpected surgical event. Medical bills totaled more than $75,000. Fortunately, I had employer-sponsored health insurance, which covered most of the expenses, leaving my family to pay approximately $400 out of pocket. Interestingly, however, the insurance company only paid out $35,000, leaving over $40,000 to disappear in "write-offs" and "negotiated savings," euphemisms for steep discounts offered to insurance companies in exchange for preferred provider arrangements. After receiving the final bill, I called the patient accounts department at the hospital where I had surgery to inquire what portion of the bill I would have been responsible for had I not had insurance. I was assured that I would have been responsible for the entire $75,000 bill and would have been sent to collections if I could not pay.

Together these three incidents were motivation to investigate the issue of workers without health insurance, to examine the practices behind these incidents, to understand the health consequences of lack of health insurance, and, most importantly, to elicit some workers' stories so that the voices of this vulnerable population can serve as a catalyst for change.

LITERATURE REVIEW

A comprehensive literature review was conducted to assess what is known about the status of workers in the United States and, in particular, those in the state of Washington who do not have health insurance. The facts are sobering and depict a broken health care system. The literature review results are presented in two parts: the first is a discussion of the prevalence and epidemiological impact of workers without health insurance, and the second is a review of the important components and relevant payment structures of our existing health care system. Aside from anecdotal stories in the lay press (Song, 2003), I found no evidence of research studies on how living without medical insurance affects the workers themselves.

Prevalence

US Census Bureau data indicate that 15.2% of the population, or 43.6 million people, were uninsured throughout 2002. This number had increased significantly over the preceding few years, with 40.9 million without insurance in 1999 and 41.2 million without insurance in 2001 (Reilly, 2003). Twenty percent (one in five) of those who are uninsured reside in rural areas. In the state of Washington, 13% of the population is without health insurance (Kaiser Family Foundation, 2003). The major reasons for not having insurance, in order of frequency, are 1) it is not offered, 2) the worker is self-employed, 3) the worker is ineligible, or 4) the worker declines it.

An important trend in the rate of uninsured Americans is the deterioration of employer-provided health coverage, the primary source of insurance for nearly two of three Americans (Kuttner, 1999). According to the National Federation of Independent Business, in 1993, 65% of employers provided insurance; today only 47% provide coverage (Guppy, 2003). Aday (1993) stated that "the majority of uninsured are in households with either full- or part-time workers." Of the number of uninsured nationwide, 75% work part-time jobs of at least 20 hours per week (Kaiser Family Foundation, 2003). In Washington State, only 52% of all employers offer medical insurance to their workers. The number of workers without health insurance is approximately 12% (Kaiser Family Foundation, 2003). Only one participant in my study had employer-sponsored insurance, and he had declined it. When interviewed he stated that if he was to take advantage of the company-offered insurance, insurance payments, deductibles, and copayments would represent 25% of his annual income. "We simply could not afford it and rely instead on our youth, hoping to forestall health-related concerns." A study by the accounting firm, KMPG Peat Marwick confirmed his assessment, finding that the high cost of health insurance relative to income is the primary reason that people forgo insurance. The estimated cost of participating in employer-sponsored insurance is 26 to 40% of total income for a family of four (Kuttner, 1999).

Epidemiology

The Institute of Medicine defines access to health care as the timely use of personal health services to achieve the best possible outcomes (Millman, 1993). These include the ability to use preventive services, manage acute and chronic conditions, and to pay for emergent conditions. Several studies cite findings that strongly associate the lack of insurance and the resulting inability to obtain services with adverse health outcomes (Andrulis, 1998). Poverty is associated with lack of health insurance, and extensive research documents that many uninsured individuals face major obstacles to care because of their inability to pay (Billings, Anderson, & Newman, 1996). Compared with those who are insured, the poor and uninsured are less likely to have a primary source of care and receive fewer services after contact with a provider (Broyles, Narine, & Brandt, 2000). A New York study found that those without insurance were more likely to receive fewer health services for medical injury, underwent fewer procedures, and had shorter hospital stays than insured persons (Burstin, Lipsitz, & Brennan 1992).

A countering argument that the uninsured are simply healthier and less in need of care is not consistent with the evidence (Moreno & Hoag, 2001). The findings of Moreno and Hoag can be found in a brief review of studies from across the nation that document disparities in care among the uninsured (Abraham, 1993; Gorey, 1999; Millman, 1993.) More importantly, the literature suggests that those without medical insurance have higher rates of morbidity and mortality. Another study compiling data from across the nation demonstrated that a lack of insurance is associated with higher rates of adverse health consequences, including late diagnosis, poorer prognosis, and less aggressive treatment as measured by deaths and longer hospital stays (Reilly, 2003). Andrulis (1998) of the New York Academy of Medicine, stated that "persons without insurance had a greater likelihood of dying." Broyels, Narine, & Brandt (2000) emphasized that the uninsured remain systematically at risk for poor-quality care.

HEALTH CARE SYSTEM

The current health care system in the United States seems to contribute to the vulnerability of the medically disenfranchised. Our system is characterized by a disjointed delivery system, a multifaceted approach to funding strategies, and a historic free market approach that sees government intervention in health care as inefficient and unnecessary.

Disjointed Delivery Structures

In the United States, the belief that there is uniform access to health care is a myth. Delivery systems are disjointed and range from communities with no services available to communities with a full ranges of services available. Patients may have access to free or reduced care at community clinics or through care provided by nurse practitioners. If the patient then needs hospitalization, for example, community-based health providers are often unable to get the uninsured patient admitted for care at for-profit institutions because there may not be agreements in place to offer reduced prices or fees for those services. Additionally, many hospitals deny admitting privileges to nurse practitioners, so patients who get care from these providers must then find others providers to care for them in the event of hospitalization. Access to specialty services may also be compromised when there are no networks established to provide that care at reduced prices. These system breakdowns result in a fractured continuum of care for patients, leaving patients and providers at risk, forced to accept patchwork care at the time of need (Gusmano, Fairbrother, & Park, 2002).

Free Market Approach to Funding

The free market approach to health coverage is a leading contributor to the number of Americans without health insurance at this time (Millman, 1993). The free market is an economic strategy that essentially allows supply and demand to drive fees and prices for goods and services, all without government intervention. Providers are allowed to charge whatever the market will bear for services.

Within the free market, health care delivery systems rely on four major sources of payment: public programs such as Medicare and Medicaid, government-owned health care systems such as the Veterans Administration or the Indian Health Service, third-party insurance reimbursement through either employer-sponsored insurance or private insurance, and private pay, individuals who are billed directly for their service usage. Historically, the cost of services was shifted among various payers, with some payers paying a higher overall cost of services than others. This resulted in huge geographical difference in prices and overall inflation.

Most organizations have charges defining the price for services rendered. With the exception of private-pay patients, however, no one pays the listed charges. Third-party payers can negotiate steep discounts through volume guarantees, and federal programs simply tell organizations what they will pay. The Community Catalyst Organization put it quite succinctly when they stated, "list prices have been described as marketing fiction designed to allow an organization to offer substantial discounts. Virtually no one pays [listed] charges except people who have no insurance" (Reilly, 2003, p. 30). Despite the common belief that, because of Medicare rules (Centers for Medicare and Medicaid Services, 2003), organizations are prevented from discounting fees, organizations are allowed to waive or reduce fees based on a person's income. Fees can be reduced if the organization has policies that state eligibility and apply criteria equally (Reilly, 2003). For the uninsured, organizational failure to adopt policies results in charges that can be as high as 60% greater than those paid by the insured (Japsen, 2003).

Despite a belief in free market approaches, numerous government attempts to control costs were employed. Toward the end of the 1990s, health care costs were out of control. Previous attempts at control had been perceived, rightly or wrongly, as being "arbitrary, inconsistent, and confusing" (C. Barnes, 2003, personal communication, Dec. 1, 2003) for providers, purchasers, and patients. Now costs are again escalating; there is no room for further cost shifting.

Demand for Universal Health Coverage

In the United States, there has historically been strong suspicion and/or rejection of a government role in what is perceived as individual private choice. Poverty and its associated lack of insurance are all too often seen as representative of individual choices. Clearly, with the uninsured representing only a small portion of the populace (15%), government efforts to mandate universal coverage will fail. Blumenthal (1999, p. 3) of Massachusetts General Hospital explains that "for a great majority of Americans, day-to-day access to healthcare may be confusing, inconvenient, or unpredictable but not personally intolerable. To cause Americans to reject market-based approaches in favor of universal health coverage and comprehensive health care reform, the problems of access would have to grow dramatically worse than they are."

A reporter for *U.S.News & World Report* agrees. Healy (2003) states that "the problems of the uninsured is [sic] partly tied to the fact that the insured are insulated from what they are spending for health care. Most [insured] people don't have a clue to what they are paying for and don't much care" (p. 72).

Impact of System Issues

The impact of health care funding strategies unfairly places disproportionate overall costs on uninsured persons (Kuttner, 1999). This leads to an increased load of medical debt, which, in turn, adversely affects a worker's health and finances (O'Toole, 2003). For the uninsured, debt or fear of debt leads to delays in seeking medical care, and this contributes to a higher degree of health risk (Andrulis, Duchon, Pryor, & Goodman, 2003). It is well documented that medical debt is devastating to families and results in ruined credit ratings, liens, foreclosures, seizures of bank accounts, and bankruptcy.

Free market strategies, too, have an adverse impact on the uninsured. Current levels of funding for public programs provide only minimal reimbursement to service providers. Cost shifting to the noninsured is the only alternative for recouping program costs. According to one study, less than 40% of physicians surveyed provide reduced fees for uninsured patients; most practitioners require full payment at the time of service. On the other hand, health systems and hospitals are less likely to accept uninsured patients (Saha & Bindman, 2001). In the meantime, uninsured people continue to face a slow erosion of health insurance coverage, a patchwork of programs, decreased access, and a higher, disproportionate share of health care costs (Kuttner, 1999). The reliance on market competition for health care reform is a political and economic experiment that is resulting in disastrous dislocations throughout society (Steen, 2003).

METHODOLOGY

After securing institutional review board approval, I selected four individuals and one couple for interviews. Participants ranged in age from 19 to over 40 years, with 4 women and 2 men. They were employed in construction (2), health care (2), the service industry (1), and education (1). One had employer-offered insurance, and five did not. I stopped seeking potential interview candidates after I had reached data saturation, i.e., when the same themes began to be repeated in each interview. Persons selected for interview were recruited through the snowballing technique. In each case, the person was screened according to the project selection criteria and interviewed after obtaining signed consent. Questions asked of every participant included the following.

- ☐ Give me an example of an experience you have had related to medical insurance.
- ☐ How do you decide how much of your income should go toward insurance?
- ☐ When you or your family needs medical care, what do you see as all of your available choices?
- ☐ Is there anything else that you would like to add?

Clarifying questions emerged as a result of the interview process. A data collection tool developed by de Chesnay (2003) was used to record field notes during the interviews. Following the interviews, data were sorted into themes that had emerged. These themes were then used as the basis for documenting the statements of the interviewees.

RESULTS

Following the often poignant interviews, three themes were consistently identified. First, the interviewees expressed a great deal of frustration with the current system of health care delivery. Second, fear regarding their current health status and fear about future health was voiced. Finally, they all shared a sense of what can only be called double jeopardy; i.e., being vulnerable in multiple arenas attributable somewhat to their lack of health insurance. One other important theme, a sense of shame, was discussed by a few contributors; however, this was not echoed across all interviewees.

Frustration

Many participants expressed their sense of frustration with the health care system. This frustration centered on three issues: access to services, affordability of services, and access to programs that provide health-related services for free or reduced prices.

Access to Services

Despite the popularity of television shows with medical themes and the plethora of services marketed in local media, many uninsured simply do not know where or how to access primary care services. These programs and advertisements "only demonstrate the gap between what others have access to that I don't," said one participant. Among the responses given when interviewees were asked how they make decisions about where to go for care when it is needed were "I guess that I would go wherever the paramedics told me I had to go," "I suppose that I would go to the emergency room at the local hospital," "Well, I hope that if I get hurt or something that it happens at work because then at least it would be covered," and, simply, "I don't know." Another person said that she would go back to the clinic where she had care prior to losing her insurance, but she was not sure they would see her without insurance.

Research supports this lack of understanding about where to access primary care services. According to an Alabama study that surveyed uninsured persons to find out what they knew about services available to them, 90% of respondents said they were unaware of available community services (Reach Out of Montgomery County, 2003).

Many of my study participants related that, although they were aware of community services, these services were not available at times they could use. Most are offered Monday through Friday during business hours. Many interviewees had jobs with hours that extended beyond traditional hours, worked two jobs in order to make ends meet, or did not get paid time off to access services. As a result, they had to access higher-cost services at hospital emergency rooms when the need arose.

Affordability of Services

Having health insurance greatly affects access to services. An estimated one third of uninsured Americans report access problems because of financial barriers, and almost two thirds report delaying care because of financial difficulties (Kaiser Commission, 1998). Numerous literature sources and research studies have documented adverse consequences associated with lack of insurance, such as individuals not seeking care when they should, failing to fill prescriptions, using emergency departments for care, and not following medical recommendations. Without exception, the participants in my interviews did not want or expect free care. What they very clearly wanted was affordable care.

My participants, like those in a study examining medical debt, pointed to specific provider practices that made it harder for them to get care. Some respondents spoke of being asked to pay cash upfront before a health care provider will serve them, often an amount they cannot afford to pay (O'Toole, 2003). One interviewee, although successful in finding services available to her at times convenient to her work schedule, stated that she felt held hostage financially by the clinic. Each concern requiring a doctor's care generated two visits to the clinic, each requiring upfront payment of fees.

> Take my high cholesterol, for example. I go to see the doctor and he takes blood. This costs me $113. Then in order to prescribe Lipitor, he requires that I come back in to review lab work. This visit costs me another $113. He refuses to talk about my blood work on the phone or to prescribe the medicine without another visit. And he only will prescribe for 3 months at a time. So, basically, even though I try to manage my health, I have to pay $226 every three months plus the cost of the medicine. I can't afford it, yet I don't want to die from a heart attack.

When asked how much of their own money should be spent on health care, most said that spending approximately 5 to 15% of their annual income on health care was reasonable. This number is consistent with estimates of the US national gross domestic product (GNP) spending on health care.

Access to Community Programs and Services

When asked about community services that offer free or reduced-price access to primary care providers, most participants were aware of programs, but they did not know how to access them or if they were qualified (because they were employed). One participant simply gave up when applying for a need-based program, stating that there were so many rules, forms, and time lines that she just could not keep up with the requirements for getting to a decision point. Another stated that after multiple attempts to seek help in paying a hospital bill she "had to give up. Besides, they had already sent me to collections at that point." Another stated that although she knew the hospital was required by law to provide care for her in an emergency, she also knew that they didn't have to do so for free. Her concern was how she would pay if forced to. According to a study conducted with the Community Catalyst Tool, hospitals and health care organizations do not routinely inform uninsured patients with low to moderate incomes that free care is available and mandated by their not-for-profit tax status (Reilly, 2003).

Fear

Living without health insurance is not unlike staring at a loaded gun. Anxiety is constant, and deferral of care is a financial necessity (Blomberg, 2003). Fear about the status of their current health and fear for their future health was a particularly poignant theme throughout the interviews. "My brain refuses to acknowledge the lumps in my breast that my fingers feel" is how one woman described her fear. She stated that even with free mammography services available, she didn't have the money to pay for follow-up care. In addition she feared that the fact that she had found a lump in her breast would limit her insurability in the future were her employer to offer insurance. Another participant, after describing her family history of diabetes, stated, "in everything I feel in my body, I just know diabetes is waiting to get me down. I can't afford to get checked because I can't afford to do anything anyway if they find it (diabetes)." Another said, "I know I don't have any real problems now because I am young, but what will I do as I get older? I suppose I'm going to need to see a doctor sooner or later." Another participant talked about how he had to limit his activities due to a fear of getting hurt. He said "I used to rollerblade, bike, and be fairly active outdoors. Now I don't do those things because I can't afford to get hurt. What if I broke my leg or needed surgery? How would I pay for it?" His concerns are not unfounded. The average outpatient cost of a broken leg is estimated at $15,401 (Agency for Healthcare Research and Quality, 2003).

Double Jeopardy

Double jeopardy was another theme that emerged from the interviews. This concept is derived from the fact that all participants voiced concern not only about the immediate effect of possible injury or poor health but the double impact that their poor health would have on their ability to be self-sufficient. Of the subjects interviewed, 100% stated that becoming ill or being injured would adversely affect their income. One said, "I don't get sick because I cannot afford to." In addition to not offering health insurance, their employers did not offer any paid days off for sick leave. Faced with the possibility of being ill or injured, they also faced the possibility of financial ruin. The interviewees went to great lengths to avoid that situation. One participant described how she had broken her foot. She worked as a cook, a job that requires standing for prolonged periods of time each day. When asked what she did about her broken foot, she responded by saying "I worked. There was no way I could get checked for the injury because I didn't have the insurance and there was no way I could take off work because I would not be paid. So I just toughed it out and worked. Mostly it is better now but it wasn't for a long time."

Yet another participant shared that, when faced with unexpected bills for a child's fractures following a bike injury, they had to miss payments on their rent, risking eviction. "When creditors are breathing down your neck you make hard choices over who gets paid each day." Another participant talked about how being sent to collections over a medical bill ruined his credit rating so that when he applied for a loan to purchase a car to replace the one he used to get to work, he was turned down.

Their fears are not unfounded. In Washington State alone, the number of individual bankruptcy cases filed in 2002 was 39,545 (Kaiser Family Foundation, 2003), and research supports the fact that personal bankruptcy due to medical reasons is increasing at an alarming rate all across the United States. One study found that about one third of bankruptcy filers reported substantial medical debt, that health care problems are a factor in half of all consumer bankruptcy filings, and that approximately 20% of those filing for bankruptcy lacked health insurance at the time of filing (Jacoby, Sullivan, & Warren, 2001).

Shame

Another theme voiced by many participants was one of shame tinged with anger. Not one of the participants wanted my pity. They all understood and accepted the responsibility for caring for themselves. They had tried to live the American dream, only to falter in a system that doesn't provide services for those members of society who do service work. One woman said, "I am 45 years old and have worked my entire adult life. I'm ashamed to find myself in this position of having no insurance or ability to provide for my health needs. I followed all the rules, you know the ones, work hard, pay your taxes, get ahead. Somehow, however, the getting ahead never happened. I don't know what happened. I don't know what the future will bring, but I worry about it constantly." Another said, "Who knew how fast those decisions [about career fields] you make as a kid catch up with you? If I had known that I'd be barely able to make it now after working all my life I might have done differently." Another said simply, "it is not supposed to work this way."

DISCUSSION

The forces at play in the American health care decreased access, fewer providers, increased numbers of uninsured, increase in chronic disease, cost containment strategies, and ill-formed policy are leading to the health care system's "perfect storm" (V. Dirksen, CEO Jefferson General Hospital, 2002 personal communication, March 20, 2002). The vulnerable population of the medically disenfranchised will face tighter access, fewer preventive services, decreased immunizations, higher morbidity, and increased mortality.

As a society we rely on the concept of herd immunity; i.e., I am protected [have insurance], so I need not be bothered by other people's situations. This belief is fundamentally flawed. Decreased immunizations among the uninsured, for example, may lead to increased incidence of preventable diseases in the community. Morbidity costs associated with lack of care for chronic conditions will lead to escalated health costs for the rest of us. More employers, facing accelerating health costs, will be forced out of being able to provide health insurance. Fewer employer-sponsored health insurance programs lead to more uninsured, resulting in escalating costs. It becomes a never ending spiral affecting us all.

After listening to what the affected workers had to say, I offer three ideas for contemplation. First, as direct care providers, we must exercise compassionate creativity in caring for our patients; second, we must be imaginative in finding ways to deliver health care so as to not disfranchise whole groups of people; and, finally, we must become advocates of local and national health system change.

Compassionate Creativity

It is easy to jump to conclusions and make assumptions when confronted with patients who do not have health insurance. Why didn't they make better job choices that would allow them to have health insurance? How could they be so irresponsible? After the interviews, the questions are easier to understand. Responsibility, or the lack of it, is not the issue. Without exception, the persons that I interviewed were deeply concerned about meeting their responsibilities, and some experienced a sense of shame associated with their lack of insurance. When viewed from a framework of Maslow's hierarchy of needs, living on poverty-level wages requires everyday choices about spending money for food, shelter, and transportation, leaving little money for the perceived luxury of paying for potential future needs. The burden then falls to providers to supply the appropriate care within the context of their lives and available choices.

In the practice setting, having clients who are uninsured requires the provider to think about their patients' care in terms of more than the disease process. The nurse practitioner has to go through a checklist, evaluating potential recommendations in terms of money.

☐ Can this patient afford a prescription?
☐ What is the likelihood of the patient returning for frequent visits?
☐ What supplies am I asking the patient to buy?
☐ How does lifestyle contribute to what I am seeing?
☐ How will the patient's lifestyle reinforce behaviors I am trying to change?

Nurse practitioners will need to be proactive in advising patients to enroll in programs that offer free or reduced prices for services. In short, the ratio of time spent treating the disease process may be far less than the time devoted to assessing and responding to the system within which they live.

The goals of the *Healthy People 2010* program include health promotion, health protection, and preventive services as means to improve health for Americans and to reduce disparities in care (Addy, 1996). Recent studies confirm that education significantly improves self-reported health and physical functioning over time (Ross & Mirowsky, 2000). Nurse practitioners, with our training that emphasizes health education, are uniquely positioned to provide care that focuses on preventive and educational health efforts and that transitions our patients away from a treat-the-sickness mentality to a focus of health education and prevention (Addy 1996).

Effective Delivery Systems

Sporadic and episodic care is not what most providers identify as appropriate care; however, this may be the only care that uninsured patients can receive. Study findings report these behaviors are not intentional efforts to sabotage health but are rather the result of being unable to afford health care and health insurance (Elliot, Beattie, & Kaitfors, 2000). It is prudent, therefore, that we build imaginative delivery systems that can facilitate the best care at each episodic visit.

With the recent legislative changes for advanced-practice registered nurses (ARNP), we have the opportunity to create new practice models. Recently a group of ARNPs in Indiana set up a practice at their neighborhood grocery store, seeking to be present where their patients are (American Academy of Nurse Practitioners Briefings, 2003). Other provider groups are boycotting any relationships with third-party payers in an attempt to align their fees with the true cost of delivering care. (Often these fees are up to 50% lower than similar peer practices because of decreased overhead associated with processing and collecting third-party fees). These clinics present attractive, affordable options for reduced-price care. Yet to be explored are ideas involving coop-type arrangements whereby patients provide services to the clinic in exchange for portions of their care. Barter-type practices or mobile clinics where "office hours" are held on site in a company lunch room present yet more options.

Regardless of the practice model chosen, we need to build community links so we can provide cost-effective, comprehensive care at the time of each episodic visit. This may entail negotiating partnerships with specialists, community health departments, parish or religious organizations, and tertiary care organizations, perhaps even exchanging services part-time.

Advocacy

The aim of public health is not to make people healthy but to assure the conditions in which people can be healthy (Steen, 2003). All interests in the health care system—patients, providers, public, and private—need to work together to resolve the problems of the system before the entire system collapses (Reilly, 2003). Analysis of the literature documents a trend of increasing empathy for single-payer, universal health care coverage for citizens of the United States. It is projected to be a long battle, however, as most voting constituents are not uninsured and not likely to be immediately affected by the crisis. In the interim, nurse practitioners can be active participants in efforts for change.

In the organization in which the nurse practitioner works, he or she should ask to see the policies that allow for waived or reduced fees for patients. If there are not policies in existence, the nurse practitioner can be instrumental in developing those policies. In the public policy arena, nurse practitioners can help to identify the current deficit of health care access and its immediate effect on the larger community. We need to become familiar with and advocate for complete availability of services for the underserved in our communities. We can and should develop nursing research that demonstrates improved nurse-driven health outcomes related to health education. We need to become public policy advocates, lobbying for change in the health care funding strategies where cost shifting and employer-sponsored health insurance are the norm. We need to advocate legislative changes to allow for innovative, independent practice models, not re-playing the familiar medical model approach to health but advocating instead from the education and prevention model our heritage provides.

Clearly, solving the problems of the medically disenfranchised worker is not going to be a simple process. At the start of the Clinton presidency, health care reform was a priority of the administration. Efforts may have succeeded at that time had it not been for political forces at play. Today there are organizations such as Community Catalyst Inc., leading grass roots efforts to change the system. In the meantime, the numbers of Americans without health insurance continues to expand.

Nurse practitioners need to be part of the solution through whatever means are at their disposal. At every patient interaction, we have the opportunity to provide compassionately creative care and to provide education about healthy self-care. As advanced-practice providers, we have the opportunity to create nursing care clinics that meet the unique needs of patient populations. Both locally and nationally we have the duty to advocate for patients by educating ourselves about the system within which we work and by making efforts for change directed toward eliminating access barriers and changing system infrastructures, such as payment strategies or delivery systems.

I want to leave the reader with a quote from William J. Clinton, former president of the United States, who said, "It is time to honor and reward people who work hard and play by the rules." As health care providers we cannot afford to ignore the issues of this growing uninsured population, many of whom provide the services we use on a daily basis.

REFERENCES

Abraham, L. (1993). *Mama might be better off dead.* Chicago, IL: University of Chicago.

Aday, L. (1993). *At risk in America.* San Francisco, CA: Jossey-Bass.

Addy, J. (1996). Issues of access: What is going on in healthcare? *Nursing Economics, 14*(5), 299–302.

Agency for Healthcare Research and Quality. (2003). *Healthcare cost and utilization project.* Retrieved November 11, 2003, from *http://www.cobracompare.com/uninsured.htm.*

American Academy of Nurse Practioners Briefings. (2003, October 15). Clinic to open in grocery store: Nurse practitioners will provide services, write prescriptions for Fort Wayne shoppers. *Indianapolis Star.*

Andrulis, D. P. (1998). Access to care is the centerpiece in the elimination of socioeconomic disparities in health. [Review]. *Annals of Internal Medicine, 129*(5), 412–416.

Andrulis, D., Duchon, L., Pryor, C., Goodman, N. (2003). *Paying for healthcare when you're uninsured: How much support does the safety net offer?* Boston, MA: The Access Project.

Billings, J., Anderson, G. M., & Newman, L. S. (1996). Recent findings on preventable hospitalizations. *Health Affairs* (Project Hope), *15*(3), 239–249.

Blomberg, M. (2003). Uninsured and vulnerable: Broken system leaves many on the margins of health care. *The Republican,* Springfield, MA, June 30. Retrieved September 30, 2003, from *http://covertheuninsuredweek.org/news/print.php?newsId=369.*

Blumenthal, D. (1999). Health care reform at the close of the 20th century. *New England Journal of Medicine, 340,* 1916–1920.

Broyels, R., Narine, L., & Brandt, E. (2000). Equity concerns with the use of hospital services by the medically vulnerable. *Journal of Health Care for the Poor and Underserved, 11*(3), 343–360.

Burstin, H. R., Lipsitz, S. R., & Brennan, T. A. (1992). Socioeconomic status and risk for substandard medical care. *Journal of the American Medical Association, 268,* 2383–2387.

Centers for Medicare and Medicaid Services (2003). *Medicare provider reimbursement manual* (Part 1, Chapter 3, Section 312). Retrieved October 2003, from *http://www.cms.hhs.gov/manuals/pub151/PUB_15_1.asp.*

Elliot, B., Beattie, K., & Kaitfors, S. (2000). Health needs of people living below poverty. *Family Medicine, 33*(5), 361–366.

Gorey, K. (1999). What is wrong with the U.S. health care system?: It does not effectively exist for one of every five Americans. *Milbank Quarterly, 77*(3).

Guppy, P. (2003, March 9). Let's legalize basic health insurance in state. *Tacoma Weekly,* A4.

Gusmano, M., Fairbrother, G., & Park, H. (2002). Exploring the limits of the safety net: Community health centers and care for the uninsured. *Health Affairs* November/December.

Healy, B. (2003). Our healthcare guilt trip. *U.S. News & World Report, 72*(2).

Jacoby, M., Sullivan, T., & Warren, E. (2001) Rethinking the debates over health care financing: Evidence from the bankruptcy courts. *NYU Law Review, 76,*v 2.

Japsen, B. (2003, January 27). Uninsured pay twice as much. *Chicago Tribune,* p. 1.

Kaiser Commission. (1998). *Uninsured in America: A chart book.* Washington, DC: Kaiser Commission on Medicaid and the Uninsured.

Kaiser Family Foundation. (2003). *The uninsured and their access to health care.* Washington, DC: Kaiser Commission on Medicaid and the Uninsured.

Kuttner, Robert. (1999). The American health care system—health insurance coverage. *New England Journal of Medicine, 340*(2), 163–168.

Millman, M. I. (Ed.). In Institute of Medicine (1993). *Access to health care in America.* Washington DC: National Academy Press.

Moreno, L., & Hoag, S. (2001, January/February). Covering the uninsured through TennCare: Does it make a difference? *Health Affairs,* 231–239.

O'Toole, T. (2003). *The consequences of medical debt: Evidence from three communities.* Boston MA: The Access Project.

Reach Out of Montgomery County. (2003). *Health care barriers and the working poor. Reach out of Montgomery County.* Retrieved September 20, 2003, from *http://www.med.wright.edu/reachout/healthcare.html.*

Reilly, P. (2003). *Not there when you need it: The search for free hospital care.* Boston MA: Community Catalyst.

Ross, C., & Mirowsky, J. (2000). Does medical insurance contribute to socioeconomic differentials in health? *Milbank Quarterly, 78*(2), 291–321.

Saha, S. & Bindman, A. B. (2001). The mirage of available health care for the uninsured. *Journal of General Internal Medicine, 10,* 714–716.

Song, K. M. (2003, April 25). Health-plan cuts will likely sting the working poor. *Seattle Times,* A11.

Steen, J. (2003). *American health policy: The perspective of the American Health Planning Association.* Retrieved November 2, 2003, from *http://www.ahpanet.org/policy.*

CHAPTER 46

Health Care for Some, but Borne on the Backs of the Poor

Beth Furlong

This chapter will discuss the factors in society and in the health care system that cause and/or contribute to people's poverty, their diminished health status, and their lack of access to health care. Examples will be given from both developed and developing countries. This chapter is based on the premise that the poor are "needed" by the middle and upper class groups in order for the latter to enjoy their economic lifestyles. Rather than viewing the poor as a problem in society, this chapter will use the lens of how society and the health care system perpetuate poverty. The chapter will close with proposed solutions that are based on a justice ethic.

CONTRIBUTING FACTORS

These four factors will be discussed in terms of the way they contribute to the causes of poverty, the diminished health status of the poor, and the lack of access to health care. The factors are 1) a life course of cumulative advantage or disadvantage, 2) inequality in social classes and nations, 3) use of language to diminish poor people, and 4) public policies at all levels: local, state, regional, national, and international.

Factor 1: Life Course

The first factor, that of the model of cumulative advantage or disadvantage, has been studied by Crystal & Shea (1990) in a population of the elderly. This model is based on the hypothesis that individuals "who are initially advantaged . . . are more likely to receive a good education, leading to good jobs, leading to better health and better pension coverage, leading to higher savings and better post-retirement benefit income" (p. 437). Their research results demonstrated this hypothesis, even given the benefit of the Social Security program. They found that as people aged, the percentage of inequality among people increased. Although the Social Security program has been an important public policy for providing a base of financial security, postretirement income sources are mainly determined by preretirement economic experiences, which, in turn, result from earlier cumulative advantage factors such as good education, a good job, good benefits, etc.

For example, if one has the ability to purchase a home rather than rent one, this has cumulative economic benefits. Another example is the cumulative advantage from education and the type of job worked, which affects benefits and salary. For example, a teacher may have received health insurance benefits during her lifetime while a construction worker may have had the same salary history, but no health insurance benefits. He may have postponed seeking medical care. Crystal, Shea, & Krishnaswami (1992) summarize this study and others they have done with this finding: "stratification established early in the life course continues at least as sharply in the later years" (pp. S220–S221). However, although Social Security has been an advantage for many, it was not effective for many African Americans. When this legislation was passed in the 1930s, it was because of the power of the southern Democrats who controlled important congressional committees (Albelda, Folbre, & The Center of Popular Ecomonics, 1996). Passage of this bill, which excluded agricultural and domestic workers (most of whom were African American), helped to keep a low-wage workforce in the southern states. "Black exclusion was the price, President Roosevelt believed, of getting the law [Social Security] through Congress" (Albelda, Folbre, & The Center of Popular Ecomonics 1996, p. 108).

Crystal et al. (1992) stress the importance of looking at many factors other than strict salary compensation when studying the life course of individuals and their cumulative advantages/ disadvantages. For example, they note the importance of education. The assets of an educated individual include 1) access to better jobs and higher pay, 2) increased income from these better jobs in the years preceding retirement, which heavily influences postretirement income, 3) better employment security and less health risk, and 4) the ability to work longer because of the fewer risks to health, thereby enhancing the educated individual's ability to save for retirement. Thus all of these aspects have contributed to some individuals' cumulative life advantage. The converse—cumulative disadvantage—is what happens to poor people.

The importance of education to one's life course can also be seen in two other examples. A recent study showed the correlation between level of education, adherence to complex medical regimens, and health outcomes (Study links education, health care, 2002). Those who had a better education had higher adherence levels to complex treatment regimens and therefore had better health outcomes. This study is important in the current health environment because of changes in the health system, such as the move from inpatient to outpatient treatment (with the patient increasingly responsible for care) and the increased complexity in treatment and/or medication regimens. A second example is the societal structure found in many southern states relative to the low tax base and availability of funds to spend on public education (S. Kay, personal correspondence, July 15, 2002; Krieger, 1999). Although southern states complied with civil rights laws and integrated public schools, it can be argued that they undermined this directive by simply not proportionately raising property taxes and also by spending relatively little on public education. Thus, there was a minimal amount of money to allocate to educate African Americans. Because southern states—the ones with relatively high proportions of black residents—had a low tax base and spent relatively less on public education, illiteracy in these states was also high among their white counterparts (Kreiger, 1999, p. 330). Therefore, the results of having received poor or no education in one's early life leads to cumulative lifetime disadvantages. Ehrenreich (2001) reported on current research into poor individuals attempting to make it in the United States today but without success.

Factor 2: Inequalities

A second factor that contributes to poverty and diminished health status, besides the model of cumulative advantage and disadvantage, is the concept of inequality among people within a society and the inequality among countries. Recent publications in both the United States and

Great Britain have addressed these concerns (Marmot & Wilkinson, 2001; Governmental Report: Whites get better quality health care, 2002). There has been extensive professional and lay publicity of these income and health disparities in the United States. The Institute of Medicine's recent report, "Unequal Treatment: Confronting Racial and Ethnic Disparities in Health Care," has raised an alarm within the health sector (Governmental Report: Whites get better quality health care, 2002). A major concern from this study is that even when the variables of insurance status, income, age, and severity of conditions are compared, racial and ethnic minorities still receive lower quality health care. Other examples of inequality are the following statistics: in 1960, chief executive officers (CEOs) made 12 times what the average factory worker made; by 1980, CEOs in the largest companies made 42 times what the average factory worker made; and in 2001, that ratio had changed to CEOs making 411 times the average worker's compensation (Albelda, Folbre, & The Center of Popular Economics, 1996; Goodman, 2002). In Great Britain there has been decreased absolute mortality; however, the mortality disparities have increased: "there is a strong relation between mortality and income inequalities. People living in countries with greater income inequality have a shorter life expectancy . . . a similar relationship has been found for geographical areas within countries" (Marmot & Wilkinson, 2001, p. 1223). These authors postulate the additive effect of psychosocial pathways on the negative health status of poor persons, in addition to the direct negative influence of decreased material living standards. Marmot & Wilkinson discuss the psychosocial effects of relative deprivation, which includes loss of control over life, anxiety, insecurity, depression, and decreased social affiliation in helping to explain decreased health status. Hemingway & Marmot's (1999) review article synthesizes the research studies that demonstrate a correlation between many of these psychosocial effects and coronary heart disease. Many other research studies show the relationship, in animals, of social status, with those experiencing downward mobility showing resultant increased atherosclerosis. To concretize and emphasize the importance that some of the these factors may have, as opposed to strictly the deprivation of material goods, Marmot & Wilkinson (2001) compared the income and life expectancy of African American men in the United States and Costa Rica in 1996. The median income for the former was $26,522 per year, and life expectancy was 66 years. For men in Costa Rica, the income was $6,410, and their life expectancy was 75 years. The authors argued that the discrepancy in life expectancy was due to the psychosocial effects of relative deprivation versus the direct effects of fewer material conditions, i.e., education disadvantage, racism, gender discrimination, social and family disruption, and fear of crime (p. 1235).

Navarro (1999) has written about global inequalities among countries because of the increased globalization of commerce, investments, and finance, which then has direct and indirect effects on all policies including health policy. He argues that individual national governments are increasingly restricted in their ability to set their own national policies because the economy is becoming increasingly internationalized and competitive.

In continuing with the theme of inequalities raised by Marmot & Wilkinson (2001), Navarro (1999) gives the example that the net worth of the world's richest 358 people is equal to the combined income of the poorest 45% of the world's population, i.e., 2.3 billion people (p. 216). Another way of understanding the inequalities is that 20% of people in high-income countries account for 86% of private consumption, and the poorest 28% of the globe consume 1.3% of the world's materials (p. 219). Navarro postulates that the inequalities within countries and among countries are due to these three factors: 1) the unprecedented growth in wealth and income from capital as opposed to labor, 2) the growing polarization of wages with a great increase in wage dispersion, and 3) decreased redistributive effect of the welfare state and the rapid deterioration of public infrastructures (p. 216). Of all countries, those in Latin America are the worst in terms of inequalities among individuals. Navarro raises concerns about globalization and addresses the arguments promoted by international organizations who dismiss globalization as isolationist, xenophobic, and protectionist. Navarro's concern is that such international organizations (whether public, private, nonprofit, governmental, or corporate) wrap their language and arguments in scientific and technical discourse with the belief that their proposals are value free. However, he sees an absence of analysis of power and politics in the policies they propose and how this contributes to poverty and decreased health status and health care for those in poverty.

One example will be given of his analysis of changes—that of the for-profit health insurance sector in Third World countries. He notes that the World Health Organization, the World Bank, the Pan American Health Organization, and US Agency for International Development (AID) "are actively promoting managed care and managed competition in Latin America" and other countries (p. 221). This integrates with the provisions of the General Agreement on Trade in Services agreement. While consulting in Armenia, a newly independent state of the former USSR, this author observed the promotion of private for-profit managed care companies. The inequalities referenced by Navarro were obvious in this country: minimal public health care infrastructure and morbidity and mortality indicators of concern. Yet this aspect of Western health care financing was being promoted for the small cohort of Armenians who might be able to pay for it. Navarro argues, "class relations, and the expression of these relations through the political, economic, and cultural institutions, are at the root of our understanding of current realities" (p. 222). Navarro compares and contrasts developed capitalist countries according to the power of capital and labor. He notes in the 35-year period from 1960 to 1995, the northern European countries, which have had a strong commitment to equity, have scored better on many indicators: greater economic growth, lower unemployment, better health indicators, and fewer inequalities (p. 223).

In other research, Navarro & Shi (2001) studied the impact of political parties in determining the level of equalities or inequalities in a country. They cite the example of the state of Kerala in southern India, which has been extensively studied for the past 40 years, because that state has been noteworthy for a major reduction in inequalities and for the improved health status of its population. As a Peace Corps volunteer serving in the contiguous state of Mysore from 1966 to 1968, I was well aware of Southern Indians frequently discussing the better social indicators of individuals in Kerala State compared with all other states of India. Navarro & Shi (2001) critique the literature because it is rare when writers report on the positive indicators being a result of the public policies implemented by Kerala's governing party, the Indian Communist Party. It is this absence of analysis, or perhaps denial, that Navarro & Shi also alluded to when discussing that many international organizations (WHO, World Bank, U.S. Agency for International Development [AID], corporations, etc.) omit such analysis when they promote globalization. Thus he posits that political parties, as well as the policies they implement, make a difference in determining the equalities or inequalities in a country. He studied major developed capitalist countries from the mid-1940s to 1980 and divided the countries into these three aspects of government: social democratic, Christian democratic, and fascist. The first group of countries (social democratic) has the best indicators: fewer inequalities, more population covered by health care, lower infant mortality rates, etc. He ascribes these indicators to the policies implemented by these political parties. In the Christian democratic countries, poverty in general and in children was greater than in social democratic countries. Furthermore, life courses and cumulative advantages and disadvantages were heavily influenced by gender roles. Caregiving was viewed as a heavier family responsibility, with fewer women employed outside the home than in social democratic countries. Thus, the male breadwinner's income and pension were especially important. Earlier content in this article by Crystal et al. (1992) on the Model of Cumulative Advantage and Disadvantage can easily be applied here by observing what happens to poor people over a lifetime. The greatest inequalities in the European Union occurred in the fascist countries (p. 18). Navarro & Shi (2001) also listed a fourth category of liberal countries, i.e., the United States, Canada, Ireland, and Great Britain. This group of countries consists of the Anglo-Saxon countries where labor has been particularly weak and the capitalist class particularly strong. These countries have been governed for the most part by parties clearly committed to a full expression of market forces, with little interference from the state as possible. (Navarro and Shi, 2001, p. 18). These countries shared the following traits: 1) they had the largest inequalities, and 2) they had low public health care expenditures. Also, the United States and Ireland had the lowest percentage of population covered by health care compared with all of the liberal countries studied. Navarro & Shi argued that the reduction of inequalities is a precondition for economic efficiency and economic growth.

Krieger (1999) also wrote about inequalities and asserted that the research on discrimination as a determinant of population health is just in its infancy. Such research is especially necessary because of the changed focus in the health care delivery system on population health status versus individual health status. Discrimination occurs when people are treated as second-class citizens because of their race, gender, sexuality, disability, and/or age. Krieger applies the model of ecosocial theory, which integrates the relationships among discrimination, inequality, and health. This theory can be summed up as follows: "taken literally the notion of 'embodiment,' this theory asks how we literally incorporate biologically—from conception to death—our social experiences and express this embodiment in population patterns of health, disease and well-being" (p. 296). She posits that the causal components of societal arrangements of power—ownership of property, patterns of production and consumption, the constraints of biology, and ecological history of populations—structure the inequalities in the exposure and susceptibility to pathogenic processes and options for resisting these processes across the life trajectories of populations of people.

Because this chapter is focused on poverty, emphasis will be given to the example Krieger (1999) gives of the embodiment of inequality in health status when the form of discrimination is social class, i.e., there is a socioeconomic gradient in morbidity and mortality with the poor at greatest risk. This is an epidemiographic finding that has been noted for decades. However, Krieger gives examples of how inequalities in health status embody other kinds of discrimination: race, gender, sexuality, disability, and age. She notes that many times people will experience multiple forms of discrimination. For example, I attended a national nursing convention where the speaker spoke to the issue of having three strikes against her: she was black, a woman, and old. Furthermore, when people experience discrimination, it can run the gamut from "everyday" discrimination to particularly horrible life-transforming events. Finally, discrimination can be obvious in an interpersonal manner or invisible and perpetuated via an institutional manner. The value of Krieger's writing is to challenge researchers to study this area because there is a paucity of research on the effect of discrimination on health status. A lack of research may reflect the dominant power structure of the health care system. When attending a hospital seminar

30 years ago on increased hypertension among African Americans, I was struck by the fact that the seminar's only focus was on the physiological aspects and that there was no attention given to societal racism as a causative factor.

Forbes (2000) sees societal structural forces as antecedents of health inequalities. He notes that power relationships and both relative and absolute economic disadvantage contribute to health status. When analyzing the social class differences in the United Kingdom, he notes that the mortality rate in social class I (highest of a V class social class) has decreased 50% in the last 20 years but has only decreased 10% for those in social class V. He also writes that those most in need of health care may not receive it, i.e., "the so-called 'inverse care law'" (p. 610).

Wagstaff (2002) reports that several major international organizations and bilateral donors are now focused on improving the health outcomes of the poor as their primary goal. On a parallel note, the United States is also concerned about this as articulated in one of the three goals of *Healthy People 2000:* to eliminate the disparities. Wagstaff states that there is increasing understanding that the disparities and inequalities are due to widely differing constraints and opportunities as opposed to the more traditional individualistic approach of what may be characterized as "blame the victim." He also agrees that these concerns constitute a social justice concern. He cites some of the same findings that several of the authors mentioned have also found, i.e., people in poor countries have worse health outcomes than people in rich countries, and within countries, there is a gradient according to social class relative to health status. He writes "poverty breeds illness, [and] ill-health maintains poverty" (p. 97).

Factor 3: Language

A third factor that has contributed to the diminished health status of poor people is how society has used language negatively against them. "Many pundits and politicians in this country [the United States] are making careers out of demonizing poor people" (Albelda, Folbre, & The Center of Popular Economics, 1996, p. 8). Numerous authors have written of how language is used against the poor (Albelda, Folbre & The Center of Popular Economics, 1996). The language phenomenon is not new; Carlson (2001) maps out the use of language from biblical times of how the unfit are perceived and classified with derogatory language. Gans (1995) has written extensively of how journalists, policy makers, experts, and others have contributed to the derogation of the poor by their choice of language in writing about the poor, policies affecting the poor, etc. For example, one frequently reads of welfare policies for the poor but less frequently reads of welfare policies for farmers in the form of subsidies and of welfare policies for corporations in the form of "bailouts." In addition to his analysis of the use of language in American society, Gans analyzes the psychological needs of Americans (and others) to "blame the victim" instead of studying the larger context of society and to understand people in that structural perspective. Furthermore, he advocates for programs that educate Americans on not stigmatizing the poor. He sees this as an indirect way to improve the health of the poor.

Factor 4: Public Policy Influence

This paper has included several examples of private and public policy at the local, state, regional, national, and international levels that have an impact on people's lives. Such policies have made differences in people's life courses, have contributed to inequalities within and among groups both nationally and internationally, and have been parts of the language used to derogate and diminish poor people.

Proposed Solutions

"Politics is 'public health in the most profound sense'" (Navarro & Shi, 2001, p. 20). Anyone interested in committing oneself to "the preferential option for the poor," which is advocated by Catholic social teaching, has to be involved in policy making. As noted in this chapter, many past and proposed policies have been harmful to the poor and have facilitated their poverty and diminished health status and lack of access to health care. One's activism in policy making can run the gamut from 1) discussion of issues with family, friends, and colleagues; 2) voting; 3) putting a policy on the agenda or blocking a policy proposal; to 4) being a candidate oneself. One policy implication from the research of Crystal & Shea (1990) on the elderly using the cumulative advantage/disadvantage model is to seriously evaluate the proposed policy of privatization of Social Security (1990). If people are living hand-to-mouth during their working years, it is questionable that they would initiate such savings. It must also be recognized that the current tax policy, which creates incentives for private pensions, salary deferral programs, IRAs, Keogh programs, etc., are, in effect, major tax subsidizations in which poor people do not participate and which contribute to their cumulative disadvantage.

A second policy implication is taken from Crystal et al.'s 1992 research, i.e., the importance of education for poor people. Promotion of state and national policies for public education is imperative. The currency of this issue is noted by debate in the Nebraska Unicameral of how best to meet the current state deficit. State cuts in public postsecondary education have been made. (Unicameral Update, 2002). Cuts in this area can have a negative impact on the life course of many poor Nebraskans.

A third policy implication can be seen from the writing of Marmot & Wilkinson (2001). One needs to recognize the societal structures that perpetuate inequalities in and among countries that lead to health disparities: racism, policies that create educational disadvantages, sexism, classism, and so forth. This is the antithesis of blaming the victim. If policy makers are unable to see and understand all these connections that create and contribute to poverty and diminished health status for people, they may want to follow the easy route and blame individuals for their poverty. The knowledge base of educated people calls us to do better than that.

A fourth policy change stems from Navarro's concern about globalization. As an example, a candidate for the U.S. Congress has raised concerns about the recent passage of a bill that allows President Bush to engage in fast track negotiations to create a North American Free Trade Agreement–style corporate trading zone to include almost all countries in the Western Hemisphere (D. Deichman, personal correspondence, July 29, 2002). Current Congressman Bernie Sanders, an independent from Vermont, has said, "When you have bad policy, why would you want to extend it?" He notes the $346 billion trade deficit of the United States and the erosion of 10% of our country's manufacturing base in the last 4 years. Rep. Sanders raises the question "When will you catch on? When all of our kids are flipping hamburgers?" (D. Deichman, personal correspondence, July 29, 2002). Many representatives have been concerned at the rapidity with which this agreement passed and the manner in which it was done. Because of the rapidity, representatives did not have time to study it well. This is but one example of policy, national in this case, in which global policy has an effect on the life course of individuals. This U.S. national policy that was enacted will have global implications, and especially for those workers in the Western Hemisphere. In the United States, the phrase "flipping hamburgers" is a code word for a low status minimum wage job with no benefits. This kind of job for large cohorts of Americans can result in cumulative disadvantage over a lifetime and be a contributing factor to poverty.

A fifth action step stemming from Navarro's research is the importance of studying power relationships and the effects of class, gender, and race domination and exploitation as it affects inequalities within and among countries. His research provides the global context to help one understand many factors contributing to poverty and decreased health status and health care. He advocates for such research as "we owe it to the millions of people who do not have health and remain voiceless . . ." (p. 225).

A sixth policy strategy is to be knowledgeable of public policy: how issues get on the formal and informal agendas, who has the power in affecting agendas, the importance of action via coalitions, and so forth. There are many current examples in the United States that reflect negative economic conditions and negative stereotypes of the poor. At the national level, President Bush has criticized the Senate welfare bill (President criticizes Senate Welfare bill, 2002). For example, one could analyze his criticisms (not appropriating as much money as requested to promote marriage, giving too much money for child care, and providing educational opportunities) as putting forth constraints on the realistic ability of people on welfare to transition to a working nonpoverty life course. Because of this proposed legislation, many poor people may experience the lived experience of cumulative life disadvantages described by the research of Crystal & Shea (1990). At the state level, governments (because of state constitutions that mandate balanced budgets) implemented Special Sessions during Summer 2002 to problem solve budget deficits (Lutey, 2002; Reed, 2002). Although both Montana and Nebraska proposed cutting funding to education, a larger concern in Nebraska was the proposed cuts to Medicaid (Kaiser Network, 2002). Nineteen thousand individuals have been dropped from the Medicaid program in Nebraska (Legislature passes Medicaid changes, 2002). This is an exemplar case of needed budget cuts affecting the most vulnerable, and again, negatively affecting their life course and cumulative disadvantage.

An educational strategy for health science students and practicing health professionals is to teach the impact of poverty on people's health status and to determine their role in moving societies to reduce poverty. Some believe reduction of poverty may be the more important strategy in reducing the burden of illness. When teaching students, I believe the more appropriate way to teach the epidemiographic aspects of disease is from a social class perspective rather than from that of a specific illness. A resource for educators to use is the Poverty Coalition (J. G. Chamberlin, personal communication, August 5, 2002). This is a group of multidisciplinary educators from universities across the United States who are interested in better educating students on the issues and problem-solving strategies of poverty.

A communicative strategy to decrease poverty is to be critically aware of language used by oneself and by others and to be sure that such language does not condemn the poor. Although it is beyond the scope of this chapter to expand on this area, I believe this to be an extremely important area. Gans (1995) has done a critical analysis of how language has been used by citizens, policy makers, journalists, health professionals, and others to condemn the poor.

For individuals working out of religious and spiritual traditions, a strategy to decrease poverty and improve health status outcomes for all emanates from their beliefs and church doctrines. For example, for Roman Catholics, there is an emphasis on social justice, a preferential option for the poor, stewardship, working for the common good, and solidarity (US Catholic Conference, 1993). As stated by the US Catholic Conference of Bishops in 1993, "The existing patterns of health care in the United States do not meet the minimal standard of social justice and the common good" (p. 1). Catholics can live out these beliefs in a number of ways. Among these are participation in problem-solving, communicative, and education strategies and participation in Church programs that promote the principles of this document. An organizational strategy that can be used is that of participation in organizations that address the challenges of poverty and health status inequalities. For example, the Bread for the World organization has many antipoverty initiatives (Bread for the World, 2002). Over the last several years, many cities have initiated and passed Living Wage ordinances (Amour, 2002). Passage of the ordinance in Omaha, Nebraska, was a result of the multifaith, multiethnic community development organization, Omaha Together One Community. Although it was passed for city employees, Omaha is one of only a few cities where the law was rescinded. However, there are now 80 communities where poor people are benefiting from this measure (Armour, 2002). When payroll taxes and earned income tax credits are calculated, this can mean an increase in earnings of about $5,000 more per year for someone. Citizens can be a part of furthering this kind of ordinance in their respective cities. At the international level, one could participate in the International Society for Equity in Health (N. Barton, personal communication, November 2, 2001). As the name suggests, health professionals from around the globe belong to this organization and are committed to decreasing health inequities.

In summary, this chapter has addressed the causes of poverty and how this leads to decreased health status and lack of access to health care for poor people. More importantly, it has identified strategies that various individuals can take to decrease poverty and increase the health status and access to health care for poor people. Such strategies are necessary for a just society and world: ". . . social justice is the foundation of public health" (Krieger, 1999, p. 296).

REFERENCES

Albelda, R., Folbre, N. & The Center For Popular Economics. (1996). *The war on the poor, a defense manual.* New York, NY: New York Press.

Armour, S. (2002, July 23). Living-wage movement takes root across nation. *USA Today,* p. 18.

Carlson, E. A. (2001). *The unfit.* Cold Spring Harbor, NY: Cold Spring Harbor Laboratory. President criticizes Senate welfare bill. (2002, July 30). *Bozeman Daily Chronicle,* p. 2.

Bread for the World. (2002). Retrieved August 9, 2002, from *www.bread.org.*

Bread for the World. (2002). *Working from poverty to promise. Bread for the World's 2002 offering of letters.* [Pamphlet]. Washington, DC: Bread for the World.

Carlson, E. A. (2001). *The Unfit.* Cold Springs Harbor, NY: Cold Springs Harbor Laboratory Press.

Crystal, S., & Shea, D. (1990). Cumulative advantage, cumulative disadvantage, and inequality among elderly people. *The Gerontologist, 30*(4), 437–443.

Crystal, S., Shea, D., & Krishnaswami, S. (1992). Educational attainment, occupational history, and stratification: Determinants of later-life economic outcomes. *Journal of Gerontology: Social Sciences, 47*(5), S213–S221.

Ehrenreich, B. (2001). *Nickel and dimed—On (not) getting by in America.* New York, NY: Henry Holt.

Gans, H. J. (1995). *The war against the poor.* New York, NY: BasicBooks.

Goodman, E. (2002, July 20). Bush Inc. blames everyone. *Omaha World-Herald,* p. A21.

Government report: Whites get better-quality healthcare. (2002). *RN, 65*(5), 16.

Hemingway, H., & Marmot, M. (1999). Psychosocial factors in the aetiology and prognosis of coronary heart disease: Systematic review of prospective cohort studies. *British Medical Journal, 318*(1), 460–467.

International Society for Equity in Health Newsletter (November 2, 2001).

Kaiser Network. (2002). *Nebraska Governor Johanns announces plan that would change Medicaid eligibility rules, end coverage for about 19,000.* Retrieved July 25, 2002, from *http://kaisernetwork.org/ dailyreports/ healthpolicy.*

Kreiger, N. (1999). Embodying inequality: A review of concepts, measures, and methods for studying health consequences of discrimination. *International Journal of Health Service, 29*(2), 295–352.

Legislature passes Medicaid changes. (2002). *Unicameral Update, XXV*(17), 7.

Lutey, T. (2002, July 25). University R & D funds targeted for cutbacks. *Bozeman Daily Chronicle,* p. 19.

Marmot, M., & Wilkinson, R. (2001). Education and debate, psychosocial and material pathways in the relation between income and health: A response to Lynch et al. *British Medical Journal, 322,* 1233–1236.

Navarro, V. (1999). Equity, health, and international relations, health and equity in the world in the era of "globalization." *International Journal of Health Services, 29*(2), 215–226.

Navarro, V., & Shi, L. (2001). The politics of policy, the political context of social inequalities and health. *International Journal of Health Services, 31*(1), 1–21.

Nichols, J. (2002). The nation on the fast track vote last night. *Online Beat of the Nation Magazine,* 1–3.

Reed, L. (2002, August 3). 60 new hires in Medicaid plan. *Omaha World-Herald,* p. B1.

Study links education, health care. (2002, July 23). *Omaha World Herald,* p. 4.

Unicameral Update. (July 30–August 15, 2002). Nebraska Legislature's Weekly Publication.

U.S. Catholic Conference. (1993, June 18). *A framework for comprehensive health care reform, protecting human life, promoting human dignity, pursuing the common good. A resolution of the Catholic Bishops of the United States.* Washington, DC: US Catholic Conference.

CHAPTER 47

Public Policy and Vulnerable Populations

Jeri A. Milstead

Government policies that target vulnerable populations may seem like an oxymoron (if we can use that word to explain a phrase). On the one hand, vulnerable populations may be difficult to define. On the other hand, vulnerable populations may not have much of a voice to articulate their plight. How and to whom in government do "populations" direct their pleas—agencies? programs? The purpose of this chapter is to define vulnerable populations, examine the policy process, and consider issues inherent in linking the two. Examples will be provided of how nurses can work within the policy process to the benefit of vulnerable populations.

DEFINITIONS

The term "vulnerable populations" is a latecomer to nursing literature and did not appear until the 1990s as a descriptor in *The Cumulative Index to Nursing and Allied Health Literature* (CINAHL). Users of the term often refer to low socioeconomic status (the poor and those out of work), the underserved (those who lack health care insurance or lack access to health care delivery), disease categories (diabetes, congestive heart failure), chronic illness (arthritis, AIDS), or those at risk for developing disease or illness. These terms are not really interchangeable; i.e., all diabetics may not be poor, and low socioeconomic status may not indicate the presence of chronic disease. These may not reflect either vulnerability or populations.

Flaskerud et al. (2002) defined vulnerable populations as "social groups who experience health disparities as a result of a lack of resources and/or increased exposure to risk" (p. 75). The CINAHL (2002) carries a category of vulnerability that is defined as "the state of being at risk or more susceptible physically, mentally or socially" (p. 405). The two major concepts appear to be the degree of risk and the experience of health problems without access to resources. However, a full understanding of vulnerable populations requires a deeper look.

Flaskerud et al. (2002) noted the evolution of knowledge about vulnerable populations from the 1950s to the early 2000s through a study of articles published in *Nursing Research*. Although the study was not comprehensive in that writings from other journals or other sources were excluded, the researchers chronicled terms that were used in investigating groups or aggregates. Only one study was published in the 1950s, and that had to do with chronically ill aged adults. Group identity was based in the 1960s on socioeconomic status, education, occupation, gender, or race. The 1970s noted "race, ethnicity and gender" (p. 76), and the beginning of research at this time focused on high-risk parents, infants, women, and immigrants. The concept of culture and its effect on the delivery of health care came into the literature in the 1980s (Leininger & McFarland, 2002). Reported as an "influence" in outcomes of social groups, culture became the context for studying a variety of societal problems that were not limited to health or health care.

The concept of health disparities did not surface until late in the 1990s, and the term reflected differences in health care and outcomes among many groups, such as adolescents and the elderly, women and infants, and low- and middle-income families. Ethnic groups also were studied as groups, often with a focus on the quality (or lack thereof) of health and health care. Quality was approached through professional accountability (vis-à-vis ethics and standards), marketing accountability (as evidenced in informed choices), and regulatory accountability (as reflected in government action) (Taub, 2002). Although the marketing method seemed prominent, the regulatory scheme used the Health Plan Employer Data and Information Set (HEDIS), hospital discharge data from the Health Care Financing Administration (HCFA), and information on the quality of managed care organizations from the National Committee for Quality Assurance. The government is the largest health care insurance company in the United States, and at least one government agency, HCFA, has measured patient satisfaction among users of managed care organizations and publishes performance measures at its Web site: *http://www.medicare.gov/mphCompare/home.asp.*

In the early years of the 21st century, many terms surfaced that referred to vulnerable populations. "Uninsured" became a blanket term for poor or low-income people, regardless of their gender, ethnicity, or employment status. Researchers discovered that the uninsured, which included the working poor, had more health problems than those who carried insurance. The homeless, as a group, were uninsured (often because they also were unemployed) and exhibited many physical and mental health problems. The range of health disparities was great. Migrants were considered "disadvantaged" (Ward, 2003), and African Americans (Plowden & Thompson, 2002; Richards, 2000) and Latinos (Campinha-Bacote, 2002) experienced much inequity related to health care. The disabled were identified as having social and physical barriers to health (Harrison, 2002). Those who lived near hazardous waste sites were considered at-risk for serious health problems (Gilden, 2003). Finally, the term "vulnerable populations" evolved to include whole populations, not just aggregates of individuals, as identifiable groups.

POLICY PROCESS

Many people think of legislation and/or laws when they hear the term "policy." Although legislation may be the most recognizable component, there are many other elements to the policy process (Milstead, 2004). When discussing public policy (as opposed to private-sector policy), it is the process of taking problems to government and obtaining a response that is being referenced. Within this broad approach, four major aspects are evident: agenda setting, government response, program and/or policy implementation, and program and/or /policy evaluation.

The process is not linear or sequential. That is, one does not always start with agenda setting and move to government response. A nurse may initially become involved during program implementation after a law has been signed. A garbage can model of organizations (Cohen, March, & Olsen, 1982) provides a foundation for considering the process of making public policy as the interweaving of streams of problems, policies, and politics. These streams mingle in government circles, often joining and breaking apart as ideas and solutions are considered, rejected, or reconsidered (Kingdon, 1995). At times, a solution hooks up with a problem, and a window of opportunity opens that results in a program that addresses the difficulty. A brief discussion of each component of the policy process will reveal opportunities for becoming involved.

Agenda Setting

The agenda is a list of items to which the president and his advisors (known as the Administration) attend. Agenda setting is the activity in which problems are brought to the attention of the Administration. If the president is not interested in a problem, it has little chance of being addressed. The issue is how to get the president's attention (Furlong, 2004). Crises can propel an issue onto the national agenda. For example, the attacks of September 11, 2001, brought immediate attention to the issue of terrorism, and funding was made available for projects and programs such as Homeland Security.

One of the issues in agenda setting is defining a problem so that it is palatable to the Administration and to the public. When HIV/AIDS was first discovered, it was defined as a problem of intravenous drug users and homosexuals. The Administration believed that the public would not support funding for research into the cause or treatment of the disease, and little funding was forthcoming. When children like Ryan White and heterosexual non-drug users began to get the disease (most often from infected blood products), the disease was redefined as a community health problem, and funding was made available. Nurses are experts at choosing words and scenarios to describe problems. Creative use of language may not be necessary in alerting an Administration to a problem, but one should know how to use key words to advantage. The point in defining a problem is to pique the interest of the Administration so that a solution can be found. Knowing that the public will scrutinize funding options is part of the context of defining the difficulty.

Government Response

The government may respond to a problem in several ways. The three most common responses are the enacting of a law, a regulation, or a program. Policy experts develop these activities in policy communities. Policy communities are loose groups of people who can provide expertise about an issue and who, for the most part, work in government agencies. Policy experts often know one another through professional associations, the literature or other media exposure, or prior experience with each other. Often legislative aides, who serve as staff in the offices of legislators, are good contacts for nurses who want to connect with "insiders." Experts discuss problems, suggest solutions, and exercise their opinions about the relative political worth of issues. Legislative aides in one legislator's office often talk informally with legislative aides in other legislators' offices and with staff in government agencies, faculty in university settings, and members of special interest groups to establish a priority list and to consider alternative solutions. Nurses who have cultivated relationships with government policy staff have a golden opportunity to be recognized as experts who are sought out to consider problems (Wakefield, 2004).

Laws are made in legislative sessions that last 2 years. Bills (potential laws) are introduced throughout the session, but bills introduced early have a better chance of action. The "how a bill becomes a law" page that can be found in nearly every basic government or political science textbook provides a simplified overview of the steps for moving a bill from introduction to signature by the president. Neither legislators nor their aides are expected to know about the myriad issues brought to them. Issues range from health to transportation to economy to defense and beyond. Nurses have a wonderful opportunity to serve as experts about many health issues. A nurse can provide a one-page overview of a problem, a summary of relevant research in ordinary language, and phone or e-mail information to pave the way for a serious contact.

Seasoned nurses understand the importance of informal processes—political processes. Many nurses shun the idea of politics, thinking that this is a tainted process that skews judgment and biases legislators. On the contrary, the political process is merely the exercise of persuasion and education to one's perspective. What nurse has not spoken informally to others before a decision was made in an effort to gather support, challenge a conclusion, or talk out a problem? The same communication techniques are used with legislators and their staffs or anyone in the policy community. Reflection, active listening, and clarification are therapeutic communication skills that are integral to how nurses approach others. The art of using talents in this way should be natural for nurses.

The legislative process must be followed carefully, and nurses must be vigilant for amendments that will help or hurt their causes. Developing strong, positive relationships with legislators, staff, and other interested parties result in a network that leads to "inside" information. Working at the subcommittee level is a more efficient use of time than letting a bill get to the committee because there are fewer members in a subcommittee. It is important to stay with a bill through passage by both houses of congress and, in many instances, a conference committee. Nurses may recommend language for inclusion in drafting a bill or an amendment and must be cognizant of amendments that could derail or inhibit passage.

Once a bill becomes a law that establishes a program, the program is assigned to a government agency for implementation. The choice of which agency is very political. Not all health programs go to agencies in the Department of Health and Human Services. Some may go to the Department of Defense (for piloting by the military), the Department of Education (school health programs), the Department of the Treasury (drug treatment or enforcement programs), or other departments and agencies. The choice may be based on past experience with similar programs, the chance for an infusion of new funding needed by an agency, rejection of a program due to lack of time or expertise, or many other reasons.

Agencies must write regulations or rules that interpret the law and provide for smooth implementation (Loquist, 2004). The regulatory process is similar to the legislative process in that legislative action is required. However, the regulatory process is governed by the Administrative Procedures Act, which dictates a specific format and course. All proposed rules require notification of the public, an established time for public comment, and public announcement of the final rule. The *Federal Register* is the vehicle for publishing information. Public comment can be in the form of letters, e-mail messages, phone calls, or in-person visits to the appropriate agency. All comments must be considered before the final rule is adopted. This is a particularly easy way for nurses to involve themselves in expressing their opinions about potential rules. Communication should be brief, focused, and identifiable (i.e., the rule on which you are commenting). Arguments should be stated clearly and prefaced by whether you are for or against the issue or section of the rule. Solutions are welcomed.

Implementation

Implementation is a fluid process that involves getting a program up and running. Agency staff may need assistance in determining eligibility. That is, who is entitled to participate? Who is excluded from participation? What are the criteria, and who monitors participation? Nurses can suggest policy tools, such as incentives (waivers, coupons), educational brochures, posters advertising a program, or learning tools (training sessions) to assist staff in operating a program (Smart, 2004).

Nurses should confer with agency personnel, known as street-level bureaucrats, who are putting the programs into operation. These street-level bureaucrats often use ideas from the program participants about how to streamline programs or make them more efficient or user-friendly. Nurses may provide tips about the population being served or thoughts about how a program could be conducted. Sometimes programs can be expanded to include broader involvement or shrunk to remain within the legislative intent and purpose. Nurses can provide concrete assistance and guidance by recommending ideas about how to alter the provision of a program.

Bardach (1977) identified games that are played by agency personnel during the implementation phase of a program. Many of the games have to do with budget, policy goals, and administrative control. For government agencies, spending funds early and requesting additional funding later is one way to increase a budget. Encouraging overspending, known as boondoggling, can be seen when consultant fees exceed the budget. Inflating costs estimated for a program is a way of padding a budget so that some of the funds can be used later (e.g., as discretionary funds) or in a way different from original intent. Some program implementors plan their work so that they do not have to spend much time at the work site.

Nurses study implementation to determine to what extent programs meet original policy goals (Wilken, 2004). They investigate any modifications that were made and seek explanations for changes. Researchers examine the level of difficulty or "tractability" of the initial problem and whether technology was accessible to address the problem. The range of services provided by a program may produce variation in program performance such that many services might dilute operations negatively. On the other hand, successful programs can become a target for piling on additional objectives. The idea is to be part of a thriving program, but too many extra activities may result in program failure.

Evaluation

Evaluation is rarely conducted and usually is not part of an original program plan, despite literature that recommends appraisal. Evaluation should be both formative and summative. Formative data can help bureaucrats determine progress during implementation. They can provide information for decisions about whether or not to continue to function as usual or to change direction. Formative data can also indicate whether resources are adequate and are being distributed appropriately.

Summative data can be useful for evaluating public programs for effectiveness or outcomes, not just efficiency or outputs. That is, what difference does it make to the public good if thousands of poor women are offered free mammograms? Has this screening method resulted in significant prevention or early treatment of breast cancer? This is not to say that efficiency is not worth assessing; a poorly run program will waste tax dollars.

Evaluative reports should be provided to agency personnel, legislators, and the public. Charts and other visual media can be used to present aggregate data, identify trends, and track progress. Reports may contain recommendations for adjusting goals and objectives or implementation strategies.

LINKING THE POLICY PROCESS WITH VULNERABLE POPULATIONS

Agenda Setting

Nurses can propel issues of vulnerable populations onto the national agenda by defining needy groups, serving as a voice for vulnerable populations, and alerting legislators to problems that affect the public health. For example, the homeless usually are not organized in any formal way and have little voice as a group. Their worries about health care go unheard unless someone, known as a policy entrepreneur, makes available his or her reputation, money, or other resources on their behalf. A nurse can serve as an entrepreneur or can mobilize the media to take up a cause. Issues of social justice are political issues. Discrimination against marginalized populations and against people based on health status, income, employment status, or type of disease or disability is unethical and unjust and may be illegal in the United States. The distribution and allocation of resources is a political process. The choice of which problems get on the national agenda is very political, and nurses are skilled in political interaction. Nurses must take up the mantle of social problems, especially health problems, for those who cannot or do not speak for themselves.

Nurses can help bureaucrats define problems in ways that help the public understand and value them. Drug users often are unemployed or financially poor and are disenfranchised in the public eye because of related crimes. (In contrast, employed drug users often go undetected by the general public and escape bias [Milstead, 1993].) Legislators ignore or shun known drug users as a group, often because the "druggies" create violence, do not vote, and are not organized politically. Social activists (including nurses) in the 1980s formed groups such as the Association for Drug Abuse Prevention and Treatment (ADAPT) and the AIDS Coalition to Unleash Power (ACT UP). Members recognized the link between gay men, intravenous drug users, and HIV/AIDS, and a few created needle exchange programs and served as policy entrepreneurs. These volunteers changed the definition from drug "addict" to drug "user" as one way to change the public's perception of a vulnerable group. Volunteers in Tacoma, Washington, and New York City educated legislators, bureaucrats, and public health officials about HIV transmission and the need for research on diagnosis and treatment (Milstead, 1993). Communications techniques such as consciousness raising and the use of sound bites were developed to a high level. Policy entrepreneurs may take years to attain their goals, and some of the first group of volunteers are still staffing exchange programs on the streets and working the state legislature to obtain legitimacy for their programs. Most needle exchange programs in the United States are still operating—and are still illegal—despite the sustained efforts of volunteers to change the laws and a legal opinion that "possession of needles was a 'medical necessity' that was intended to prevent a greater societal harm, AIDS" (*New York Times,* 1991).

Government Response

Laws are composites of language that reflect the wishes and priorities of those who craft them. Laws often are the result of negotiation and compromise among many people with disparate philosophies and values. Nurses can help shape laws by means of their expertise in health care and health care delivery. Congressional representatives usually do not know much about diseases such as diabetes or tuberculosis. A nurse who has nurtured relationships with elected officials by becoming a contact for health issues and providing understandable explanations of medical terminology has a great opening to contribute to language as a bill is being constructed. A nurse's knowledge of current issues can be a tremendous help to a legislator or his staff. Nurses also bring anecdotes to the policy community that put a personal face on an issue.

The elderly are often considered a vulnerable population. The designation may be confusing because the term does not necessarily refer to low socioeconomic status, the underserved, or disease categories. "Elderly" cuts across all types of categories and, as a vulnerable population, there is inference of risk and lack of resources for health care, specifically in relation to an increased danger of suffering disease or disability and a lack of resources because of fixed incomes. The elderly have a strong, organized lobby through the American Association of Retired Persons (AARP). During the early years of the 21st century, AARP waged a campaign in the US Congress to create protection for members (aged 50 years or older) in the form of a program for funding prescription drugs.

The Medicare Prescription Drug Improvement and Modernization Act of 2003 amended Title XVIII (Medicare) of the Social Security Act to add a new part D (Voluntary Prescription Drug Benefit Program) under which each individual who is entitled to benefits under Medicare part A (hospital insurance) or Medicare part B (supplemental medical insurance) is entitled to obtain qualified prescription drug coverage. The law was passed by both the House of Representatives and the Senate and became public law 108-173 on December 8, 2003 (*http://www.thomas. loc.gov*).

Nurses, physicians, and other health care providers participated in a focused assault on legislators in an effort to effect this law. Senators and representatives held hearings, met with lobbyists and AARP members, talked with constituents, and discussed issues within the policy community. The issue evolved into a hotly debated partisan battle, but compromise language created a bill that was acceptable enough to pass the Republican-dominated House and Senate. Herein lies a caveat: although the bill has been signed into law, there are many changes that probably will be made as the program is implemented. Nurses have an occasion to become knowledgeable about the current law and can peruse the law and how it came into being through the Web site previously noted (*http://www.thomas.loc.gov*). The Medicare prescription plan is an example of how the streams of agenda setting, government response, and implementation interconnect. During efforts to move the issue of prescription costs onto the national agenda, work already was in process to determine alternative solutions, and the basic rudiments of a program were already being conceived.

Implementation

An example of a purely symbolic policy action is the Stewart B. McKinney Act of 1987. Vladeck (1990) studied the homeless: characteristics, causes of homelessness, and health status. He chronicled the evolution of a joint initiative between the Robert Wood Johnson Foundation and the Pew Charitable Trusts that became a model for a program that would provide federal support for the homeless. Even though there was agreement among policy makers that homelessness was a problem worthy of government intervention, authorization of funding did not eliminate the problem or even address most of the social, economic, health care, and other issues.

A brief search for initiatives about the homeless in the 108th Congress shows a plethora of attempts in which bills were introduced but stalled in committee or subcommittee. These attempts include House of Representatives (H.R.) 1941, a bill to convert the voucher system to state-administered block grants to help low-income families find safe and affordable housing; H.R. 1256, to place memorials (e.g., wreaths) at the graves of homeless or indigent veterans; H.R. 2897, to end homelessness in the United States; HR 3459, to improve the health of minorities; and Senate (S.) bill 100, to expand access to affordable health care and make more services available in rural and underserved areas (*http://www.thomas.loc.gov.*). Symbolic efforts are important and may keep an issue from fading from the agenda. Symbolism is important because it is just that—symbolic or representative or illustrative that someone or some agency hears pleas for help. This "splinting" (Ebersole, 2002) helps to keep up spirits and encourages perseverance, especially when the effort expended has not produced an implementable program.

Sometimes a lack of federal policy results in a local project. A symposium held at the University of Miami (Florida) School of Law in 1990 (Symposium: Law and the Homeless, 1991) served as a mechanism to discuss medical and other problems of the homeless that were addressed without federal assistance.

Evaluation

Evaluation of health policy that affects vulnerable groups does not occur often at the program level. Rather, policy itself has been evaluated through research. Nurse-led studies in the 1990s and the early 2000s reported in *Nursing Research* (Flaskerud et al., 2002) evaluated resources available for Hispanics, African Americans, Filipinos, lesbians, low-income families and age-related groups, and the homeless. Disease categories included mental illness (including depression), chronic illness, addictive disease, pregnancy, injuries, and specific populations with asthma, hypertension, HIV/AIDS, lung and heart disease, sexually transmitted diseases, and tuberculosis. The discovery of health disparities between vulnerable groups and the general population indicated levels of risk and lack of access to health care providers and resources.

Research uncovered problems in defining vulnerable populations, specifically in relation to issues of race and ethnicity. The Institute of Medicine challenged the National Institutes of Health (NIH) to replace the term "race" with "ethnic group" (Oppenheimer, 2001). The Office of Management and Budget sets policy about which racial and ethnic classes are to be referenced by any federal agency, although OMB recognizes that these terms are based on ill-defined social or political types, not scientific categories. The American Anthropological Association approves the concept of race/ethnicity as an interim combined term until race is eliminated in the next census. Researchers will have to take care to define race or ethnicity clearly as they study various groups. Vulnerable groups will be subject to scrutiny, and federal agencies that authorize programs, initiate policies, and appropriate funds must take into consideration the legal, governmental, cultural, and historic implications of terms.

Sudduth (2004) asserts that nurses "are not strangers to evaluation" (p. 194). She urges advanced-practice nurses to transfer the skills they use to determine outcomes in a health care setting to evaluation of government programs. "Social programs are public policy made visible" (p. 197), and nurses are well equipped to determine the worth, efficacy, and efficiency of many programs.

CONCLUSION

Nurses work with vulnerable populations in the provision, administration, and evaluation of health care. Public officials design policies in response to problems that rise to the agenda-setting attention of the president and his advisors. The policy community is involved in defining problems, prioritizing their value, and seeking and considering alternative solutions. Legislators, their staff, interest groups, and others in the community of interest draft government responses to the problems, often in the form of laws, regulations, and programs.

Nurses must integrate political knowledge and skill into their professional lives. Nurses can identify problems, bring them to the Administration, keep them from fading, suggest re-definitions, and propose alternative solutions. Nurses must persevere throughout the process by using their expertise to help legislators choose policy tools and implement and evaluate programs and policies. Public officials are not used to nurses participating actively in the process of policy making; therefore, nurses must initiate the contacts, provide information that a lay person can understand, and acknowledge those legislators or bureaucrats who respond positively and move government to action.

References

Bardach, E. (1977). *The implementation game: What happens after a bill becomes a law.* Cambridge, MA: MIT.

Campinha-Bacote, J. (2002). The process of cultural competence in the delivery of healthcare services: A model of care. *Journal of Transcultural Nursing, 13*(3), 181–184.

Cohen, M., March, J., & Olsen, J. (1982). A garbage can model of organizational choice. *Administrative Science Quarterly, 17,* 1–25.

People of the State of New York v. Bordowitz, et al., No. 90N0248423 (June 25, 1991). In J. A. Milstead. (1993). *The advancement of policy implementation theory: An analysis of three needle exchange programs.* University of Georgia.

Ebersole, P. (2002). Situational vulnerability. *Geriatric Nursing, 23*(1), 4.

Flaskerud, J. H., Lesser, J., Dixon, E., Anderson, N., Conde, F., Kim, S., et al. (2002). Health Disparities among vulnerable populations. *Nursing Research, 51*(2), 74–85.

Furlong, E. A. (2004). Agenda Setting. In J. A. Milstead (Ed.). *Health policy and politics: A nurse's guide* (2nd ed., pp. 37–66). Sudbury, MA: Jones and Bartlett.

Gilden, R. C. (2003). Community involvement at hazardous waste sites: A review of policies from a nursing perspective. *Policy, Politics, & Nursing Practice, 4*(1), 29–35.

Harrison, T. C. (2002). Has the Americans with Disabilities Act made a difference? A policy analysis of quality of life in the post-Americans with Disabilities Act era. *Policy, Politics, & Nursing Practice, 3*(4), 333–347.

Kingdon, J. W. (1995). *Agendas, alternatives, and public policies* (2nd ed.). New York, NY: Harper Collins.

Leininger, M., & McFarland, M. R. (2002). *Transcultural nursing: Concepts, theories, research and practice* (3rd ed.). New York, NY: McGraw-Hill.

Loquist, R. S. (2004). Government regulation: Parallel and powerful. In J. A. Milstead (Ed.). *Health policy and politics: A nurse's guide* (2nd ed., pp. 89–127). Sudbury, MA: Jones and Bartlett.

Manhattan Criminal Court Judge Laura E. Drager. (1991, June 26). New York Times, p. 1. In Milstead, J. A. (1993). The advancement of policy implementation theory: An analysis of three needle exchange programs. Doctoral dissertation. Athens, GA: University of Georgia.

Medicare Prescription Drug and Modernization Act of 2003. Retrieved December 31, 2003, from *http://www.thomas.loc.gov.*

Milstead, J. A. (1993). The advancement of policy implementation theory: An analysis of three needle exchange programs. Doctoral dissertation. Athens, GA: University of Georgia.

Milstead, J. A. (2004). Advanced practice nurses and public policy, naturally. In J. A. Milstead (Ed.). *Health policy and politics: A nurse's guide* (2nd ed., pp. 1–36). Sudbury, MA: Jones and Bartlett.

Oppenheimer, G. M. (2001). Paradigm lost: Race, ethnicity, and the search for a new population taxonomy. *American Journal of Public Health, 91*(7), 1049–1054.

Plowden, K. O., & Thompson, L. S. (2002). Sociological perspectives of Black American health disparity: Implications for social policy. *Policy, Politics, & Nursing Practice, 3*(4), 325–332.

Richards, H. (2000). And miles to go before we sleep: Rising to meet the challenges of ending health care disparities among African-Americans. *Journal of National Black Nurses Association, 11*(2), 2.

Smart, P. (2004). Policy design. In J. A. Milstead (Ed.). *Health policy and politics: A nurse's guide* (2nd ed., pp. 129–160). Sudbury, MA: Jones and Bartlett.

Sudduth, A. L. (2004). Policy evaluation. In J. A. Milstead (Ed.). *Health policy and politics: A nurse's guide* (2nd ed., pp. 193–228). Sudbury, MA: Jones and Bartlett.

Symposium: Law and the Homeless. (1991). In *University of Miami Law Review, 45*(N1990/Ja): 261–736.

Taub, L.F. M. (2002). A policy analysis of access to health care inclusive of cost, quality, and scope of services. *Policy, Politics, & Nursing Practice, 3*(2), 167–176.

Vladeck, B. (1990). Health care and the homeless: A political parable for our time. *Journal of Health Politics, Policy and Law, 15*(2), 305–317.

Wakefield, M. (2004). Government Response: Legislation. In J. A. Milstead (Ed.). *Health policy and politics: A nurse's guide* (2nd ed., pp. 67–88). Sudbury, MA: Jones and Bartlett.

Ward, L. S. (2003). Migrant health policy: History, analysis, and challenge. *Policy, Politics, & Nursing Practice, 4*(1), 45–52.

Wilken, M. (2004). Policy implementation. In J. A. Milstead (Ed.). *Health policy and politics: A nurse's guide* (2nd ed., pp. 161–192). Sudbury, MA: Jones and Bartlett.

Index